Core Concepts in the Disorders of Fluid, Electrolytes and Acid-Base Balance

David B. Mount • Mohamed H. Sayegh
Ajay K. Singh
Editors

Core Concepts in the Disorders of Fluid, Electrolytes and Acid-Base Balance

Springer

Editors
David B. Mount, MD
Renal Division
VA Boston Healthcare System
Brigham and Women's Hospital
Harvard Medical School
Boston, MA, USA

Mohamed H. Sayegh, MD
Renal Division
Brigham and Women's Hospital
Harvard Medical School
Boston, MA, USA

Ajay K. Singh, MB, FRCP (UK)
Renal Division
Brigham and Women's Hospital
Harvard Medical School
Boston, MA, USA

ISBN 978-1-4614-3769-7 ISBN 978-1-4614-3770-3 (eBook)
DOI 10.1007/978-1-4614-3770-3
Springer New York Heidelberg Dordrecht London

Library of Congress Control Number: 2012941302

Printed on acid-free paper

Springer is part of Springer Science+Business Media (www.springer.com)

To my wife and children; Erika, Julia, and Nicholas

–DBM

Preface

Fluid, electrolyte, and acid–base disorders are central to the day-to-day practice of almost all areas of patient-centered medicine, both medical and surgical. Despite the steep learning curve for trainees, the underlying pathophysiology and/or management is often viewed as "settled," with the perception that there is little in this field that is new. However, there have been significant recent developments in all aspects of these important disorders. This book encompasses these new findings in comprehensive reviews of both pathophysiology and clinical management, meant for both the nephrologist and the nonspecialist physician or medical trainee.

Virtually every subject in this textbook has witnessed major developments in the last decade. New pathophysiology includes the molecular identification of "pendrin" (SLC26A4) as the apical Cl^-/HCO_3^- exchanger in β[beta]-intercalated cells [1, 2]; this transporter functions in distal chloride and bicarbonate transport, with evolving roles in the pathophysiology of hypertension and metabolic alkalosis. A host of previously uncharacterized genetic tubular disorders have recently yielded to molecular genetics, with major impact of this gene identification on the understanding of renal physiology and pathophysiology. In particular, the identification in 2001 [3] of causative mutations in the WNK1 (With No K/Lysine) and WNK4 kinases in familial hypertension with hyperkalemia (Gordon's syndrome) led to a still-evolving cascade of insight into the role of these and associated signaling proteins in the coordination of aldosterone-dependent and aldosterone-independent regulation of distal potassium, sodium, and chloride transport [4]. Characterization of multiple genes for familial hypomagnesemia led to the identification of novel magnesium transport pathways [5] and to the identification of cell-associated epidermal growth factor as a major paracrine regulator of distal tubular magnesium transport [6]. Finally, characterization of FGF23 (fibroblast growth factor-23) as the disease gene for autosomal dominant hypophosphatemic rickets [7] uncovered a major new regulatory hormone in calcium and phosphate balance [8, 9].

At the clinical level, the spectrum of the acquired causes of electrolyte disorders continues to expand. Examples include hypokalemia due to the activation of colonic potassium secretion in Ogilvie's syndrome [10], and hypomagnesemia, with or without associated hypokalemia, after treatment with the EGF antagonist cetuximab [6, 11, 12]. The management of electrolyte disorders has also evolved considerably in the last decade. Nowhere is this more evident than in hyponatremia, with the recent availability of vasopressin antagonists [13, 14] and the increasing familiarity with relowering of serum sodium concentration in patients who have corrected too quickly [15].

The integrated analysis and management of fluid, electrolyte, and acid–base disorders can be a daunting challenge, especially for trainees. With this in mind, the last chapter includes ten real-life clinical vignettes that provide a step-by-step analysis of the pathophysiology, differential diagnosis, and management of selected clinical problems.

Boston, MA, USA

David B. Mount
Mohamed H. Sayegh
Ajay K. Singh

References

1. Royaux IE, Wall SM, Karniski LP, et al. Pendrin, encoded by the Pendred syndrome gene, resides in the apical region of renal intercalated cells and mediates bicarbonate secretion. Proc Natl Acad Sci U S A. 2001;98:4221–6.
2. Verlander JW, Hassell KA, Royaux IE, et al. Deoxycorticosterone upregulates PDS (Slc26a4) in mouse kidney: role of pendrin in mineralocorticoid-induced hypertension. Hypertension 2003;42:356–62.
3. Wilson FH, Disse-Nicodeme S, Choate KA, et al. Human hypertension caused by mutations in WNK kinases. Science 2001;293:1107–12.
4. Welling PA, Chang YP, Delpire E, Wade JB. Multigene kinase network, kidney transport, and salt in essential hypertension. Kidney Int. 2010;77:1063–9.
5. Schlingmann KP, Weber S, Peters M, et al. Hypomagnesemia with secondary hypocalcemia is caused by mutations in TRPM6, a new member of the TRPM gene family. Nat Genet. 2002;31:166–70.
6. Groenestege WM, Thebault S, van der Wijst J, et al. Impaired basolateral sorting of pro-EGF causes isolated recessive renal hypomagnesemia. J Clin Invest. 2007; 117:2260–7.
7. Consortium A. Autosomal dominant hypophosphataemic rickets is associated with mutations in FGF23. The ADHR Consortium. Nat Genet. 2000;26:345–8.
8. Wolf M. Forging forward with 10 burning questions on FGF23 in kidney disease. J Am Soc Nephrol. 2010;21:1427–35.
9. Alon US. Clinical practice. Fibroblast growth factor (FGF)23: a new hormone. Eur J Pediatr. 2011;170:545–54.
10. Blondon H, Bechade D, Desrame J, Algayres JP. Secretory diarrhoea with high faecal potassium concentrations: a new mechanism of diarrhoea associated with colonic pseudo-obstruction? Report of five patients. Gastroenterol Clin Biol. 2008;32:401–4.
11. Cao Y, Liao C, Tan A, Liu L, Gao F. Meta-analysis of incidence and risk of hypomagnesemia with cetuximab for advanced cancer. Chemotherapy 2010;56:459–65.
12. Cao Y, Liu L, Liao C, Tan A, Gao F. Meta-analysis of incidence and risk of hypokalemia with cetuximab-based therapy for advanced cancer. Cancer Chemother Pharmacol. 2010;66:37–42.
13. Schrier RW, Gross P, Gheorghiade M, et al. Tolvaptan, a selective oral vasopressin V2-receptor antagonist, for hyponatremia. N Engl J Med. 2006;355:2099–112.
14. Zeltser D, Rosansky S, van Rensburg H, Verbalis JG, Smith N. Assessment of the efficacy and safety of intravenous conivaptan in euvolemic and hypervolemic hyponatremia. Am J Nephrol. 2007;27:447–57.
15. Perianayagam A, Sterns RH, Silver SM, et al. DDAVP is effective in preventing and reversing inadvertent overcorrection of hyponatremia. Clin J Am Soc Nephrol. 2008; 3:331–6.

Contents

Contributors

Tomas Berl, MD Department of Medicine, University of Colorado, Aurora, CO, USA

David H. Ellison, MD Division of Nephrology and Hypertension, Department of Medicine, Oregon Health and Science University, Portland, OR, USA

F. John Gennari, MD Department of Medicine, University of Vermont, Burlington, VT, USA

Ali Hariri, MD Section of Nephrology, Department of Medicine, Yale School of Medicine, New Haven, CT, USA

John T. Herrin, MBBS, FRACP Attending Nephrology, Division of Nephrology, Department of Medicine, Children's Hospital, Boston, MA, USA

Jeffrey A. Kraut, MD Dialysis Unit and Department of Nephrology, VHAGLA Healthcare System, David Geffen School of Medicine at UCLA, Los Angeles, CA, USA

Ira Kurtz, MD, FRCP(C) Department of Medicine, Division of Nephrology, University of California at Los Angeles, Los Angeles, CA, USA

Harold E. Layton, PhD Department of Mathematics, Duke University, Durham, NC, USA

Orson W. Moe, MD Internal Medicine/Nephrology and Charles and Jane Pak Center for Mineral Metabolism and Clinical Research, UT Southwestern Medical Center, Dallas, TX, USA

David B. Mount, MD Renal Division, VA Boston Healthcare System, Brigham and Women's Hospital, Harvard Medical School, Boston, MA, USA

Biff F. Palmer, MD Internal Medicine, UT Southwestern Medical Center, Dallas, TX, USA

Asghar Rastegar, MD Department of Internal Medicine, Yale School of Medicine, New Haven, CT, USA

Jeff M. Sands, MD Department of Medicine, Renal Division, Emory University, Atlanta, GA, USA

Mohamed H. Sayegh, MD Renal Division, Brigham and Women's Hospital, Harvard Medical School, Boston, MA, USA

Alan Segal, MD Division of Nephrology, Department of Medicine, University of Vermont, Burlington, VT, USA

Ajay K. Singh, MB, FRCP (UK) Renal Division, Brigham and Women's Hospital, Harvard Medical School, Boston, MA, USA

Arohan R. Subramanya, MD Department of Medicine, Renal-Electrolyte Division, University of Pittsburgh School of Medicine, Pittsburgh, PA, USA

Joshua M. Thurman, MD Department of Internal Medicine, University of Denver School of Medicine, Aurora, CO, USA

Jill W. Verlander, DVM College of Medicine Core Electron Microscopy Lab, Division of Nephrology, Hypertension and Transplantation, Department of Medicine, University of Florida College of Medicine, Gainesville, FL, USA

I. David Weiner, MD Department of Medicine, University of Florida College of Medicine and North Florida/South Georgia Veterans Health System, Gainesville, FL, USA

Michael R. Wiederkehr, MD Department of Nephrology, Baylor University Medical Center, Dallas, TX, USA

Charles S. Wingo, MD Division of Nephrology, Department of Medicine, University of Florida, Gainesville, FL, USA
North Florida/South Georgia Vetrans Health System, Gainesville, FL, USA

The Physiology of Water Homeostasis

1

Jeff M. Sands, David B. Mount, and Harold E. Layton

Introduction

Water is the most abundant constituent in the body, comprising approximately 50 % of body weight in women and 60 % in men. Total body water is distributed in two major compartments: 55–75 % is intracellular (intracellular fluid, ICF), and 25–45 % is extracellular (extracellular fluid, ECF). The ECF is further subdivided into intravascular (plasma water) and extravascular (interstitial) spaces, in a ratio of 1:3. Fluid movement between the intravascular and interstitial spaces occurs across the capillary wall and is determined by Starling forces. The solute or particle concentration of a fluid is known as its osmolality, expressed as milliosmoles per kilogram (mOsm/kg) of water. Water easily diffuses across most cell membranes to achieve osmotic equilibrium (ECF osmolality = ICF osmolality). Water homeostasis is therefore critical to the maintenance of both circulatory integrity and the normal osmolality of body fluids.

J.M. Sands, M.D. (✉)
Department of Medicine, Renal Division, Emory University, 1639 Pierce Drive, NE, WMB Room 338, Atlanta, GA 30322, USA
e-mail: jeff.sands@emory.edu

D.B. Mount, M.D.
Renal Division, VA Boston Healthcare System, Brigham and Women's Hospital, Harvard Medical School, Boston, MA, USA
e-mail: dmount@rics.bwh.harvard.edu; david.mount2@va.gov

H.E. Layton, Ph.D.
Department of Mathematics, Duke University, Box 90230, Durham, NC 27708-0320, USA

Vasopressin secretion, water ingestion, and the renal concentrating mechanism collaborate to maintain human body fluid osmolality between 280 and 295 mOsm/kg. The primary hormonal control of renal water excretion is by arginine vasopressin (AVP; also named antidiuretic hormone, ADH). Under normal circumstances, vasopressin's circulating level is determined by osmoreceptors in the hypothalamus, which trigger increases in vasopressin secretion (by the posterior pituitary gland) when the osmolality of the blood rises above a threshold value, about 292 mOsm/kg H_2O; thirst and thus water intake also increase above this threshold. The kidney responds to changes in vasopressin levels by varying urine flow (i.e., water excretion).

The mammalian kidney maintains blood plasma osmolality and sodium concentration nearly constant by means of mechanisms that independently regulate water and sodium excretion. Since many mammals do not have continuous access to water, the ability to vary water excretion can be essential for survival. Sodium and its anions are the principal osmotic constituents of blood plasma, and since stable electrolyte concentrations are also essential, water excretion must be regulated by mechanisms that decouple it from sodium excretion. The urine concentrating mechanism plays a fundamental role in regulating water and sodium excretion. When water intake is large enough to dilute blood plasma, a urine that is more dilute than blood plasma is

D.B. Mount et al. (eds.), *Core Concepts in the Disorders of Fluid, Electrolytes and Acid-Base Balance*, DOI 10.1007/978-1-4614-3770-3_1, © Springer Science+Business Media New York 2013

produced. When water intake is so small that blood plasma is concentrated, a urine that is more concentrated than blood plasma is produced. In both cases, the total urinary solute excretion rate and the urinary sodium excretion rates are small and normally vary within narrow bounds.

In contrast to solute excretion, urine osmolality varies widely in response to changes in water intake. Following several hours without water intake, such as occurs overnight during sleep, human urine osmolality may rise to ~1,200 mOsm/kg H_2O, about four times plasma osmolality (~290 mOsm/kg H_2O). Conversely, urine osmolality may decrease rapidly following the ingestion of large quantities of water, such as commonly occurs at breakfast; human (and other mammals) urine osmolality may decrease to ~50 mOsm/kgH_2O. Most physiologic studies relevant to the urine concentrating mechanism have been conducted in species (rodents, rabbits) that can achieve higher maximum urine osmolalities than humans. For example, rabbits can concentrate to ~1,400 mOsm/kg H_2O, rats to ~3,000 mOsm/kg H_2O, mice and hamsters to ~4,000 mOsm/kg H_2O, and chinchillas to ~7,600 mOsm/kg H_2O (reviewed in [1, 2]).

Osmoreception

Regulation of Vasopressin Release

Vasopressin is synthesized in magnocellular neurons within the hypothalamus; the distal axons of these neurons project to the posterior pituitary or neurohypophysis, from which vasopressin is released into the circulation (see Fig. 1.1). Vasopressin secretion is stimulated as osmolality increases above a threshold level, beyond which there is a linear relationship between circulating osmolality and vasopressin (Fig. 1.2). The *X* intercept of this relationship in healthy humans is ~285 mOsm/kg H_2O; vasopressin levels are essentially undetectable below this threshold.

Changes in blood volume and blood pressure are also potent stimuli for vasopressin release, albeit with a more exponential response profile. Of perhaps greater relevance to the pathophysiology of hyponatremia, ECF volume strongly modulates the relationship between circulating osmolality and vasopressin release, such that hypovolemia reduces the osmotic threshold and increases the slope of the response curve to osmolality; *hypervolemia* has an opposite effect, increasing the osmotic threshold and reducing the slope of the response curve (Fig. 1.2) [3]. Similar modulation of the osmotic response occurs in heart failure, with both higher baseline vasopressin levels and an exaggerated response to hypertonic IV contrast [4]. A number of other stimuli have potent positive effects on vasopressin release, including nausea, angiotensin II, acetylcholine, relaxin, serotonin, cholecystokinin, and a variety of drugs [5] (see also *Regulation of osmoreceptor function*).

There are considerable male–female differences in the sensitivity of vasopressin release to osmolality, with a greater male sensitivity compared with women in both the follicular and luteal phase of the menstrual cycle [6]. Pregnancy is also associated with a 6 mOsm/kg H_2O drop in the osmotic threshold for vasopressin release, in addition to an 11 mOsm/kg H_2O drop in the osmotic threshold for thirst [7]. The physiology of these relationships is very complex and often contradictory due to a variety of genomic and non-genomic effects of gonadal steroids [8]. In males, testosterone appears to increase synthesis and osmotic release of vasopressin [9]. Human magnocellular neurons express both estrogen receptor-β (ER-β) and estrogen receptor-α (ER-α) [8]; activation of these homologous receptors can have opposing effects on gene expression, consistent perhaps with the complex and sometimes contradictory effects of estrogen. Several lines of evidence suggest that activation of ER-α increases vasopressin expression and release, whereas ER-β attenuates vasopressin expression and release [8]. In particular, ER-β is drastically reduced in vasopressin-positive neurons by both hypertonicity and hypovolemia [10], suggesting inhibitory effects of ER-β on vasopressin expression and release.

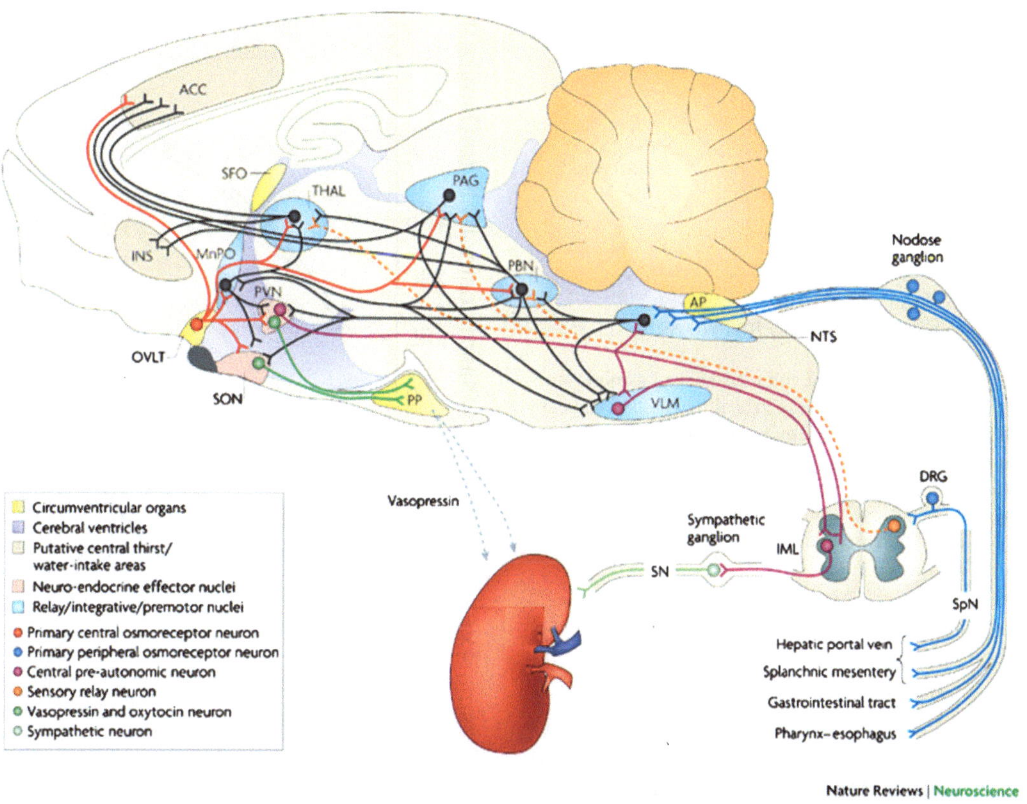

Fig. 1.1 Osmoregulatory circuits in the mammalian nervous system. Sagittal illustration of the rat brain, in which the relative positions of relevant structures and nuclei have been compressed into a single plane. Neurons and pathways are color coded to distinguish osmosensory, integrative, and effector areas. Vasopressin (AVP) is synthesized in magnocellular neurons within the supraoptic (SON) and paraventricular (PVN) nuclei of the hypothalamus; the distal axons of these neurons project to the posterior pituitary (PP) from which vasopressin is released into the circulation. *ACC* anterior cingulate cortex, *AP* area postrema, *DRG* dorsal root ganglion, *IML* intermediolateral nucleus, *INS* insula, *MnPO* median preoptic nucleus, *NTS* nucleus tractus solitarius, *OVLT* organum vasculosum laminae terminalis, *PAG* periaqueductal grey, *PBN* parabrachial nucleus, *PP* posterior pituitary, *PVN* paraventricular nucleus, *SFO* subfornical organ, *SN* sympathetic nerve, *SON* supraoptic nucleus, *SpN* splanchnic nerve, *THAL* thalamus, *VLM* ventrolateral medulla. Adapted from Bourque [12] with permission

Regulation of Thirst

Classically, the onset of thirst, defined as the conscious need for water, was considered to have a threshold of ~295 mOsm/kg H_2O, i.e., ~10 mOsm/kg H_2O *above* that for vasopressin release [6]. However, more recent studies using semiquantitative visual analog scales to assess thirst suggest that the osmotic threshold is very close to that of vasopressin release, with a steady increase in the intensity of thirst as osmolality increases above this threshold [11] (see Fig. 1.3). Thirst and vasopressin release share a potent "off" response to drinking, with a rapid drop that precedes any change in circulating osmolality (see Fig. 1.3). Teleologically, this reflex response serves to prevent over-hydration [11]. Although the mechanisms involved are still somewhat obscure, peripheral osmoreceptors in the oropharynx, upper gastrointestinal (GI) tract, and/or portal vein are postulated to sense the rapid change in local osmolality and relay the information back through the vagus nerve and splanchnic nerves [12].

As with vasopressin release, thirst is stimulated by hypovolemia, although this requires a

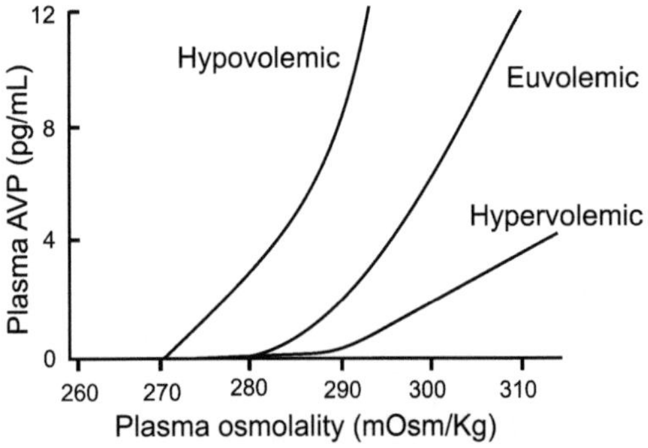

Fig. 1.2 The influence of volume status on osmotic stimulation of vasopressin release in healthy adults. The heavy oblique line in the center depicts the relationship of plasma vasopressin to osmolality in normovolemic, normotensive subjects. *Labeled lines* to the left or right depict the relationship when blood volume and/or pressure are acutely decreased or increased, in hypovolemia or hypervolemia, respectively

deficit of 8–10 % in plasma volume, versus the 1–2 % increase in tonicity that is sufficient to stimulate osmotic thirst [13]. Angiotensin II is a particularly potent dipsogenic agent, especially when infused directly into the brain or, more recently, overproduced in the subfornical organ (SFO) in transgenic mice [14]. Double-transgenic mice that express human renin from a neuronal promoter and human angiotensinogen from its own promoter were thus found to exhibit marked increases in water and salt intake. This phenotype is evidently caused by a marked increase in angiotensin II generation in neurons within the SFO due to the neuronal overexpression of human renin. Intracerebroventricular delivery of losartan blocked this polydipsic phenotype, as did inactivation of a "floxed" allele of angiotensinogen within the SFO, using adenoviral delivery of Cre recombinase [14]. Transgenic mice that overexpress brain angiotensin II type Ia (AT1a) receptors from a neuronal promoter also demonstrate increased intake of water and salt [15]. Finally, mice lacking angiotensin II due to targeted deletion of the murine angiotensinogen gene do not show impaired osmotic stimulation of thirst, but do have impaired thirst response to various hypovolemic stressors [16]. Therefore, the neuronal

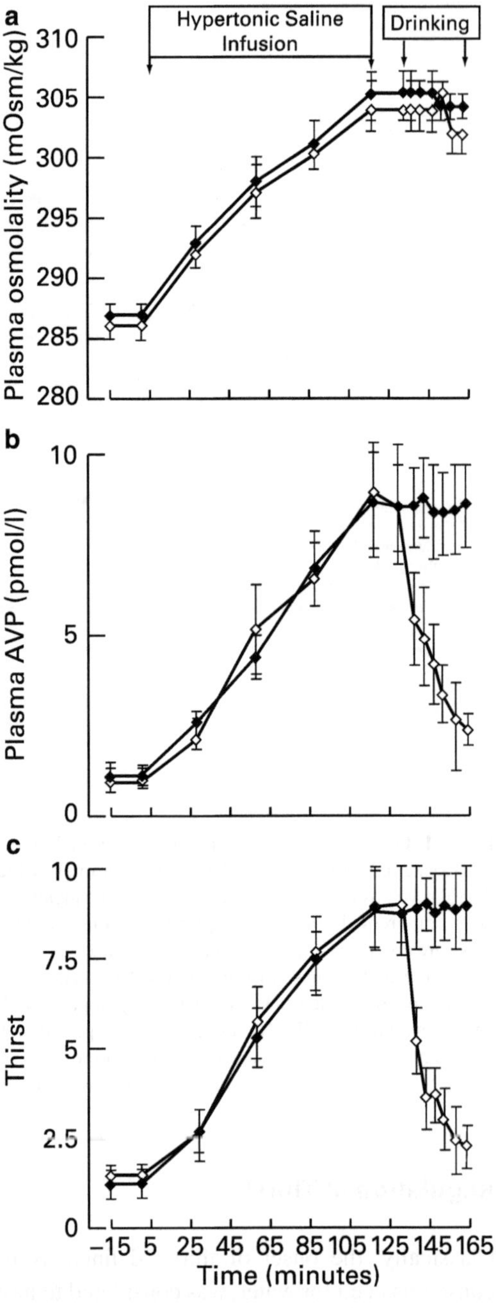

Fig. 1.3 The response of (**a**) plasma osmolality, (**b**) circulating vasopressin, and (**c**) thirst to hypertonic saline followed by drinking (*open diamonds*) or water deprivation (*filled diamonds*). Thirst and vasopressin steadily increase in response to increased osmolality, with a rapid drop in both parameters after drinking (**b** and **c**) despite the lack of acute change in osmolality (**a**). From McKenna et al. [11], with permission

effects of angiotensin II are evidently required for hypovolemic thirst, but not osmotic thirst [16].

Angiotensin II-dependent thirst has been demonstrated in a number of mammalian and non-mammalian species [13], but seems to be somewhat less potent in humans [17]. Although the experimental physiology is suggestive of a role for angiotensin II in thirst associated with heart failure and other disorders, much of the evidence is understandably indirect [13]. Perhaps the most compelling clinical evidence is the profound polydipsia that can accompany high-renin states such as renal artery stenosis or renin-secreting tumors [13]. In addition, a number of studies have implicated increased levels of angiotensin II in dialysis-associated thirst, with reduced thirst after angiotensin converting enzyme (ACE) inhibition [6].

Several ACE inhibitors (lisinopril, enalapril, cilazapril, benazepril, and captopril) have been associated with the development of the Syndrome of Inappropriate Anti-Diuresis (SIAD, formerly named Syndrome of Inappropriate Anti-Diuretic Hormone Secretion, SIADH) and/or hyponatremia [6], which is superficially paradoxical given the potent effect of angiotensin II on both vasopressin secretion and thirst. The pathogenesis of hyponatremia in these patients is not entirely clear. However, ACE inhibition in these patients may have had much less effect on the generation of angiotensin II within the central nervous system (CNS), compared to *systemic* angiotensin II, with central stimulation of both vasopressin and thirst. Notably, ACE inhibitors can be strongly polydipsic in both animals and patients [6]. This polydipsia appears to be dependent on bradykinin generation by ACE inhibition, with blockade of the effect by the bradykinin antagonist B-9430 [18].

Finally, in SIAD, one could postulate that thirst is also subject to abnormal regulation, with a decreased threshold and/or altered relationship to osmolality; indeed, the simple *persistence* of water intake in SIAD, at osmolalities lower than the typical threshold for thirst, is demonstrative of such an abnormality. In a landmark study, Smith et al. recently demonstrated that the osmotic threshold for thirst is in fact reduced in patients with SIAD, with thresholds that were almost identical to the corresponding osmotic thresholds for vasopressin release [19]. This suggests a shared pathophysiology for the abnormal vasopressin release and thirst in SIAD, perhaps due to alteration in osmoreceptor function (see below). Of interest, the act of drinking reduced thirst in the patients with SIAD, but did not attenuate vasopressin levels [19], versus the normal response of vasopressin to drinking (see Fig. 1.3).

Osmoreceptive Neural Networks

Seminal canine experiments some 60 years ago, correlating the effect of carotid infusion of various osmolytes on urine output, led to the prescient postulation of a central "osmoreceptor" [20]. The primary, dominant "osmostat" is encompassed within the organum vasculosum of the lamina terminalis (OVLT); this small periventricular region lacks a blood–brain barrier, affording direct sensing of the osmolality of circulating blood. However, osmoreceptive neurons are widely distributed within the CNS, such that vasopressin release and thirst are controlled by overlapping osmosensitive neural networks [12, 21–23] (see Fig. 1.1). Osmosensitive neurons are thus found in the SFO and the nucleus tractus solitarii, centers which help integrate regulation of circulating osmolality with that of related phenomena, such as ECF volume [12, 21, 22]. As discussed above, angiotensin II generation in the SFO has a very potent dipsogenic effect [6]. Finally, the "magnocellular" neurons of the hypothalamus, which synthesize and secrete vasopressin, are located in the supraoptic and paraventricular nuclei (Fig. 1.1) and are also directly sensitive to changes in osmolality [24].

Experimental ablation of the OVLT and adjacent circumventricular regions leads to variable defects in water intake and vasopressin release, in a number of different species [25, 26]. In sheep, ablation of the OVLT or SFO alone does not affect osmotic-induced drinking; combined ablation of both regions is more effective, but with some residual response. Complete abolition of thirst is however seen after combined ablation of the OVLT, the adjacent median preoptic nucleus (MnPO), and much of the SFO (see Fig. 1.1) [27]. Similar observations can be made in respect to vasopressin release, in that combined ablation of the OVLT, SFO, and MnPO is required to fully abolish osmotic-induced release of vasopressin; notably, "non-osmotic" stimuli such as hemorrhage and fever are still effective in inducing vasopressin release in these animals [26].

In humans, functional magnetic resonance imaging (fMRI) studies have revealed thirst-associated activation of the anterior wall of the third ventricle, encompassing the OVLT, in two out of four subjects treated with a rapid infusion of hypertonic saline [28]. Clinically, a variety of infiltrative, neoplastic, vascular, congenital, and traumatic processes in this circumventricular region can be associated with abnormalities in thirst and vasopressin release. Patients with this "adipsic" or "essential" hypernatremia generally exhibit combined defects in both vasopressin release and thirst [29]. In some cases, however, thirst is impaired but not vasopressin release [29], underscoring the functional redundancy and/or plasticity of the osmosensitive neuronal network; alternatively, the intrinsic osmosensitivity of the magnocellular neurons that synthesize and secrete vasopressin may preserve a residual osmotic-induced vasopressin release [26].

Increases in systemic tonicity cause electrophysiological activation of a subset of neurons within the OVLT, MnPO, and SFO [12, 26]. This is accompanied by increased expression of the immediate-early transcription factor c-fos, a marker of calcium-dependent neuronal activation [12, 26]. Distinct subsets of neurons in the OVLT and SFO project to magnocellular neurons within the supraoptic and paraventricular nuclei (SON and PVN); the pattern of c-fos induction corresponds to the known distribution of these same neurons, indicating that the OVLT/SFO osmosensitive neurons are upstream activators of the magnocellular neurons that release vasopressin [26, 30]. Direct identification of bona fide osmoreceptive neurons, i.e., neurons that translate changes in tonicity into alterations in action-potential discharge [12, 22], has been achieved using isolated neurons or explants from the OVLT, the SFO, the PVN, and the SON [6]. These neurons are generally activated by hypertonic conditions, i.e., exhibiting an increased action-potential discharge, and inhibited by hypotonic conditions [12, 22].

Molecular Physiology of Osmosensitive Neurons

Osmosensitive neurons from the SON differ dramatically from hippocampal neurons in that they demonstrate exaggerated changes in cell volume during cell shrinkage (hypertonic media) or cell swelling (hypotonic media) [31]. In hippocampal neurons, cell swelling evokes a rapid regulatory volume decrease (RVD) response, whereas cell shrinkage evokes a regulatory volume increase (RVI) response. In consequence, if external tonicity is slowly increased or decreased these RVD and RVI mechanisms are sufficient to prevent any change in the cell volume of hippocampal neurons; in contrast, osmosensitive neurons exhibit considerable changes in cell volume during such osmotic ramps [31]. This relative lack of volume regulatory mechanisms maximizes the mechanical effect of extracellular tonicity and generates an ideal osmotic sensor.

Osmosensitive neurons also depolarize after cell shrinkage induced by exposure to hypertonic stimuli, with a marked increase in neuronal spike discharges; the associated current is unaffected by anion substitution but is affected by substituting Na^+ with K^+, suggesting involvement of a nonselective cation channel [24]; more recent studies indicate a fivefold higher permeability for Ca^{2+} over Na^+ [32]. Hypotonic stimuli in turn hyperpolarize the cells and essentially abolish spike discharges [24]. Depolarization and spike discharges, in the absence of hypertonicity, can also be evoked by suction-induced changes in cell volume during whole-cell voltage recording, suggesting involvement of a stretch-inactivated cation channel [24]. Furthermore, the external blockade of stretch-sensitive cation channels with gadolinium inhibits depolarization and spike discharges induced by hypertonic stimuli, without affecting cell shrinkage [6]. Mechanosensitive, stretch-inactivated cation channels are evidently a key component of the osmoreceptor complex.

Members of the transient receptor potential (TRP) gene family of cation channels have recently been implicated in neuronal osmosensing. A *Caenorhabditis elegans* (worm) TRP channel was initially identified as OMS-9, a gene involved in osmotic-avoidance responses, with expression in osmoreceptor neurons [33]. Liedtke et al. demonstrated expression of the homologous mammalian TRPV4 transcript in osmoreceptor neurons in the OVLT and MnPO [34]; subsequent immunohistochemistry revealed expression of the TRPV4 protein in circumventricular neurons [35]. The nonselective TRPV4 cation channel is osmotically sensitive when expressed in mammalian cells [34, 36]. However, it functions as a *swelling*-activated channel, inhibited by cell shrinkage, the opposite behavior expected of the *shrinkage*-activated and stretch-inactivated channel implicated in neuronal osmoreceptor function [24, 37, 38]. Notably, however, mammalian TRPV4 is capable of rescuing the avoidance response to hypertonicity in *C. elegans* OSM-9 mutant worms, suggesting a critical in vivo role in the osmotic response to hypertonicity [39].

The physiological characterization of TRPV4 knockout mice has yielded somewhat contradictory findings [35, 39], which nonetheless indicate a role in central osmosensing. Liedtke et al. demonstrated reduced drinking in single-caged TRPV4–/– mice, with an associated mild increase in serum osmolality [39]. The mice also had an exaggerated increase in serum osmolality after water deprivation or intraperitoneal hypertonic saline, with a blunted increase in vasopressin [39]. The induction of c-fos after intraperitoneal hypertonic saline was also attenuated in OVLT neurons of these TRPV4–/– mice [39]. Finally, TRPV4 knockout mice became hyponatremic during treatment with the V2 agonist dDAVP (Desmopressin), with a relative failure to reduce drinking after the development of systemic hypotonicity. Consistent with an anti-dipsogenic effect of TRPV4, the intracerebroventricular infusion of a TRPV4 agonist reduces spontaneous drinking and drinking induced by angiotensin II; however, drinking induced by water deprivation or hypertonic infusion was unaffected [40].

Using a separate TRPV4 knockout strain to that of Liedtke et al., Mizuno et al. did not detect abnormalities in baseline water intake or serum osmolality [35], perhaps since this seems to require housing in single cages to reduce group behavioral influences [39]. With respect to vasopressin release, Mizuno detected an *exaggerated* response to hypertonic stress in TRPV4 knockout mice, compared to wild-type mice [35]; notably, however, they only measured this response in one mouse from each genotype [35], versus fourteen mice per genotype in Liedtke et al. [39]. However, using brain slices from five mice in each genotype, Mizuno et al. also demonstrated an exaggerated secretion of vasopressin in TRPV4 knockout mice sections, during graded increases in tonicity [35].

More recently, Bourque et al. have implicated TRPV1, a related member of the TRP channel gene family, in the activation of osmoreceptor neurons by hypertonic stimuli [41, 42]. These authors detected the expression of TRPV1 C-terminal exons by RT-PCR in neurons from the SON, without detectable expression of N-terminal exons; vasopressin-positive neurons also stained positive with a C-terminal TRPV1 antibody. Given prior data on a mechanosensitive, shrinkage-activated TRPV1-TRPV4 cDNA [43], generated by fusion of N-terminal truncated TRPV1 sequence to the TRPV4 C-terminus [42], the authors went on to characterize TRPV1 knockout mice; the hypothesis was that an N-terminal truncated isoform of TRPV1 was the osmoreceptor channel. Isolated magnocellular and OVLT neurons from these mice lack the usual depolarization and spike discharges induced by hypertonic stress, indicating a critical role for TRPV1 [41, 42]. TRPV1 knockout mice also show a marked decrease in the slope of the curve that relates systemic osmolality to circulating vasopressin, suggesting impairment but not abolition of osmotic-induced vasopressin release [42]. In addition, TRPV1–/– mice challenged with intraperitoneal hypertonic saline showed a 20 % reduction in drinking compared to wild-type control mice [41], indicating impairment but not abolition of osmotic-induced thirst. Again, however, as in the case of TRPV4 knockout mice [35, 39], there is a substantial discrepancy in the reported phenotypes of TRPV1 knockout mice [41, 42, 44]. In a more extensive study, Taylor et al. have reported that TRPV1−/− mice have *no* abnormality in water intake induced by hypovolemic or osmotic stimuli, with no detectable difference in the c-fos induction by hypertonicity within OVLT neurons [44].

To summarize, shrinkage-activated, mechanosensitive cation channels [37, 38] appear to depolarize osmoreceptor neurons under hypertonic conditions, leading to increased spike discharges and downstream activation of thirst and vasopressin release. A relative lack of volume regulatory mechanisms in osmoreceptor neurons also maximizes the cellular and mechanical effect of extracellular tonicity [31]. The swelling-activated TRPV4 channel is expressed in osmoreceptor neurons, where it may play an inhibitory role, limiting the thirst response in hypotonicity and perhaps downregulating osmotic-induced vasopressin release; however, there are substantial differences in the reported phenotypes of TRPV4 knockout mice [35, 39], such that the exact role of this channel is still unclear. TRPV1 appears to be a critical component of the mechanosensitive osmoreceptor, with loss of osmoreceptive neuronal depolarization and neuronal activation after hypertonic stimuli in TRPV1−/− mice [41, 42]. However, the primary structure of the putative N-terminal splice form of TRPV1 that mediates this activity is not yet known; the reported TRPV1–TRPV4 chimeric transcript that generates the only known shrinkage-activated, stretch-inhibited TRP channel activity [43] is evidently a cDNA cloning artifact [42]. Finally, the reported phenotypes of TRPV1 knockout mice differ considerably [41, 42, 44].

A major unresolved issue is why the loss of TRPV1 expression completely abrogates osmoreceptive neuronal activation [41, 42], yet has only modest effects on thirst and vasopressin release [41, 42, 44]. It is conceivable that other channel subunits are capable of substituting for TRPV1 or modulating the endogenous mechanosensitive channels, perhaps in neuronal subtypes that are distinct from those that have been tested thus far. It is notable in this regard that TRPV2, a swelling-activated TRP channel, is also expressed in osmoreceptor neurons [45], along with TRPV1 and TRPV4. A related issue is whether osmoreceptive neuronal activation is directly affected by loss of TRPV4 function, given the lack of equivalent electrophysiology to that of TRPV1 mice [41, 42] in TRPV4 knockout mice; conceivably these mice have a *gain* in osmoreceptor sensitivity, should TRPV4 function as a tonic or swelling-activated inhibitor of osmosensitive neuronal activity. Regardless, despite the many remaining questions and controversies, the identification of TRPV1 and TRPV4 as components of the osmoreceptor mechanism(s) is a major advance.

Regulation of Osmoreceptor Sensitivity

Vasopressin release and thirst are regulated by a number of hormones and neurotransmitters, via effects on the inhibitory and excitatory interactions between osmoreceptor neurons in the OVLT and downstream magnocellular neurons within the PVN/SON, modulatory effects on glial–neuronal interactions, and direct effects on osmoreceptor gain in the various osmosensitive neuronal subtypes [12, 26, 46]. Hypotonic inhibition of magnocellular neurons is thus due to a combination of a decrease in synaptic excitation by glutamatergic inputs from the OVLT, glycine receptor activation and neuronal hyperpolarization in response to taurine release from surrounding astrocytes, and hyperpolarizing effect of swelling-induced inhibition of the stretch-inhibited osmoreceptor channel [46]. Hypertonic activation of magnocellular neurons is in turn the net effect of an increase in glutamatergic excitation by OVLT neurons, a reduction in the hyperpolarizing effect of glycinergic receptors due to decreased taurine release from astrocytes, and direct neuronal depolarization due to shrinkage activation of the stretch-inhibited osmoreceptor channel [46].

Several factors directly influence the sensitivity of the stretch-inhibited osmoreceptor channel in magnocellular neurons and presumably other osmosensitive neurons in the OVLT and SFO [6]. In particular, extracellular Na^+ potentiates the response of magnocellular neurons to hypertonic stimuli, such that the number of spike discharges evoked by a 30 mOsm/kg H_2O pulse of NaCl is ~600 % higher

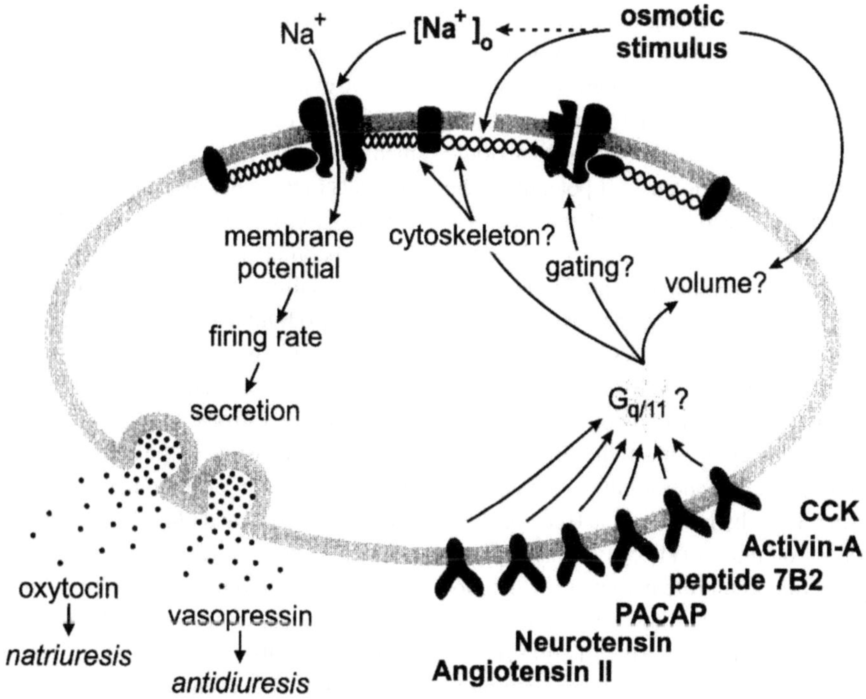

Fig. 1.4 Modulation of intrinsic osmosensitivity in magnocellular neurons. Changes in osmolality cause changes in cell volume that alter the probability of opening of stretch-inhibited (SIC) channels. In turn, changes in SIC channel activity alter the membrane potential and firing rate of magnocellular neurons and other osmoreceptor neurons, leading to vasopressin secretion and thirst (see text for details). Changes in $[Na^+]_0$ modulate osmoreceptor currents by affecting the driving force through the channel and by altering the relative permeability to Na^+ ions. Osmotic stimuli are normally associated with proportional changes in cerebrospinal $[Na^+]$ (*dashed line*). Numerous excitatory peptides, particularly those mediating their actions through Gq/lh appear to enhance osmosensory gain. This effect might be mediated by peptide-evoked changes in cell volume, cytoskeleton properties, and/or SIC channel gating. From Bourque et al. [46] with permission

than that induced by a 30 mOsm/kg H_2O pulse of mannitol [47]. Increases in extracellular Na^+ concentration appear to enhance the relative Na^+ permeability of the stretch-inhibited osmoreceptor channel, thus amplifying the electrophysiological response to hypertonicity [47]. This phenomenon provides an attractive explanation for the long-standing observation that vasopressin release can be modulated by changes in the osmolality and/or Na^+ concentration of cerebral spinal fluid (CSF); for example, intraventricular infusion of hypertonic sucrose has no evident effect on vasopressin release in the absence of concomitant Na^+, whereas parallel changes in Na^+ concentration and osmolality have a synergistic effect [48]. Rather than separate central Na^+ and osmoreceptors, as previously hypothesized [48], the response of the stretch-inhibited osmoreceptor channel is modulated by changes in extracellular $[Na^+]$ (see also Fig. 1.4).

A host of peptide and non-peptide hormones directly modulate the response of osmoreceptor neurons to hypertonicity. Treatment of magnocellular neurons with angiotensin II, cholecystokinin, and other excitatory peptides causes depolarization and an increase in excitatory discharges due to activation of a stretch-inactivated cation channel that is inhibited by gadolinium, i.e., the stretch-inhibited osmoreceptor channel [49]. In addition, these peptides potentiate the excitatory effect of hypertonicity, such that their stimulatory effect on vasopressin release is due, at least in part, to an increase in the "gain" of the osmoreceptor mechanism [46, 49]. Many of the receptors for these peptides signal through the

Gq/11 G protein, suggesting a shared signaling pathway [46, 49] (see also Fig. 1.4). Angiotensin II does not affect the volume responses of magnocellular neurons, i.e., the quantitative change in cell volume induced by hypotonic or hypertonic stimuli [50]. Rather, angiotensin II potentiates the cellular mechanosensitivity of these neurons, increasing the change in membrane conductance in response to mechanical or osmotic shrinkage [50]. This is associated with an increase in cortical F-actin density, perhaps due to Gq/11-dependent activation of the RhoA GTP-ase protein [50]. Regardless of the mechanism involved, the potentiation of osmoreceptor sensitivity by this and other hormones likely underlies the modulation of vasopressin release by ECF volume (see Fig. 1.2).

Finally, serotonin (5-HT, 5-hydroxytryptamine) plays an important role in regulating magnocellular neurons, such that serotonin itself, serotoninergic precursors, serotoninergic releasers, selective serotonin reuptake inhibitors (SSRIs), and serotonin agonists induce vasopressin release [6]. Vasopressin release induced by serotonin appears to be mediated by 5-HT2C, 5-HT4, and 5-HT7 receptors [6], and is associated with c-fos induction in magnocellular neurons [51]. Although the effect of serotonin on the stretch-inhibited osmoreceptor channel has not been reported, it directly depolarizes and excites magnocellular neurons [52]. This direct excitatory effect of serotonin on magnocellular neurons provides a mechanistic explanation for the common association between SSRIs and SIAD [6]. In addition, the recreational drug ecstasy (MDMA, 3.4-methylenedioxymethamphetamine) has potent serotoninergic effects, leading to induction of c-fos in magnocellular neurons [53], vasopressin release [54], and perhaps thirst [6]; these effects explain the association between ecstasy use and acute hyponatremia [55].

General Features of the Concentrating Mechanism

All mammalian kidneys maintain an osmotic gradient that increases from the cortico-medullary boundary to the tip of the medulla (papillary tip). This osmotic gradient is sustained even in diuresis, although its magnitude is diminished relative to antidiuresis [56, 57]. NaCl is the major constituent of the osmotic gradient in the outer medulla, while NaCl and urea are the major constituents in the inner medulla [56, 57]. The cortex is nearly isotonic to plasma, while the inner medullary (papillary) tip is hypertonic to plasma, and has osmolality similar to urine during antidiuresis [58]. Sodium and potassium, accompanied by univalent anions and urea are the major urinary solutes; urea is normally the predominant urinary solute during a strong antidiuresis [56, 57].

The mechanisms for the independent control of water and sodium excretion are mostly contained within the renal medulla. The medullary nephron segments and vasa recta are arranged in complex but specific anatomic relationships, both in terms of three-dimensional configuration and in terms of which segments connect to which segments. The production of concentrated urine involves complex interactions among the medullary nephron segments and vasculature [59, 60]. In the outer medulla, the thick ascending limbs of the loops of Henle actively reabsorb NaCl. This serves two vital functions: it dilutes the luminal fluid and it provides NaCl to increase the osmolality of the medullary interstitium, pars recta, descending limbs, vasculature, and collecting ducts. Both the nephron segments and vessels are arranged in a countercurrent configuration, thereby facilitating the generation of a medullary osmolality gradient along the cortico-medullary axis. In inner medulla, osmolality continues to increase, although the source of the concentrating effect remains controversial. The most widely accepted mechanism remains the passive reabsorption of NaCl, in excess of solute secretion, from the thin ascending limbs of the loops of Henle [61, 62].

Perfused tubule studies provided the basis for many of the theories of how concentrated urine is produced (reviewed in [2]). The cloning of many of the proteins that mediate urea, sodium, and water transport in nephron segments that are important for urinary concentration and dilution has provided additional insights into the urine concentrating mechanism (Fig. 1.5). In general, the urea, sodium, and water transport proteins are

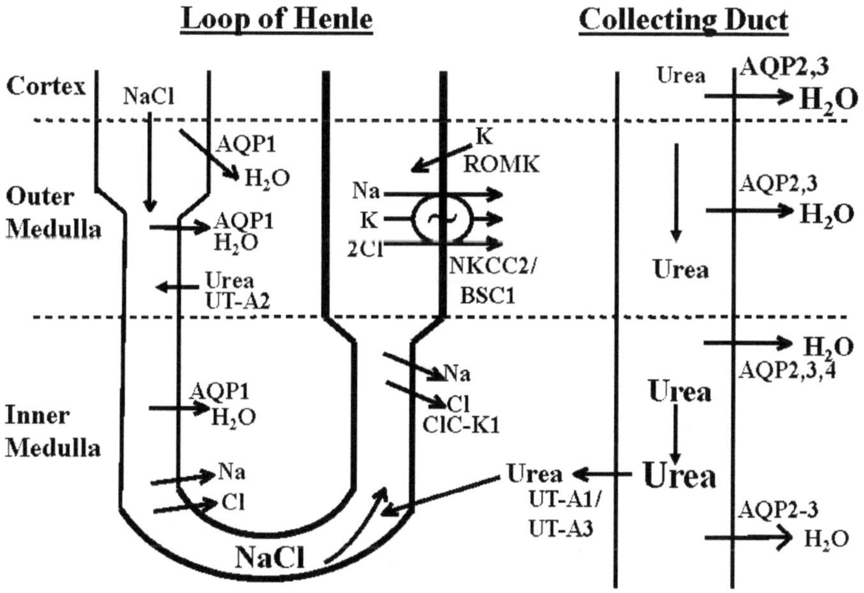

Fig. 1.5 Molecular identities and locations of the sodium, urea, and water transport proteins involved in the passive mechanism hypothesis for urine concentration in the inner medulla [61, 62]. The major kidney regions are indicated on the *left*. NaCl is actively reabsorbed across the thick ascending limb by the apical plasma membrane Na-K-2Cl cotransporter (NKCC2/BSC1), and the basolateral membrane Na/K-ATPase (not shown). Potassium is recycled through an apical plasma membrane channel, ROMK. Water is reabsorbed across the descending limb segments by AQP1 water channels in both apical and basolateral plasma membranes. Water is reabsorbed across the apical plasma membrane of the collecting duct by AQP2 water channels in the presence of vasopressin. Water is reabsorbed across the basolateral plasma membrane by AQP3 water channels in the cortical and outer medullary collecting ducts and by both AQP3 and AQP4 water channels in the inner medullary collecting duct (IMCD). Urea is concentrated within the collecting duct lumen (by water reabsorption) until it reaches the terminal IMCD where it is reabsorbed by the urea transporters UT-A1 and UT-A3. According to the passive mechanism hypothesis (see text), the fluid that enters the thin ascending limb from the contiguous thin descending limb has a higher NaCl and a lower urea concentration than the inner medullary interstitium, resulting in passive NaCl reabsorption and dilution of the fluid within the thin ascending limb. *AQP* aquaporin, *UT* urea transporter

highly specific and appear to eliminate a molecular basis for solvent drag; this specifically suggests that the reflection coefficients should be 1. For a detailed review of the transport properties, the reader is referred to [2].

Countercurrent Multiplication

Countercurrent multiplication refers to the process by which a small osmolality difference, at each level of the outer medulla, between fluid flows in ascending and descending limbs of the loops of Henle, is multiplied by the countercurrent flow configuration to establish a large axial osmolality difference. This axial difference is frequently referred to as the cortico-medullary osmolality gradient, as it is distributed along the cortico-medullary axis. Figure 1.7 illustrates the principle of countercurrent multiplication. The figure panels show a schematic of a short loop of Henle; the left channel represents the descending limb while the right channel represents the thick ascending limb. A water-impermeable barrier separates the two channels. Vertical arrows indicate flow down the left channel and up the right channel. Horizontal arrows (left-directed) indicate active transport of solute from the right channel to the left channel. Local fluid osmolality is indicated by the numbers within the channels. Successive panels represent the time course of the multiplication process.

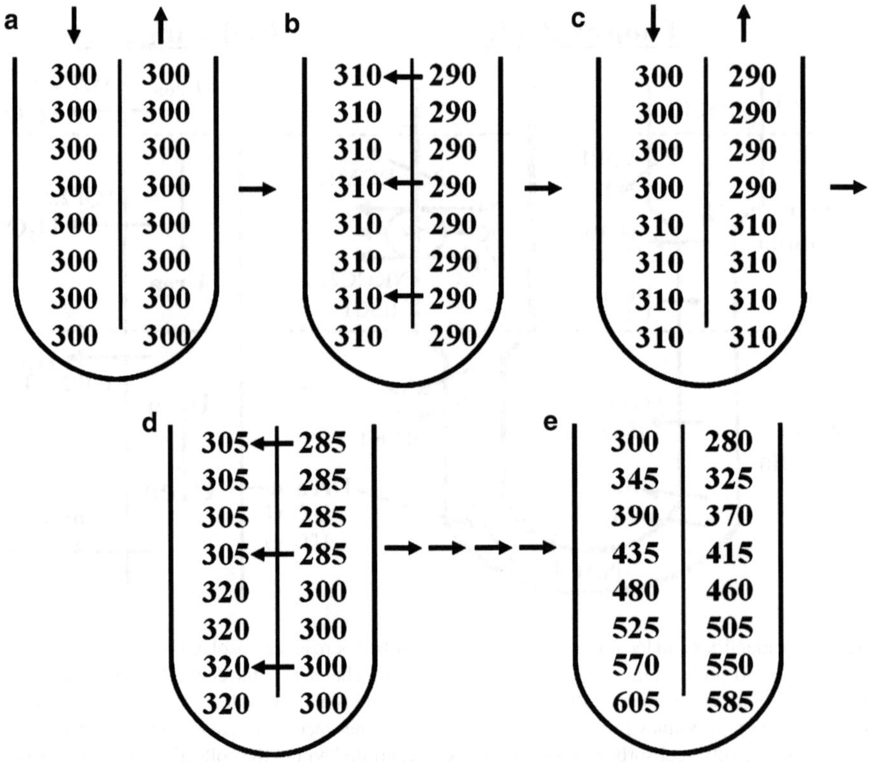

Fig. 1.6 Countercurrent multiplication of a single effect in a diagram of the loop of Henle in the outer medulla. (**a**) Process begins with isosmolar fluid throughout both limbs. (**b**) Active solute transport establishes a 20 mOsm/kg H_2O transverse gradient (single effect) across the boundary separating the limbs. (**c**) Fluid flows halfway down the descending limb and up the ascending limb. (**d**) Active transport reestablishes a 20 mOsm/kg H_2O transverse gradient. Note that the luminal fluid near the bend of the loop achieves a higher osmolality than loop-bend fluid in (**b**). (**e**) As the processes in (**c, d**) are repeated, the bend of the loop achieves a progressively higher osmolality so that the final axial osmotic gradient far exceeds the transverse 20 mOsm/kg H_2O gradient generated at any level

The schematic loop starts with isosmolar fluid throughout (Fig. 1.6a). In panel Fig. 1.6b, enough solute has been pumped by an active transport mechanism to establish a 20 mOsm/kg H_2O osmolality difference between the ascending and descending flows at each level. This small osmolality difference, transverse to the flow, is called the "single effect." Osmolality values after the fluid has convected the solute halfway down the left channel and halfway up the right channel are illustrated in Fig. 1.6c. In Fig. 1.6d, a 20 mOsm/kg H_2O osmolality difference has been reestablished by the active transport mechanism, and the luminal fluid near the bend of the loop has attained a higher osmolality than in Fig. 1.6a. A progressively higher osmolality is attained at the loop bend by successive iterations of this process. A large osmolality difference is generated along the flow direction, as illustrated in Fig. 1.6e, where the osmolality at the loop bend is nearly 300 mOsm/kg H_2O above the osmolality of the fluid entering the loop. Thus, a 20 mOsm/kg H_2O difference, the "single effect," has been multiplied axially down the length of the loop by the process of countercurrent multiplication.

In short loops of Henle, the process of countercurrent multiplication is similar to the process shown in Fig. 1.6. The tubular fluid emerging from the end of the proximal tubule and entering the outer medulla is isotonic to plasma (about 290 mOsm/kg H_2O). That tubular fluid is concentrated as it passes through the proximal straight tubule (pars recta) and on into the thin descending limb of the loop of Henle. The tubular fluid osmolality attains an osmolality about twice that of blood plasma at the bend of the loop of Henle. The fluid is then diluted as it flows up the medullary thick ascending limb of the loop of Henle, so that the tubular fluid emerging from this nephron segment is hypo-osmotic to plasma. The thick ascending limb is nearly impermeable to water and no aquaporin proteins have been detected in this nephron segment (reviewed in [1, 2]). The thick ascending limb has a low NaCl permeability, but it vigorously transports NaCl from the tubular lumen to the medullary interstitium by an active transport mechanism.

Countercurrent Exchange

The blood supply to the medulla, the descending and ascending vasa recta, is arranged in a counterflow configuration connected by a capillary plexus. Vasa recta achieve osmotic equilibration through a combination of water absorption and solute secretion, as they are freely permeable to water, urea, and sodium [63]. Descending vasa recta lose water and gain solute while ascending vasa recta gain water and lose solute. The exchange of water and solute between the descending and ascending vasa recta and the surrounding interstitium is called "countercurrent exchange."

Countercurrent exchange must be highly efficient to produce a concentrated urine since hypotonic fluid carried into the medulla and hypertonic fluid carried away from the medulla will each tend to dissipate the work of countercurrent multiplication. Thus, fluid flowing through the vasa recta must achieve near osmotic equilibrium with the surrounding interstitium at each medullary level, and fluid entering the cortex from the ascending vasa recta must have an osmolality close to that of blood plasma, in order to minimize wasted work. Conditions that decrease medullary blood flow, such as volume depletion, improve urine concentrating ability and the efficiency of countercurrent exchange by allowing more time for blood in the ascending vasa recta to lose solute and achieve osmotic equilibration [63]. Conversely, conditions that increase medullary blood flow, such as osmotic diuresis, decrease urine concentrating ability and impair the efficiency of countercurrent exchange [63]. For a more detailed treatment of countercurrent exchange, the reader is referred to [64].

Urine Concentrating Mechanism: History and Theory

Overview

One may divide the conceptual history of the concentrating mechanism into three periods. The first period (1942–1971) was inaugurated by a study by Kuhn and Ryffel [65] that proposed that the production of a concentrated urine results from the countercurrent multiplication of a "single effect." Kuhn and Ryffel [65] constructed a working apparatus that exemplified the principles of countercurrent multiplication. This first period saw the further development of the theory of the countercurrent multiplication hypothesis and the generation of experimental evidence that supported the hypothesis as the explanation for the urine concentrating mechanism of the outer medulla [66]. In particular, active transport of NaCl from thick ascending limbs of the loops of Henle was identified as the source of the outer medullary single effect [67, 68].

The second period (1972–1992) was inaugurated by the simultaneous publication of two seminal papers, one by Kokko and Rector and one by Stephenson, proposing that a "passive mechanism" provides the single effect for countercurrent multiplication in the inner medulla [61, 62]. According to the passive mechanism hypothesis, a net solute efflux from thin ascending limbs of the loops of Henle results from favorable transepithelial urea and NaCl gradients; these gradients arise from the separation of urea and NaCl, which is driven by the outer medullary concentrating mechanism.

Although a large body of experimental evidence initially appeared to support the passive mechanism, findings from several subsequent studies are difficult to reconcile with this hypothesis [69–71]. Moreover, when the measured transepithelial permeabilities were incorporated into mathematical models, the models failed to predict a significant inner medullary concentrating effect [72–74]. The discrepancy between the very effective inner medullary concentrating effect and the consistently negative results from mathematical modeling studies has persisted through more than three decades. The discrepancy has helped to stimulate the formulation of several highly sophisticated mathematical models (notably, [75]) and research on the transport properties of the renal tubules of the inner medulla, but no model study has resolved the discrepancy to the general satisfaction of modelers and experimentalists.

A third period of conceptual thought may be considered to have begun in 1993 as new hypotheses for the inner medullary concentrating mechanism began to receive serious consideration. In 1993, a key role for the peristalsis of the papilla was proposed by Knepper and colleagues [70, 76]. In 1994, the principle of "externally driven" countercurrent multiplication, arising, e.g., by the net production of osmotically active particles in the interstitium, was considered by Jen and Stephenson [77]. At about the same time, experimental measurements in perfused tubules from chinchillas, which can produce very highly concentrated urine, provided evidence that the passive mechanism, as originally proposed, cannot explain the inner medullary urine concentrating mechanism [78]. Recent studies have sought to further develop hypotheses involving the potential generation of osmotically active particles, especially lactate [79, 80], and peristalsis of the papilla [81]. In 2004, hypotheses related to the passive mechanism were reconsidered due to experimental evidence suggesting an absence of significant urea transport proteins in loops of Henle reaching deep into the inner medulla [82]. Recently, Pannabecker and colleagues [59] proposed that the spatial arrangements of loop of Henle subsegments and the identification of multiple countercurrent systems in the inner medulla, along with their initial mathematical model, are most consistent with a solute-separation, solute-mixing mechanism for the inner medullary urine concentrating mechanism.

Urine Concentrating Mechanism in the Outer Medulla

The urine concentrating mechanism is believed to operate as follows in the outer medulla. NaCl is actively transported from the tubular fluid of thick ascending limbs of the loops of Henle into the surrounding interstitium, mediated by the Na-K-2Cl cotransporter NKCC2/BSC1 in the apical plasma membrane and Na-K-ATPase in the basolateral plasma membrane. This active NaCl reabsorption raises the osmolality of interstitial fluid and promotes the osmotic reabsorption of water from the tubular fluid of descending limbs and collecting ducts. Because of the reabsorption of fluid from descending limbs of the loops of Henle, the fluid delivered to the ascending limbs has a high NaCl concentration that favors transepithelial NaCl transport from ascending limb fluid. (There may also be some NaCl diffusion into descending limb fluid.) NaCl reabsorption dilutes the thick ascending limb tubular fluid, so that at each medullary level the fluid osmolality is less than that in the other tubules and vessels, and so that the fluid delivered to the cortex is dilute relative to blood plasma. The ascending limb fluid that enters the cortex is further diluted by active NaCl reabsorption from cortical thick ascending limbs, so that its osmolality is less than the osmolality of blood plasma. In the presence of vasopressin (antidiuretic hormone), cortical collecting ducts are highly water permeable, and sufficient water is reabsorbed to return the fluid to isotonicity with blood plasma. This cortical water reabsorption greatly reduces the load that is placed on the urine concentrating mechanism by the fluid that reenters the medulla via the collecting ducts. In the absence of vasopressin, the entire collecting duct system has very limited water permeability, and even though some water is reabsorbed due to the very large osmotic pressure gradient, fluid that is dilute relative to plasma is delivered by the collecting ducts to the border of the outer and inner medulla.

This modern conceptual formulation of the outer medullary urine concentrating mechanism (which is very similar to the proposal of Hargitay and Kuhn as modified by Kuhn and Ramel

[83, 84]) is supported by recent mathematical modeling studies using parameters compatible with perfused tubule and micropuncture experiments (reviewed in [2]). In particular, the outer medullary osmotic gradients predicted by mathematical simulations [85, 86] are consistent with the gradients reported in tissue slice experiments, where osmolality is increased by a factor of 2–3 [87, 88].

The Passive Mechanism Hypothesis for the Inner Medulla

In contrast to the outer medulla, in which active NaCl transport from thick ascending limbs generates the single effect, isolated perfused tubule experiments in rabbit thin ascending limbs demonstrated no significant active NaCl transport [67, 89]. Instead, the thin ascending limb had relatively high permeabilities to sodium and urea while being impermeable to water [90]. In contrast, the inner medullary thin descending limb is highly water permeable but has low urea and sodium permeabilities [91, 92]. Moreover, it had long been known that urea administration enhances maximum urine concentration in protein-deprived rats and humans [93], and evidence from some species showed that urea tended to accumulate in the inner medulla, with concentrations similar to those of NaCl [57]. Several inner medullary concentrating mechanism models were published that failed to gain general acceptance (reviewed in [2]).

In 1972, two independent papers, one by Kokko and Rector and one by Stephenson (appearing in the same issue of *Kidney International*), proposed that the single effect in the inner medulla arises from a "passive mechanism" [61, 62]. The urea concentration of collecting duct fluid is increased by active absorption of NaCl from the thick ascending limb and the subsequent absorption of water from the cortical and outer medullary collecting ducts. In the highly urea-permeable terminal IMCD, urea diffuses down its concentration gradient into the inner medullary interstitium; urea is trapped in the inner medulla by countercurrent exchange in the vasa recta. Fluid entering thin ascending limbs has a high NaCl concentration relative to urea, and the thin ascending limb is hypothesized to have a high NaCl permeability, relative to urea. In addition, due to inner medullary interstitial accumulation of urea, the NaCl concentration in the thin ascending limb exceeds the NaCl concentration in the interstitium, and consequently NaCl diffuses down its concentration gradient into the interstitium. If the urea permeability of the thin ascending limb is sufficiently low, the rate of NaCl efflux from the thin ascending limb will exceed the rate of urea influx, resulting in dilution of thin ascending limb fluid and the flow of relatively dilute fluid up the thin ascending limb at each level and into the thick ascending limb. Thus, dilute fluid is removed from the inner medulla, as required by mass balance, and the interstitial osmolality is progressively elevated along the tubules of the inner medulla. Water will be drawn from the thin descending limbs by the elevated osmolality, thus raising the NaCl concentration of the descending limb flow that enters thin ascending limbs. In addition, the elevated osmolality of the inner medullary interstitium will draw water from the water-permeable IMCD, raising the concentration of urea in collecting duct fluid; accumulation of NaCl in the interstitium will tend to sustain a transepithelial urea concentration gradient favorable to urea reabsorption from the terminal IMCD.

Several matters regarding the passive mechanism merit discussion. First, this process should be thought of as a continuous, steady-state process, even though it is described above in stepwise fashion. Second, even though the mechanism is characterized as "passive," it depends on the separation of urea and NaCl that is sustained by active NaCl reabsorption by thick ascending limbs. The separated high-concentration flows of NaCl (in the loops of Henle) and of urea (in the collecting ducts) constitute a source of potential energy that is used to effect a net transport of solute from the thin ascending limbs. Thus, there is no violation of the laws of thermodynamics. Third, the description above speaks rather loosely of NaCl and urea as solutes having equal standing, but NaCl is nearly completely dissociated into Na and Cl ions, so that each NaCl molecule has nearly twice the osmotic effect of each urea molecule. Formal mathematical descriptions must represent this distinction. Fourth, the passive mechanism hypothesis is very similar to the outer medullary urine concentrating mechanism inasmuch as it depends on net solute absorption from the thin ascending limb to dilute thin ascending limb fluid and raise the osmolality in vasa recta and collecting ducts. Thus, the production of a small amount of highly concentrated urine is balanced by a larger amount of slightly dilute flow in the thin ascending limbs. Although the osmolality gradient along the inner medulla depends on countercurrent exchange, especially exchange between descending and ascending vasa recta, equilibration in countercurrent flows is incomplete. Hence the achievable urine osmolality is limited by the dissipative effect of ascending flows that are slightly concentrated relative to descending flows.

The passive mechanism hypothesis, as described above, closely follows the Kokko and Rector formulation [61], which made use of key ideas in a largely experimental study by Kokko [92]. Kokko and Rector [61] acknowledged Niesel and Rosenbleck [94] for the idea that IMCD urea reabsorption contributes to the inner medullary osmolality gradient. Kokko and Rector presented a conceptual model of the passive mechanism hypothesis, and although it was accompanied by a plausible set of solute fluxes, concentrations, and fluid flow rates that are consistent with the requirements of mass balance, it did not demonstrate that measured loop of Henle permeabilities were consistent with the hypothesis, and their presentation did not include a mathematical treatment. Stephenson's formulation of the passive mechanism hypothesis [62] introduced the highly influential central core assumption and included a more mathematical treatment, but it also did not contain a mathematical reconciliation of tubular transport properties with the hypothesis.

In recent years, mathematical simulations of the urine concentrating mechanism have become increasingly comprehensive and sophisticated in the representation of medullary architecture [72, 75, 95–97] and tubular transport [98–100]. This evolution is a consequence of faster computers with increased computational capacity, the increasing body of experimental knowledge, and the sustained failure of simulations to exhibit a significant inner medullary concentration gradient.

Studies by Pannabecker, Dantzler, and coworkers, conducted by means of immunohistochemical labeling and computer-assisted reconstruction, have revealed much new detail about the functional architecture of the rat inner medulla (see recent review [59]). In particular, their findings indicate that descending thin limbs (DTLs) of loops of Henle turning within the upper first millimeter of the IM do not have significant aquaporin-1 (AQP1), whereas DTLs of loops turning below the first millimeter have three discernible functional subsegments: the upper 40 % of these DTLs expresses AQP1, whereas the lower 60 % does not; moreover, the final ~165 μm expresses ClC-K1, as does the contiguous thin ascending limb (Fig. 1.7).

Layton et al. [82] proposed two hypotheses closely related to the passive mechanism; these hypotheses were motivated by implications of recent studies in rat by Pannabecker et al. [101, 102]. One hypothesis is based directly on principles of the passive mechanism: thin limbs of loops of Henle were assumed to have low urea permeabilities because no significant labeling for urea transport proteins was found in loops reaching deep into the inner medulla [82]. A second, more innovative hypothesis assumed very high urea loop of Henle urea permeabilities, but limited NaCl permeability and zero water permeability in thin descending limbs reaching deep into the inner medulla. Thus in the deepest portion of the inner medulla, tubular fluid urea concentration in loops of Henle would nearly equilibrate with the local interstitial urea concentration; thin descending limb fluid osmolality would be raised by urea secretion; and substantial NaCl reabsorption would occur in the prebend segment and early thin ascending limb. The role of the decreasing loop of Henle population is emphasized in both hypotheses, which facilitates a spatially distributed NaCl reabsorption along the inner medulla, from prebend segments and early thin

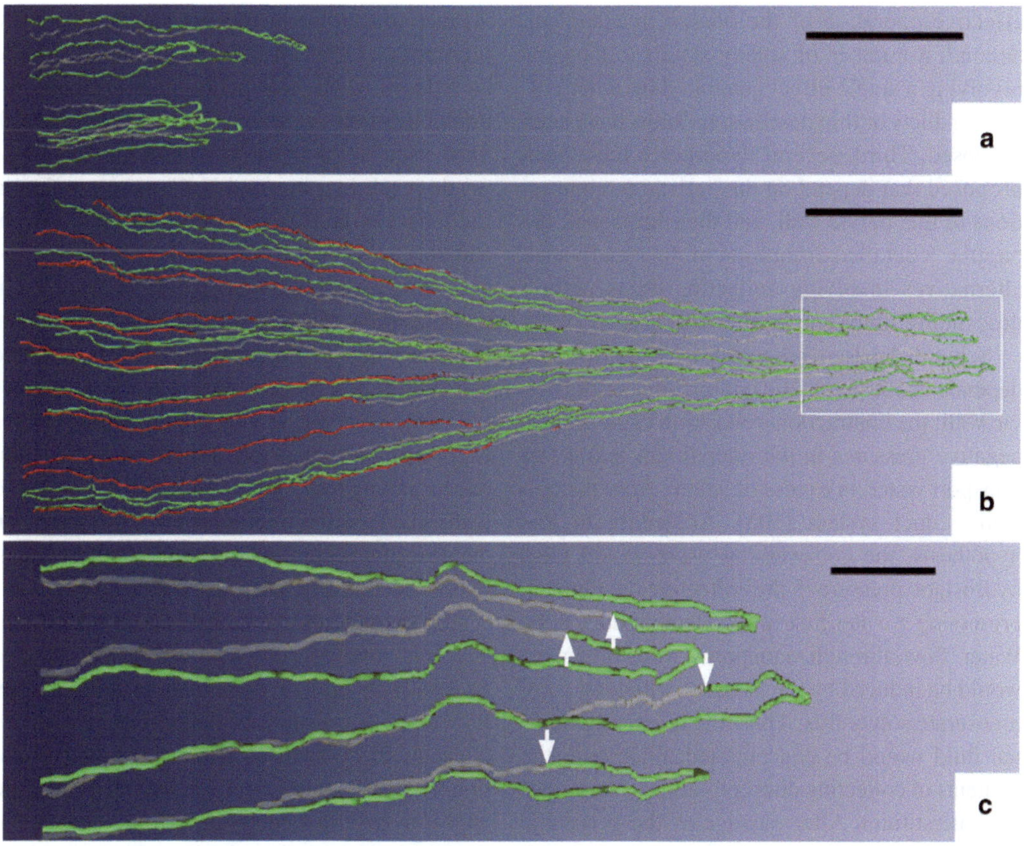

Fig. 1.7 Reconstruction of loops of Henle from rat inner medulla (IM). *Red* indicates expression of aquaporin-1 (AQP1); *green*, ClC-K1; *gray*, both AQP1 and ClC-K1 are undetectable. (**a**) Loops that turn within the first millimeter beyond the outer medulla. Descending thin limbs (DTLs) lack detectable AQP1; ClC-K1 is expressed along prebend segments and ascending thin limbs (ATLs). (**b**) Loops that turn beyond the first millimeter of the IM. DTLs express AQP-1 along the initial ~40 %; ClC-K1 is expressed along the prebend segments and ATLs. (**c**) Enlargement of near-bend regions from *box* in (**b**). Prebend ClC-K1 expression, on average, begins ~165 μm before the loop bend (*arrows*). Scale bars: 500 μm (**a**, **b**); 100 μm (**c**). From [82]; used with the permission of the American Physiological Society

ascending limbs. A distinctive aspect of both hypotheses is an emphasis on NaCl reabsorption from the IMCDs as an important active transport process that separates NaCl from tubular fluid urea and that indirectly drives water and urea reabsorption from the collecting ducts. Computer simulations for both hypotheses predicted urine flow, concentrations, and osmolalities consistent with urine from moderately antidiuretic rats. The first hypothesis has a critical dependence on low loop of Henle urea permeabilities and is subject to the criticism that urea transport may be paracellular rather than transepithelial: that hypothesis depends on more conclusive experiments to determine urea transport properties in rat. The second hypothesis may contribute to understanding the chinchilla urine concentrating mechanism, in which high loop urea permeabilities have been measured [78].

Alternatives to the Passive Mechanism

Alternatives to the original passive mechanism hypothesis fall into three categories. First, many simulation studies have attempted to show that a better representation of medullary anatomy or transepithelial transport is required for the effective operation of the passive mechanism. Second, a number of steady-state mechanisms involving a single effect generated in either collecting ducts or thin descending limbs have been proposed. Third, several hypotheses have been proposed that depend on the peristaltic contractions of the pelvic wall, and their impact on the papilla. A detailed discussion of the steady-state alternatives involving collecting ducts or thin descending limbs can be found in [2].

Schmidt-Nielsen proposed a hypothesis that depends on the peristaltic contractions of the pelvic wall: the contraction–relaxation cycle creates negative pressures in the interstitium that act to transport water, in excess of solute, from the collecting duct system [103]. According to this hypothesis, the compression wave would raise hydrostatic pressure in the collecting duct lumen, promoting a water flux into collecting duct cells. Water flow through aquaporin water channels would be induced by the pressure without a commensurate solute flux. Thus, the remaining luminal fluid would be concentrated, relative to the contents of collecting duct cells and the surrounding interstitium. After passage of the peristaltic wave, the collecting ducts would be collapsed. The papilla, transiently narrowed and lengthened by the wave, would rebound and a negative hydrostatic pressure would develop in the elastic interstitium, which is rich in glycosamine glycans and hyaluronic acid. Water would be withdrawn from the collecting duct cells (through aquaporins) by the negative pressure and enters into the vasa recta, which reopen during the relaxation phase of the contraction and carry reabsorbate toward the cortex. This hypothesis appears to provide no role for long loops of Henle or the special role of urea in producing concentrated urine [93], and it does not explain the large NaCl gradient generated in the papilla [57, 104].

Knepper and colleagues [81] hypothesized that hyaluronic acid, which is plentiful in the rat inner medullary interstitium, could serve as a mechano-osmotic transducer, i.e., the intrinsic viscoelastic properties of hyaluronic acid could be utilized to transform the mechanical work of papillary peristalsis into osmotic work that could be used to concentrate urine. They proposed three distinct concentrating mechanisms arising from peristalsis. (1) Interstitial sodium activity would be reduced in the contraction phase through the immobilization of cations by their pairing with fixed negative charges on hyaluronic acid. This would result in a lowered NaCl concentration in fluid that can be expressed from the interstitium, and that relatively dilute fluid would enter the ascending vasa recta. Water would be absorbed in the relaxation phase from descending thin limbs (2) as a result of decreased interstitial pressure (previously proposed by Knepper and colleagues [70, 76]) and (3) as a result of elastic forces exerted by the expansion of the elastic interstitial matrix arising from hyaluronic acid. If water is so reabsorbed, without proportionate solute, then the descending limb tubular fluid would be relatively concentrated relative to other flows.

The hypotheses that depend on peristaltic contractions involve complex, highly coordinated cycles, with critical combinations of pressure, flow rates, permeabilities, compliances, and frequencies of peristalsis. Moreover, a determination of the adequacy of these hypotheses would appear to require a comprehensive knowledge of the physical properties of the renal inner medulla and a demonstration that the energy input from the contractions, plus any other sources of harnessed energy, is sufficient to account for the osmotic work performed. Thus the evaluation of these hypotheses, whether by means of mathematical models or experiments, presents a daunting technical challenge.

Role of the Collecting Duct

Water Transport

The collecting duct, under the influence of vasopressin, is the nephron segment that, by regulating water reabsorption, is responsible for the control of water excretion. Countercurrent multiplication in the loops of Henle generates the cortico-medullary osmotic gradient necessary for water reabsorption, and countercurrent exchange in the vasa recta minimizes the dissipative effect of vascular flows. However, water excretion requires another structural component, the collecting duct system, which starts in the cortex and ends at the papillary tip. In the absence of vasopressin, all collecting duct segments are nearly water impermeable, except for the terminal IMCD, which has a moderate water permeability even in the absence of vasopressin [105, 106]. Excretion of dilute urine only requires that not much water be absorbed nor much solute be secreted along the collecting duct since the fluid that leaves the thick ascending limb and enters the cortical collecting duct is dilute relative to plasma.

The entire collecting duct becomes highly water permeable in the presence of vasopressin. This occurs as follows. When blood plasma osmolality is elevated, as, e.g., by water deprivation, hypothalamic osmoreceptors, which can sense an increase of only 2 mOsm/kg H_2O, stimulate vasopressin secretion from the posterior pituitary gland (see *Osmoregulation*). Vasopressin binds to V2-receptors in the basolateral plasma membrane of collecting duct principal cells and IMCD cells. The binding stimulates adenylyl cyclase to produce cAMP, which in turn activates protein kinase A, phosphorylates aquaporin 2 (AQP2) at serines 256, 261, 264, and 269, inserts AQP2 water channels into the apical plasma membrane, and increases water absorption across the collecting duct ([107–110] and reviewed in [111]). The major mechanism by which vasopressin acutely regulates water reabsorption is regulated trafficking of AQP2 between subapical vesicles and the apical plasma membrane (reviewed in [111]). This "membrane shuttle hypothesis," originally advanced by Wade and colleagues [112], proposes that water channels are stored in vesicles and inserted exocytically into the apical plasma membrane in response to vasopressin. Subsequent to the cloning of AQP2, the shuttle hypothesis was confirmed experimentally in rat inner medulla (reviewed in [111]). Subsequent studies have elucidated the role of vesicle targeting proteins (SNAP/SNARE system), several signal transduction pathways that are involved in regulating AQP2 trafficking (insertion and retrieval of AQP2), and the role of the cytoskeleton (reviewed in [111]).

In the presence of vasopressin, water is reabsorbed across the collecting ducts at a sufficiently high rate for collecting duct tubular fluid to attain near-osmotic equilibrium with the hyperosmotic medullary interstitium; the reabsorbed water is returned to the systemic circulation via the ascending vasa recta. Most of the water is reabsorbed from collecting ducts in the cortex and outer medulla. Although the inner medulla has a higher osmolality than the outer medulla, its role in water reabsorption is important only when maximal water conservation is required. The IMCD reabsorbs more water during diuresis than antidiuresis, owing to the large transepithelial osmolality difference during diuresis [113].

Urea Transport

Urea plays a special role in the urinary concentrating mechanism. Urea's importance has been appreciated since 1934 when Gamble and colleagues described "an economy of water in renal function referable to urea" [93]. Many studies show that maximal urine concentrating ability is decreased in protein-deprived or malnourished mammals, and urea infusion restores urine concentrating ability (reviewed in [1, 2]). Recently, a UT-A1/UT-A3 knockout mouse, a UT-A2 knockout mouse, and a UT-B knockout mouse were each shown to have urine concentrating defects (reviewed in [114]). Thus, an effect derived from urea or urea transporters must play a role in any solution to the question of how the inner medulla concentrates urine.

The initial IMCD has a low urea permeability that is unaffected by vasopressin [105, 106]. In contrast, the terminal IMCD has a higher basal urea permeability than other portions of the collecting duct; either vasopressin or hypertonicity can each increase urea permeability by a factor of 4–6, and together they can increase urea permeability by a factor of 10. In the 1980s, three groups showed that vasopressin could increase passive urea permeability in isolated perfused rat IMCDs (reviewed in [1, 2]). In 1987, a specific facilitated or carrier-mediated urea transport process was first proposed in rat and rabbit terminal IMCDs [106]. Subsequent physiologic studies identified the functional characteristics for a vasopressin-regulated urea transporter. To date, two urea transporter genes have been cloned in mammals: the UT-A (*Scl14A2*) gene encodes six protein and nine cDNA isoforms; the UT-B (*Scl14A1*) gene encodes two protein isoforms (reviewed in [1, 2]).

UT-A1 is expressed in the apical plasma membrane of the IMCD (reviewed in [1, 2]). Urea transport by UT-A1 is stimulated by vasopressin when stably expressed in UT-A1-MDCK cells [115] or UT-A1-mIMCD3 cells [116] and by cAMP when expressed in *Xenopus* oocytes [117–121]. UT-A3 is also expressed in the IMCD and has been detected in both the basolateral and apical plasma membranes in different studies [122–124]. Urea transport by UT-A3 is stimulated by cAMP analogs when expressed in MDCK cells, human embryonic kidney (HEK) 293 cells, or *Xenopus* oocytes (reviewed in [1, 2]). UT-A2, the first urea transporter to be cloned [125], is expressed in thin descending limbs and urea transport by UT-A2 is not stimulated by cAMP analogs when expressed in either *Xenopus* oocytes or HEK-293 cells (reviewed in [1, 2]).

UT-B is also the Kidd blood group antigen (in humans) and was initially cloned from a human erythroid cell line [126] and then from rodents (reviewed in [1, 2]). UT-B protein and phloretin-inhibitable urea transport are present in descending vasa recta (reviewed in [1, 2]). Several studies tested whether UT-B transports urea only, or both water and urea [127–129]. Red blood cells from a UT-B/AQP1 double knockout mouse show that UT-B can function as a water channel. However, the amount of water transported under physiologic conditions through UT-B is small (in comparison to AQP1) and is probably not physiologically significant to the urine concentrating mechanism [130].

Rapid Regulation of Facilitated Urea Transport in the IMCD

The perfused rat IMCD has been the primary method for investigating the rapid regulation of urea transport. While this method provides physiologically relevant functional data, it cannot determine which urea transporter isoform is responsible for a specific functional effect in rat terminal IMCDs since both UT-A1 and UT-A3 are expressed in this nephron segment. Vasopressin increases both the phosphorylation and the apical plasma membrane accumulation of both UT-A1 and UT-A3 in freshly isolated suspensions of rat IMCDs [124, 131]. Vasopressin phosphorylates UT-A1 at serines 486 and 499 [132]. Mutation of both serine residues eliminates vasopressin stimulation of UT-A1 apical plasma membrane accumulation and urea transport [132]. Antibodies to phospho-serine 486 show that vasopressin increases UT-A1 phosphorylation at serine 486 [116, 133]. UT-A chimera proteins in which the loop region of UT-A1 (aa 460–532) containing serines 486 and 499 is attached to UT-A2, which normally lacks these amino acids, show that this section confers vasopressin sensitivity to UT-A2 [134].

Vasopressin phosphorylates both UT-A1 and UT-A3 at serine 84 in rat, based upon studies utilizing an antibody to phospho-serine 84 [133]. However, using site-directed mutagenesis, the equivalent serine in mouse UT-A3, serine 85, was shown not to be a PKA phosphorylation site [135]. The latter study also found that serine 92 was not a PKA phosphorylation site [135].

UT-A1 is linked to the SNARE machinery via snapin in rat IMCD and this interaction may be functionally important for regulating urea transport [121]. Both UT-A1 and UT-A3 proteins can be ubiquitinated, i.e., the abundance of these proteins is increased when the ubiquitin–proteasome proteolytic pathway has been inhibited [136, 137]. However, only UT-A1 has been rigorously shown to have high-molecular-weight ubiquitinated forms by immunoprecipitation and western analysis, mediated by the ubiquitin ligase MDM2 [137].

Increasing osmolality, either by adding NaCl or mannitol, to high physiological values as occur during antidiuresis acutely increases urea permeability in rat terminal IMCDs, even in the absence of vasopressin, suggesting that hyperosmolality is an independent activator of urea transport (reviewed in [1, 2]). Increasing osmolality with vasopressin present has an additive stimulatory effect on urea permeability. Hyperosmolality-stimulated urea permeability is inhibited by the urea analogue thiourea and by phloretin [138]. Kinetic studies show that hyperosmolality, like vasopressin, increases urea permeability by increasing V_{max} rather than K_m. However, hyperosmolality stimulates urea permeability via increases in activation of PKC and intracellular calcium while vasopressin stimulates urea permeability via increases in adenylyl cyclase (reviewed in [1, 2]). Hypersomolality, like vasopressin, increases the phosphorylation and the plasma membrane accumulation of UT-A1 and UT-A3 [124, 131, 139, 140].

Long-Term Regulation of Urea Transporters

Vasopressin

Administering vasopressin to Brattleboro rats (which lack vasopressin and have central diabetes insipidus) for 5 days decreases UT-A1 protein abundance in the inner medulla (reviewed in [1, 2]). However, 12 days of vasopressin administration increases UT-A1 protein abundance. This delayed increase in UT-A1 protein abundance is consistent with the time course for the increase in inner medullary urea content following vasopressin administration in Brattleboro rats [141]. Suppressing endogenous vasopressin levels by 2 weeks of water diuresis in normal rats decreases UT-A1 protein abundance [142]. Analysis of UT-A promoter I may explain this time course since the 1.3 kb that has been cloned does not contain a cAMP response element (CRE) and cAMP does not increase promoter activity [143, 144]. However, a tonicity enhancer (TonE) element is present in promoter I and hyperosmolality increases promoter activity [143, 144]. Thus, vasopressin may first directly increase the transcription of the Na-K-2Cl cotransporter NKCC2/BSC1 in the thick ascending limb; the increase in NaCl reabsorption will increase inner medullary osmolality, which will then increase UT-A1 transcription (reviewed in [1, 2]).

Genetic Knockout of Urea Transporters

Humans with genetic loss of UT-B (Kidd antigen) are unable to concentrate their urine above 800 mOsm/kg H_2O, even following overnight water deprivation and exogenous vasopressin administration [145]. UT-B knockout mice also have mildly reduced urine concentrating ability that is not improved by urea loading [128, 146]. UT-A1 and UT-A3 abundances are unchanged in UT-B knockout mice, but UT-A2 protein abundance is increased [147]. The up-regulation of UT-A2 may partially compensate for the loss of urea recycling through UT-B, thereby contributing to the mild phenotype observed in humans lacking UT-B/Kidd antigen and in UT-B knockout mice. The absence of UT-B is also predicted (by mathematical modeling studies) to decrease the efficiency of small solute trapping within the renal medulla, thereby decreasing urine concentrating ability and the efficiency of countercurrent exchange [148–150]. Thus, UT-B protein expression in descending vasa recta and/or red blood cells is necessary for the production of maximally concentrated urine (reviewed in [2]).

UT-A1/UT-A3 knockout mice have reduced urine concentrating ability, reduced inner medullary interstitial urea content, and lack vasopressin-stimulated or phloretin-inhibitable urea transport in their IMCDs [71, 114]. However, when these mice are fed a low-protein diet, they are able to concentrate their urine almost as well as wild-type mice [71], which supports the hypothesis that IMCD urea transport contributes to urine concentrating ability by preventing urea-induced osmotic diuresis [151]. Inner medullary tissue urea content was markedly reduced after water restriction, but there was no measurable difference in NaCl content between UT-A1/UT-A3 knockout mice and wild-type mice [71]. While this latter finding was initially interpreted as being inconsistent with the predictions of the passive mechanism, a recent mathematical modeling analysis of these data concludes that the results found in the UT-A1/UT-A3 knockout mice are precisely what one would predict for the passive mechanism [59, 114, 152].

Urea Recycling

The inner medulla contains several urea recycling pathways that contribute to its high interstitial urea concentration (reviewed in [1, 2]). The major urea recycling pathway is reabsorption from the terminal IMCD, mediated by UT-A1 and UT-A3, and secretion into the thin descending limb and, especially, the thin ascending limb (Fig. 1.8, line 1). In the inner medulla, collecting ducts and thin ascending limbs are virtually contiguous [101, 102, 153, 154]. The urea that is secreted into the thin ascending limb is carried distally through several nephron segments having very low urea permeabilities until it reaches the urea-permeable terminal IMCD.

Two other urea recycling pathways (Fig. 1.8, lines 2 and 3) exist in the medulla. One involves urea reabsorption from terminal IMCDs through ascending vasa recta and secretion into thin descending limbs of short-looped nephrons, mediated by UT-A2, or into descending vasa recta, mediated by UT-B. The other involves urea reabsorption from cortical thick ascending limbs and secretion into proximal straight tubules. All three urea recycling pathways would limit the loss of urea from the inner medulla where it is needed to increase interstitial osmolality (reviewed in [1, 2, 155]).

In addition to urea's role in the urine concentrating mechanism, urea is the major source for excretion of nitrogenous waste and large quantities of urea need to be excreted daily. The kidney's ability to concentrate urea reduces the need to excrete water simply to excrete nitrogenous waste. A high interstitial urea concentration also serves to osmotically balance urea within the collecting duct lumen. The interstitial NaCl concentration would have to be much higher if interstitial urea were unavailable to offset the osmotic effect of luminal urea destined for excretion [71, 151].

Summary

The renal medulla produces concentrated urine through the generation of an osmotic gradient extending from the cortico-medullary boundary to the inner medullary tip. This gradient is generated in the outer medulla by the countercurrent multiplication of a comparatively small transepithelial difference in osmotic pressure. This small difference, called a single effect, arises from active NaCl reabsorption from thick ascending limbs, which dilutes ascending limb flow relative to flow in vessels and other tubules. In the inner medulla, the gradient may also be generated by the countercurrent multiplication of a single effect, but the single effect has not been definitively identified. Although the passive mechanism, proposed by Kokko and Rector [61] and by Stephenson [62] in

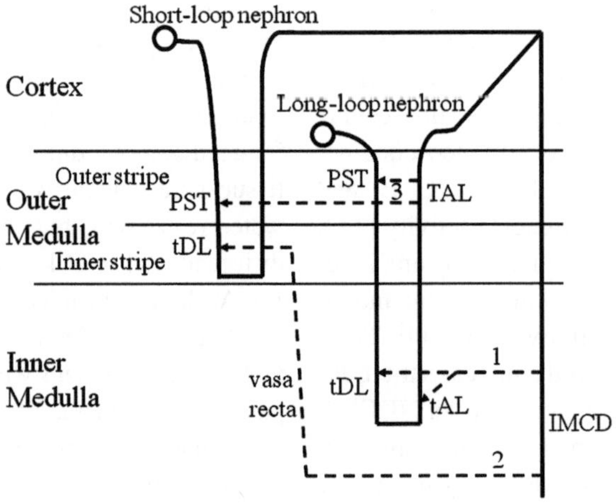

Fig. 1.8 Urea recycling pathways in the medulla. Diagram shows a long-looped nephron (*right*) and a short-looped nephron (*left*). *Dotted lines* labeled *1*, *2*, and *3* show urea recycling pathways. *PST* proximal straight tubule, *tDL* thin descending limb of Henle's loop, *tAL* thin ascending limb of Henle's loop, *TAL* thick ascending limb of Henle's loop, and *IMCD* inner medullary collecting duct

1972, remains the most widely accepted hypothesis for the inner medullary single effect, much of the evidence from perfused tubule and micropuncture studies is either inconclusive or at variance with the passive mechanism. Moreover, the passive mechanism has not been supported when measured transepithelial transport parameters are used in mathematical simulations.

Nevertheless, there have been important recent advances in our understanding of key components of the urine concentrating mechanism, in particular, the identification and localization of key transport proteins for water, urea, and sodium, elucidation of the role and regulation of osmoprotective osmolytes, better resolution of the anatomical relationships in the medulla, and improvements in mathematical modeling of the urine concentrating mechanism. Continued experimental investigation of transepithelial transport and its regulation, both in normal animals and in knockout mice, and incorporation of the resulting information into mathematical simulations, may help to more fully elucidate the inner medullary urine concentrating mechanism.

Acknowledgments This chapter is an expanded version of two articles published originally as Sands JM, Layton HE. The physiology of urinary concentration: an update. Semin Nephrol. 2009;29(3):178–95, copyright Elsevier Inc.; and Mount DB. The brain in hyponatremia: both culprit and victim. Semin Nephrol. 2009;29(3):196–215, copyright Elsevier Inc., 2009.

This work was supported by National Institutes of Health grants R01-DK41707 to J.M.S., R01-DK42091 to H.E.L., and PO1-DK070756 to D.B.M.

References

1. Sands JM, Layton HE. The physiology of urinary concentration: an update. Semin Nephrol. 2009;29(3): 178–95.
2. Sands JM, Layton HE. The urine concentrating mechanism and urea transporters. In: Alpern RJ, Hebert SC, editors. The Kidney: Physiology and Pathophysiology. 4th ed. San Diego: Academic Press; 2008. p. 1143–78.
3. Robertson GL, Aycinena P, Zerbe RL. Neurogenic disorders of osmoregulation. Am J Med. 1982;72(2):339–53.
4. Uretsky BF, Verbalis JG, Generalovich T, Valdes A, Reddy PS. Plasma vasopressin response to osmotic and hemodynamic stimuli in heart failure. Am J Physiol. 1985;248(3 Pt 2):H396–402.
5. Verbalis JG, Berl T. Disorders of water balance. In: Brenner BM, editor. The Kidney. 8th ed. Philadelphia, PA: Saunders; 2008. p. 459–549.
6. Mount DB. The brain in hyponatremia: both culprit and victim. Semin Nephrol. 2009;29(3):196–215.
7. Davison JM, Gilmore EA, Durr J, Robertson GL, Lindheimer MD. Altered osmotic thresholds for vasopressin secretion and thirst in human pregnancy. Am J Physiol. 1984;246(1 Pt 2):F105–9.
8. Sladek CD, Somponpun SJ. Estrogen receptors: their roles in regulation of vasopressin release for maintenance of fluid and electrolyte homeostasis. Front Neuroendocrinol. 2008;29(1):114–27.
9. Pak TR, Chung WC, Hinds LR, Handa RJ. Estrogen receptor-beta mediates dihydrotestosterone-induced stimulation of the arginine vasopressin promoter in neuronal cells. Endocrinology. 2007;148(7): 3371–82.
10. Somponpun SJ, Sladek CD. Depletion of oestrogen receptor-beta expression in magnocellular arginine vasopressin neurones by hypovolaemia and dehydration. J Neuroendocrinol. 2004;16(6):544–9.
11. McKenna K, Thompson C. Osmoregulation in clinical disorders of thirst appreciation. Clin Endocrinol (Oxf). 1998;49(2):139–52.
12. Bourque CW. Central mechanisms of osmosensation and systemic osmoregulation. Nat Rev Neurosci. 2008;9(7):519–31.
13. Fitzsimons JT. Angiotensin, thirst, and sodium appetite. Physiol Rev. 1998;78(3):583–686.
14. Sakai K, Agassandian K, Morimoto S, Sinnayah P, Cassell MD, Davisson RL, et al. Local production of angiotensin II in the subfornical organ causes elevated drinking. J Clin Invest. 2007;117(4):1088–95.
15. Lazartigues E, Sinnayah P, Augoyard G, Gharib C, Johnson AK, Davisson RL. Enhanced water and salt intake in transgenic mice with brain-restricted overexpression of angiotensin (AT1) receptors. Am J Physiol Regul Integr Comp Physiol. 2008;295(5): R1539–45.
16. McKinley MJ, Walker LL, Alexiou T, Allen AM, Campbell DJ, Di NR, et al. Osmoregulatory fluid intake but not hypovolemic thirst is intact in mice lacking angiotensin. Am J Physiol Regul Integr Comp Physiol. 2008;294(5):R1533–43.
17. Phillips PA, Rolls BJ, Ledingham JG, Morton JJ, Forsling ML. Angiotensin II-induced thirst and vasopressin release in man. Clin Sci (Lond). 1985; 68(6):669–74.
18. Cadnapaphornchai MA, Rogachev B, Summer SN, Chen YC, Gera L, Stewart JM, et al. Evidence for bradykinin as a stimulator of thirst. Am J Physiol Renal Physiol. 2004;286(5):F875–80.
19. Smith D, Moore K, Tormey W, Baylis PH, Thompson CJ. Downward resetting of the osmotic threshold for thirst in patients with SIADH. Am J Physiol Endocrinol Metab. 2004;287(5):E1019–23.
20. Verney EB. The antidiuretic hormone and the factors which determine its release. Proc R Soc Lond B Biol Sci. 1947;135(878):25–106.

21. McKinley MJ, Denton DA, Oldfield BJ, De Oliveira LB, Mathai ML. Water intake and the neural correlates of the consciousness of thirst. Semin Nephrol. 2006;26(3):249–57.
22. Bourque CW, Ciura S, Trudel E, Stachniak TJ, Sharif-Naeini R. Neurophysiological characterization of mammalian osmosensitive neurones. Exp Physiol. 2007;92(3):499–505.
23. Sewards TV, Sewards MA. The awareness of thirst: proposed neural correlates. Conscious Cogn. 2000;9(4):463–87.
24. Oliet SH, Bourque CW. Mechanosensitive channels transduce osmosensitivity in supraoptic neurons. Nature. 1993;364(6435):341–3.
25. McKinley MJ, Cairns MJ, Denton DA, Egan G, Mathai ML, Uschakov A, et al. Physiological and pathophysiological influences on thirst. Physiol Behav. 2004;81(5):795–803.
26. McKinley MJ, Mathai ML, McAllen RM, McClear RC, Miselis RR, Pennington GL, et al. Vasopressin secretion: osmotic and hormonal regulation by the lamina terminalis. J Neuroendocrinol. 2004;16(4): 340–7.
27. McKinley MJ, Mathai ML, Pennington G, Rundgren M, Vivas L. Effect of individual or combined ablation of the nuclear groups of the lamina terminalis on water drinking in sheep. Am J Physiol Regul Integr Comp Physiol. 1999;276(3):R673–83.
28. Egan G, Silk T, Zamarripa F, Williams J, Federico P, Cunnington R, et al. Neural correlates of the emergence of consciousness of thirst. Proc Natl Acad Sci U S A. 2003;100(25):15241–6.
29. Baylis PH, Thompson CJ. Osmoregulation of vasopressin secretion and thirst in health and disease. Clin Endocrinol (Oxf). 1988;29(5):549–76.
30. Shi P, Martinez MA, Calderon AS, Chen Q, Cunningham JT, Toney GM. Intra-carotid hyperosmotic stimulation increases Fos staining in forebrain organum vasculosum laminae terminalis neurones that project to the hypothalamic paraventricular nucleus. J Physiol. 2008;586(Pt 21):5231–45.
31. Zhang Z, Bourque CW. Osmometry in osmosensory neurons. Nat Neurosci. 2003;6:1021–2.
32. Zhang Z, Bourque CW. Calcium permeability and flux through osmosensory transduction channels of isolated rat supraoptic nucleus neurons. Eur J Neurosci. 2006;23(6):1491–500.
33. Colbert HA, Smith TL, Bargmann CI. OSM-9, a novel protein with structural similarity to channels, is required for olfaction, mechanosensation, and olfactory adaptation in Caenorhabditis elegans. J Neurosci. 1997;17(21):8259–69.
34. Liedtke W, Choe Y, Marti-Renom MA, Bell AM, Denis CS, Sali A, et al. Vanilloid receptor-related osmotically activated channel (VR-OAC), a candidate vertebrate osmoreceptor. Cell. 2000;103(3): 525–35.
35. Mizuno A, Matsumoto N, Imai M, Suzuki M. Impaired osmotic sensation in mice lacking TRPV4. Am J Physiol Cell Physiol. 2003;285(1):C96–C101.
36. Strotmann R, Harteneck C, Nunnenmacher K, Schultz G, Plant TD. OTRPC4, a nonselective cation channel that confers sensitivity to extracellular osmolarity. Nat Cell Biol. 2000;2(10):695–702.
37. Oliet SH, Bourque CW. Gadolinium uncouples mechanical detection and osmoreceptor potential in supraoptic neurons. Neuron. 1996;16(1):175–81.
38. Qiu DL, Shirasaka T, Chu CP, Watanabe S, Yu NS, Katoh T, et al. Effect of hypertonic saline on rat hypothalamic paraventricular nucleus magnocellular neurons in vitro. Neurosci Lett. 2004;355(1–2): 117–20.
39. Liedtke W, Friedman JM. Abnormal osmotic regulation in trpv4–/– mice. Proc Natl Acad Sci U S A. 2003;100(23):13698–703.
40. Tsushima H, Mori M. Antidipsogenic effects of a TRPV4 agonist, 4alpha-phorbol 12,13-didecanoate, injected into the cerebroventricle. Am J Physiol Regul Integr Comp Physiol. 2006;290(6):R1736–41.
41. Ciura S, Bourque CW. Transient receptor potential vanilloid 1 is required for intrinsic osmoreception in organum vasculosum lamina terminalis neurons and for normal thirst responses to systemic hyperosmolality. J Neurosci. 2006;26(35):9069–75.
42. Sharif NR, Witty MF, Seguela P, Bourque CW. An N-terminal variant of Trpv1 channel is required for osmosensory transduction. Nat Neurosci. 2006;9(1): 93–8.
43. Suzuki M, Sato J, Kutsuwada K, Ooki G, Imai M. Cloning of a stretch-inhibitable nonselective cation channel. J Biol Chem. 1999;274(10):6330–5.
44. Taylor AC, McCarthy JJ, Stocker SD. Mice lacking the transient receptor vanilloid potential 1 channel display normal thirst responses and central Fos activation to hypernatremia. Am J Physiol Regul Integr Comp Physiol. 2008;294(4):R1285–93.
45. Wainwright A, Rutter AR, Seabrook GR, Reilly K, Oliver KR. Discrete expression of TRPV2 within the hypothalamo-neurohypophysial system: Implications for regulatory activity within the hypothalamic-pituitary-adrenal axis. J Comp Neurol. 2004;474(1): 24–42.
46. Bourque CW, Voisin DL, Chakfe Y. Stretch-inactivated cation channels: cellular targets for modulation of osmosensitivity in supraoptic neurons. Prog Brain Res. 2002;139:85–94.
47. Voisin DL, Chakfe Y, Bourque CW. Coincident detection of CSF Na^+ and osmotic pressure in osmoregulatory neurons of the supraoptic nucleus. Neuron. 1999;24(2):453–60.
48. McKinley MJ, Denton DA, Weisinger RS. Sensors for antidiuresis and thirst—osmoreceptors or CSF sodium detectors? Brain Res. 1978;141(1):89–103.
49. Chakfe Y, Bourque CW. Excitatory peptides and osmotic pressure modulate mechanosensitive cation channels in concert. Nat Neurosci. 2000;3(6):572–9.
50. Zhang Z, Bourque CW. Amplification of transducer gain by angiotensin II-mediated enhancement of cortical actin density in osmosensory neurons. J Neurosci. 2008;28(38):9536–44.

51. Mikkelsen JD, Hay-Schmidt A, Kiss A. Serotonergic stimulation of the rat hypothalamo-pituitary-adrenal axis: interaction between 5-HT1A and 5-HT2A receptors. Ann N Y Acad Sci. 2004;1018:65–70.
52. Ho SS, Chow BK, Yung WH. Serotonin increases the excitability of the hypothalamic paraventricular nucleus magnocellular neurons. Eur J Neurosci. 2007;25(10):2991–3000.
53. Stephenson CP, Hunt GE, Topple AN, McGregor IS. The distribution of 3,4-methylenedioxymethamphetamine "Ecstasy"-induced c-fos expression in rat brain. Neuroscience. 1999;92(3):1011–23.
54. Fallon JK, Shah D, Kicman AT, Hutt AJ, Henry JA, Cowan DA, et al. Action of MDMA (ecstasy) and its metabolites on arginine vasopressin release. Ann N Y Acad Sci. 2002;965:399–409.
55. Campbell GA, Rosner MH. The agony of ecstasy: MDMA (3,4-methylenedioxymethamphetamine) and the kidney. Clin J Am Soc Nephrol. 2008;3(6): 1852–60.
56. Knepper MA, Stephenson JL. Urinary concentrating and diluting processes. In: Andreoli TE, Hoffman JF, Fanestil DD, Schultz SG, editors. Physiology of membrane disorders. 2nd ed. New York: Plenum; 1986. p. 713–26.
57. Hai MA, Thomas S. The time-course of changes in renal tissue composition during lysine vasopressin infusion in the rat. Pfleugers Arch. 1969;310:297–319.
58. Knepper MA. Measurement of osmolality in kidney slices using vapor pressure osmometry. Kidney Int. 1982;21:653–5.
59. Pannabecker TL, Dantzler WH, Layton HE, Layton AT. Role of three-dimensional architecture in the urine concentrating mechanism of the rat renal inner medulla. Am J Physiol Renal Physiol. 2008;295(5):F1271–85.
60. Kriz W. Der architektonische und funktionelle Aufbau der Rattenniere. Z Zellforsch. 1967;82: 495–535.
61. Kokko JP, Rector FC. Countercurrent multiplication system without active transport in inner medulla. Kidney Int. 1972;2:214–23.
62. Stephenson JL. Concentration of urine in a central core model of the renal counterflow system. Kidney Int. 1972;2:85–94.
63. Zimmerhackl BL, Robertson CR, Jamison RL. The medullary microcirculation. Kidney Int. 1987;31(2): 641–7.
64. Pallone TL, Turner MR, Edwards A, Jamison RL. Countercurrent exchange in the renal medulla. Am J Physiol Regul Integr Comp Physiol. 2003;284(5): R1153–75.
65. Kuhn W, Ryffel K. Herstellung konzentrierrter Lösungen aus verdünnten durch blosse Membranwirkung: Ein Modellversuch zur Funktion der Niere. Hoppe Seylers Z Physiol Chem. 1942;276:145–78.
66. Gottschalk CW, Mylle M. Micropuncture study of the mammalian urinary concentrating mechanism: evidence for the countercurrent hypothesis. Am J Physiol. 1959;196:927–36.
67. Rocha AS, Kokko JP. Sodium chloride and water transport in the medullary thick ascending limb of Henle. Evidence for active chloride transport. J Clin Invest. 1973;52:612–23.
68. Ullrich KJ, Schmidt-Nielsen B, O'Dell R, Pehling G, Gottschalk CW, Lassiter WE, et al. Micropuncture study of composition of proximal and distal tubular fluid in rat kidney. Am J Physiol. 1963;204:527–31.
69. Jamison RL, Kriz W. Urinary concentrating mechanism. Structure and function. New York: Oxford University Press; 1982.
70. Chou C-L, Knepper MA, Layton HE. Urinary concentrating mechanism: the role of the inner medulla. Semin Nephrol. 1993;13(2):168–81.
71. Fenton RA, Chou C-L, Stewart GS, Smith CP, Knepper MA. Urinary concentrating defect in mice with selective deletion of phloretin-sensitive urea transporters in the renal collecting duct. Proc Natl Acad Sci U S A. 2004;101(19):7469–74.
72. Layton HE, Knepper MA, Chou C-L. Permeability criteria for effective function of passive countercurrent multiplier. Am J Physiol. 1996;270(1):F9–F20.
73. Moore LC, Marsh DJ. How descending limb of Henle's loop permeability affects hypertonic urine formation. Am J Physiol. 1980;239:F57–71.
74. Wexler AS, Kalaba RE, Marsh DJ. Passive, one-dimensional countercurrent models do not simulate hypertonic urine formation. Am J Physiol. 1987;253:F1020–30.
75. Wexler AS, Kalaba RE, Marsh DJ. Three-dimensional anatomy and renal concentrating mechanism. I. Modelling results. Am J Physiol. 1991;260: F368–83.
76. Knepper MA, Chou C-L, Layton HE. How is urine concentrated by the renal inner medulla? Contrib Nephrol. 1993;102:144–60.
77. Jen JF, Stephenson JL. Externally driven countercurrent multiplication in a mathematical model of the urinary concentrating mechanism of the renal inner medulla. Bull Math Biol. 1994;56(3):491–514.
78. Chou C-L, Knepper MA. In vitro perfusion of chinchilla thin limb segments: urea and NaCl permeabilities. Am J Physiol Renal Physiol. 1993;264: F337–43.
79. Thomas SR. Inner medullary lactate production and accumulation: a vasa recta model. Am J Physiol Renal Physiol. 2000;279:F468–81.
80. Hervy S, Thomas SR. Inner medullary lactate production and urine-concentrating mechanism: a flat medullary model. Am J Physiol Renal Physiol. 2003;284(1):F65–81.
81. Knepper MA, Saidel GM, Hascall VC, Dwyer T. Concentration of solutes in the renal inner medulla: interstitial hyaluronan as a mechano-osmotic transducer. Am J Physiol Renal Physiol. 2003;284(3): F433–46.
82. Layton AT, Pannabecker TL, Dantzler WH, Layton HE. Two modes for concentrating urine in rat inner medulla. Am J Physiol Renal Physiol. 2004;287(4): F816–39.

83. Hargitay B, Kuhn W. Das Multiplikationsprinzip als Grundlage der Harnkonzentrierung in der Niere. Z Elektrochem. 1951;55:539–58.
84. Vehaskari VM, Hering-Smith KS, Moskowitz DW, Weiner ID, Hamm LL. Effect of epidermal growth factor on sodium transport in the cortical collecting tubule. Am J Physiol. 1989;256:F803–9.
85. Layton AT, Layton HE. A region-based mathematical model of the urine concentrating mechanism in the rat outer medulla. I. Formulation and base-case results. Am J Physiol Renal Physiol. 2005;289(6): F1346–66.
86. Layton AT, Layton HE. A region-based mathematical model of the urine concentrating mechanism in the rat outer medulla. II. Parameter sensitivity and tubular inhomogeneity. Am J Physiol Renal Physiol. 2005;289(6):F1367–81.
87. de Rouffignac C. The urinary concentrating mechanism. In: Kinne RKH, editor. Urinary concentrating mechanisms. Comparative physiology. Basel: Karger; 1990. p. 31–102.
88. Macri P, Breton S, Marsolais M, Lapointe JY, Laprade R. Hypertonicity decreases basolateral K^+ and Cl^- conductances in rabbit proximal convoluted tubule. J Membr Biol. 1997;155(3):229–37.
89. Morgan T, Berliner RW. Permeability of the loop of Henle, vasa recta, and collecting duct to water, urea, and sodium. Am J Physiol. 1968;215:108–15.
90. Imai M, Kokko JP. Sodium, chloride, urea, and water transport in the thin ascending limb of Henle. J Clin Invest. 1974;53:393–402.
91. Kokko JP. Sodium chloride and water transport in the descending limb of Henle. J Clin Invest. 1970;49:1838–46.
92. Kokko JP. Urea transport in the proximal tubule and the descending limb of Henle. J Clin Invest. 1972;51:1999–2008.
93. Gamble JL, McKhann CF, Butler AM, Tuthill E. An economy of water in renal function referable to urea. Am J Physiol. 1934;109:139–54.
94. Niesel W, Röskenbleck H. Konzentrierung von Lösungen unterschiedlicher Zusammensetzung durch alleinige Gegenstromdiffusion und Geggenstromosmose als möglicher Mechanismus der Harnkonzentrierung. Pflfiegers Arch. 1965;283: 230–41.
95. Layton HE, Davies JM. Distributed solute and water reabsorption in a central core model of the renal medulla. Math Biosci. 1993;116:169–96.
96. Wang X, Wexler AS, Marsh DJ. The effect of solution non-ideality on membrane transport in three-dimensional models of the renal concentrating mechanism. Bull Math Biol. 1994;56(3):515–46.
97. Thomas SR. Cycles and separations in a model of the renal medulla. Am J Physiol Renal Physiol. 1998;275(5):F671–90.
98. Stephenson JL, Zhang Y, Eftekhari A, Tewarson RP. Electrolyte transport in a central core model of the renal medulla. Am J Physiol. 1989;253:F982–97.
99. Stephenson JL, Zhang Y, Tewarson RP. Electrolyte, urea, and water transport in a two-nephron central core model of the renal medulla. Am J Physiol. 1989;257:F388–413.
100. Thomas SR, Wexler AS. Inner medullary external osmotic driving force in a 3D model of the renal concentrating mechanism. Am J Physiol. 1995;269: F159–71.
101. Pannabecker TL, Dantzler WH. Three-dimensional lateral and vertical relationships of inner medullary loops of Henle and collecting ducts. Am J Physiol Renal Physiol. 2004;287(4):F767–74.
102. Pannabecker TL, Abbott DE, Dantzler WH. Three-dimensional functional reconstruction of inner medullary thin limbs of Henle's loop. Am J Physiol Renal Physiol. 2004;286(1):F38–45.
103. Schmidt-Nielsen B. The renal concentrating mechanism in insects and mammals: a new hypothesis involving hydrostatic pressures. Am J Physiol. 1995;268:R1087–100.
104. Tomita K, Pisano JJ, Knepper MA. Control of sodium and potassium transport in the cortical collecting duct of the rat. Effects of bradykinin, vasopressin, and deoxycorticosterone. J Clin Invest. 1985;76:132–6.
105. Sands JM, Knepper MA. Urea permeability of mammalian inner medullary collecting duct system and papillary surface epithelium. J Clin Invest. 1987;79: 138–47.
106. Sands JM, Nonoguchi H, Knepper MA. Vasopressin effects on urea and H_2O transport in inner medullary collecting duct subsegments. Am J Physiol. 1987;253:F823–32.
107. Hoffert JD, Fenton RA, Moeller HB, Simons B, Tchapyjnikov D, McDill BW, et al. Vasopressin-stimulated Increase in Phosphorylation at Ser269 Potentiates Plasma Membrane Retention of Aquaporin-2. J Biol Chem. 2008;283(36): 24617–27.
108. Hoffert JD, Pisitkun T, Wang GH, Shen RF, Knepper MA. Dynamics of aquaporin-2 serine-261 phosphorylation in response to short-term vasopressin treatment in collecting duct. Am J Physiol Renal Physiol. 2007;292(2):F691–700.
109. Hoffert JD, Pisitkun T, Wang G, Shen R-F, Knepper MA. Quantitative phosphoproteomics of vasopressin-sensitive renal cells: regulation of aquaporin-2 phosphorylation at two sites. Proc Natl Acad Sci U S A. 2006;103(18):7159–64.
110. Fenton RA, Moeller HB, Hoffert JD, Yu MJ, Nielsen S, Knepper MA. Acute regulation of aquaporin-2 phosphorylation at Ser-264 by vasopressin. PNAS. 2008;105(8):3134–9.
111. Nielsen S, Frokiaer J, Marples D, Kwon ED, Agre P, Knepper M. Aquaporins in the kidney: from molecules to medicine. Physiol Rev. 2002;82:205–44.
112. Wade JB, Stetson DL, Lewis SA. ADH action: evidence for a membrane shuttle mechanism. Ann N Y Acad Sci. 1981;372:106–17.

113. Jamison RL, Buerkert J, Lacy FB. A micropuncture study of collecting tubule function in rats with hereditary diabetes insipidus. J Clin Invest. 1971;50: 2444–52.
114. Fenton RA, Knepper MA. Urea and renal function in the 21st century: insights from knockout mice. J Am Soc Nephrol. 2007;18(3):679–88.
115. Fröhlich O, Klein JD, Smith PM, Sands JM, Gunn RB. Urea transport in MDCK cells that are stably transfected with UT-A1. Am J Physiol Cell Physiol. 2004;286(6):C1264–70.
116. Klein JD, Blount MA, Fröhlich O, Denson C, Tan X, Sim J, et al. Phosphorylation of UT-A1 on serine 486 correlates with membrane accumulation and urea transport activity in both rat IMCDs and cultured cells. Am J Physiol Renal Physiol. 2010;298(4):F935–40.
117. Shayakul C, Steel A, Hediger MA. Molecular cloning and characterization of the vasopressin-regulated urea transporter of rat kidney collecting ducts. J Clin Invest. 1996;98(11):2580–7.
118. Promeneur D, Rousselet G, Bankir L, Bailly P, Cartron JP, Ripoche P, et al. Evidence for distinct vascular and tubular urea transporters in the rat kidney. J Am Soc Nephrol. 1996;7(6):852–60.
119. Fenton RA, Stewart GS, Carpenter B, Howorth A, Potter EA, Cooper GJ, et al. Characterization of the mouse urea transporters UT-A1 and UT-A2. Am J Physiol Renal Physiol. 2002;283(4):F817–25.
120. Chen G, Fröhlich O, Yang Y, Klein JD, Sands JM. Loss of N-linked glycosylation reduces urea transporter UT-A1 response to vasopressin. J Biol Chem. 2006;281(37):27436–42.
121. Mistry AC, Mallick R, Fröhlich O, Klein JD, Rehm A, Chen G, et al. The UT-A1 urea transporter interacts with snapin, a snare-associated protein. J Biol Chem. 2007;282(41):30097–106.
122. Terris JM, Knepper MA, Wade JB. UT-A3: localization and characterization of an additional urea transporter isoform in the IMCD. Am J Physiol Renal Physiol. 2001;280(2):F325–32.
123. Stewart GS, Fenton RA, Wang W, Kwon TH, White SJ, Collins VM, et al. The basolateral expression of mUT-A3 in the mouse kidney. Am J Physiol Renal Physiol. 2004;286(5):F979–87.
124. Blount MA, Klein JD, Martin CF, Tchapyjnikov D, Sands JM. Forskolin stimulates phosphorylation and membrane accumulation of UT-A3. Am J Physiol Renal Physiol. 2007;293(4):F1308–13.
125. You G, Smith CP, Kanai Y, Lee W-S, Stelzner M, Hediger MA. Cloning and characterization of the vasopressin-regulated urea transporter. Nature. 1993;365:844–7.
126. Olives B, Neau P, Bailly P, Hediger MA, Rousselet G, Cartron JP, et al. Cloning and functional expression of a urea transporter from human bone marrow cells. J Biol Chem. 1994;269(50):31649–52.
127. Yang BX, Verkman AS. Urea transporter UT3 functions as an efficient water channel—Direct evidence for a common water/urea pathway. J Biol Chem. 1998;273(16):9369–72.
128. Yang B, Bankir L, Gillespie A, Epstein CJ, Verkman AS. Urea-selective concentrating defect in transgenic mice lacking urea transporter UT-B. J Biol Chem. 2002;277:10633–7.
129. Sidoux-Walter F, Lucien N, Olivès B, Gobin R, Rousselet G, Kamsteeg EJ, et al. At physiological expression levels the Kidd blood group/urea transporter protein is not a water channel. J Biol Chem. 1999;274(42):30228–35.
130. Yang B, Verkman AS. Analysis of double knockout mice lacking aquaporin-1 and urea transporter UT-B. J Biol Chem. 2002;277(39):36782–6.
131. Zhang C, Sands JM, Klein JD. Vasopressin rapidly increases the phosphorylation of the UT-A1 urea transporter activity in rat IMCDs through PKA. Am J Physiol Renal Physiol. 2002;282(1):F85–90.
132. Blount MA, Mistry AC, Fröhlich O, Price SR, Chen G, Sands JM, et al. Phosphorylation of UT-A1 urea transporter at serines 486 and 499 is important for vasopressin-regulated activity and membrane accumulation. Am J Physiol Renal Physiol. 2008;295(1):F295–9.
133. Hwang S, Gunaratne R, Rinschen MM, Yu M-J, Pisitkun T, Hoffert JD, et al. Vasporessin increases phosphorylation of ser84 and ser486 in Slc14a2 collecting duct urea transporters. Am J Physiol Renal Physiol. 2010;299(3):F559–67.
134. Mistry AC, Mallick R, Klein JD, Sands JM, Froehlich O. Functional characterization of the central hydrophilic linker region of the urea transporter UT-A1: cAMP activation and snapin binding. Am J Physiol Cell Physiol. 2010;298:C1431–7.
135. Smith CP, Potter EA, Fenton RA, Stewart GS. Characterization of a human colonic cDNA encoding a structurally novel urea transporter, UT-A6. Am J Physiol Cell Physiol. 2004;287(4):C1087–93.
136. Stewart GS, O'Brien JH, Smith CP. Ubiquitination regulates the plasma membrane expression of renal UT-A urea transporters. Am J Physiol Cell Physiol. 2008;295:C121–9.
137. Chen G, Huang H, Fröhlich O, Yang Y, Klein JD, Price SR, et al. MDM2 E3 ubiquitin ligase mediates UT-A1 urea transporter ubiquitination and degradation. Am J Physiol Renal Physiol. 2008;295(5):F1528–34.
138. Gillin AG, Sands JM. Characteristics of osmolarity-stimulated urea transport in rat IMCD. Am J Physiol. 1992;262:F1061–7.
139. Blessing NW, Blount MA, Sands JM, Martin CF, Klein JD. Urea transporters UT-A1 and UT-A3 accumulate in the plasma membrane in response to increased hypertonicity. Am J Physiol Renal Physiol. 2008;295(5):F1336–41.
140. Klein JD, Fröhlich O, Blount MA, Martin CF, Smith TD, Sands JM. Vasopressin increases plasma membrane accumulation of urea transporter UT-A1 in rat inner medullary collecting ducts. J Am Soc Nephrol. 2006;17:2680–6.
141. Harrington AR, Valtin H. Impaired urinary concentration after vasopressin and its gradual correction in hypothalamic diabetes insipidus. J Clin Invest. 1968;47:502–10.

142. Kim D-U, Sands JM, Klein JD. Role of vasopressin in diabetes mellitus-induced changes in medullary transport proteins involved in urine concentration in Brattleboro rats. Am J Physiol Renal Physiol. 2004;286:F760–66.
143. Nakayama Y, Naruse M, Karakashian A, Peng T, Sands JM, Bagnasco SM. Cloning of the rat Slc14a2 gene and genomic organization of the UT-A urea transporter. Biochim Biophys Acta. 2001;1518: 19–26.
144. Nakayama Y, Peng T, Sands JM, Bagnasco SM. The TonE/TonEBP pathway mediates tonicity-responsive regulation of UT-A urea transporter expression. J Biol Chem. 2000;275(49):38275–80.
145. Sands JM, Gargus JJ, Fröhlich O, Gunn RB, Kokko JP. Urinary concentrating ability in patients with Jk(a-b-) blood type who lack carrier-mediated urea transport. J Am Soc Nephrol. 1992;2:1689–96.
146. Bankir L, Chen K, Yang B. Lack of UT-B in vasa recta and red blood cells prevents urea-induced improvement of urinary concentrating ability. Am J Physiol Renal Physiol. 2004;286(1):F144–51.
147. Klein JD, Sands JM, Qian L, Wang X, Yang B. Upregulation of urea transporter UT-A2 and water channels AQP2 and AQP3 in mice lacking urea transporter UT-B. J Am Soc Nephrol. 2004;15(5): 1161–7.
148. Layton AT. Role of UTB urea transporters in the urine concentrating mechanism of the rat kidney. Bull Math Biol. 2007;69(3):887–929.
149. Edwards A, Pallone TL. Facilitated transport in vasa recta: Theoretical effects on solute exchange in the medullary microcirculation. Am J Physiol Renal Physiol. 1997;272(4):F505–14.
150. Edwards A, Pallone TL. A multiunit model of solute and water removal by inner medullary vasa recta. Am J Physiol Heart Circ Physiol. 1998;274(4): H1202–10.
151. Berliner RW, Levinsky NG, Davidson DG, Eden M. Dilution and concentration of the urine and the action of antidiuretic hormone. Am J Med. 1958;24:730–44.
152. Sands JM. Critical role of urea in the urine-concentrating mechanism. J Am Soc Nephrol. 2007;18(3): 670–1.
153. Lemley KV, Kriz W. Cycles and separations: the histotopography of the urinary concentrating process. Kidney Int. 1987;31:538–48.
154. Pannabecker TL, Dantzler WH. Three-dimensional architecture of inner medullary vasa recta. Am J Physiol Renal Physiol. 2006;290(6):F1355–66.
155. Knepper MA, Roch-Ramel F. Pathways of urea transport in the mammalian kidney. Kidney Int. 1987;31:629–33.

2 Disorders of Water Metabolism

Joshua M. Thurman and Tomas Berl

Introduction

Disorders of water balance and serum Na (S_{Na}) are very common in hospitalized patients [1]. In health, water balance and plasma osmolality, and thereby S_{Na}, are tightly regulated by the kidney, which makes minute-by-minute adjustments to the composition of urine in order to maintain a near-constant plasma osmolality. The development of hyponatremia or hypernatremia may therefore reflect serious underlying illness and both conditions often suggest a poor prognosis for the underlying causative disease. Hypo- and hypernatremia are associated with increased morbidity and, equally vexing to the clinician, inappropriate correction may itself cause serious morbidity or mortality. A careful therapeutic approach as well as close attention to the patient's response are therefore important for the clinician caring for patients with these conditions.

Hypo- and hypernatremia are each the common manifestation of several distinct underlying diseases. Effective therapy depends upon an accurate evaluation of the underlying process and different treatment strategies are often necessary, even when patients present with the same serum sodium level. A patient presenting with a S_{Na} of 115, for example, may be benefited or harmed by hydration with saline, depending upon whether the hyponatremia was caused by volume contraction, congestive heart failure, or the syndrome of inappropriate secretion of anti discretion hormone (SIADH). Furthermore, water handling by the kidney can change quickly as the patient's condition changes. A patient who is volume contracted and is concentrating his or her urine at presentation may subsequently start excreting free water in response to rehydration. This patient's urine osmolality would initially be high but would fall in response to volume resuscitation. Perhaps the most important aspect of therapy, then, is continuous reassessment of patients and their response to therapy.

Normal Regulation of Water Balance

The serum sodium is determined by the total body sodium plus potassium and the total body water. Sodium is the primary extracellular osmole, so the serum sodium concentration usually reflects the osmolality of the extracellular fluid, and patients with disorders of water handling often present as hypo- or hypernatremic. Potassium is the primary intracellular osmole, and water equilibrates across cell membranes such that the intra- and extracellular osmolality will balance. The serum sodium concentration is,

J.M. Thurman, M.D. (✉)
Department of Internal Medicine,
University of Denver School of Medicine,
1775 Aurora Ct., M20-3103, Aurora, CO 80111, USA
e-mail: joshua.thurman@ucdenver.edu

T. Berl, M.D.
Department of Medicine, University of Colorado,
12700 E. 19th Ave., C281, Aurora, CO 80045, USA

D.B. Mount et al. (eds.), *Core Concepts in the Disorders of Fluid, Electrolytes and Acid-Base Balance*,
DOI 10.1007/978-1-4614-3770-3_2, © Springer Science+Business Media New York 2013

therefore, primarily determined by the total body sodium, potassium, and water (2.1):

$$S_{Na} = \frac{(TB_{Na} + TB_K)}{TBW}. \quad (2.1)$$

While this empirically derived relationship has undergone careful reanalysis by Nguyen and Kurtz [2], in large measure it predicts well changes in serum sodium concentration under most clinical circumstances. In the steady state each of these components is maintained. Therefore, daily losses must equal daily intake. The intake of both water and solute are inconstant, however. The average person consumes approximately 700–800 mOsm of solute and 1–3 L of water each day, but consumption is episodic. Water is also contained in food and generated by the oxidation of carbohydrates. In addition to their excretion in urine,water and solute are lost through the gastrointestinal tract, sweat, and water is lost through respiratory processes. In spite of variations in the intake and extra-renal losses of water and solute, the plasma osmolality is tightly maintained within 275–290 mOsm/kg. The primary mechanism by which the body maintains water balance in spite of variations in intake and losses is by adjusting the urine osmolality. The average daily U_{Osm} is determined by the intake of osmoles and the intake of water (2.2):

$$U_{Osm} = \frac{\text{Daily intake of osmoles}}{\text{Daily urine output}\left(\text{daily intake of water} - \text{non-renal losses}\right)}. \quad (2.2)$$

The kidney can generate urine as dilute as 40–100 mOsm/kg [3] and as concentrated as 900–1,200 mOsm/kg [4]. Although this range tends to narrow with age, it still permits great flexibility in the renal response to the intake of food and water. If, however, the ratio of consumed osmoles and water exceeds this range, steady state can no longer be maintained and the total body water will increase or decrease (Fig. 2.1).

Serum sodium is determined by total body Na plus K and total body water (2.1), and the kidney could maintain serum sodium through its handling of either component. The active regulation of osmolality is primarily accomplished by regulation of the total body water, and it is useful to consider the renal handling of solute and water as separate functions. As water is gained or lost in relation to total body osmoles—decreasing or increasing the net plasma osmolality—the kidneys decrease or increase water reabsorption in the collecting duct. This response involves precise sensing of the plasma osmolality by osmoreceptors in the hypothalamus, which control the production and release of the antidiuretic hormone, arginine vasopressin (AVP). AVP regulates insertion of water channels in the principal cells of the collecting duct [5]. As the number of channels increases and the cells become more freely permeable to water, it passes from the urine to the hypertonic medulla, thereby concentrating the urine and returning free water to the circulation.

Sodium handling by the kidney, in contrast, is regulated by the renin-angiotensin aldosterone system and by atrial natriuretic peptide, which respond to changes in the effective arterial blood volume. Retention or excretion of sodium in response to these systems is accompanied by retention or excretion of water, such that the net change is an isosmotic change of volume. However, changes in salt handling will affect the amount of filtered osmoles. Given the limits to the osmolality that the kidney can achieve, changes in the net amount of filtered osmoles will affect the limits of free water that the kidney is able to excrete (Fig. 2.1).

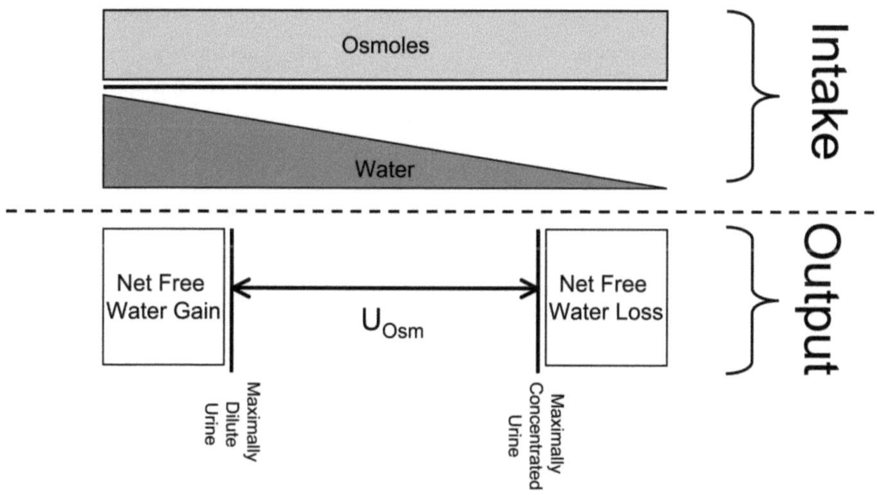

Fig. 2.1 Daily balance of solute and water. The body maintains water and solute balance by excreting an amount equal to the daily oral intake. As non-renal losses are fairly fixed, the concentration of the urine is adjusted so as to keep the net excretion equal to net intake. The amount of overall solute and water consumed will therefore determine the concentration of the urine. If the balance of solute to water is too low or too high it may exceed the range of concentrations that the kidney can achieve, and hyponatremia or hypernatremia will ensue

Hyponatremia and Hypoosmolar States

Mechanisms of Hyponatremia

All patients with hyponatremia have consumed or received water in excess of the kidneys' ability to excrete it. If renal function is normal, this imbalance can occur because:

- AVP or, less commonly, an intrarenal AVP-independent mechanism limits the degree to which urine can be diluted.
- Inadequate intake and/or excretion of osmoles limits the amount of water that can be excreted.
- Water consumption exceeds even normal urinary dilution.

Because the kidneys can ordinarily excrete such a large volume of free water (approximately 20 L for normally functioning kidneys), hyponatremia due exclusively to polydipsia is rare, and hyponatremia usually occurs in patients with some limitation to their ability to excrete a water load. This may be due to a decrease in GFR, decreased NaCl reabsorption in the diluting segment of the nephron, or the presence of AVP [6].

Non-osmotic and Inappropriate Release of AVP

Typically, hypoosmolality causes full suppression of AVP release. For patients in whom the U_{Osm} is not maximally diluted (e.g., >100 mOsm/kg) one can assume that there is some AVP being released. Its presence in the setting of hyponatremia/hypoosmolality reflects that it is being released due to non-osmotic factors (i.e., decreased effective arterial blood volume) or it is being inappropriately released. By increasing the U_{Osm}, AVP limits the amount of water relative to solute that one can take in without retaining free water. For hyponatremic patients who are not maximally diluting their urine, the urine sodium concentration can help in the determination of the stimulus for AVP release as well as help guide therapy (Table 2.1). Urine sodium below 20 mEq/L is suggestive of a low effective arterial blood volume and non-osmotic release of AVP. Patients with a low urine sodium will likely retain sodium which is administered as part of their therapy. A urine sodium higher than 20 mEq/L, on the other hand, is more suggestive of SIADH. These patients are effectively euvolemic and will excrete administered sodium.

Table 2.1 Use of urinary osmolality and urinary Na in the evaluation of the hyponatremic patient

Volume status	Clinical setting	U_{Osm} (mOsm/kg)	U_{Na}
Hypovolemic	Renal salt wasting • Diuretics • Mineralocorticoid deficiency • Salt-losing nephropathy • Bicarbonaturia • Ketonuria • Osmotic diuresis	>100	>20 mEq/L
	Extrarenal Losses • Diarrhea • Vomiting • "Third space"	>100	<10 mEq/L
Euvolemic	Polydipsia or Potomania Low solute intake	<100	↔
	SIADH Glucocorticoid deficiency Hypothyroidism Drugs	>100	>20 mEq/L
Hypervolemic	Congestive heart failure Nephrotic syndrome Cirrhosis	>100	<20
	Renal failure	>100	>20 mEq/L

Measurement of the urine electrolytes also helps to gauge how much free water is being lost in the urine. The main electrolytes in urine are sodium and potassium, and their total concentration relative to the plasma sodium is used to measure the tonicity of the urine relative to plasma (2.3):

$$\text{Tonicity of urine relative to plasma} = \frac{(U_{Na} + U_K)}{S_{Na}}. \tag{2.3}$$

If this ratio is less than one the urine is hypotonic relative to the plasma and electrolyte free water is being excreted, tending to correct the hyponatremia. Alternatively, if the ratio is greater than one the urine is hypertonic relative to plasma. This concentrated urine reflects a gain of electrolyte free water and will tend to exacerbate the hyponatremia (see (2.1)).

The urine can also be thought of as comprising two fractions—an isotonic fraction and a water fraction. For example, if the ratio described by (2.3) is 0.5, the urine would be 50 % isotonic fluid and 50 % electrolyte free water. Together these fractions make a whole that has an electrolyte concentration half that of plasma. The rate of urine flow can then be measured to determine the electrolyte free water clearance and find the rate of electrolyte free water gain or loss. The electrolyte free water that is being excreted or retained is also a function of urine flow and defined by the following equation (2.4):

$$\text{Electrolyte - free water clearance} = \text{Urine flow x} \tag{2.4}$$

For example, in the patient whose $U_{Na} + U_K$ is equal to 0.5 of the S_{Na}, half of the urine flow is electrolyte free water. If this patient is making 100 mL of urine an hour, the electrolyte free water clearance is 50 mL an hour. This calculation allows one to predict the hourly change in total body water and plasma sodium.

As can be seen from (2.4), if the $U_{Na} + U_K > S_{Na}$, the electrolyte free water clearance will actually be negative. In this case, the urinary losses of electrolytes exceed urinary losses of water and the production of urine is tending to exacerbate the hyponatremia even in the absence of water consumption. If one administered normal saline to a euvolemic patient with these urinary indices, the administered sodium would eventually be excreted (since the patient is euvolemic) in a more concentrated urine. This would result in a negative electrolyte free water clearance or a net gain in free water, further decreasing the serum sodium concentration.

Polydipsia and Inadequate Solute Intake

The kidney has a broad range of achievable osmolality, and regulation of the sense of thirst will also help maintain a balanced intake and excretion of solute and water. However, continued ingestion of too much water relative to intake of solute will exceed the diluting capacity of the kidneys, eventually leading to accumulation of total body water and hyponatremia (Fig. 2.1). Patients in whom hyponatremia is caused by excessive consumption of water should have a very dilute urine with full suppression of endogenous AVP. As can be deduced from (2.2) and Fig. 2.1, inadequate solute intake also limits the ability to excrete free water and can contribute to hyponatremia [7]. As with primary polydipsia, hyponatremia caused by inadequate solute intake (potomania) is also characterized by full suppression of AVP and maximally dilute urine. These two disorders can be distinguished by history or by collecting the urine and measuring the total osmoles.

Complications of Hypotonic Hyponatremia

Severe hyponatremia can cause significant morbidity. However, aggressive therapy is also associated with complications. The primary mechanism of injury during both the generation and the resolution of the hypoosmolar state is caused by the passage of water into or out of cells whose membranes are impermeable to some solutes but are freely permeable to water. Changes in the tonicity of the extracellular fluid cause an osmotic gradient across cell membranes and passage of water into or out of the cells. Because the cells of the brain are contained within the fixed confines of the skull they are at great risk of injury and most of the symptoms of hyponatremia are neurologic.

Some adaptation to changes in tonicity can occur within 1–3 h. As plasma osmolality drops and cellular volume expands, interstitial pressure increases and forces extracellular fluid into the cerebrospinal fluid. The transfer of this extracellular fluid effectively relieves some of the elevation in intracranial pressure (ICP). This mechanism protects against mild, acute changes in hyponatremia but likely does not defend against more severe and long-standing hypotonicity. A second protective mechanism involves a reduction in intracellular solutes, a process that starts approximately 3 h after the onset of hypotonicity with the loss of cellular potassium. Adaptation proceeds through a decrease in the intracellular levels of organic solutes including glutamate, taurine, myo-inositol, and glutamine [8]. Although some of the decrease in the intracellular osmolytes occurs within 24 h, the loss of such solutes becomes more marked over the next several days and accounts for almost complete restoration of cerebral water. Because of the time required for full compensation, however, acute changes in the extracellular osmolality cause significant changes in cell volume.

Cerebral Edema

Severe acute hyponatremia is a medical emergency. If plasma osmolality drops too quickly the intracranial cells cannot adequately decrease the intracellular osmolytes, and water then crosses into the cells causing cerebral edema. This can be aggravated by the hypoxemia brought about by coexistant neurogenic pulmonary edema [9]. Precipitous changes in plasma osmolality can cause tentorial herniation and death. Even in otherwise healthy patients, failure to aggressively correct these patients is associated with high mortality rates [10]. Symptoms of hyponatremia, such as gastrointestinal complaints, lethargy, apathy, agitation, and cramps, most commonly occur with rapid decreases in serum sodium to below 125 mEq/L. Seizures and coma usually result from acute decreases to levels of approximately 110 mEq/L or less [11, 12]. When choosing goals of therapy the clinician must weight the risks of overly rapid correction with those of inadequate correction. Patients with signs, symptoms, and risk factors for cerebral edema should be corrected more aggressively than those without.

The patients at greatest risk for cerebral edema are those in whom hyponatremia has developed over less than 48 h. This is because full adaptation to changes in tonicity requires 48–72 h. The magnitude of hyponatremia and its duration are, therefore, the most important factors to consider in planning the treatment goals.

Risk Factors for Severe Cerebral Edema

Hypoxia. The combination of hyponatremia and hypoxia may be particularly dangerous [9]. In experimental animals, hypoxia abrogates the volume adaptive response to hyponatremia, therefore resulting in increased brain edema [13].

Hospital-acquired hyponatremia in premenopausal women. Several reports suggest that menstruating women who develop acute hyponatremia while hospitalized are at greater risk of developing neurologic complications than men [10, 12, 14]. The incidence of hyponatremia appears to be similar for men and women in this setting, but women are more likely to develop symptoms or neurologic deficits. In a report in which 307 men developed postoperative hyponatremia, only one man had an outcome of permanent cerebral dysfunction or death [15]. In contrast, 33 of 367 women with hyponatremia had severe neurologic complications. The susceptibility of women to complications from hyponatremia may be due to differences in cellular adaptation to changes in osmolality in part related to hormonal differences [16].

Thiazide diuretics. Thiazide diuretics may predispose to the development of hyponatremia, and patients who develop thiazide-induced hyponatremia may be at higher risk for the development of neurologic complications. In one reported series, 12 of 129 patients who developed thiazide-induced hyponatremia died [17], highlighting the potential severity of thiazide-induced hyponatremia. Thiazides reduce sodium chloride reabsorption in the distal tubule, the primary site for urinary dilution, thus decreasing the amount of electrolyte free water delivered to the collecting duct. Diuretics may also stimulate thirst. Loop diuretics may also induce volume depletion, but by interfering with the transfer of NaCl into the medullary interstitium they also reduce the gradient driving water reabsorption from the collecting tubules and thus are less likely to induce hyponatremia [18]. Certain patients seem to be particularly predisposed to develop hyponatremia on thiazides and develop recurrent hyponatremia when rechallenged. The patients most likely to develop hyponatremia due to thiazides appear to be the elderly, those with low body weight, and those with hypokalemia [19].

Children. Children are at risk for the development of hyponatremia in response to the administration of excessive hypotonic fluid [10]. Hyponatremia can result from overestimation of the fluid requirement as well as concurrent nonosmotic stimuli for the release of AVP, further limiting the patient's capacity for excretion of free water [20]. The susceptibility of children to neurologic sequelae may be due to limitation of space within the skull to accommodate brain edema, an inadequate degree of compensation, and delay in diagnosis and treatment.

Osmotic Demyelination Syndrome

In contrast to the risk of cerebral edema in the setting of acute hyponatremia, the correction of hyponatremia of longer duration (>48 h) is associated with an increased risk of osmotic demyelination syndrome (ODS). ODS is a life-threatening neurologic abnormality caused by demyelination, classically within the central basis pontis, but occurring also in extrapontine sites. Just as the rapid development of hypotonicity causes passage of water into the cells of the brain, overly rapid correction of hypotonicity induces an osmotic passage of water out of these same cells. Cells require several days to decrease intracellular osmolytes in response to a fall in extracellular tonicity. Rapid correction causes cerebral dehydration by drawing water out of cells. This dehydration is enhanced by the delay in the aforementioned osmolytes' return to the brain. The downregulation of transporters during hypotonicity, such as SNAT2, may partially be responsible for this delayed restoration of solutes [21]. The overly rapid correction has been linked with the development of ODS [22]. Clinicians treating patients with hyponatremia thus face the dilemma of correcting hyponatremia quickly enough to avoid morbidity from cerebral edema without precipitating ODS.

Patients who are corrected overly rapidly may initially improve during therapy but show subsequent deterioration. In fact, the development of ODS can occur several days after the hyponatremia has been corrected [23]. The signs and symptoms of ODS classically include motor abnormalities potentially progressing to quadriplegia and respiratory paralysis, pseudobulbar palsy, lethargy, altered mental status, and coma, and it is often but not always fatal [24]. The diagnosis of ODS is confirmed by the presence of foci of demyelination on head magnetic resonance imaging (MRI), but these findings may lag behind clinical findings by several weeks. Thus early imaging may not reveal any pathology, and even later imaging may show no lesions. The diagnosis is primarily made on clinical grounds.

Risk Factors for Development of ODS

The risk of development of ODS is related to the severity and chronicity of the hyponatremia and the rate and magnitude of the correction. ODS is rarely observed in patients presenting with serum sodium greater than 120 mEq/L, and patients probably need to have been hyponatremic for at least 48 h [24]. Other risk factors for the development of ODS include alcoholism, malnutrition, hypokalemia, and severe hyponatremia (<105 mEq/L), as well as thiazide-induced hyponatremia in the elderly [24]. Catabolic patients, such as those with burns, may also be at increased risk [25].

Complications of Hyponatremia in CHF and Cirrhosis

Hyponatremia is a poor prognostic sign in both CHF [26] and cirrhosis [27]. This is probably because it reflects neurohormonal activation and thus reflects underlying circulatory derangements and disease severity. In patients with CHF, free water retention contributes to overall volume overload [28]. The development of hyponatremia may also limit the use of diuretics, thus impeding treatment. In addition to being a marker of disease, there is also evidence that hyponatremia itself contributes to worse outcomes. In a study in which patients were treated with a standard diuretic regimen versus high-dose furosemide combined with hypertonic saline, those that received the latter regimen achieved similar improvement in congestion but had improved serum sodium concentrations [29]. This group had fewer symptoms and had decreased mortality, indicating that correction of the serum sodium concentration may be of benefit in patients who achieve similar reductions in volume overload.

In patients with cirrhosis it is also difficult to distinguish whether hyponatremia is simply a marker of worse disease or whether it contributes to the development of complications and worse outcomes. There is some evidence that the adaptation of brain cells with cirrhosis and hyponatremia adversely affects cell function, and that hyponatremia predisposes patients with cirrhosis to the development of hepatic encephalopathy [30].

Treatment of Symptomatic Hyponatremia

Calculation of the Free Water Excess

As can be surmised from (2.1) hyponatremia can occur either by decrements in solutes (the numerator) or increments in total body water (the denominator). In most instances the predominant process is one that leads to an increase in total body water with a modest decrease in total body sodium.

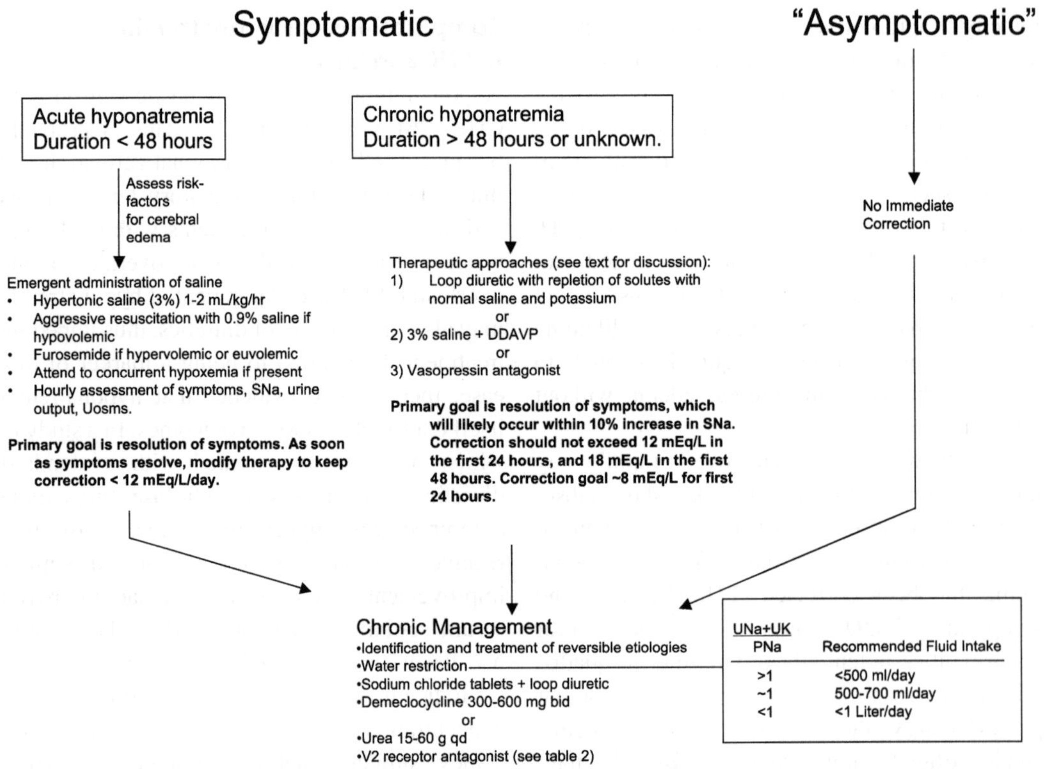

Fig. 2.2 Treatment of the patient with severe hyponatremia. Adapted with permission from Therapy of dysnatremic disorders, Joshua M. Thurman, Tomas Berl. In: Wilcox CS, editor. Therapy in nephrology and hypertension, 3rd ed. WB Saunders; 2008

Even in hypovolemic states that are characterized by a decrease in body sodium, there is a relative excess of body water. The free water excess can therefore be calculated as follows (2.5):

$$\text{Free water excess} = 0.6 \times \text{weight(kg)}\left[1 - \frac{(S_{Na})}{(\text{desired } S_{Na})}\right], \tag{2.5}$$

where $0.6 \times$ weight is taken as the total body water. For women the total body water may be approximated as $0.5 \times$ weight.

In a 70 kg patient an increase in the S_{Na} by 10 % can be accomplished by removing the free water excess which can be estimated to be $0.6 \times 70\ \text{kg} \times (1 - 0.9) \approx 4$ L. To accomplish this over 10 h will require 400 mL/h of electrolyte free water excretion.

Acute Hyponatremia

In view of the potentially life-threatening complication of acute hyponatremia as described above there is a wide consensus that rapid correction of hyponatremia is indicated in patients in whom hyponatremia has developed over less than 48 h (Fig. 2.2). Generally, the presence of symptoms indicates that hyponatremia has developed too quickly for the adaptive mechanisms to compensate, and symptomatic patients have probably developed hyponatremia over a short period. Because patients who have acutely developed hyponatremia have not had time to adapt to the change in tonicity they also are at less risk of developing complications from correction of the hyponatremia (ODS) [24].

Goals of Therapy

Therapy should be initiated immediately in symptomatic patients, particularly in those at increased risk of complications, such as those with hypoxia, in whom, if present, intubation should be considered. For patients with hyponatremia of less than 48-h duration and/or risk factors for the development of cerebral edema, treatment is aimed at achieving a rapid increase in serum sodium.

Initial sodium administration should increase the serum sodium by approximately 2 mEq/L/h. A rapid increase in the serum sodium can be achieved by administering hypertonic saline (3 % saline contains 513 mEq/L of Na). Hypertonic saline is often started at 1–2 mL/kg/h. Studies in patients with impending trans-tentorial herniation have revealed that an increase in serum sodium by 5–6 mEq/L is sufficient to reverse the herniation and reduce ICP by 40 % [31]. This was achieved with 30 mL of 23.4 % saline. The primary goal for the administration of hypertonic saline is not the restoration of a sodium deficit but the rapid reversal of potentially life-threatening cerebral edema.

It must be noted that if the urine electrolyte free water clearance (2.4) is negative, the excretion of urine represents a net gain in free water. This point is critical to consider in the treatment of patients with euvolemic hyponatremia. Although normal saline is hypertonic relative to the plasma, it will eventually be excreted in a more concentrated form and will exacerbate the hyponatremia. Even if the urine electrolyte free water clearance (2.4) is negative, as long as $U_{Na}+U_K<513$ mEq/L (the sodium concentration of 3 % saline) the urine is more dilute than 3 % saline. The ultimate excretion of the sodium will then result in a net decrease in total body water. If $U_{Na}+U_K=250$ mEq/L, for example, the sodium in any administered 3 % saline will be excreted in a urine only half as concentrated, and half of the resultant urine volume will be a free water loss.

Chronic Symptomatic Hyponatremia

For patients in whom the duration of hyponatremia is unknown or is longer than 48 h, or in whom there are risk factors for the development of ODS, initial therapy is aimed at achieving rapid resolution of symptoms, but care must be taken not to exceed well-defined goals [24]. Several general principles should guide the therapeutic approach.

- For patients with chronic hyponatremia cerebral water is increased by approximately 10 %, so a 10 % increase in serum sodium (or 10 mEq/L) should be sufficient for resolution of symptoms.
- If the duration is unknown or is longer than 48 h, as soon as symptoms resolve care should be taken not to overcorrect the serum sodium. At that point the hourly correction rate should not exceed 0.5 mEq/L/h. The cumulative limit of correction should be no more than 12 mEq/L/day or 18 mEq/L over 2 days, and a more appropriate goal of correction is approximately 8 mEq/L over 24 h.
- If patients exceed these goals, or if the rate and osmolality of the urine indicate that they will overcorrect (e.g., if the patient is making a large volume of hypotonic urine), then hypotonic fluid or dDAVP should be administered to control the rate of change and even to lower the S_{Na} concentration and keep the net correction within the desired range [32, 33].
- Restriction of free water: While patients with symptomatic hyponatremia should have free water restriction, the rate of correction achieved by this means is too slow in the symptomatic patient and other corrective measures must also be employed.

Therapeutic Approach

The overall goal of therapy is to remove free water from the patient with chronic symptomatic hyponatremia, and to prevent ODS. Several different strategies can be employed to achieve this, each with certain advantages. We describe three general approaches below.

Loop diuretics with sodium and potassium repletion. Loop diuretics cause excretion of electrolyte free water with a salt concentration approximating half-normal saline (e.g., ~75 mEq/L of Na^++K^+). Therefore, in patients who are euvolemic and receiving intravenous saline, furosemide can be used to prevent exacerbation of volume overload and to also increase electrolyte free water excretion. If the $U_{Na}+U_K$ after furosemide is ~75 mEq/L, for example, one could titrate the dose to maintain approximately 300 mL/h of urine output. This urine would contain 150 mL/h of electrolyte free water. Depending upon the free water excess, one could increase or decrease these rates to change the rate of correction.

This approach offers control over the balance of water and electrolytes. It is, however, labor intensive as it involves frequent monitoring of urine volume and sodium and potassium losses. Likewise, it necessitates equally frequent decisions regarding the composition of the repletion fluid in order to achieve the desired rate of correction. It can also cause over-correction of hyponatremia, although this can be countered by the administration of free water. When properly conducted this approach results in neutral solute balance and net negative water balance, resulting in an increase in the serum sodium concentration.

Hypertonic saline and DDAVP. Hypertonic saline (e.g., 3 % saline at 1–2 mL/kg/h) will increase the S_{Na}. If reversible causes of hyponatremia (e.g., dehydration) are concurrently reversed, resulting in a water diuresis, the correction may be overly rapid. Some investigators, therefore, have recommended administering hypertonic saline concurrently with DDAVP to patients with chronic symptomatic hyponatremia [34, 35]. This approach addresses the concern of overly rapid correction, particularly in settings in which hyponatremia is transient. On the other hand, it runs the risk of worsening the underlying hyponatremia if the patient is not carefully monitored. Because this approach could lead to positive sodium balance, it may not be advisable for patients with marginal cardiac function. Furthermore, it does not directly address the need to achieve negative water balance.

Vasopressin antagonists. A third therapeutic approach is to give patients with chronic symptomatic hyponatremia a vasopressin antagonist. These drugs are likely to result over the ensuing hours in the excretion of a dilute urine. The S_{Na} should therefore be monitored at least every 4 h after administering these agents. Once the S_{Na} has increased by 6–8 mEq/L the urine output can be matched with D5W to prevent further correction. Two vasopressin antagonists are currently available on the market [36, 37]. In a report on 18 patients who received conivaptan, the drug resulted in a mean increase in S_{Na} of 8 mEq/L in 24 h [37].

In general, all patients must be monitored closely for evidence of over- or under-correction. If the rise in S_{Na} indicates over-correction, the serum sodium exceeds the noted limits, and the serum sodium should be lowered. As a general rule, the S_{Na} should be monitored frequently. The urine output and vital signs should also be continually monitored. The U_{Osm} and urine electrolytes can be monitored periodically, particularly if DDAVP or a vasopressin antagonist is used.

Hypovolemic patients. Therapy can begin with the rapid administration of normal saline to achieve volume resuscitation. This will achieve partial correction of the serum sodium and may also stop the release of AVP leading to self-correction of the hyponatremia. These patients also need to be monitored to prevent excessively rapid correction. The same caution as to correction rates described in euvolmic patients needs to be exercised in this population.

Hypervolemic patients. The primary goal in hypervolemic patients is removal of free water. However, symptomatic patients require Na administration as well as water restriction to ensure a timely correction. Saline should typically be accompanied by furosemide to achieve a negative salt balance. If salt balance is maintained, the loss of free water in the urine will be the mechanism of correction of the S_{Na}.

Treatment of "Asymptomatic" Hyponatremia

At the outset it should be noted that some have questioned whether there are hyponatremic patients who are truly asymptomatic, as even mild hyponatremia may be associated with subtle neurologic impairments. A study of 122 such patients revealed that they frequently had gait unsteadiness, attention deficits, and a 67-fold increased risk for falls [38]. The recently described association of hypontremia with osteoporosis [39] may also contribute to the increased risk of fractures in this population [40]. The initial assessment of "asymptomatic" patients with hyponatremia involves consideration of the same issues—the duration of hyponatremia, underlying cause of hyponatremia, patient's volume status, and quantitative assessment of how the patient is currently handling sodium and water. Since these patients almost always have chronic hyponatremia there is no urgency to treat them rapidly. Even without symptoms some risk stratification must be done. Hyponatremia is often a sign of underlying disease severity. Furthermore, the clinical manifestations may be subtle, such as mild gait imbalance. Even the asymptomatic patient, therefore, warrants careful consideration. In general, patients with $S_{Na} < 125$ or elderly patients who are at risk of falls should probably be treated. Patients with $S_{Na} < 120$ should be observed in the hospital with their labs repeated frequently enough to feel comfortable that the sodium level is correcting at the desired rate.

Hypovolemic Hyponatremia

Patients are classified as hypovolemic based upon their clinical history, physical examination, and a low urine sodium (e.g., <20 mEq/L). Hypovolemic patients with asymptomic hyponatremic should receive volume resuscitation with normal saline. The saline will be hypertonic relative to the patient's serum, but several liters of normal saline will not cause a rapid rise in the serum sodium level as the change in tonicity will be equilibrated through the total body water. The other, perhaps more significant, effect on the serum sodium will be the fall in non-osmotic release of AVP. As patients become volume replete they may then begin excreting hypotonic urine resulting in autocorrection of the serum sodium. This can result in overly rapid correction of the serum sodium and necessitate administration of hypotonic fluids or dDAVP. Patients with other causes of hyponatremia, such as SIADH, may become volume depleted, thus presenting with two stimuli for AVP release. This should become apparent if the patient remains hyponatremic after the volume resuscitation is complete. In that case they can subsequently be managed as euvolemic hyponatremia.

Hypervolemic Hyponatremia

Patients can appear clinically hypervolemic yet have non-osmotic release of AVP. This can occur because of a low effective arterial blood volume as is seen in patients with advanced heart failure or advanced cirrhosis. The hyponatremia reflects neurohormonal activation due to the hemodynamic abnormalities seen with both diseases, and this is often indicated by a low urine sodium (e.g., <20 mEq/L). Consequently, hyponatremia due to either congestive heart failure or cirrhosis signifies severe underlying disease and is a poor prognostic sign. By definition, these patients have an excess of total body sodium and administration of saline is often not a therapeutic option. These patients frequently require natriuretic agents. In this regard, loop diuretics are preferable as they increase electrolyte free water clearance, while thiazides limit free water clearance. Some patients may present after being overdiuresed or after developing relative hypovolemia due to other causes such as diarrhea, however, and the clinical decision may be made to administer saline to a patient who is hypervolemic. The patients may be hypotensive or have an elevated creatinine. In those circumstances the administered volume may also improve the serum sodium concentration just as it does for hypovolemic patients.

The S_{Na} in patients with hypervolemic hyponatremia does not usually fall below 120 mEq/L. Chronic therapies are often unpleasant for patients, and there is no clear evidence to support a specific target. Most commonly therapy involves limiting intake of free water. The non-osmotic release of AVP in these patients limits their ability to excrete free water. One can calculate the electrolyte free water losses in the urine (2.4). Limiting the free water intake to less than the losses results in a net free water loss, correcting the hyponatremia, but adherence to this regimen is difficult and variable.

Table 2.2 Non-peptide AVP receptor antagonists

	Tolvaptan	Lixivaptan	Satavaptan[a]	Conivaptan
Receptor	V_2	V_2	V_2	V_{1a}/V_2
Route of administration	Oral	Oral	Oral	IV
Urine volume	↑	↑	↑	↑
Urine osmolality	↓	↓	↓	↓
Na excretion	⇔	⇔ low dose ⇔↑ high dose	⇔	⇔

Adapted with permission from Ellison D, Berl T. N Engl J Med. 2007;356(20):2064–72
[a]Not under further development

Table 2.3 Chronic medical therapy for diabetes insipidus

Etiology	Drug	Dose
Complete central diabetes insipidus	dDAVP	10–20 μ(mu)g intranasally every 12–24 h Start at 0.05 at bid, and titrate dose to effect
Partial central diabetes insipidus	dDAVP	
	Aqueous vasopressin	5–10 U SQ every 4–6 h
	Chlorpropamide	250–500 mg/day
	Clofibrate	500 mg tid–qid
	Carbamazepine	400–600 mg/day
Nephrogenic diabetes insipidus	Thiazide diuretics	Conventional doses
	NSAIDs	Conventional doses
	Amiloride (for lithium-induced DI)	5 mg qid

Adapted with permission from Thurman JM, Berl T. Therapy of dysnatremic disorders. In: Wilcox CS, editor. Therapy in nephrology and hypertension, 3rd ed. WB Saunders; 2008

Vasopressin Antagonists

Because free water restriction can be difficult for patients and may not be effective in all settings, the recent development of vasopressin antagonists may provide a more easily tolerated treatment (Table 2.2). The vasopressin antagonists are a group of small molecule antagonists that block the action of AVP at its receptors. One of the antagonists, conivaptan, antagonizes both the V_{1a} and V_2 receptors. The others currently available selectively block the V_2 receptor. Blockade of both the V_{1a} and V_2 receptors causes a vasodilatory effect (through antagonism of V_{1a}) and an aquaretic effect (through antagonism of V_2). This could make conivaptan appropriate for the treatment of congestive heart failure, where the vasodilatory effect may be beneficial [41], but inappropriate for disorders such as cirrhosis. Conivaptan has been shown to decrease pulmonary capillary wedge pressure but the effect could be related to volume loss rather than a change in cardiac function [42]. Because the action of the other antagonists is limited to the V_2 receptor, and given that non-osmotic release of vasopressin is the primary cause of free water excess in these conditions, the V_2 selective antagonists specifically target the underlying cause of hyponatremia in these diseases. The oral V_2 antagonists Lixivaptan [43] and Tolvaptan [44, 45] have been used effectively to induce a water diuresis in patients with CHF (Table 2.3).

A number of studies have reported that the vasopressin antagonists raise the serum sodium in patients with cirrhosis. Lixivaptan has been used by several different investigators, all of whom reported increases in the serum sodium [46–48]. While the drug may have a small effect on sodium excretion in these patients, it seems to raise the S_{Na} in patients with cirrhosis primarily through its aquaretic effects [48]. Dilutional hyponatremia in cirrhotic patients may predispose them to hepatic encephalopathy, and a worse outcome before and after liver transplantation [49, 50], but no studies have yet demonstrated a clinical benefit from treatment with V_2 antagonists.

Euvolemic "Asymptomatic" Hyponatremia

Hyponatremia in clinically euvolemic patients is usually caused by the SIADH, drugs, or endocrinopathies (see Table 2.1). The discontinuation of the drugs and treatment of the underlying endocrine disorder is necessary. Normally functioning kidneys have a very large capacity to excrete free water, so hyponatremia usually involves factors limiting the full excretion of water. Conversely, even patients with severe SIADH require the intake of water in order to become hyponatremic. For these reasons, therapy of patients with asymptomatic euvolemic hyponatremia begins with free water restriction. Measurement of the urine osmolality and calculation of the electrolyte free water clearance permit assessment of whether AVP is present, the rate at which the patient will correct their serum sodium if they stop oral intake of water, and estimation of the free water restriction necessary to start correcting their serum sodium. Alternatively, empiric free water restriction can be instituted based upon urine free water clearance (Fig. 2.2). In addition to the compliance limitation, it is evident that when $U_{Na} + U_K$ exceeds S_{Na} essentially no degree of water restriction is likely to be beneficial [51].

In "asymptomatic" patients, the acute administration of intravenous saline is unnecessary. For chronic control of the serum sodium, increasing the intake of dietary osmoles increases the amount of free water a patient can safely consume (2.2). This can be achieved with salt tablets or with urea tablets, although salt tablets induce thirst and urea tablets are considered unpleasant and frequently unpalatable. Loop diuretics induce production of a dilute urine and can increase patients' ability to excrete free water, but may cause hypovolemia in patients who present as euvolemic. Thus, concurrent NaCl administration is necessary.

Lithium and demeclocycline cause nephrogenic diabetes insipidus. By impeding the renal response to AVP these drugs can be useful in the treatment of SIADH. Demeclocycline is usually started at 300–600 mg twice a day, and achieves its maximum aquaretic effect in about 2 weeks. Free water restriction can be eased during this time period, and rechecking the urine electrolytes permits a revised determination of the amount of free water that a patient can safely consume. Demeclocycline is not recommended in pregnant women or children, and it can cause photosensitivity. It can also cause gastrointestinal discomfort and renal dysfunction, particularly if there is concomitant hepatic disease.

The vasopressin antagonists specifically correct the mechanism that causes hyponatremia in SIADH. Most of the experience with these agents is in patients with SIADH. Several studies have demonstrated efficacy of these agents at inducing aquaresis and increasing the S_{Na} [45, 46, 52]. In the largest trial reported to date (SALT I and II) more than half of the 223 patients who received Tolvaptan were euvolemic and they increased their S_{Na} consistently [42].

Patients with SIADH often have much lower S_{Na} values than patients with cirrhosis or CHF. The rationale for a treatment that increases the S_{Na} is therefore greater, although the absolute goals of therapy are still not certain. The V2 antagonists are an important emerging option for chronic treatment of patients with SIADH. Those agents with selective activity at the V2 receptor should be used in order to avoid hypotension. As there is not yet much experience with these agents, they should be initiated at the lowest available dose, when they become available. The urine osmolality can be monitored, and the dose can gradually be increased. These drugs should permit easing of the free water restriction, and may increase the achievable S_{Na}. Long-term administration of a V2 antagonist has proven to be safe and effective [53], and ODS has not been reported with these agents. However, with further experience possible adverse affects may emerge as the use of the drug widens.

Hypernatremic States

Hypernatremia results from an increase in total body Na plus K or a decrease in total body water. Because sodium is the main plasma electrolyte, hyperosmolarity that is caused by a fall in total body water is marked by an increased plasma sodium concentration. Free water can be lost in urine, in gastrointestinal tract, through respiration, or through insensible losses. Hypernatremia, or hyperosmolarity, occurs in patients whose intake of free water is insufficient to match these losses. The addition of osmoles that cannot pass freely into cells into the extracellular compartment—such as sodium, glucose, or mannitol—will cause water to shift out of the cells until osmotic balance is established. In the cases of glucose or mannitol this shift of water decreases the S_{Na} even though the net serum osmolality is increased. Patients with severe hyperglycemia, for example, often present with decreased S_{Na} levels, although they have an increased serum osmolarity. As insulin is administered and the glucose level falls, the S_{Na} will increase. Furthermore, these patients often also have a net loss in total body water due to osmotic diuresis induced by the hyperglycemia, and after normalization of the serum glucose the S_{Na} is often increased.

Even in patients with severe defects in their ability to concentrate urine, thirst and increased oral intake can usually compensate for free water losses. Therefore, a rise in S_{Na} usually occurs when there is also limited access to free water. For example, if a patient whose maximum U_{Osm} is 200 mOsm/kg eats 800 mOsm/day, he or she only needs to take in 4 L of free water (plus enough to compensate for insensible losses) to stay in balance (Fig. 2.1). If this patient becomes impaired and maintains a near-normal intake of solute but cannot maintain this intake of free water, however, he or she will become hypernatremic.

Mechanisms of Hypernatremia

The addition of sodium or loss of water may cause hypernatremia (2.1). As stated above, however, the maintenance of hyperosmolarity requires impaired access to free water. Awareness of clinical settings in which this commonly occurs aids in its prevention. Predisposing factors include high free water losses, an impaired sense of thirst or impaired sensorium, or lack of access to water.

A decrease of the maximal urine concentration that the kidneys can achieve obligates an increase in the minimal intake of water required to stay in balance (Fig. 2.1). Concentration of the urine requires (1) release of AVP from the hypothalamus, (2) response of the collecting ducts to the AVP, and (3) a hypertonic renal medulla that favors reabsorption of water from the urine [6]. Failure of the hypothalamus to release AVP sufficiently to maintain the P_{Osm} is referred to as central diabetes insipidus (DI). Failure to concentrate the urine in response to AVP is referred to as nephrogenic DI. The therapeutic importance of this distinction is that administration of vasopressin will reverse the defect and increase the U_{Osm} in patients with central DI, but it will have little effect in patients with nephrogenic DI.

Complications of Hypernatremic States

The complications of hyperosmolar states are primarily caused by the shift of water out of cells. As with hypoosmolar states, the most serious complications occur due to injury to neurons, or traumatic injury to the central nervous system caused by cell shrinkage [54]. Symptoms of hyperosmolarity can include lethargy, seizures, hyperreflexia, nausea, vomiting, seizures, and coma [55]. Mortality may be as high as 70 % in acute hyperosmolar states and long-term sequelae are common [56].

Cells adapt to hyperosmolarity by increasing the intracellular osmolarity, essentially by the reverse process of that used to decrease intracellular osmolarity in response to hypoosmolarity. As with the response to hypoosmolality, adaptation starts within hours but probably continues over several days before approaching normalization of the intracellular water content [11]. The initial response is to increase the cellular content of sodium, potassium, and chloride [57]. With more prolonged hyperosmolarity, the intracellular content of glutamine, glutamate, myoinositol, taurine, and urea increases [57]. Given the lag in adaptation, acute hyperosmolarity causes a greater degree of cellular dehydration and poses a greater risk of neurologic injury. Severe hyperosmolarity is associated with myelinolysis [25, 58].

Correction of hyperosmolarity can cause water to shift back intracellularly, and can cause cerebral edema if performed too rapidly. Patients with chronic hypernatremia are less likely to be symptomatic from the hypernatremia as they will have more fully adapted. However, they are also at greater risk of complications from therapy. Thus, correction of hyperosmolarity should be more gradual in these patients.

Treatment of Hypernatremia

Treatment of hypernatremia and hyperosmolarity must emphasize prevention as there are well-defined groups at risk, and it is commonly iatrogenic [59, 60]. Furthermore, even when the S_{Na} is measured and found to be elevated, treatment is often delayed [59, 60]. Patients at greatest risk of developing hypernatremia include infants and the elderly, hospitalized patients who are receiving hypertonic solutions such as high-protein nutritional supplements, patients receiving loop diuretics, those with altered cognition, and those incapable of drinking ad libitum. Patients who are polyuric or who have urinary concentrating defects are at risk of developing hypernatremia. Diabetics as a group are also at increased risk of free water depletion since hyperglycemia induces an osmotic diuresis. Patients receiving lactulose frequently have hypotonic stool losses.

The treatment of hypernatremia has two central goals:

- Restoration of water deficit
- Decrease of ongoing water losses

Estimation of Free Water Deficit

Correction of hypernatremia and restoration of water losses involve the administration of free water, and the amount of free water necessary to normalize the S_{Na} can be estimated. In determining how much free water to administer one needs to account for the free water deficit and the ongoing free water losses. If one calculates the free water deficit without accounting for these losses, the therapy will undershoot its target.

From (2.1) and (2.5), one can see that an increase of the S_{Na} above normal by a given percentage indicates a decrease of total body water by the same percentage. The water deficit can therefore be calculated as follows (2.6):

$$\text{Free water deficit} = 0.6 \times \text{weight(kg)}\left[\frac{(S_{Na})}{140} - 1\right], \tag{2.6}$$

where $0.6 \times$weight is taken as the total body water and 140 mEq/L is the normal S_{Na}.

For women the total body water may be approximated as $0.5 \times$weight. The percentage of body weight that is water may be lower in the elderly. Also, in patients with a large free water deficit the free water comprises a smaller fraction of the body weight. Calculation of the free water deficit in patients who are severely hyperosmolar can therefore be performed using $0.4 \times$weight as the estimate of total body water [61].

Ongoing urinary water losses can be estimated using (2.4), the formula for electrolyte free water clearance. If, for example, a patient is excreting 200 mL of urine each hour, and half of it is electrolyte free water, then the patient must receive 100 mL/h of free water just to maintain his or her current S_{Na}. The loss of free water from extrarenal sources must be estimated, but measurement of the change in S_{Na} (either up or down) can be used to estimate the change in total body water (2.6). The change in total body water should roughly equal the amount of free water taken minus that lost in the urine and that lost from extrarenal sources. Thus, extrarenal losses can be deduced.

Rate of Correction

To minimize the risk of cerebral edema hypernatremia should be corrected in a controlled fashion, particularly in those in whom the condition has been present for more than 48 h. In contrast, in patients whose S_{Na} has risen rapidly the correction

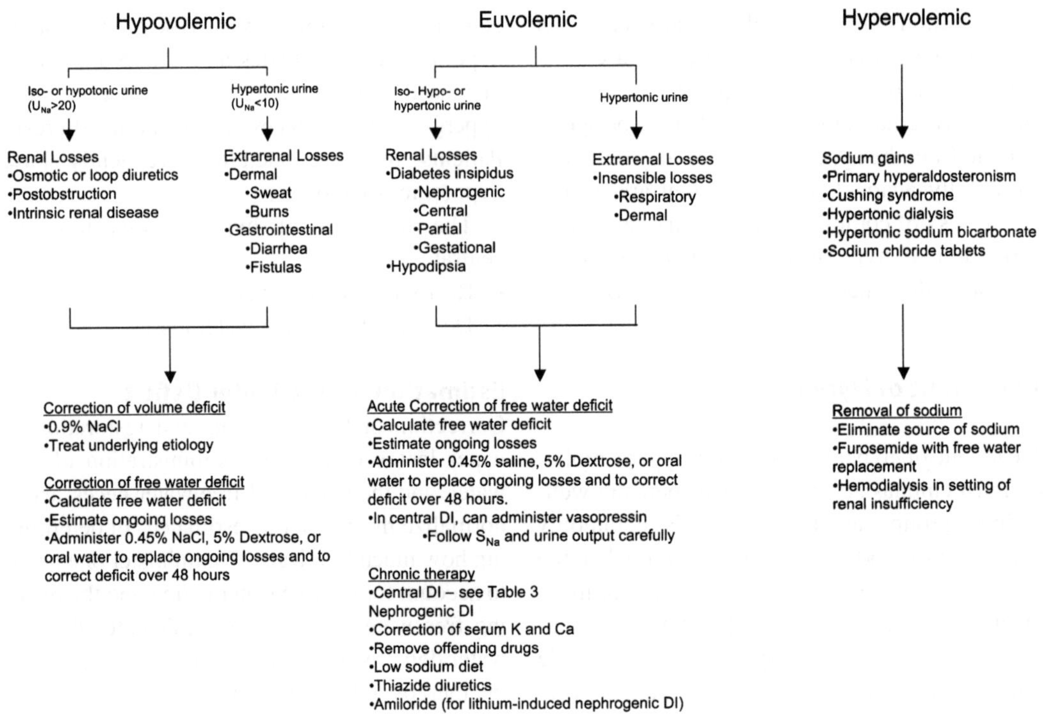

Fig. 2.3 Diagnostic approach to the patient with hyponatremia based upon clinical volume status. Adapted with permission from Therapy of dysnatremic disorders, Joshua M. Thurman, Tomas Berl. In: Wilcox CS, editor. Therapy in nephrology and hypertension, 3rd ed. WB Saunders; 2008

can also probably proceed rapidly as cerebral adaptation is less likely to be complete. Correction of the free water deficit should occur over 48 h, with the rate of correction not exceeding 2 mEq/L/h. A slower rate is appropriate, however, if the patient is not symptomatic. For example, two studies in children found that outcomes were better when the rate of correction was ≤ 0.5 mEq/L/h [62, 63], and no complications were seen in patients corrected at this rate.

Volume Status

Assessment of the hyperosmolar patient includes clinical estimation of volume status, and measurement of urine osmolality, sodium, potassium, and urine flow rate. Perturbations in the total body water may also be accompanied by perturbations in the total body osmoles, and treatment is guided by the patient's volume status and urine sodium (Fig. 2.3).

Hypovolemic Hypernatremia

Patients who lose hypotonic fluids and do not adequately replace them can become hypovolemic and hypernatremic. Therapy should usually begin with isotonic fluid such as normal saline. Volume resuscitation with isotonic fluids will restore the extracellular fluid and hemodynamic stability. This fluid will be relatively hypotonic compared to the patient's plasma and will cause a slight decrease in the S_{Na}, although this will be modest. Once the patient is euvolemic, hypotonic fluid (such as 0.45 % saline or D5) can be used to correct the free water deficit.

Euvolemic Hypernatremia

Initial therapy of patients with euvolemic hypernatremia is the repletion of free water—either intravenously or orally. As described above, the amount of water administered should aim to match ongoing losses and correct the free water deficit

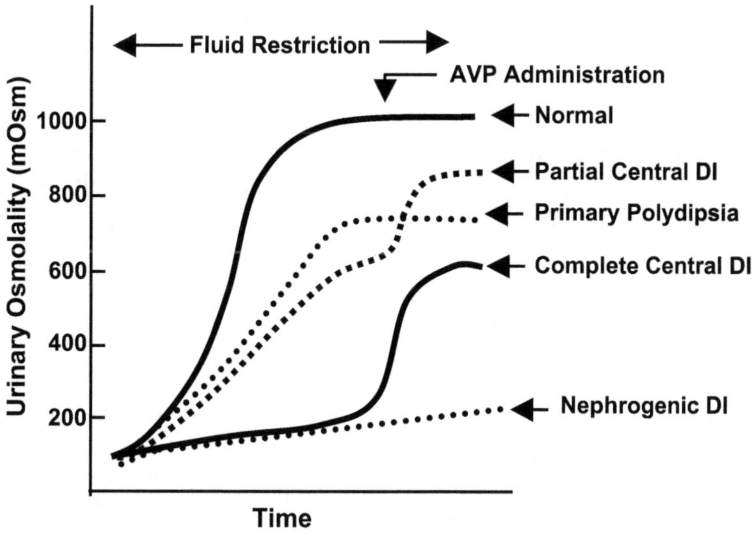

Fig. 2.4 Diagnostic approach to patients with diabetes insipidus based upon the response of the urine osmolality to exogenous AVP. Adapted with permission from Robertson G. Am J Med. 2006;119(7 Suppl 1): S36–42

over 48 h. It is important, but sometimes difficult, to determine the source of free water losses. Polyuria, a submaximally concentrated urine, or a positive electrolyte free water clearance indicates ongoing urinary losses of free water. In hypernatremic patients with polyuria and/or an inappropriately dilute urine there must be a defect in urinary concentration as the hypernatremic state should induce AVP-mediated concentration of the urine. These patients have effectively failed a water deprivation test. The distinction, then, is whether urinary water losses are caused by central diabetes insipidus, nephrogenic diabetes insipidus, or an osmotic diuresis. This last possibility would be indicated by an elevated U_{Osm} (indicating an intact AVP axis) but a positive electrolyte free water clearance (2.4). Such patients can concentrate their urine, but large quantities of nonelectrolyte solute (such as glucose, urea, or mannitol) obligate the loss of water.

In patients with polydipsia and polyuria who present with a normal serum sodium it can be difficult to differentiate whether the polydipsia is causing the polyuria or vice versa. The response of a polyuric patient to exogenous vasopressin helps distinguish primary polydipsia, central DI, and nephrogenic DI (Fig. 2.4). Administration of AVP can be as aqueous vasopressin or dDAVP. Aqueous vasopressin has a shorter half-life and may be preferential in the acute setting. It is an agonist for the V_1 receptor, however, and is contraindicated in patients with vascular disease. Patients with central DI should respond to the exogenous AVP by decreasing their urine flow and increasing their urine osmolarity [64]. An increase in the U_{Osm} of more than 10 % is diagnostic of at least a component of central DI.

Ongoing treatment with exogenous vasopressin reverses the primary defect of central DI and decreases the free water requirement (nn). Aqueous vasopressin has a very short half-life and because of its vasoconstrictive action should not be given intravenously; it is mainly used in transient postoperative DI. dDAVP has a longer half-life (8–12 h) and has less activity at the V_1 receptor. It is less likely, therefore, to cause vasoconstriction. It can also be administered intranasally or orally. The intranasal preparation provides 10 μ(mu)g/0.1 mL. The oral preparation is available as 0.1 or 0.2 mg tablets. When prompt antidiuresis is needed a parenteral route should be considered and is effective at 1–2 μ(mu)g every 8–12 h. dDAVP should be started at a low dose and can be titrated to achieve a decreased urine output. The lowest effective dose should be used in order to minimize cost and the risk of hyponatremia. Events such as a CVA can cause transient central DI. Patients should therefore be periodically reassessed to determine whether they still need the dDAVP (e.g., by reducing the dose and observing for a significant increase in urinary volume) and the S_{Na} should be monitored periodically. Care should also be taken if the patient is receiving large volumes of free water replacement. Continued replacement in addition to dDAVP may cause an overly rapid fall in the S_{Osm}. Vasopressin does not, itself, lower the S_{Osm}, however; it only decreases urinary losses. One hour after administration of vasopressin, the urine volume and urine osmolarity should be measured.

Alternative therapies for central DI include chlorpropamide, clofibrate, and carbamazepine. These drugs are not as effective as vasopressin, but they may be useful when vasopressin is unavailable. These agents potentiate the release and/or response to endogenous AVP. Chlorpropamide may also increase water intake. Thiazide diuretics (and amiloride for lithium-induced DI) may also be effective at decreasing free water losses. By inducing volume depletion these drugs enhance proximal sodium and water reabsorption. Thiazides also reduce the absorption of NaCl at the distal tubule without decreasing the osmolarity in the medulla, and may also increase expression of aquaporin-2 [65]. Loop diuretics, in contrast, should not be used in patients with DI as they can decrease the medullary tonicity and reduce free water reabsorption in the collecting ducts. Potential future therapies for DI include manipulation of the chaperone proteins that enable insertion of aquaporin-2 in the epithelial cell membrane [66].

Hypervolemic Hypernatremia

Patients who are clinically hypervolemic and also have hypernatremia have an increase in TBW but also a greater proportional increase in total body Na (2.1). Hypervolemic hypernatremia may, in fact, not be uncommon, particularly in intensive care unit settings [67, 68]. Administration of free water will cause a volume expansion, so treatment to increase natriuresis should also be employed. Thiazide diuretics may be useful, but are not as potent as loop diuretics. Loop diuretics, on the other hand, will increase free water losses, likely increasing the need for free water replacement.

References

1. Waikar SS, Mount DB, Curhan GC. Mortality after hospitalization with mild, moderate, and severe hyponatremia. Am J Med. 2009;122:857–65.
2. Nguyen MK, Kurtz I. New insights into the pathophysiology of the dysnatremias: a quantitative analysis. Am J Physiol Renal Physiol. 2004;287:F172–80.
3. Schoen EJ. Minimum urine total solute concentration in response to water loading in normal men. J Appl Physiol. 1957;10:267–70.
4. Lindeman RD, Van Buren HC, Raisz LG. Osmolar renal concentrating ability in healthy young men and hospitalized patients without renal disease. N Engl J Med. 1960;262:1306–9.
5. Nielsen S, Frokiaer J, Marples D, Kwon TH, Agre P, Knepper MA. Aquaporins in the kidney: from molecules to medicine. Physiol Rev. 2002;82:205–44.
6. Berl T, Schrier RW. Disorders of Water Homeostasis. In: Schrier RW, editor. Renal and electrolyte disorders. 6th ed. Philadelphia, PA: Lippincott Williams & Wilkins; 2010. p. 1–44.
7. Berl T. Impact of solute intake on urine flow and water excretion. J Am Soc Nephrol. 2008;19:1076–8.
8. Sterns RH, Silver SM. Brain volume regulation in response to hypo-osmolality and its correction. Am J Med. 2006;119:S12–6.
9. Ayus JC, Arieff AI. Noncardiogenic pulmonary edema in marathon runners. Ann Intern Med. 2000;133:1011.
10. Arieff AI, Ayus JC, Fraser CL. Hyponatraemia and death or permanent brain damage in healthy children. BMJ. 1992;304:1218–22.
11. Pollock AS, Arieff AI. Abnormalities of cell volume regulation and their functional consequences. Am J Physiol. 1980;239:F195–205.
12. Arieff AI. Hyponatremia, convulsions, respiratory arrest, and permanent brain damage after elective surgery in healthy women. N Engl J Med. 1986;314:1529–35.
13. Ayus JC, Armstrong D, Arieff AI. Hyponatremia with hypoxia: effects on brain adaptation, perfusion, and histology in rodents. Kidney Int. 2006;69:1319–25.
14. Ayus JC, Arieff AI. Brain damage and postoperative hyponatremia: the role of gender. Neurology. 1996;46:323–8.
15. Ayus JC, Wheeler JM, Arieff AI. Postoperative hyponatremic encephalopathy in menstruant women. Ann Intern Med. 1992;117:891–7.
16. Fraser CL, Kucharczyk J, Arieff AI, Rollin C, Sarnacki P, Norman D. Sex differences result in increased morbidity from hyponatremia in female rats. Am J Physiol. 1989;256:R880–5.
17. Sonnenblick M, Friedlander Y, Rosin AJ. Diuretic-induced severe hyponatremia. Review and analysis of 129 reported patients. Chest. 1993;103:601–6.
18. Szatalowicz VL, Miller PD, Lacher JW, Gordon JA, Schrier RW. Comparative effect of diuretics on renal water excretion in hyponatraemic oedematous disorders. Clin Sci (Lond). 1982;62:235–8.

19. Chow KM, Szeto CC, Wong TY, Leung CB, Li PK. Risk factors for thiazide-induced hyponatraemia. QJM. 2003;96:911–7.
20. Durward A, Tibby SM, Murdoch IA. Hyponatraemia can be caused by standard fluid regimens. BMJ. 2000;320:943.
21. Franchi-Gazzola R, Dall'Asta V, Sala R, Visigalli R, Bevilacqua E, Gaccioli F, Gazzola GC, Bussolati O. The role of the neutral amino acid transporter SNAT2 in cell volume regulation. Acta Physiol (Oxf). 2006;187:273–83.
22. Norenberg MD. Central pontine myelinolysis: historical and mechanistic considerations. Metab Brain Dis. 2010;25:97–106.
23. Berl T, Rastegar A. A patient with severe hyponatremia and hypokalemia: osmotic demyelination following potassium repletion. Am J Kidney Dis. 2010;55:742–8.
24. Sterns RH, Cappuccio JD, Silver SM, Cohen EP. Neurologic sequelae after treatment of severe hyponatremia: a multicenter perspective. J Am Soc Nephrol. 1994;4:1522–30.
25. McKee AC, Winkelman MD, Banker BQ. Central pontine myelinolysis in severely burned patients: relationship to serum hyperosmolality. Neurology. 1988;38:1211–7.
26. Sica DA. Hyponatremia and heart failure—pathophysiology and implications. Congest Heart Fail. 2005;11:274–7.
27. Heuman DM, Abou-Assi SG, Habib A, Williams LM, Stravitz RT, Sanyal AJ, Fisher RA, Mihas AA. Persistent ascites and low serum sodium identify patients with cirrhosis and low MELD scores who are at high risk for early death. Hepatology. 2004;40: 802–10.
28. Schrier RW. Role of diminished renal function in cardiovascular mortality: marker or pathogenetic factor? J Am Coll Cardiol. 2006;47:1–8.
29. Licata G, Di Pasquale P, Parrinello G, Cardinale A, Scandurra A, Follone G, Argano C, Tuttolomondo A, Paterna S. Effects of high-dose furosemide and small-volume hypertonic saline solution infusion in comparison with a high dose of furosemide as bolus in refractory congestive heart failure: long-term effects. Am Heart J. 2003;145:459–66.
30. Cardenas A, Gines P. Management of complications of cirrhosis in patients awaiting liver transplantation. J Hepatol. 2005;42(Suppl):S124–33.
31. Koenig MA, Bryan M, Lewin 3rd JL, Mirski MA, Geocadin RG, Stevens RD. Reversal of transtentorial herniation with hypertonic saline. Neurology. 2008;70:1023–9.
32. Soupart A, Ngassa M, Decaux G. Therapeutic relowering of the serum sodium in a patient after excessive correction of hyponatremia. Clin Nephrol. 1999;51: 383–6.
33. Oya S, Tsutsumi K, Ueki K, Kirino T. Reinduction of hyponatremia to treat central pontine myelinolysis. Neurology. 2001;57:1931–2.
34. Perianayagam A, Sterns RH, Silver SM, Grieff M, Mayo R, Hix J, Kouides R. DDAVP is effective in preventing and reversing inadvertent overcorrection of hyponatremia. Clin J Am Soc Nephrol. 2008;3: 331–6.
35. Sterns RH, Hix JK, Silver S. Treating profound hyponatremia: a strategy for controlled correction. Am J Kidney Dis. 2010;56:774–9.
36. Greenberg A, Verbalis JG. Vasopressin receptor antagonists. Kidney Int. 2006;69:2124–30.
37. Velez JC, Dopson SJ, Sanders DS, Delay TA, Arthur JM. Intravenous conivaptan for the treatment of hyponatraemia caused by the syndrome of inappropriate secretion of antidiuretic hormone in hospitalized patients: a single-centre experience. Nephrol Dial Transplant. 2010;25:1524–31.
38. Renneboog B, Musch W, Vandemergel X, Manto MU, Decaux G. Mild chronic hyponatremia is associated with falls, unsteadiness, and attention deficits. Am J Med. 2006;119(71):e71–8.
39. Verbalis JG, Barsony J, Sugimura Y, Tian Y, Adams DJ, Carter EA, Resnick HE. Hyponatremia-induced osteoporosis. J Bone Miner Res. 2010;25:554–63.
40. Gankam Kengne F, Andres C, Sattar L, Melot C, Decaux G. Mild hyponatremia and risk of fracture in the ambulatory elderly. QJM. 2008;101:583–8.
41. Sica DA. Hyponatremia and heart failure—treatment considerations. Congest Heart Fail. 2006;12:55–60.
42. Udelson JE, Smith WB, Hendrix GH, Painchaud CA, Ghazzi M, Thomas I, Ghali JK, Selaru P, Chanoine F, Pressler ML, Konstam MA. Acute hemodynamic effects of conivaptan, a dual V(1A) and V(2) vasopressin receptor antagonist, in patients with advanced heart failure. Circulation. 2001;104:2417–23.
43. Abraham WT, Shamshirsaz AA, McFann K, Oren RM, Schrier RW. Aquaretic effect of lixivaptan, an oral, non-peptide, selective V2 receptor vasopressin antagonist, in New York Heart Association functional class II and III chronic heart failure patients. J Am Coll Cardiol. 2006;47:1615–21.
44. Gheorghiade M, Niazi I, Ouyang J, Czerwiec F, Kambayashi J, Zampino M, Orlandi C. Vasopressin V2-receptor blockade with tolvaptan in patients with chronic heart failure: results from a double-blind, randomized trial. Circulation. 2003;107:2690–6.
45. Schrier RW, Gross P, Gheorghiade M, Berl T, Verbalis JG, Czerwiec FS, Orlandi C. Tolvaptan, a selective oral vasopressin V2-receptor antagonist, for hyponatremia. N Engl J Med. 2006;355:2099–112.
46. Wong F, Blei AT, Blendis LM, Thuluvath PJ. A vasopressin receptor antagonist (VPA-985) improves serum sodium concentration in patients with hyponatremia: a multicenter, randomized, placebo-controlled trial. Hepatology. 2003;37:182–91.
47. Gerbes AL, Gulberg V, Gines P, Decaux G, Gross P, Gandjini H, Djian J. Therapy of hyponatremia in cirrhosis with a vasopressin receptor antagonist: a randomized double-blind multicenter trial. Gastroenterology. 2003;124:933–9.

48. Guyader D, Patat A, Ellis-Grosse EJ, Orczyk GP. Pharmacodynamic effects of a nonpeptide antidiuretic hormone V2 antagonist in cirrhotic patients with ascites. Hepatology. 2002;36:1197–205.
49. Gines P, Cardenas A, Arroyo V, Rodes J. Management of cirrhosis and ascites. N Engl J Med. 2004;350: 1646–54.
50. Londono MC, Guevara M, Rimola A, Navasa M, Taura P, Mas A, Garcia-Valdecasas JC, Arroyo V, Gines P. Hyponatremia impairs early posttransplantation outcome in patients with cirrhosis undergoing liver transplantation. Gastroenterology. 2006;130: 1135–43.
51. Furst H, Hallows KR, Post J, Chen S, Kotzker W, Goldfarb S, Ziyadeh FN, Neilson EG. The urine/plasma electrolyte ratio: a predictive guide to water restriction. Am J Med Sci. 2000;319:240–4.
52. Soupart A, Gross P, Legros J, Alfoldi S, Annane D, Heshmati H, Decaux G. Successful long-term treatment of hyponatremia in syndrome of inappropriate antidiuretic hormone secretion with satavaptan (SR121463B), an orally active nonpeptide vasopressin V2-receptor antagonist. CJASN. 2006;1: 1154–60.
53. Berl T, Quittnat-Pelletier F, Verbalis JG, Schrier RW, Bichet DG, Ouyang J, Czerwiec FS. Oral tolvaptan is safe and effective in chronic hyponatremia. J Am Soc Nephrol. 2010;21:705–12.
54. Finberg L, Luttrell C, Redd H. Pathogenesis of lesions in the nervous system in hypernatremic states. II. Experimental studies of gross anatomic changes and alterations of chemical composition of the tissues. Pediatrics. 1959;23:46–53.
55. Arieff AI, Guisado R. Effects on the central nervous system of hypernatremic and hyponatremic states. Kidney Int. 1976;10:104–16.
56. Morris-Jones PH, Houston IB, Evans RC. Prognosis of the neurological complications of acute hypernatraemia. Lancet. 1967;2:1385–9.
57. Lien YH, Shapiro JI, Chan L. Effects of hypernatremia on organic brain osmoles. J Clin Invest. 1990;85:1427–35.
58. Brown WD, Caruso JM. Extrapontine myelinolysis with involvement of the hippocampus in three children with severe hypernatremia. J Child Neurol. 1999;14:428–33.
59. Palevsky PM, Bhagrath R, Greenberg A. Hypernatremia in hospitalized patients. Ann Intern Med. 1996;124:197–203.
60. Polderman KH, Schreuder WO, Strack van Schijndel RJ, Thijs LG. Hypernatremia in the intensive care unit: an indicator of quality of care? Crit Care Med. 1999;27:1105–8.
61. Rose BD, Post TW. Clincial physiology of acid-base and electrolyte disorders. New York: McGraw Hill; 2001.
62. Kahn A, Brachet E, Blum D. Controlled fall in natremia and risk of seizures in hypertonic dehydration. Intensive Care Med. 1979;5:27–31.
63. Blum D, Brasseur D, Kahn A, Brachet E. Safe oral rehydration of hypertonic dehydration. J Pediatr Gastroenterol Nutr. 1986;5:232–5.
64. Miller M, Dalakos T, Moses AM, Fellerman H, Streeten DH. Recognition of partial defects in antidiuretic hormone secretion. Ann Intern Med. 1970;73:721–9.
65. Kim GH, Lee JW, Oh YK, Chang HR, Joo KW, Na KY, Earm JH, Knepper MA, Han JS. Antidiuretic effect of hydrochlorothiazide in lithium-induced nephrogenic diabetes insipidus is associated with upregulation of aquaporin-2, Na-Cl co-transporter, and epithelial sodium channel. J Am Soc Nephrol. 2004;15:2836–43.
66. Fujiwara TM, Bichet DG. Molecular biology of hereditary diabetes insipidus. J Am Soc Nephrol. 2005;16:2836–46.
67. Hoorn EJ, Betjes MG, Weigel J, Zietse R. Hypernatraemia in critically ill patients: too little water and too much salt. Nephrol Dial Transplant. 2008;23:1562–8.
68. Lindner G, Kneidinger N, Holzinger U, Druml W, Schwarz C. Tonicity balance in patients with hypernatremia acquired in the intensive care unit. Am J Kidney Dis. 2009;54:674–9.

Potassium and the Dyskalemias

3

Alan Segal

Physiological Overview of Potassium Homeostasis: The Lion, the Wildebeest, and the Potassium

As the sun rises on the Serengeti, a lion yawns and quickly realizes it is time for breakfast. Not far away, a blue wildebeest grazes on short green grasses, unaware that life will be over within the hour. Eating the "lion's share," the successful predator pulls at the flesh and rapaciously devours 8-kg of beast meat. At about 50 mmol of potassium (K^+) per kg of wildebeest, the lion ingests ~400 mmol of K^+, more than threefold the total amount of K^+ normally in the lion's extracellular fluid (ECF)! Now it is the lion's turn to be blissfully unaware of potentially life-threatening hyperkalemia. Happily for the lion, several physiological mechanisms are set in motion to ensure that the lion will live to hunt tomorrow (see Fig. 3.1).

First, the carbohydrates ingested along with the K^+ provide a signal that the fasted state has given way to the fed state, stimulating *insulin* release from pancreatic β[beta] islet cells. Independent of carbohydrates, an increase in extracellular [K^+] also stimulates insulin secretion. Among the myriad actions of insulin, stimulation of the Na^+/K^+-ATPase pump promotes the prompt transfer of K^+ into the cells, primarily muscle, fat, and liver. Secondly, activation of the sympathetic nervous system during the chase increases circulating levels of *catecholamines*, which also promote cellular K^+ uptake via the *Na^+/K^+-ATPase*, not only in the tissues mentioned, but also into the cells of the distal nephron, the predominant site for K^+ secretion. However, it is likely that this signal becomes attenuated as eating commences and parasympathetic nervous activity begins to dominate. Potassium in excess of that needed to maintain intracellular fluid (ICF) [K^+] will be temporarily stored within these cells for subsequent excretion.

The majority (up to 92 %) of the K^+ load will ultimately be excreted in the urine via K^+ secretion along the connecting tubule and collecting duct. The most important determinants of K^+ secretion are the *peritubular [K^+]* and processes directly or indirectly regulated by *aldosterone*. The major factors controlling aldosterone secretion from the zona glomerulosa of the adrenal cortex are (1) physiological levels of renin and angiotensin II (Ang II) reflective of ECF volume status and (2) the plasma [K^+]. As will be seen, the control of aldosterone by both ECF volume and [K^+] is no accident. On the contrary, it is likely that such dual control evolved under substantial selective pressure as volume-depleted predators had to chase their prey.

The overall effect of eating on aldosterone levels depends on the relative balance between volume repletion and plasma [K^+]. The beauty of the

A. Segal, M.D. (✉)
Division of Nephrology, Department of Medicine, University of Vermont, 1 South Prospect St., Burlington, VT 05401, USA
e-mail: alan.segal@uvm.edu

D.B. Mount et al. (eds.), *Core Concepts in the Disorders of Fluid, Electrolytes and Acid-Base Balance*, DOI 10.1007/978-1-4614-3770-3_3, © Springer Science+Business Media New York 2013

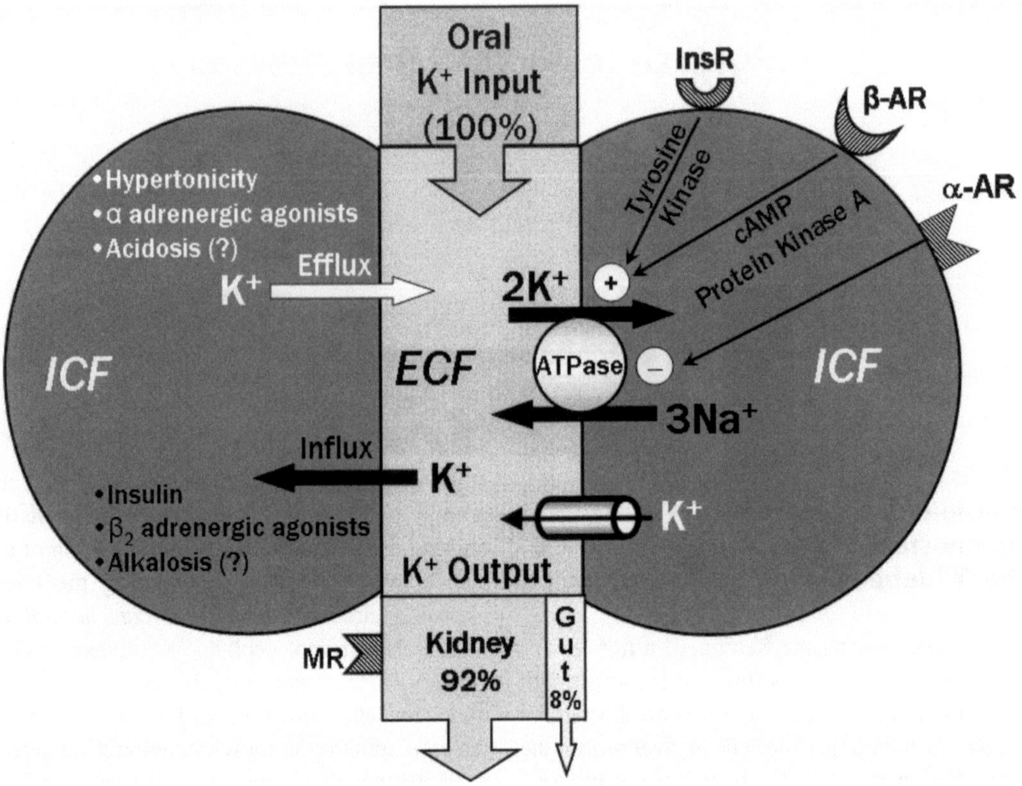

Fig. 3.1 Overview of potassium homeostasis. The center of the diagram shows "external" K^+ balance where the K^+ output equals the oral K^+ input in the steady state. The kidney excretes 92 % of the daily load, and major factors that increase K^+ secretion include peritubular [K^+] and aldosterone, which activate cytoplasmic mineralocorticoid receptors (MR) in collecting duct cells. The *left side* shows overall "internal" K^+ homeostasis between the ECF and ICF and the major factors associated with K^+ efflux and K^+ influx. The *right side* shows the major cellular elements involved in "internal" K^+ homeostasis. Factors that promote cellular K^+ uptake by the Na^+/K^+-ATPase pump include (1) insulin acting via the insulin receptor (InsR) and tyrosine kinase signaling and (2) β_2[beta2]-adrenergic agonists acting via the β[beta]-adrenergic receptor (β[beta]-AR) and cAMP/PKA signaling. In contrast, α[alpha]-adrenergic agonists (α[alpha2]-AR) act to inhibit the pump

dual control now becomes evident: as sodium is reabsorbed to restore euvolemia, the driving force for K^+ secretion increases and thereby prevents a serious level or duration of hyperkalemia from developing.

This story highlights the "divide and conquer" strategy used to maintain overall K^+ homeostasis (see Fig. 3.1). Namely, to first transfer K^+ from ECF to ICF (e.g., via the ancient Na^+/K^+-ATPase pump under the influence of *insulin* and *catecholamines*) for temporary storage; followed by the secretion of K^+ by the principal cells (PCs) of the collecting duct, assisted by *aldosterone*, the *plasma [K^+]* level itself, and an increase in urine flow rate. A final reason that the lions avoid sustained hyperkalemia is probably because they tend to develop less congestive heart failure and/or chronic kidney disease (CKD) than humans, and they rarely ingest substances that interfere with K^+ excretion.

Clinical Significance of Dyskalemia

The total amount of potassium in the average 70-kg man is ~4,000 mmol, yielding an average of ~57 mmol K^+ per kg of body weight. Over 98 % of total body K^+ is within cells, and the intracellular [K^+] is 140–150 mM. Clinically, the extracellular [K^+] is assessed by measurements of serum [K^+]; the normal range is from 3.5–3.6 mM to 5.0–5.1 mM, depending on the laboratory or institution. Patients with an ECF [K^+] <3.5 mM are said to have hypokalemia; those with an ECF [K^+] >5.1 mM are said to have hyperkalemia. It is important to keep in mind that the status of total body K^+ stores may not be altered in the same direction as the dyskalemia. Because of derangements in transcellular movements of K^+, some patients with hypokalemia may not have a deficit of total body K^+. The converse also holds; a patient with hyperkalemia may not have excess total body K^+. An important example of the latter includes diabetic ketoacidosis, a condition in which patients can present with hyperkalemia despite total body K^+ depletion [1].

Symptoms and Signs of Dyskalemia

Maintenance of the appropriate ratio of ECF [K^+]:ICF [K^+] is vital for the proper function of electrically excitable tissues because the resting potential is in large part determined by the K^+ conductance that dominates in most cells at rest. Alterations in this ratio that develop rapidly or are of sufficient magnitude are most likely to produce symptoms and/or signs, most of which are related to disturbances in neuromuscular transmission and cardiac conduction.

Hypokalemia

In hypokalemia, a decrease in the ratio of ECF [K^+]:ICF [K^+] causes hyperpolarization of the resting membrane potential, which more fully removes inactivation from voltage-gated Na^+ channels and thereby promotes membrane excitability. Effects on skeletal muscle include weakness, discomfort, cramps, and if severe (ECF [K^+] <2.0 mM), flaccid paralysis, respiratory muscle insufficiency, and rhabdomyolysis [2]. Weakness typically begins in the legs. Effects on gut smooth muscle can produce constipation, and if severe, ileus. Effects of hypokalemia on the heart relate to an increase in the excitability of cardiomyocytes, and include increased cardiac automaticity and delayed ventricular repolarization. These in turn can promote reentrant arrhythmias including ventricular tachycardia and fibrillation. Cardiac arrhythmias are common in hypokalemia, especially in patients with heart disease and those on digoxin [3]. Electrical abnormalities such as delayed repolarization due to hypokalemia can produce characteristic patterns on the surface electrocardiogram (ECG) including ST segment depression, QT prolongation, flattening of the T waves, and the appearance of prominent U waves [4]. Significant K^+ depletion and hypokalemia can also lead to a urinary concentrating defect with resultant polyuria [5].

Hyperkalemia

In hyperkalemia, an increase in the ratio of ECF [K^+]:ICF [K^+] causes depolarization of the resting membrane potential, which initially activates voltage-gated Na^+ channels. Ultimately however, this leads to a decrease in membrane excitability because inactivation is not fully removed from these channels, which then become refractory. Unless the rise is rapid, symptoms and signs may not be seen until ECF [K^+] exceeds 7.0 mM. Effects on skeletal muscle are similar to those seen with hypokalemia, and include weakness (again often beginning in the legs) and, if severe, flaccid paralysis. The effects of hyperkalemia on the cardiac conduction system are more complex and potentially life-threatening. In addition to the inactivating effect of hyperkalemia on voltage-gated Na^+ channels, it also appears that some cardiac K^+ channels are activated by extracellular K^+, potentiating repolarization (as evidenced by taller T waves). The classical sequence of surface ECG changes occurring as hyperkalemia worsens is (1) peaked and tented T waves with shortening of the QT interval, (2) an increase in the PR interval, (3) widening of the QRS complex, (4) loss of P waves with further widening of the QRS complex that (5) merges with the T wave to give the appearance of a sine wave [4]. The overall disruption of the coordinated integrity of voltage-gated cardiac channels in hyperkalemia can be highly arrhythmogenic, including generation of ventricular fibrillation and cardiac standstill. That said, it is important for the clinician to appreciate the relative insensitivity of the ECG in the diagnosis and management of hyperkalemia. Although the likelihood of ECG changes increases with the degree of hyperkalemia, such changes may be absent even in severe hyperkalemia [6].

It should also be mentioned that hyperkalemia can mimic the so-called Brugada pattern on the ECG [7]. The Brugada syndrome is a distinct genetic entity most often due to a mutation in the *SCN5A* gene, which encodes the alpha subunit of the cardiac voltage-gated sodium channel. The genetic syndrome, which is associated with a high risk of sudden death in otherwise healthy people, is characterized by a specific ST-segment elevation in the right precordial leads (V1 and V2). The hyperkalemic Brugada pattern usually (but not always [8]) differs from the pattern seen in genetic Brugada syndrome in several ways: the absence of P waves, abnormal QRS axis, and widening of the QRS not seen in the genetic syndrome. Moreover, those with the genetic syndrome are neither hyperkalemic nor critically ill, which are features of the hyperkalemic variant [7].

Origins and Evolutionary Physiology

The introductory vignette alluded to the evolutionary significance of maintaining normal K^+ balance, and the foregoing section pointed to the central importance of maintaining a proper transmembrane K^+ gradient. But how did these circumstances develop?

Origin of High Intracellular [K^+]

Potassium is the dominant ion in virtually all living cells, and every mammalian cell has a high intracellular [K^+]. How this came about is not known with certainty, but any proposed model of the origin of life should be able to take this into account. The fact that K^+ resides in cells indicates that an inorganic environment high in K^+ was more conducive to organic biochemistry than the alternatives available under primeval conditions. This in turn, suggests that early life forms may have originated on a substrate composed mainly of clays and their analogs such as argillites high in silica.

Consistent with this notion, it is interesting to consider the following: In present day seawater, the [Na^+]:[K^+] ratio is ~30 [9], which is very similar to the [Na^+]:[K^+] ratio in mammalian ECF. In contrast, the average [K^+] of the Earth's crust is ~65 times higher than in seawater [9], which is comparable to the mammalian ICF:ECF ratio of [K^+]. Measurements made on sedimentary rocks of the Baltic shield from the Rhyacian period (2.2 billion years ago) show the highest ratio of potassium to sodium content. Therefore, primitive cells (or protocells) may have first emerged on a mineral substrate of K^+-rich clay silicates in shallow puddles of Na^+-rich medium. From that point forward, the ICF became inextricably associated with a high [K^+] cytoplasm in which the biochemical reactions required for cellular life and replication could occur.

Eventually, a plasma membrane to separate the ICF (*the 1st space*) from the ECF (*the 2nd space*) became mandatory. Further requirements of this membrane included that it be generally impermeant to water (i.e., comprised of lipids) and possess transport elements for regulated transfer of ions (e.g., pumps, exchangers, and channels) and water (i.e., aquaporins) across the membrane. Unregulated water permeability was a must to avoid because all cells contain membrane-impermeant substances (e.g., proteins, nucleic acids, etc.), which constitute an osmotic driving force favoring water influx that would otherwise flood the cell. Animal cells solved the problem by making use of ancient P-type ATPase pumps, at the cost of energy expenditure.

The use of ATP as an energy molecule appears to be as old as life itself, as cyanobacteria from 3.5 billion years ago were able to use photosynthesis to convert energy from the sun into ATP by removing electrons from hydrogen sulfide [10]. ATP powers the ubiquitous Na^+/K^+-ATPase pump in the plasma membrane. This pump acts to maintain the high [K^+] of the ICF of cells constantly immersed in a high [Na^+], low [K^+] of the ECF. The pump subserves multiple physiological functions [11]; in addition to pumping two K^+ ions into the cell with each turn, the three Na^+ ions pumped out of the cell contribute to the control of cell volume [12]. The activity of the pump is intrinsically regulated by an internal binding site that has a high affinity for Na^+ and a low affinity for K^+. This intrinsic negative feedback mechanism allows for inhibition of the pump when the intracellular $[K^+]$:$[Na^+]$ ratio is optimal. For continued operation of this pump, an efflux pathway for K^+ recycling is necessary, which may explain why there are >1,000 different types of ion channels that conduct K^+ [13].

In this light, it is not surprising that potassium plays a number of important roles in cell biology, including regulation of intracellular volume, pH, nucleic acid and protein synthesis, cell growth, and biochemical and enzyme function [14, 15].

Ontogeny of Total Body K^+

The cytoplasmic $[K^+]$ of a human oocyte is about 140 mM. Following fertilization, the process of cell division commences. At this point, nature has a problem to solve: how to maintain the intracellular $[K^+]$ in both daughter cells, and each subsequent cell. The mechanistic details of how this occurs are not known with precision, but include transport events such as increased activity of the Na^+/K^+-ATPase and K^+ influx via inwardly rectifying K^+ channels, which increase the amount of cytoplasmic K^+ prior to cell division. In fact, there is evidence that an increase in cellular K^+ (or $[K^+]$) is one of the signals involved in the control of mitosis [16].

The additional K^+ necessary as the embryo and placenta grow must come from maternal intake, which is easily achieved with the typical dietary K^+ of 60–120 mmol/day. For example, a new-born infant weighing 3.5 kg (with a 0.5-kg placenta) would require at least 8-g (200 mmol) of elemental K^+ (atomic mass 39.1 mg/mmol). This is based on an estimate of 2-g K^+ per kilogram body weight and an average of ~50 mmol K^+ per kilogram body weight and ~70 mmol K^+ per kilogram of fat-free mass. Integrated over the human gestation period of 280 days, a woman would only have to maintain a net positive K^+ balance of ~0.7 mmol/day.

Following birth, ingestion of K^+ in breast milk or infant formula is required to maintain total body K^+ stores and to replace losses from the skin (in sweat), gut, and kidney (in urine).

Discovery of Potassium

Sir Humphry Davy (1778–1829) was the first to isolate metallic potassium. Davy succeeded in isolating two new alkali metals using electrolysis. On October 6, 1807 he made the landmark discovery of potassium from molten caustic potash (KOH). Davy named it "potassium" because he used potash as the starting material. A few days later, he isolated sodium from molten caustic soda (NaOH) [17].

Potassium has an atomic number of 19, an atomic weight of 39.1 g/mol, and is denoted in the periodic table of elements by the symbol K^+ from the Latin word *kalium*, which itself is derived from the English word "alkali" based on the Arabic, *al qalīy*. For this reason, the clinical disorders of ECF $[K^+]$ are known as hypokalemia and hyperkalemia.

Electrophysiological Significance of Transmembrane $[K^+]$

The distribution of both Na^+ and K^+ ions across the cell membrane is maintained by the Na^+/K^+-ATPase pump. The driving (electromotive) force for transport of an ionic species across a membrane is given by the Nernst potential, which is a relationship that depends on the temperature, valence, and the ratio of ionic concentrations (or activities) on each side of the membrane. For an ion X, the Nernst potential (in volts) is: $E_X = (RT/z_X F) \times \ln([X]_{out}/[X]_{in})$, where:

- R is the universal gas constant, 8.314 J/mol K^+
- T is the absolute temperature in Kelvin (K^+ = °C + 273.15)
- z_X is the valence of ion X (e.g., +1 for K^+, −1 for Cl^-, +2 for Ca^{2+})
- F is Faraday's constant (the amount of electrical charge in one mole of an entity with a single charge), 96,485.34 C/mol
- $[X]_{out}$ is the concentration of X outside the cell
- $[X]_{in}$ is the concentration of X inside the cell

At body temperature of 37 °C (310.15 K^+), E_X (in mV) = $(26.725/z_X) \times \ln([X]_{out}/[X]_{in})$. Using typical concentrations of the ECF ($[K^+]$ = 4 mM; $[Na^+]$ = 140 mM) and ICF ($[K^+]$ = 140 mM;

$[Na^+] = 15$ mM), yields $E_{K^{++}} \cong -95$ mV and $E_{Na^{++}} \cong +60$ mV.

Net *transport* is determined by the product of *driving force* and *permeability*. Establishing driving forces requires time and energy, and cannot be rapidly changed. So one motif commonly found in nature is to regulate passive permeabilities (e.g., ion channels) in the presence of constant driving forces (e.g., Nernst potentials). At any moment, the cell membrane potential (V_m) varies between E_{K^+} and E_{Na^+} depending on the prevailing permeability ratio (p_{K^+}:p_{Na^+}). The resting membrane potential of cells is negative (e.g., −70 mV) because the membrane conductance for K^+ (due to K^+-selective ion channels in the membrane) dominates over all other conductances at rest. This natural system may constitute the earliest example of digital signal processing. The ability of V_m to change abruptly from a highly negative potential (i.e., p_{K^+} high; p_{Na^+} low) to a highly positive potential (i.e., p_{K^+} low; p_{Na^+} high) during an action potential constitutes the high fidelity digital signaling system of the nervous system.

Against this background, it becomes transparent how and why perturbations in ECF $[K^+]$ can have profound effects on cellular activity, particularly in excitable tissues such as nerve, muscle, and especially the heart. Most of the adverse effects of dyskalemia are related to alterations in (1) the relationship between the resting membrane potential and the "threshold" voltage (V_T) and (2) the behavior of voltage-gated channels.

Distribution and Disposition of Potassium

Steady-State Distribution

Assuming that total body fluid (TBF) is 60 % of body weight and consists of 2/3 resides in the ICF and 1/3 in the ECF, a 70-kg man has a TBF of 42 L with 28 L of ICF and 14 L of ECF. The ICF has a $[K^+]$ of ~140 mM, which yields a total intracellular content of 3,920 mmol K^+. The ECF has a $[K^+]$ of ~4 mM, which yields a total extracellular content of 56 mmol K^+. Notice that 98.6 % of total body K^+ is inside the cells, which is a major reason that estimating deficits in total body K^+ is difficult.

Integrated over a day, the amount of K^+ leaving the body equals the amount of K^+ entering the body, which maintains total body K^+ stores at a steady-state level. However, the actual ECF K^+ level will—in the steady-state—vary with intake. If a person who consumes 80 mmol of K^+ per day and consistently has an ECF $[K^+]$ of 4.0 mM makes a step increase (or *decrease*), for example, and ingests 100 mmol (or *60 mmol*) of K^+ per day for the next several weeks, the ECF $[K^+]$ will rise (or *fall*) to a level above (or *below*) 4.0 mM. The actual increment by which the $[K^+]$ will rise or fall will vary, but should be fairly consistent for a given person in the absence of other factors that could perturb the way the kidney handles potassium.

The Na^+/K^+-ATPase Pump

The Na^+/K^+-ATPase pumps three Na^+ ions out of the cell and two K^+ ions into the cell against an electrochemical gradient [18] (for review, see [11]). As might be expected, the activity of the pump is affected by deficits and surfeits of body K^+. This change in activity promotes a net release of intracellular K^+ and represents an adaptive mechanism to maintain E_{K^+} in the face of hypokalemia [11]. Important activators of the pump include insulin, insulin growth factor-1 (IGF-1) catecholamines (e.g., epinephrine, norepinephrine), β_2 [beta-2]-agonists, adrenal steroids, and ECF $[K^+]$ itself [11, 19].

Insulin

This peptide hormone plays a major role in extrarenal K^+ homeostasis by promoting K^+ uptake into muscle, liver, and fat cells via activation of the Na^+/K^+-ATPase (see Fig. 3.1). Insulin activates the Na^+/K^+-ATPase by increasing its affinity for intracellular Na^+. That insulin promotes cellular uptake of K^+ also makes physiological sense; during a meal, ingestion of K^+ is usually coupled with carbohydrates, and both stimulate insulin release. This effect occurs within the physiological range of ECF $[K^+]$, and is probably an adaptive response to defend against hyperkalemia. For example, an increase in ECF $[K^+]$ of 1.0–1.5 mM results in a two- to threefold increase in circulating insulin levels [20].

Catecholamines

Adrenergic receptor agonists play an important role in extrarenal K^+ homeostasis via circulating catecholamines and the sympathetic nervous system [21]. For K^+ homeostasis, β_2[beta-2]-adrenoreceptors play the major physiological role (see Fig. 3.1) [22]. In healthy individuals given intravenous KCl (0.5 mmol/kg), the ECF [K^+] rose by 0.6 mM under control conditions, but the level rose to 0.9 mM in the presence of propranolol, a nonselective β[beta]-blocker [21]. When the K^+ load was infused along with epinephrine, the rise in ECF [K^+] was reduced to only 0.1 mM. These effects occurred without significant changes in plasma aldosterone and insulin levels, and without a change in renal K^+ excretion. Similar results were obtained in healthy subjects given intravenous KCl (0.75 mmol/kg over 2 h), KCl with propranolol (1.43 μg/kg per minute), KCl with epinephrine (0.05 μg/kg per minute), and KCl with both propranolol and epinephrine [23]. Nearly half of the K^+ load was excreted in the urine when KCl was given alone; urinary K^+ excretion was markedly blunted by epinephrine, an effect reversed by propranolol.

Alpha adrenergic agonists impair the activity of the Na^+/K^+-ATPase in skeletal muscle [24]. ECF [K^+] rose by 0.64 mM in healthy subjects infused with KCl (0.5 mmol/kg) alone, but by 0.93 mM in the presence of an α[alpha]-agonist (phenylephrine). Inclusion of an α[alpha]-antagonist (phentolamine) with the α[alpha] agonist (phenylephrine) abrogated the latter increase in ECF [K^+] [25].

Healthy subjects performing maximal exercise developed a peak rise in ECF [K^+] of 1.23 mM in the absence of drugs. ECF [K^+] rose by 1.89 mM (+54 %) when exercise was preceded by β[beta]-blockade and then remained elevated for at least 30 min after exercise. Serum insulin and aldosterone levels increased significantly during β[beta]-blockade. Treatment with an α[alpha]-blocker (5 mg of intravenous phentolamine) led to a 43 % reduction in the rise of ECF [K^+]. The opposing effects of β_2[beta-2]—agonists (to ↓ECF [K^+]) and α[alpha]-agonists (to ↑ECF [K^+]) probably operate to allow adaptation to rapid changes in activity, such as with exercise [26].

Methylxanthines

Many of the world's most popular beverages contain a significant amount of caffeine, which can cause hypokalemia if taken in large doses [27–29]. A 5 oz (150 mL) cup of coffee typically contains 60–180 mg of caffeine, and there are 46 mg in a 12 oz (355 mL) can of Coca-Cola® [30]. The biological effects of caffeine result from its ability to block adenosine receptors [30]. Caffeine can cause a shift of K^+ from the ECF to the ICF by inhibiting the adenosine-mediated decrease in catecholamine release [30]. In the kidney, block of adenosine receptors promotes kaliuresis. In one case, consumption of large volumes of Coca-Cola® produced severe hypokalemia (serum [K^+] of 1.4 mM) in an otherwise healthy man [29]. Recently, two cyclists presented with symptomatic acute hypokalemia (serum [K^+] ~2.4 mM) due to caffeine-loading equivalent to ~18 cups of coffee per day for a week before a race [27]. Theophylline is three to five times more potent than caffeine at blocking adenosine receptors [30], and hypokalemia is found in ~85 % of patients with acute theophylline toxicity. The well-known ability of methylxanthines to inhibit cyclic nucleotide phosphodiesterases may also promote hypokalemia [26].

Thyroid Hormone

Thyroid hormones are the main endocrine factor regulating the content of Na^+/K^+-ATPase pumps in the plasma membrane of muscle cells. They stimulate Na^+/K^+-ATPase activity in rat skeletal muscle and intestinal epithelia, reducing ECF [K^+]. As will be discussed, hypokalemic periodic paralysis (HypoPP) can develop as a complication of thyrotoxicosis.

Hypertonicity

An increase in plasma tonicity is associated with a rise in ECF [K^+], and hyperkalemia has been observed in association with the administration of hypertonic saline and mannitol [31]. The use of mannitol, particularly in neurosurgery, has been associated with clinically significant hyperkalemia. In patients with advanced kidney disease, hypertonicity induced by the administration of large doses of radiocontrast can cause hyperkalemia [32].

Translocational hyperkalemia has also been reported in patients receiving intravenous immunoglobulin.

Under certain conditions, hyperglycemia, the most common cause of hypertonicity, is associated with hyperkalemia. Glucose infusions and hyperglycemia exacerbated hyperkalemia in diabetic patients who have low aldosterone levels and underlying hyperkalemia [33]. In contrast, glucose infusions are associated with a fall in serum [K^+] in control individuals. Some have speculated that the mechanism of hyperkalemia might involve the paradoxical increase in glucagon observed in these patients [34], which may release K^+ sequestered with glycogen stores. Although such a process would increase intracellular K^+, the mechanism and efflux pathway leading to hyperkalemia remains unexplained.

Clinically, patients who develop hypertonicity usually have coexisting conditions that affect K^+ homeostasis, such as: insulinopenia, ECF volume depletion, osmotic diuresis, acid–base disturbances, hypoaldosteronism, and impaired kidney function. Diabetic ketoacidosis (DKA) is one condition where all these factors can be present, and it is not uncommon for such patients to present with *hyper*kalemia despite total body K^+ depletion [1].

To be sure that hypertonicity itself is responsible for an abnormal increase in ECF [K^+], it is important that hyperglycemia due to insulin deficiency, or changes in insulin levels, not be confounding factors [35, 36]. In summary, hypertonicity is associated with an increase in ECF [K^+], which most likely is related to K^+ efflux through ion channels. However, the mechanisms by which hypertonicity (caused by the addition of an effective osmole to the ECF) *alone* produces an increase in ECF [K^+] remain elusive, and whether such an increase is of a magnitude sufficient to cause hyperkalemia remains uncertain.

Systemic pH. Acute respiratory acidosis is associated with a modest increase in ECF [K^+] [37]. Interestingly, a careful study suggested that acute respiratory alkalosis is also associated with rise in ECF [K^+]; ~0.3 mM when pCO_2 fell by ~20 mmHg [38]. It is thought that $\downarrow pCO_2 \rightarrow \downarrow HCO_3^- \rightarrow \uparrow$alpha-adrenergic tone$\rightarrow\uparrow$ ECF [K^+]. On the other hand, chronic respiratory alkalosis is associated with a modest decrease in ECF [K^+] in humans [37].

Metabolic alkalosis from any etiology causes a shift of H^+ from the ICF to the ECF, which appears to be associated with a K^+ shift from ECF to ICF [37]. Total body K^+ depletion causes a specific type of metabolic alkalosis that requires only K^+ repletion for correction. K^+ depletion metabolic alkalosis is generally attributed to an increase in ammoniagenesis [39]. K^+ depletion is also associated with increased HCO_3^- reabsorption in the proximal tubule [40], through the combined action of the apical Na^+/H^+ exchanger (NHE3) and the basolateral Na^+/HCO_3^- cotransporter (NBC-1) [41].

Infusion of mineral acid (i.e., HCl or NH_4Cl) consistently leads to an increase in ECF [K^+], albeit over a wide range (Δ[delta]K^+/Δ[delta]pH varied from 1.7 to 16.7 mmol K^+ per each unit fall in pH) [37]. In contrast, ECF [K^+] is not affected in organic acidoses (e.g., ketoacidosis, lactic acidosis) [42]. The most likely cause for this difference is that infusion of mineral acid creates a driving force for H^+ entry into cells (e.g., via a H^+/K^+-ATPase), whereas in an organic acidosis, the opposite is true. Although it is clear that inorganic acidemia is often associated with an increase in ECF [K^+] and inorganic alkalemia is often associated with a decrease in ECF [K^+], this correlation does not indicate that a direct cause and effect relationship exists and there are important exceptions. For example, diarrhea often leads to hypokalemia despite metabolic acidosis, as do certain forms of distal RTA. In the only study in which acute metabolic acidosis was studied in humans [43], volunteers were given and infusion of NH_4Cl into the duodenum, which caused plasma bicarbonate concentration to decrease by 5.8 mM over 3 h. The plasma [K^+], however, did not change. Whether this is due to a lack of acidosis-associated K^+ movement between the ICF and ECF, K^+-efflux (e.g., via a H^+/K^+-ATPase) that equals K^+-influx (e.g., via the Na^+/K^+-ATPase), or a confounding effect of the experimental protocol remains to be determined [36, 43].

Potassium Handling Along the Nephron

As illustrated in Fig. 3.1, potassium homeostasis and ECF [K^+] is kept in a steady state by matching daily K^+ excretion to daily K^+ intake. The kidney excretes more than 90 % of the daily K^+ load, and excretion varies intake. Virtually, all K^+ excreted by the kidney occurs via K^+ secretion beyond the early distal tubule [44].

Proximal Nephron to the Early Distal Tubule

Regardless of dietary K^+ intake, the majority of filtered K^+ (70–80 %) is reabsorbed along the proximal tubule, as shown by micropuncture and microperfusion experiments [45]. An additional 10–20 % of filtered K^+ is reabsorbed between the end of the proximal tubule and initial early distal tubule [45]. Remarkably, the fraction of filtered K^+ that reaches the earliest part of the distal tubule accessible to micropuncture remains about 10 % regardless of K^+ intake and despite the fact that subsequent K^+ excretion can range from 2 to 180 % of the filtered load [45].

Distal Nephron

Potassium secretion is the dominant process beyond the early distal tubule, and this is the process underlying the regulation of potassium homeostasis. The first direct evidence to support distal K^+ secretion came from the classic micropuncture experiments performed in rat nephron by Malnic, Klose, and Giebisch in the 1960s [45].

Electrophysiological Model of the Connecting Tubule and Collecting Duct

This part of the nephron contains aldosterone receptors and two major cell types: [46, 47] the PCs, which reabsorb Na^+ via ENaC and secrete K^+ via ROMK; and α[alpha]-intercalated cells (α[alpha]-ICs), which secrete acid primarily via an H^+-ATPase. There is also an apical H^+/K^+-ATPase, which is activated by K^+ depletion and hypokalemia. The ROMK channels are exclusively localized to the PCs (see Fig. 3.2), whereas the maxi-K or BK channels are found in both PCs and α[alpha]-ICs (see Fig. 3.3). [48, 49] The BK channel is composed of two subunits; the channel in the PC is BK-alpha/beta1 and the channel in the IC is BK-alpha/beta4 [50]. The BK-alpha/beta1 channel is in the apical membrane of connecting tubule PCs, where it plays a role in K^+ secretion; and in the basolateral membrane (BLM) of collecting duct PCs, where it appears to help maintain the driving force for Na^+ reabsorption under conditions of a low sodium diet [51]. In contrast, the BK-alpha/beta4 channel is in the apical membrane of the ICs, where it has been proposed to regulate cell volume and contribute to potassium adaptation [50]. The idea is that a high K^+ diet→↑activity of BK-alpha/beta4 channels→↓IC cell volume→↑luminal diameter and distal urine flow rate→↑K^+ secretion [50].

The major pathway for K^+ secretion in the collecting duct is via ROMK channels in the apical membrane of PCs (see Fig. 3.2). This membrane contains two important conductances: a Na^+-selective conductance (G_{Na^+}) due to ENaC, and a K^+-selective conductance (G_{K^+}) due to ROMK channels. The apical membrane potential (V^{AP}) is determined by the instantaneous status of G_{Na^+} and G_{K^+} assuming relatively constant values of intracellular and luminal [Na^+] and [K^+]. If $[K^+]_{cell} > [K^+]_{lumen}$, which is the usual case, then E_{K^+} will be negative and opening of ROMK channels (↑G_{K^+}) will hyperpolarize V^{AP}.

Unlike E_{K^+}, which will always be negative, E_{Na^+} may be positive (when $[Na^+]_{lumen} > [Na^+]_{cell}$) or negative (when $[Na^+]_{lumen} < [Na^+]_{cell}$). The former condition ($[Na^+]_{lumen} > [Na^+]_{cell}$) can occur when either aldosterone levels are suppressed (e.g., Na^+ ingestion is high or in hypoaldosteronism) or when aldosterone levels are elevated (e.g., Na^+ excretion is high due to diuretics or genetic salt-wasting disorders). In these cases, E_{Na^+} will be positive and opening of ENaC channels (↑G_{Na^+}) will depolarize V^{AP}. However, the magnitude of G_{Na^+} will directly correlate with aldosterone levels, and will be low when aldosterone is suppressed and limit K^+ secretion under

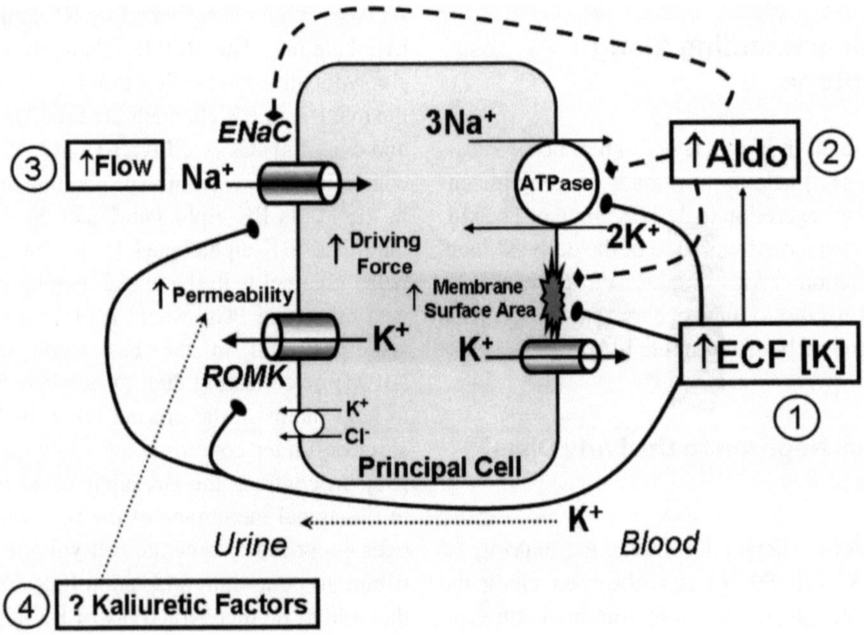

Fig. 3.2 Physiology of K^+ transport in principal cells of the collecting duct. K^+ enters the cell across the basolateral membrane (BLM) via the Na^+/K^+-ATPase. Sodium is reabsorbed across the luminal membrane through ENaC Na^+ channels, with the resultant cellular depolarization increasing the electrical driving force for K^+ secretion through ROMK K^+ channels. (1) Elevation of peritubular $[K^+]$ (*circular arrows*) increases the density of luminal ENaC and ROMK channels, which both promote K^+ secretion by increasing the electrical driving force and K^+ permeability, respectively. Increases in peritubular $[K^+]$ also activate the Na^+/K^+-ATPase pump in the BLM and stimulate aldosterone release. (2) Aldosterone (*diamond arrows*) increases the density of ENaC (but not ROMK) channels and activates the Na^+/K^+-ATPase pump, both of which increase the driving force for K^+ secretion. The surface area of the BLM containing the Na+/K^+-ATPase pump undergoes amplification during prolonged exposure to either increased peritubular $[K^+]$ or aldosterone. (3) Increases in urine flow rate may activate ENaC, promoting K^+ secretion. (4) Kaliuretic factors, including K^+ itself, have been proposed that somehow directly increase K^+ secretion. For example, high luminal $[K^+]$ may directly increase the activity of ROMK channels

these conditions. This helps explain why (1) normal potassium homeostasis is maintained when Na^+ ingestion is high, (2) the development of hyperkalemia in hypoaldosteronism, and (3) hypokalemia in the setting of loop and thiazide diuretics or the genetic syndromes of Bartter and Gitelman. The one exception is Liddle syndrome, when K^+ wasting and hypokalemia occur despite negligible aldosterone levels. However, this is easily explained because the defect in Liddle syndrome relates to a direct increase in G_{Na^+} that is independent of aldosterone.

On the other hand, situations where $[Na^+]_{lumen} \leq [Na^+]_{cell}$ are possible under conditions of volume depletion, renal hypoperfusion, or low dietary Na^+ intake. When this occurs, E_{Na^+} can be zero ($[Na^+]_{lumen} = [Na^+]_{cell}$) or negative, which means that V^{AP} will not depolarize no matter how many ENaC channels are activated by elevated aldosterone levels. This prevents the lumen from becoming more electronegative, which inhibits K^+ secretion. This explains why potassium homeostasis is maintained under these conditions despite elevated aldosterone levels.

These considerations also help distinguish between the effects of distal Na^+ delivery versus luminal $[Na^+]$ on K^+ secretion. As will be discussed, most of the kaliuretic effect of "increased distal Na^+ delivery" probably relates more to the opening of flow-dependent maxi-K channels,

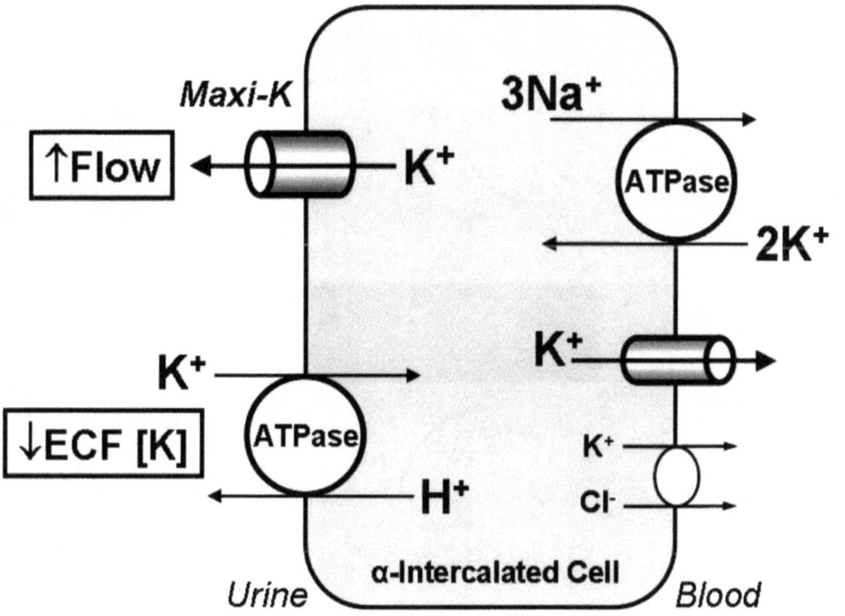

Fig. 3.3 Physiology of K^+ transport in alpha-intercalated cells of the collecting duct. As in the principal cell, K^+ secretion is a two-step process: K^+ enters the cell across the basolateral membrane (BLM) via the Na^+/K^+-ATPase, and exits across the apical membrane via maxi-K channels, which are activated by an increase in urine flow rate. Under conditions of hypokalemia and/or total body K^+ depletion, this cell can also reabsorb K^+ via an apical H^+/K^+-ATPase

whereas the effect of luminal [Na^+] is explained by the mechanism just discussed. Similarly, the "K^+-sparing" effect of agents that block ENaC (e.g., amiloride, triamterene) or aldosterone (e.g., spironolactone, eplerenone) is directly related to the decrease in G_{Na^+}, which predictably inhibits K^+ secretion irrespective of E_{Na^+}.

In summary, secretion of K^+ via ROMK is controlled by the weighted balance between the G_{Na^+} and E_{Na^+} system and the G_{K^+} and E_{K^+} system. An increase in G_{Na^+} (e.g., due to increased aldosterone levels or Liddle syndrome) will tend to move V^{AP} toward E_{Na^+}, which is usually (but not always) a depolarizing force that increases lumen electronegativity and promotes K^+ secretion. A decrease in G_{Na^+} (e.g., due to amiloride) will tend to prevent V^{AP} from moving toward E_{Na^+}, preventing depolarization and attenuating K^+ secretion. Although K^+ secretion along the collecting duct is primarily mediated by the ROMK channel in the apical membrane of PCs, recent findings have provided evidence that K^+ secretion also occurs via flow-dependent maxi-K channels and K^+-Cl cotransport [52].

Mechanisms Underlying K^+ Handling Along the Distal Nephron

As shown in Figs. 3.2 and 3.3, the predominant pathways mediating K^+ secretion are apical ion channels; ROMK in PCs and maxi-K in both principal and intercalated cells (ICs). Some K^+ secretion also occurs via a K-Cl cotransporter in PCs and the electronegative lumen may also drive some K^+ through the paracellular pathway [52]. The major factors that regulate K^+ secretion are: (1) *peritubular [K^+]*, which reflects ECF [K^+]; (2) *aldosterone level*, which affects K^+ secretion through its effects on Na^+ reabsorption; (3) *urinary flow rate*, which affects K^+ secretion by its effects on ENaC and the maxi-K channel; (4) *alkalosis and alkalemia,* which increase the activity of ROMK; (5) any other factor that brings about an *increase in the electronegativity of the lumen or lowers luminal chloride*, including exogenous mineralocorticoids, impermeant (nonreabsorbable) anions, and Mg^{2+} deficiency; and (6) *Ang II*, which decreases K^+ secretion. Insulin, which has an anti-natriuretic effect, may be a factor that has not been fully appreciated.

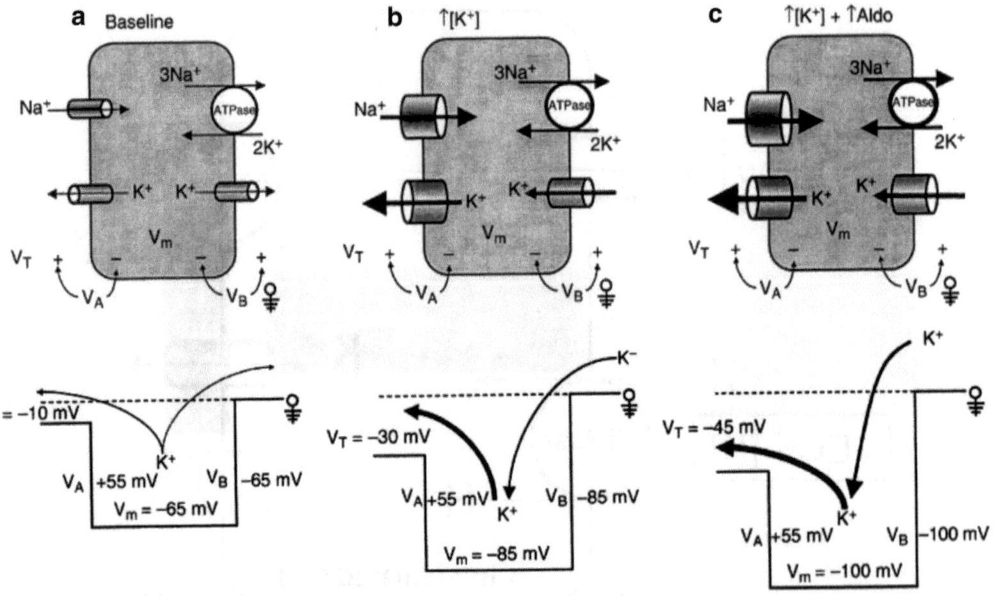

Fig. 3.4 Electrophysiological profile of K^+ secretion and K^+ adaptation in principal cells of the collecting duct. The apical membrane has ENaC Na channels and ROMK K^+ channels, and the peritubular membrane has K^+ channels and Na^+/K^+-ATPase pumps. The thickness of the *arrow* though a channel is proportional to the driving force and the size of the channel is proportional to the conductance. Stimulation of the pump is denoted by increased thickness. (**a**) At baseline, K^+ entering across the BLM via the Na^+/K^+-ATPase pump is subsequently secreted across the apical membrane into an electronegative lumen while some K^+ recycles back into the blood. (**b**) An increase in peritubular $[K^+]$ activates the pump and leads to an increase in the K^+ conductance in the BLM, resulting in hyperpolarization of VB. When VB becomes more negative than EKBLM, the direction of K^+ current reverses, and K^+ enters the cell. An elevation of peritubular $[K^+]$ also increases the density of apical membrane conductances; more Na current via ENaC increases lumen electronegativity (VT) and therefore the driving force for K^+ secretion through a higher density of ROMK channels. (**c**) The combination of increased peritubular $[K^+]$ and mineralocorticoids further augments the changes described in panel **b**. Note that aldosterone leads to an increase in the driving force for K^+ secretion through ROMK channels, but does not increase the density of these channels

The collecting duct is also capable of K^+ reabsorption via the H^+/K^+-ATPase in the apical membrane of α[alpha]-ICs, which appears to be most active under conditions of K^+ depletion [53]. Chronic hypokalemia appears to be the most important activator of the H^+/K^+-ATPase ($HK\alpha_2$[alpha2] type), which probably contributes to the maintenance of the metabolic alkalosis associated with hypokalemia.

Peritubular [K+]

Potassium secretion by PCs along the collecting duct is a two-step process consisting of (1) active K^+ entry across the BLM via the Na^+/K^+-ATPase pump, and (2) passive K^+ exit across the apical membrane via K^+ channels that, when open, allow diffusion of K^+ down a favorable electrochemical gradient [19]. In adrenalectomized rats, a rise in ECF $[K^+]$ increases K^+ secretion regardless of whether the aldosterone secretion rate is fixed at a high or low level [54]. These results indicate a specific effect of peritubular $[K^+]$ on K^+ secretion because urine flow rate, Na^+ delivery, pH, and transepithelial voltage were all held constant.

Experiments using isolated perfused rabbit collecting ducts have shown that the proximate signal is peritubular $[K^+]$ [55]. An increase in peritubular $[K^+]$ leads to (1) immediate activation of the Na^+/K^+-ATPase, (2) an increase in the apical Na^+ conductance (i.e., ENaC), and (3) an increase in the K^+ conductance of both the apical (i.e., ROMK) and basolateral membranes (see Figs. 3.2 and 3.4).

Aldosterone

This endogenous mineralocorticoid plays a major role in the regulation of both ECF volume and ECF [K^+] homeostasis, and is secreted in response to either hypovolemia or hyperkalemia. Aldosterone signaling affects both the apical and BLM of collecting duct epithelia. Effects in the apical membrane lead to an overall increase in Na^+ (ENaC) conductance, whereas basolateral effects include an increase in the activity of the Na^+/K^+-ATPase pump and amplification of membrane area [19]. The increase in Na^+/K^+-ATPase activity may be mediated by aldosterone-induced proteins (AIPs) [56] and/or may be secondary to the increase in apical ENaC conductance [55]. Additional gain is built into the system because aldosterone enhances the effect of increased peritubular [K^+] on K^+ secretion (see Figs. 3.2 and 3.4). The overall effect is an increase in K^+ entry across the BLM (↑Na^+/K^+-ATPase activity) and an increase in K^+ exit across the apical membrane (↑electronegative lumen).

SGK1 Is an Aldosterone-Induced Protein that Indirectly Promotes K^+ Secretion

Serum- and glucocorticoid-induced kinase 1 (SGK1) is an AIP that plays an important and complex role in regulating ENaC [57, 58] and ROMK [59] channels along the connecting tubule and collecting duct. Aldosterone regulation of SGK1 leads to increased reabsorption of Na^+ via ENaC by increasing its open probability, lifetime in the apical membrane, and gene transcription [58]. SGK1-associated increases in ENaC conductance depolarize the cell and increase the electronegativity of the lumen, which increases the net driving force for K^+ secretion.

Nedd4–2 Is a Natural Inhibitor of ENaC Trafficking

Nedd4–2 is a ligase that interacts with the C-terminus of ENaC, resulting in the retrieval and internalization of ENaCs off the membrane. Mutations in the carboxy terminal of ENaC that interfere with membrane retrieval increase the membrane lifetime of ENaC. The resultant hyperreabsorption of Na^+ (with consequent increase in K^+ secretion in PCs and H^+ secretion in α[alpha]-ICs) causes hypertension with hypokalemia and metabolic alkalosis, which is seen in patients with Liddle syndrome (pseudohyperaldosteronism) [60].

WNK4 as a Differential Regulator of Aldosterone Signaling

WNK4, a member of the with-no-lysine (*wnk*) family of serine–threonine protein kinases [61], has emerged as a diverse regulatory protein involved in the control of several transport processes in the distal nephron. Mutations in WNK4 (and WNK1) cause pseudohypoaldosteronism type II (PHA-II) [61]. PHA-II is characterized by hypertension (due to increased Na^+ reabsorption via NCC, the thiazide-sensitive cotransporter, and ENaC), metabolic acidosis (due to decreased H^+ secretion by α[alpha]-ICs), and hyperkalemia (due to decreased K^+ secretion by PCs).

WNK4 appears to act as a "molecular switch" that modifies the downstream signaling of aldosterone and associated proteins [62], including SGK1 [59]. Serine 1169 on WNK4 is a phosphorylation site for SGK1. Under normal steady-state conditions of euvolemia and normokalemia, aldosterone (and SGK1) levels are relatively low. Therefore, most WNK4 proteins will be unphosphorylated at S1169 and exert an inhibitory effect on multiple transport elements including the thiazide-sensitive cotransporter [62], ENaC [63], and ROMK [62]. In contrast, when hyperkalemia causes aldosterone (and SGK1) levels to be high, S1169 on WNK4 will be phosphorylated by SGK1, leading to loss of inhibition of ENaC and ROMK, which synergistically promotes K^+ secretion.

In summary, WNK4 can exist in at least three distinct states: (1) unphosphorylated at S1169, which dominates under normal conditions of euvolemia and normokalemia, (2) phosphorylated by SGK1 at S1169 under conditions of aldosterone secretion stimulated by hyperkalemia, and (3) loss-of-function mutations in WNK4, which produce PHA-II because basal inhibition of NCC and ENaC is relieved, resulting in increased ECF volume, hypertension, and suppression of aldosterone secretion. Relative hypoaldosteronism and low SGK1 lead to decreased H^+ secretion by α[alpha]-ICs and K^+

secretion by PCs, resulting in metabolic acidosis and hyperkalemia, respectively. Although the molecular pathophysiology appears to be complex, the available studies suggest the PHA-II mutations predominately lead to a gain-of-function of NCC. The resultant increase in ECF volume tends to suppress the RAA system and predispose to hyperkalemia.

Potassium Adaptation

Human history has seen cultures featuring a diet very high in K^+, so it stands to reason that mechanisms have developed to effectively manage such a situation. Adaptation to high ECF [K^+] involves (1) increases in the apical conductances for both Na^+ and K^+, (2) an increase in activity and density of the Na^+/K^+-ATPase pumps in the BLM, and (3) amplification of the BLM of the distal tubule epithelial cells responsible for K^+ secretion. Together, these changes generate an increase in the lumen electronegativity of the distal nephron, which promotes K^+ secretion [19, 64]. The mechanisms involved in potassium adaptation are summarized in Figs. 3.2 and 3.4 [19].

Distal Na^+ Delivery and Urine Flow Rate

These two factors, although often presented together as a single concept, promote K^+ secretion by separate mechanisms.

Distal Na^+ delivery. In vivo microperfusion studies of rat distal tubule have demonstrated that changing luminal [Na^+] (between 40 and 100 mM) or increasing distal Na^+ delivery or absorption did *not* affect K^+ secretion if flow rate was held constant [65]. Interestingly, lowering luminal [Na^+] to 15 mM did not significantly decrease K^+ secretion even though Na^+ reabsorption was completely abrogated. However, replacement of high luminal [Na^+] with an impermeant cation (tetramethylammonium, TMA) halved both the electronegativity of the lumen and K^+ secretion [66].

How can these results be interpreted and reconciled with the traditional view that an increase in distal Na^+ delivery promotes K^+ secretion? This writer offers the explanation that, rather than Na^+ delivery or reabsorption, the interplay between the driving force for Na^+ (E_{Na^+}) and the apical Na^+ conductance (G_{Na^+}, total activity of ENaC) is key. For example, when the luminal [Na^+] is high, E_{Na^+} will be positive, but this will lead to significant depolarization of the apical membrane (and significant K^+ secretion) only when G_{Na^+} increases relative to G_{K^+} (i.e., when aldosterone levels are high). But aldosterone levels are not likely to be high when luminal [Na^+] is high. Conversely, when luminal [Na^+] is low and approaches the intracellular [Na^+] (i.e., 10–15 mM), the driving force for K^+ secretion remains low even if G_{Na^+} is maximal (i.e., when aldosterone levels are high).

Consider what happens to these parameters under conditions of hypervolemia, hypovolemia, and initial treatment with loop or thiazide diuretics. In hypervolemia, K^+ secretion is limited despite an increase in distal Na^+ delivery (and [Na^+]) because aldosterone is suppressed, which lowers G_{Na^+}. In hypovolemia, the traditional view is that despite high aldosterone levels, K^+ secretion is limited by low distal Na^+ delivery. However, the major factors that probably limit K^+ secretion in hypovolemia are low urine flow rate and the likelihood that E_{Na^+} is low despite a large aldosterone-induced increase in G_{Na^+}. During initial treatment with a thiazide diuretic, high luminal [Na^+] and elevated aldosterone levels will coexist. The former will increase the driving force for Na^+ (↑E_{Na^+}) while the latter will increase the Na^+ conductance (↑G_{Na^+}), which together with the increase in urine flow rate will markedly stimulate K^+ secretion.

Urine flow rate. High urine flow rates can occur under conditions where Na^+ delivery is high (e.g., initial diuretic treatment or saline infusions), or under conditions of aquaresis where distal Na^+ delivery may be low (e.g., as in diabetes insipidus or with high water intake). With an aquaresis, the dominant pathway for increased K^+ secretion is probably via flow-stimulated maxi-K channels [67]. These maxi-K channels, which are thought to be predominately localized to ICs, are calcium-activated and mechanosensitive [68].

Studies using perfused tubules of rabbit cortical collecting duct have provided evidence that both ENaC [69] and the maxi-K channel [67] are regulated by flow (see Figs. 3.2 and 3.3). Therefore, the following paradigm can now be proposed: Under conditions of aquaresis (high flow rates but low Na^+ delivery), K^+ secretion would be stimulated by flow-dependent activation of the maxi-K channel and low luminal [K^+]. On the other hand, under conditions of natriuresis (high flow rate and high Na^+ delivery), K^+ secretion would be stimulated not only by these two factors, but also by any increase in lumen electronegativity resulting from Na^+ reabsorption via ENaC (i.e., an increase in G_{Na^+}).

Relationship between distal Na^+ delivery, urine flow rate, and aldosterone. Although distal Na^+ delivery probably does not play a major role as a direct luminal factor affecting K^+ secretion, it has indirect effects important for K^+ homeostasis.

Under conditions of decreased effective arterial blood volume (EABV), distal Na^+ delivery and tubule flow rate decrease, which would tend to decrease K^+ secretion and predispose to hyperkalemia (e.g., a major risk in patients with oliguria). However, these same factors provide signals that act to correct the situation. Low Na^+ and Cl^- delivery is sensed at the macula densa, which leads to renin release from juxtaglomerular (JG) cells and subsequent activation of the renin-angiotensin-aldosterone system (RAAS). This, in turn, increases Na^+ reabsorption via ENaC and the Na^+/K^+-ATPase, which increases the electronegativity of the lumen, promoting K^+ secretion as the volume deficit is repaired.

The converse situation obtains when EABV increases: increased distal Na^+ delivery will be accompanied by increased tubule flow rate, which could lead to flow-dependent K^+ wasting and hypokalemia. However, high Na^+ and Cl^- at the macula densa lead (via tubuloglomerular feedback) to constriction of the afferent arteriole and decreased renin release from JG cells. Together, these effects will limit K^+ wasting, so K^+ balance is maintained as the excess volume is excreted.

Alkalosis and Alkalemia

Both respiratory and metabolic alkalosis are associated with hypokalemia. Acute respiratory alkalosis has often been associated with a prompt kaliuresis and hypokalemia [70]. However, the kaliuresis is quickly curtailed so that, even in chronic respiratory alkalosis, the total K^+ deficit is small and easily repaired [70]. In contrast, respiratory alkalosis has also been associated with an initial rise in ECF [K^+] [38]. When acute respiratory alkalosis was induced in humans by voluntary hyperventilation, the ECF [K^+] increased by about 0.3 mM and was associated with a rise in plasma catecholamines [38]. The increase in [K^+] was enhanced by β[beta]-adrenergic receptor blockade, and abrogated by α[alpha]-adrenergic receptor blockade, suggesting that the hyperkalemic response is due to predominance of α[alpha]-adrenergic activity over β[beta]-adrenergic activity.

In normal human volunteers undergoing nasogastric (NG) suction to produce selective depletion of HCl, renal K^+ secretion is increased and hypokalemia is induced despite adequate dietary K^+ intake [71]. In these studies, ECF volume was maintained by precise replacement of all water and electrolytes except for H^+ and Cl^-. ECF [K^+] decreased from 4.1 to 3.2 mM, while ECF [Cl] decreased from 100 to 88 mM and ECF [HCO_3] increased from 28.6 to 37.5 mM. The mean K^+ loss in these subjects was 128 mmol.

Other Factors that Increase in the Electronegativity of the Lumen or Lowers Luminal Chloride

A semiquantitative analysis of how electrophysiological events along the collecting duct affect K^+ secretion is presented in Fig. 3.4. Here, the effects of impermeant anions and Mg^{2+} deficiency will be considered.

Impermeant (nonresorbable) anions. Cl^- and HCO_3^- are the only monovalent anions the distal nephron is designed to reabsorb. Because the bulk of HCO_3^- is reabsorbed indirectly (via luminal H^+ secretion), Cl^- is essentially the only anion directly reabsorbed from the lumen (interestingly, bromide and thiocyanate can also be reabsorbed). The major transport elements used for Cl^- reabsorption are the furosemide-sensitive Na-K^+-2Cl cotransporter in the TALH and the thiazide-sensitive Na-Cl cotransporter in the early distal tubule.

These transport proteins possess high affinity Cl^- binding sites that do not bind other anions such as sulfate, gluconate, and acetate.

Clinically, the impermeant anion effect has been reported to occur with large doses of certain antibiotics such as carbenicillin [72]. K^+ secretion is significantly increased in the collecting duct when impermeant anions are present in the lumen. Traditionally, hypokalemia due to these anions has been attributed solely to increased luminal electronegativity, but continuous microperfusion experiments have shown that replacement of luminal chloride with gluconate in rat distal tubule increased K^+ secretion by 44 % without a significant change in transepithelial potential [73]. The increase in K^+ secretion persisted in the presence of luminal amiloride (blocker of ENaC) or barium [73].

Similarly, studies using stationary microperfusion of rat superficial nephrons showed that, compared to perfusion with high luminal chloride, K^+ secretion was increased 32 % by sulfate, 37 % by acetate, and 62 % by bicarbonate [74]. For sulfate and bicarbonate, these increases occurred in without a significant increase in lumen electronegativity (the transepithelial potential was −37.6 mV with chloride, −35.1 mV with sulfate, and −39.1 mV with bicarbonate). The significant exaggeration of luminal bicarbonate to increase K^+ secretion is thought to be due to the combination of low luminal Cl^- plus enhanced K^+-Cl cotransport at higher pH.

In summary, hypokalemia occurring with "impermeant anions" appears to relate more to the fact that the distal nephron is not equipped to reabsorb monovalent anions other than chloride than to an increase in lumen electronegativity. For example, this may explain (in part) the pronounced kaliuretic effect associated with carbonic anhydrase inhibitors (CAIs).

Magnesium depletion and hypomagnesemia. It has long been appreciated that magnesium depletion predisposes to increased urinary K^+ excretion that can cause hypokalemia [75, 76]. Magnesium plays a key role as a cofactor in the interaction of ATP with the Na^+/K^+-ATPase complex; therefore, a decrease in Na^+/K^+-ATPase activity due to Mg^{2+} depletion can result in concomitant cellular K^+ depletion [77]. In addition to Mg^{2+} depletion reducing the movement of K^+ into the cell, decreased intracellular Mg^{2+} can also increase cellular K^+ efflux though inwardly rectifying K^+ channels because it is well established that a voltage-dependent block of outward K^+ current by intracellular Mg^{2+} ions underlies the inward rectification of many K^+ channels [78] including ROMK [79, 80]. The mechanism by which magnesium depletion causes total body K^+ depletion with hypokalemia was recently reviewed [81].

Angiotensin II

Recent electrophysiological studies have shown that Ang II inhibits the ROMK1 channels found in the apical membrane of PCs along the connecting tubule and collecting duct [82]. Ang II inhibits ROMK1 channels via losartan-sensitive angiotensin type 1 receptors, both by promoting WNK4-induced inhibition and by increasing tyrosine phosphorylation of the channel [83]. It is speculated that Ang II-induced inhibition of ROMK1 may limit K^+ secretion in states of volume depletion. Clinically, this effect may also act to mitigate the hyperkalemic response to angiotensin receptor blockers (ARBs).

Diuretic-Induced Hypokalemia

The pathophysiology of how diuretics that act proximal to the cortical collecting duct can lead to hypokalemia follows from the foregoing discussion. Acutely, these diuretics stimulate flow-dependent K^+ secretion, which causes an initial component of K^+ depletion. Chronically, a subsequent component of K^+ loss occurs due to ECF volume contraction with secondary activation of aldosterone resulting in increased luminal electronegativity of the collecting duct, and chronic metabolic alkalosis. Loop diuretics may cause additional K^+ loss as they decrease the lumen-positivity of the thick ascending loop of Henle (TALH), which decreases paracellular K^+ reabsorption in that nephron segment. Loop diuretics also inhibit the Na-K^+-2Cl cotransporter in the cells of the macula densa, leading to loss of tubuloglomerular feedback mechanisms [84], which can lead to additional K^+ loss.

Diuretic-induced hypokalemia is problematic because of: (1) decreased insulin sensitivity, which is diabetogenic; (2) increased risk of arrhythmias for patients on cardiac glycosides; (3) increased cardiovascular risks due to loss of the benefits that have been associated with higher ECF [K^+] levels [85]. However, giving these patients supplemental K^+ can also be problematic because they often have a decreased GFR and/or hypoaldosteronism associated with diabetes and/or medications that interfere with the RAAS, which puts them at risk of developing hyperkalemia. Indeed, numerous studies have shown that a significant percentage (up to a third) of patients who develop hyperkalemia are actually on K^+ supplements [86]; most of the remainders are on one or more medications that interfere with K^+ secretion.

Antidiuretic Hormone

As noted above, urine flow rate has an important influence on cation transport in the distal nephron, with flow-dependent increases in both Na^+ reabsorption ad K^+ secretion (reviewed in [87]). However, it is important to distinguish between high flow rates associated with an increase in distal sodium delivery, and those due to an inability to reabsorb water due to suppression or absence of antidiuretic hormone (ADH). Infusion of ADH into experimental animals with central diabetes insipidus reduced the urine flow rate sevenfold yet increased the fractional excretion of potassium by nearly 80 % [88]. The increase in K^+ clearance following ADH was all attributable to K^+ secretion in the late distal tubule, and this occurred under the conditions of a low urinary flow rate. This experiment suggests that ADH has a direct effect to promote K^+ secretion independent of its ability to increase tubular water permeability [88].

Pharmacological Inhibitors of Na^+ Transporters Along the Nephron

CAIs lead to a decrease in the kinetics of the Na^+/H antiporter (NHE3) in the proximal tubule, resulting in transient natriuresis and bicarbonaturia. CAIs have a potent kaliuretic effect, which leads to K^+ depletion [89]. This effect is presumably due to an increase in both Na^+ delivery and luminal flow in the collecting duct.

Loop diuretics inhibit the Na^+-K^+-2Cl triple cotransporter in the thick ascending limb of Henle's loop. This has at least two effects that promote hypokalemia by increasing K^+ secretion via ROMK: (1) secondary aldosteronism due to volume depletion, (2) the subsequent increase in distal solute and flow rate, (3) increased luminal [Na^+] in the collecting duct, and (4) generation of metabolic alkalosis.

Thiazide diuretics inhibit the Na^+-Cl cotransporter in the apical membrane of the early distal tubule, and promote hypokalemia by the same mechanisms as loop diuretics.

Amiloride is a specific blocker of ENaC in the apical membrane of PCs in the collecting duct, the same site as the ROMK potassium channel. Although each channel is highly ion selective, the activity of ENaC has important effects on secretion of K^+ through ROMK due to the special properties of this part of the nephron. By decreasing the electronegativity of the lumen, blockade of ENaC will also reduce proton secretion by the α[alpha]-ICs, which tends to lower systemic pH and therefore the open probability of ROMK. Therefore, amiloride promotes hyperkalemia by decreasing the net electrical driving force for K^+ secretion, and decreasing the net K^+ permeability of the apical membrane. Other agents that can block ENaC and thus predispose to hyperkalemia include triamterene, trimethoprim, pentamidine, and metabolites of nafamostat [90].

Aldosterone Receptor Agonists and Antagonists

Aldosterone binds to the intracellular mineralocorticoid (steroid) receptor, which can lead to diverse downstream signaling due to the production of AIPs, such as the serum- and glucocorticoid-regulated kinase (SGK). Both aldosterone receptor agonists and antagonists are clinically available. The classic agonist is fludrocortisone acetate (Florinef™), a synthetic steroid with potent mineralocorticoid activity, and is used in the treatment of adrenal insufficiency. The classic antagonist is spironolactone, a synthetic steroid that competes with aldosterone for the mineralocorticoid receptor. Once relegated as a niche "K^+-sparing diuretic" in the treatment of cirrhotic ascites, the use of spironolactone exploded after it was shown to significantly reduce morbidity and mortality in the Randomized Aldactone Evaluation Study (RALES) [91] of patients with severe congestive heart failure. As one might expect, hyperkalemia does develop in a subset of such patients [92].

Oral contraceptives such as Yaz and Yasmin-28 contain 3-mg of the synthetic progestin drospirenone, which has anti-mineralocorticoid effects equivalent to about 25-mg of spironolactone. These medications are therefore contraindicated in women with kidney disease or adrenal insufficiency, and should be avoided in those taking NSAIDs, ACEIs, ARBs, amiloride, spironolactone, eplerenone, heparin, or K^+ supplements [93, 94].

Dietary Considerations

Dietary K^+

The diet of early humans was very rich in fruits and vegetables, resulting in the ingestion of 10 g (256 mmol) or more potassium per day. In contrast, the typical intake of potassium (39.1 mg/mmol) in the modern Western diet is only 40–120 mmol/day, which corresponds to only 1.6–4.7 g of K^+ per day. A dietary survey in the United States revealed that the average daily potassium intake is ~2.3 g (59 mmol) for adult women and ~3.1 g (79 mmol) for adult men [95]. The Food and Nutrition Board of the Institute of Medicine (IOM) has recently established the adequate daily intake of potassium for adults (with normal kidney function, see Table 3.1) to be 4.7 g/day, which corresponds to 120 mmol/day [96]. This recommendation is based on studies that have found higher K^+ intake levels to be associated with lower blood pressure and improved cardiovascular outcomes.

Table 3.1 Adequate intake for potassium by age

Life stage group	Age	Males (g/day)	Females (g/day)
Infants	0–6 months	0.4	0.4
Infants	7–12 months	0.4	0.7
Children	1–3 years	3.0	3.0
Children	4–8 years	3.8	3.8
Children	9–13 years	4.5	4.5
Adolescents	14–18 years	4.7	4.7
Adults	>18 years	4.7	4.7
Pregnancy	14–50 years	–	4.7
Breastfeeding	14–50 years	–	5.1

Low-K^+ diets. Under normal circumstances, K^+ homeostasis will be maintained as long as K^+ intake is above a certain minimum level. In the absence of vomiting or diarrhea, gastrointestinal K^+ loss is typically about 5–10 mmol/day. In the absence of ECF volume depletion and mineralocorticoids, secretion of K^+ into the urine will be minimized, but some obligate renal loss of K^+ will occur. The H^+/K^+-ATPase pumps along the collecting duct will help reabsorb K^+ under these K^+-depleted conditions, but complete cessation of K^+ secretion may not be possible given the combination of any ROMK channel activity (K^+ permeability) in the presence of the lumen electronegativity (K^+ driving force) of the collecting duct. Obligatory renal K^+ loss is around 15 mmol/day, so it is reasonable to consider the minimal K^+ intake necessary to maintain an ECF [K^+] within the normal range to be at least 25 mmol/day. There are two situations where this obligate requirement is not met:

1. *Fasting.* Under fasting conditions, the lack of K^+ intake will of course be accompanied by a lack of salt (NaCl) and carbohydrates. The former will lead to activation of the RAAS, while the latter will keep insulin levels low. The low insulin level will decrease K^+ transport into cells (although catecholamines, if elevated, may cause some K^+ influx), which will mitigate against hypokalemia. At least initially, there will be some obligate K^+ loss via renal K^+ secretion because of increased aldosterone levels promoting Na^+ reabsorption. If water is available or allowed during the fast, additional renal K^+ loss could occur if

any apical K^+ channels are open. Taken together, fasting will lead to a decrease in total body K^+ and some degree of hypokalemia.

2. *Zero-K^+ diet.* If an artificial zero-K^+ diet is given, the degree of hypokalemia depends mainly on how much insulin-mediated K^+ transfer from ECF→ICF occurs due to ingested carbohydrates. Renal K^+ loss should be minimized as long as ECF volume remains replete. Again, a defense against hypokalemia is mounted, but will be overcome as the zero K^+ diet continues.

High-K^+ diets. Primitive cultures subsisting on mostly fruits and vegetables consumed a diet much higher in K^+ (and considerably lower in Na^+) than in modern industrialized cultures. Daily consumption of K^+ may have exceeded 250 mmol, yet (presumably) significant or at least symptomatic hyperkalemia did not develop.

Possible Kaliuretic Signaling in the Gut

Experiments in sheep have demonstrated that food intake is associated with enhanced renal K^+ excretion that does not appear to be attributable to changes to the rise in ECF [K^+], an increase in aldosterone, or the level of Na^+ excretion. These experiments led to the hypothesis that a "feed-forward kaliuretic reflex" exists [97].

Additional evidence in support of a gut-based kaliuretic signal was recently obtained in a study in rats [98]. These experiments showed that urinary disposal of a K^+ load was significantly enhanced when overnight-fasted rats were given a K^+-deficient intragastric meal. Regardless of whether the K^+ load was given via a systemic vein, the portal vein, or directly placed in the stomach, the time course of the plasma [K^+] level in rats given the K^+-deficient meal showed significantly less area under the curve than rats not given a meal. Moreover, renal K^+ excretion increased significantly above baseline despite almost no change in rats who received intragastric K^+ along with a meal. The investigators suggest this finding is consistent with the operation of a kaliuretic gut factor leading to increased efficiency of renal K^+ excretion (see Fig. 3.2) via a feed-forward system.

The identity of such a putative K^+ sensor in the gut remains unknown, but it is worth noting that a possible role for insulin has not been excluded. Insulin can stimulate distal reabsorption of Na^+ via ENaC [58], which promotes K^+ secretion in the collecting duct.

Hypokalemia: Extrarenal Causes

Urinary K^+ excretion less than 20 mmol/day in the presence of hypokalemia suggests that the etiology involves extrarenal K^+ losses.

Inadequate K^+ Intake, Alcoholism, and Eating Disorders

The development of hypokalemia due to fasting or a K^+-deficient diet was discussed above. Patients with eating disorders are at risk to develop a variety of biochemical disturbances and are quite prone to serious hypokalemia due to a combination of inadequate intake, vomiting, metabolic alkalosis, and laxative or diuretic abuse (see below). Low ECF [K^+] levels are seen in up to 15 % of all patients with eating disorders, and a higher percentage of those with bulimia, abusing laxatives, or with lower body weights [99]. Patients with alcoholism are at risk for K^+ depletion and hypokalemia for a number of reasons, including inadequate dietary intake, vomiting, and hypomagnesemia [100].

Treatment

Repletion of total body K^+ should be relatively straightforward in patients with inadequate K^+ intake who do not have an eating disorder. It is important to insure that any coexisting magnesium deficiency (e.g., in alcoholism) is treated, as hypomagnesemia complicates effective treatment of K^+ depletion. In patients with eating disorders, the key is oral K^+ repletion combined with effective multidisciplinary therapy of the underlying psychological or psychiatric issues. Patients who develop serious hypokalemic metabolic alkalosis are at risk for cardiac arrhythmias, and require monitoring and more aggressive K^+ repletion [101].

Pathological Transcellular Shift (ECF→ICF)

Hypokalemic Periodic Paralysis

The two major causes of HypoPP are autosomal dominant HypoPP and thyrotoxic HypoPP. The clinical manifestations are the same in all forms of HypoPP, so it is crucial to exclude hyperthyroidism [102].

The familial periodic paralysis syndromes result from inherited defects in specific voltage-gated ion channels found in skeletal muscle [103]. These "channelopathies" are characterized by episodes of muscle weakness lasting hours to days that can progress to severe flaccid paralysis. HypoPP is caused by mutations in the genes coding for the α1-subunit of the L-type voltage-dependent calcium channel (*CACN1AS*; HypoPP1, ~60–70 % of cases) or the α[alpha]-subunit of the voltage-gated type IV sodium channel (*SCN4A*; HypoPP2, ~20–30 % of cases) [104]. The prevalence is ~1 case per 100,000 people. The clinical features are the same with either mutation, and include onset of symptoms before the age of 20, with focal or generalized episodes of weakness often triggered by a carbohydrate load, resting after vigorous exercise, or β_2[beta2]-agonists. These triggers suggest that the probability of an episode is increased by insulin- and/or catecholamine-induced cellular K^+ uptake. The attacks are always associated with hypokalemia, which may be severe, and is often attended by hypomagnesemia and hypophosphatemia [105]. The hypokalemia is entirely due to transfer of K^+ from the ECF→ICF because there is no change in total body K^+.

Pathogenesis

In familial HypoPP, the pathogenesis of the muscle weakness relates to an abnormal level of myocyte membrane depolarization, which leads to inactivation of voltage-gated sodium channels and loss of muscle excitability [103]. The mechanism underlying the hypokalemia remains a mystery, but it is possible that the increase in intramyocyte [Na^+] activates muscle Na^+/K^+-ATPase to a degree that transiently depletes ECF [K^+].

Thyrotoxic HypoPP, which also appears to result from abnormal myocyte membrane polarization, may be due to hormone-induced increases in the content and activity of Na^+/K^+-ATPase pump, resulting in excessive cellular uptake of K^+. Patients can have severe hypokalemia with ECF [K^+] <1.5 mM, which can be associated with life-threatening cardiac arrhythmias [102].

The recent discovery of the *KCNJ18* gene—the transcription of which is regulated by thyroid hormone and whose gene product (Kir2.6) is a novel inwardly rectifying K^+ channel found in skeletal muscle—has shed light on the pathogenesis of thyrotoxic HypoPP [106]. When Kir2.6 was cloned and sequenced from 30 patients from the United States, Brazil, and France known to have thyrotoxic HypoPP, five mutations (R399X, Q407X, T354M, K366R, and T140M) were found. In contrast, no mutations were found in 281 healthy controls.

Patients from Asia were also tested, and although none of 31 patients from Thailand and only one of 83 patients from Hong Kong harbored a sixth mutation (R205H), 7 of 27 patients from Singapore had the R399X mutation. No mutations were found in 98 patients from Hong Kong who were thyrotoxic but without a history of HypoPP.

When functionally expressed, one of these mutations (T140M) was associated with loss of channel function, and one (T354M) with decreased K^+ currents. Thyrotoxicosis increases PKC activity, which may also have differential effects on the mutant Kir2.6 channels compared to wild-type channels.

These results indicate not only that mutations in Kir2.6 genetically predispose ~25–30 % of thyrotoxic patients to HypoPP, but also that other genes—that vary in different ethnic populations—play a role in other patients [106].

Diagnosis

For patients with hypokalemia and paralysis, the first diagnostic step is to differentiate HypoPP from renal K^+ wasting by making use of the transtubular K^+ gradient (TTKG): a TTKG greater than four suggests renal K^+ wasting, while a TTKG less than three is highly suggestive of HypoPP [107].

This distinction has important therapeutic implications because those with renal K^+ wasting require aggressive K^+ repletion, whereas even a small amount of K^+ given to those with HypoPP can result in rebound hyperkalemia.

In those with a low TTKG, a next diagnostic step is to differentiate non-thyrotoxic HypoPP from thyrotoxic HypoPP. The tendency of patients with thyrotoxic HypoPP to be both hypercalciuric and hypophosphaturic suggests the clinical utility of a urinary calcium to phosphate ratio. It has been shown that a calcium:phosphate ratio greater than 1.7 in a spot urine is 100 % sensitive and 96 % specific for thyrotoxic HypoPP [108].

Treatment

First, hyperthyroidism must be excluded. Patients with inherited HypoPP should be counseled on how to avoid the factors and situations that increase the probability of triggering an attack (e.g., high carbohydrate meals, vigorous exercise), how to recognize that an attack is imminent, and what medications to have on hand (e.g., acetazolamide, KCl, propranolol). Although the total body content of K^+ is not depleted in HypoPP, treatment with oral K^+ is effective in shortening the episode and attenuating the weakness. Oral K^+ (20–30 mmol) at the onset of symptoms and then every 30–60 min as long as symptoms persist can be effective, but one must be mindful of the risk of rebound hyperkalemia [109]. The frequency of attacks may be decreased by CAIs (e.g., acetazolamide 250–500 mg/day). The mechanism of action of CAIs is not dependent on inhibition of carbonic anhydrase activity, and may relate to activation of calcium-activated K^+ (maxi-K) channels.

Patients with thyrotoxicosis require antithyroid therapy. Propranolol, a nonselective beta-blocker that blocks β_2[beta-2]-receptors, has been shown to reverse acute attacks of thyrotoxic HypoPP with prompt improvement of both the hypokalemia and hypophosphatemia without causing rebound hyperkalemia [110, 111]. Agents that reduce renal K^+ excretion (e.g., spironolactone, amiloride, triamterene) have been tried, but their utility is questionable because the amount of K^+ excreted by the kidney during attacks has not been shown to be significant. Moreover, CAIs are proven effective in HypoPP despite their ability to promote kaliuresis.

Drugs

The most important endogenous agents affecting the distribution of K^+ between the ECF and ICF are insulin and catecholamines. Obviously, exogenous insulin is also a critically important medication for many patients with diabetes. Exogenous β_2[beta-2]-adrenergic agonists are used clinically as well, mostly in the form of inhaled agents (e.g., albuterol) in the treatment of asthma and chronic lung disorders. As will be discussed, both insulin and inhaled albuterol are used in the emergency treatment of serious hyperkalemia. Other drugs that promote a shift of K^+ into cells include theophylline, ritodrine, and terbutaline.

Clenbuterol

This agent deserves special mention because it is a long-acting β_2[beta-2]-agonist recently implicated in a number of accidental poisoning cases. It has not been approved for use in humans in the United States, but has been used in other countries to treat patients with pulmonary disease. Clenbuterol usually accumulates in the liver—but not the muscle—of treated animals. Nonetheless, 15 people in Italy became ill after eating meat from these animals [112]. Symptoms included tremors, palpitations, headache, hyperglycemia, and hypokalemia. In a separate case, a young woman who ingested a "small amount" of the drug developed tachycardia (140 bpm), marked hypokalemia (2.4 mM), hypomagnesemia (1.52 mg/dL), and hypophosphatemia (0.9 mg/dL). She was treated with metoprolol and supplemental K^+, but remained symptomatic for nearly a day. In 2005, an outbreak occurred among heroin users (26 people in five states) who presented with tachycardia and palpitations. The cause was found to be heroin adulterated with clenbuterol.

Barium Intoxication

The form of barium used in radiology is barium sulfate, which forms insoluble complexes in the gut that are not resorbed. However, acid-soluble barium salts are resorbed. Barium intoxication is usually a result of a suicide attempt [113], but can be accidental. Symptoms include abdominal pain, cardiac arrhythmias (ventricular bigeminy and fibrillation), and weakness that can progress to flaccid paralysis. Patients can develop rhabdomyolysis and death can occur.

Though barium intoxication dates to the late 1940s, the hypokalemia, which can be severe and is resistant to K^+ supplementation, became more widely appreciated in 1964 when some cases occurred from accidental barium carbonate food poisoning in the United Kingdom. The mechanisms of hypokalemia are not fully understood but barium is the classic blocker of K^+ channels, which would decrease whole cell K^+ conductance and depolarize the cell membrane potential. The former will tend to decrease passive efflux of K^+. The latter, through the opening of voltage-gated calcium channels, will increase intracellular calcium, activate Na^+/Ca exchange and increase intracellular sodium, stimulating the Na^+/K^+-ATPase pump. Increased cellular loading of K^+ by the pump combined with a decrease in K^+ efflux both favor hypokalemia. Many patients also develop significant diarrhea and barium may also produce a kaliuresis, both of which will contribute to hypokalemia.

Therapy for barium intoxication is mainly supportive, including ventilatory support, gastric lavage, enteral sodium sulfate to precipitate barium and prevent absorption, and hemodialysis [113]. Patients may require up to 500 mmol of supplemental K^+ to replete total body stores, indicating that K^+ losses occur in addition to shifts of K^+.

Other Causes

Some miscellaneous causes of hypokalemia due to shift into cells include anabolism (e.g., during treatment for pernicious anemia, rapidly growing leukemias and lymphomas), chloroquine overdose, cesium (which also blocks K^+ channels), and hypothermia.

Skin K^+ Losses via Sweat

It is possible for K^+ depletion to result from profuse losses of sweat, but hypokalemia is quite rare because such losses are usually temporary and decreased urine flow rate limits renal K^+ excretion. However, if aldosterone levels are high [114] or in the setting of intensive exercise [115], K^+ depletion occurred. One study of healthy volunteers engaged in vigorous physical conditioning during the hot summer months sustained a K^+ deficit of over 500 mmol in the face of a K^+ intake of 100 mmol/day [115]. In this case, renal excretion of K^+ (50–75 mmol/day) due to high aldosterone levels contributed to total body K^+ depletion. When the same training was performed under cooler conditions, K^+ depletion did not occur.

Gastrointestinal K^+ Losses

The most common underlying etiology of K^+ depletion and hypokalemia relates to gastrointestinal dysfunction because: (1) K^+ intake normally occurs by oral ingestion, which is impaired in conditions of anorexia or nausea; (2) K^+ is secreted into the lumen of the gut, leading to K^+ depletion if excessive fluid is lost via vomiting, diarrhea, nasogastric suction, high output ileostomy, or fistulae; and (3) loss of HCl and fluid from the upper GI tract generates metabolic alkalosis and ECF volume depletion, both of which promote excretion of K^+ in the urine.

Upper Gastrointestinal K^+ Losses

Loss of gastric fluid due to vomiting or NG drainage is the most common situation for upper GI processes to produce hypokalemia. Some of the K^+ loss occurs primarily from the gut because the $[K^+]$ of gastric fluid is 10–15 mM, but most of the K^+ loss (up to 200 mmol/day) occurs through urinary losses secondary to the effects of metabolic alkalosis, ECF volume depletion with hyperaldosteronism, and chloride depletion [116]. Therefore, a high urine K^+ is usually a key laboratory finding in distinguishing upper GI losses from lower GI losses, in which the urine K^+ will be low.

Differential Diagnosis

The diagnosis is straightforward in all patients with NG drainage and most patients who have been vomiting. In patients with hypokalemic metabolic alkalosis and elevated urine K^+ who deny vomiting, the differential diagnosis is that of "renal K^+ wasting," which includes covert vomiting, diuretic (ab)use, Gitelman syndrome (mimics thiazide diuretic use), Bartter syndrome (mimics loop diuretic use), magnesium deficiency, and syndromes of apparent mineralocorticoid excess (AME) (e.g., Conn syndrome, Liddle syndrome). The latter can be easily differentiated from vomiting because of the presence of ECF volume expansion and/or hypertension rather than the ECF volume depletion that accompanies vomiting. Magnesium deficiency or hypomagnesemia is not a very specific finding because it may coexist with hypokalemic metabolic alkalosis in patients with eating disorders or alcoholism, and is also seen in Gitelman syndrome and those (ab)using diuretics [117]. On the other hand, the absence of hypomagnesemia helps point away from these diagnoses.

Classically, the most difficult differential diagnosis was to distinguish covert vomiting from furosemide abuse and Bartter syndrome [118, 119]. However, in light of the elucidation of the molecular genetics of Bartter syndrome [120, 121], most adults thought to possibly have Bartter syndrome were either covertly vomiting or abusing furosemide. The five known forms of Bartter syndrome all involve mutations in transport elements in the thick ascending limb of Henle's loop, and occur almost exclusively in the neonatal and pediatric population [122].

Clinical Approach

Discerning covert vomiting from furosemide abuse is a challenge, although a positive diuretic screen is helpful. One must consider, however, that a patient may be doing both. Of course, a diuretic screen may also yield a false-negative result. Fortunately, there are other means that help suggest a person has been vomiting, such as characteristic changes in the teeth and some useful investigations. In the period just after vomiting, the filtered load of bicarbonate will increase, which will obligate the loss of a cation such as sodium. Therefore, a disparity between the urinary sodium and chloride (i.e., a high urine sodium and a low urine chloride) suggests recent vomiting. Indeed, the urine chloride will virtually always be low in a hypovolemic patient who has been vomiting, but may vary in a patient abusing diuretics.

Lower Gastrointestinal K^+ Losses

Normally, the loss of K^+ from the GI tract is less than 10 mmol/day. Although K^+ is reabsorbed along the small intestine, K^+ secretion occurs along the aldosterone-sensitive portion of the large intestine. Therefore, large lower GI tract losses or other processes that increase colonic K^+ secretion can cause hypokalemia. The increase in aldosterone due to concomitant ECF volume depletion can exacerbate K^+ loss through both the colon and the kidney, although the decrease in urine flow rate will diminish the latter.

A clinically accepted definition of diarrhea is a stool weight of more than 200 g/day, which is reasonable given that the stool weight in healthy volunteers is ~160 g/day for men and ~90 g/day for women. Analysis of fecal fluid using in vivo dialysis on healthy subjects shows a $[K^+]$ of about 75 mM [123]. The typical amount of K^+ loss from the GI tract is about 7.5–9 mmol because the usual amount of fecal fluid excreted per day is about 100–120 mL. Interestingly, with large lower GI losses, the fecal fluid $[K^+]$ falls sharply to <15 mM, and the electrolyte loss is tenfold lower for potassium (14.2 mM fecal fluid per day) than it is for sodium (142 mM fecal fluid per day). Therefore, a patient with cholera sustaining a fecal fluid loss of 8 L/day would lose 1,136 mmol of Na^+ per day, but only 113.6 mmol of K^+ per day via the GI tract [124]. Indeed, it is the inability of the colon to reabsorb Na^+ and increase the electronegativity of the lumen that limits secretory K^+ losses in acute diarrheal states.

This is not the case with losses in chronic GI disorders (e.g., associated with AIDS, inflammatory bowel disease, neoplasia, laxative abuse). The lower flow rate occurring with smaller, but more frequent diarrhea over long periods of time, can lead to marked potassium losses in these conditions. Secondary hyperaldosteronism due to coexistent hypovolemia will exacerbate K^+-depletion by augmenting K^+ secretion in the colon.

Differential Diagnosis

The clinical spectrum of disorders featuring diarrhea is extensive. Chronic diarrhea can be classified as watery diarrhea, inflammatory diarrhea, or fatty diarrhea. Watery diarrhea can be further broken down as *osmotic* (e.g., due to osmotic laxatives or carbohydrate malabsorption) or *secretory* (e.g., due to stimulant laxatives, inflammatory bowel disease, colonic pseudo-obstruction, endocrinopathies, neoplasia, infections, toxins, or medications). Inflammatory diarrhea includes infectious causes (e.g., AIDS-associated, *Clostridium difficile*, *E. coli*), noninfectious causes (e.g., IBD, diverticulitis, ischemia, hyperthyroidism), neoplastic causes (e.g., colon cancer, lymphoma, villous, adenoma, carcinoid, VIPoma, gastrinoma, pheochromocytoma), and drugs (e.g., laxative abuse). In nearly all of these disorders, the loss of K^+ in the urine will be minimal unless the patient has concomitant metabolic alkalosis from vomiting, nasogastric suction, or kaliuretic agents.

The global AIDS epidemic and the myriad etiologies of chronic diarrhea that can occur in AIDS predispose these patients to K^+ depletion and hypokalemia. Up to 50 % of AIDS patients develop hypokalemia referable to the GI tract at some point.

Laxative Abuse

Perhaps the most difficult diagnostic challenge is presented by individuals who surreptitiously (ab) use laxatives [125]. Laxative abuse can play a part in eating disorders, disorders of body image, and various forms of Munchausen syndrome [125]. The clinical presentation is typically complex and confusing, leading to expensive diagnostic "wild-goose chases" and time-consuming therapeutic procedures. Patients may appear to have an enteropathy suggestive of a malabsorption syndrome, irritable bowel syndrome, or IBD. The differential diagnosis usually also includes endocrinopathies and nephropathies. Metabolic disturbances include metabolic acidosis or alkalosis, total body K^+-depletion with hypokalemia, and hypomagnesemia. A low urinary K^+ excretion should suggest the potassium loss is enteral, although this sign may be confounded if loop or thiazide diuretics are also being (ab)used.

The vast majority of individuals who habitually (ab)use laxatives use bisacodyl (the active ingredient in Dulcolax®, Correctol®, and Ex-Lax®) and/or senna (the active ingredient in Castoria® and Senokot®). The biochemical assay used to detect these drugs in urine or stool is based on the thin layer chromatography (TLC) method developed by de Wolff and colleagues [126]. Apparently, specimens for all patients are currently analyzed in only one clinical reference laboratory (CRL) in the United States, and the reliability of the assay has been recently scrutinized [127]. Healthy volunteers with no history of laxative use were given a single dose of either bisacodyl, senna, or a control laxative (polyethylene glycol, castor oil, or milk of magnesia). Specimens of both urine and stool were sent to that CRL. In contrast to the CRL reported sensitivity of 99 % for bisacodyl in urine, these investigators found a sensitivity of only 73 % for bisacodyl in urine (but 91 % sensitivity in stool). Senna was not detected either in the urine or stool from *any* of the 11 volunteers who had ingested it, a result that flies in the face of the 100 % sensitivity reported by the CRL. This study underscores the importance of using all available clinical data when working up the possibility of factitious disease such as laxative abuse, rather than excluding the possibility based on a single laboratory test [127].

Clinical Approach

Patients with hypokalemia due to lower GI losses almost always have minimal urinary K^+ loss unless they are also (ab)using loop or thiazide diuretics. Consideration of habitual use or abuse of laxatives should always be kept in mind for any patient with hypokalemia not explained by inadequate intake or urinary K^+ losses. Because the reliability of detecting laxatives, particularly senna, in urine or stool, such testing must be combined with a complete history. Finally, it should be kept in mind that the prevalence of surreptitious bisacodyl use is ~2.5 % among patients with diarrhea of uncertain origin, although the prevalence of factitious diarrhea rises to ~25 % in the subset of those patients in which a diagnosis is not identified after an extensive workup [127].

Clay Ingestion

The ingestion of clay (geophagia), either due to a pica or a cultural practice, can cause hypokalemia or hyperkalemia depending on the type of clay. Red (riverbed) clay is high in K^+ (about 1 mmol/g), so can lead to hyperkalemia, especially in patients with CKD or ESKD. Other clays do not contain much K^+, but are able to bind K^+ in the gut, which can lead to marked hypokalemia. In either case, discontinuation of the geophagia leads to correction of the dyskalemia.

Congenital Chloridorrhea

This rare autosomal recessive disorder causes hypokalemia due to an increase in stool volume and an increased lumen electronegativity of the gut, both of which promote K^+ losses. The defect involves Cl^-/HCO_3^- exchange in the distal ileum and colon, which leads to decreased resorption of chloride [128]. Retention of bicarbonate results in metabolic alkalosis. An acquired, transient, variant has also been described in children presenting with voluminous diarrhea high in chloride, and associated hypokalemia, hypochloremia, and metabolic alkalosis. Any attendant volume contraction and secondary aldosteronism will increase K^+ secretion in the collecting duct, and exacerbate the hypokalemia. Treatment is aimed at complete oral replacement of the electrolytes and water lost in the stool.

VIPoma

These are rare pancreatic endocrine tumors that secrete excess vasoactive intestinal polypeptide, which leads to a profuse watery secretory diarrhea, hypovolemia, hypokalemia, and metabolic acidosis. The hypokalemia is due to passive and VIP-induced active secretion of potassium by colonic epithelial cells. Other than replacement of electrolytes and water, patients can be treated with synthetic somatostatin analogues before surgery if definitive surgical removal is not possible.

Colonic Pseudo-Obstruction

Patients with colonic pseudo-obstruction (Ogilvie syndrome) can develop profound hypokalemia due to profuse secretory diarrhea with an abnormally high fecal [K^+]. In a recent study of five consecutive patients with Ogilvie syndrome, the fecal [K^+] was 100–180 mmol/L (compared to less than 50 mmol/L in typical secretory diarrhea), suggesting the presence of active colonic K^+ secretion [129]. Support for this hypothesis was provided by a case of secretory diarrhea in a dialysis patient who developed recurrent colonic pseudo-obstruction from ischemic colitis [130]. Following colectomy, immunohistochemistry showed overexpression of BK (maxi-K) channels in the apical membrane of colonic epithelial cells as compared to colon from control subjects and other dialysis patients. Overexpression of colonic BK channels—leading to increased active K^+ secretion and passive luminal water entry—could explain the development of colonic pseudo-obstruction and profound hypokalemia seen in Ogilvie syndrome and other causes of secretory diarrhea due to colonic secretion of K^+ rather than Cl^- [131, 132].

Hypokalemia: Renal Causes Along the Nephron

Urinary K^+ excretion exceeding 20 mmol/day in the presence of hypokalemia suggests that the etiology involves renal K^+ losses.

Proximal Renal Tubular Acidosis

Any process that impairs bicarbonate reabsorption in the proximal tubule causes an increase in renal K^+ excretion as a result of alkalinization along the collecting duct, which is a potent stimulus for K^+ secretion. CAIs produce drug-induced proximal RTA. Patients with familial (primary) Fanconi syndrome and acquired (secondary) Fanconi syndrome develop hypokalemia, which worsens if such patients are treated with exogenous bicarbonate [133]. Proximal RTA can also result from the deposition of certain light chains, particularly certain kappa (κ) light chains [134]. These κ[kappa] light chains, which are thought to be resistant to proteolysis, accumulate in the proximal tubule and cause cellular dysfunction.

Loop of Henle

Anything that disrupts transport in the TALH can increase kaliuresis and produce hypokalemia. Under normal circumstances, the lumen of the TALH is electropositive (+8 to +10 mV), and the positive voltage is a major driving force for the reabsorption of not only Ca^{2+} and Mg^{2+}, but also K^+.

Loop Diuretics

These agents promote volume loss (i.e., natriuresis and chloruresis) via inhibition of the Na-K^+-2Cl triple cotransporter in the apical membrane of the TALH including the cells of the macula densa. This action also decreases the electropositivity of the lumen and causes calciuria, magnesuria, and some kaliuresis. Inhibition of the triple cotransporter at the macula densa blocks tubuloglomerular feedback (TGF), producing significant increases in natriuresis and distal urinary flow rate. Therefore, enhanced K^+ secretion occurs along the collecting duct due to (1) flow-dependent maxi-K channels in the apical membrane of α[alpha]-ICs, (2) secondary hyperaldosteronism, and (3) increased luminal [Na] in the presence of increased ENaC channel activity, which increases lumen electronegativity.

Bartter Syndrome

Hereditary disorders that affect transport elements in the apical or basolateral membranes of the TALH cause Bartter syndrome [121]. Hypokalemia develops whether the molecular defect involves the triple cotransporter (Type 1), the ROMK channel in the apical membrane (Type 2), or the ClC-Kb channel in the BLM (Type 3). There are two ClC chloride channels (i.e., ClC-Ka and ClC-Kb) in the BLM of the TALH, and both are closely associated with a protein called Barttin [135]. A fourth type of Bartter syndrome due to mutations in Barttin and associated with sensorineural deafness has been described [136]. A fifth type of Bartter syndrome, also associated with sensorineural deafness but with normal Barttin, is due to digenic defects in ClC-Ka and ClC-Kb [137]. All these forms of Bartter syndrome are autosomal recessive. Finally, an autosomal dominant form of Bartter syndrome is due to an activating mutation of the calcium sensing receptor in the BLM of the TALH [138]. Patients with this Bartter-like syndrome have hypocalcemia in addition to hypokalemic metabolic alkalosis.

Affected individuals usually present in the perinatal period or early in life. The pathogenesis of hypokalemic metabolic alkalosis in all forms of Bartter syndrome is essentially identical to that occurring with loop diuretics.

Early Distal Tubule

By mechanisms similar to those just described, inhibited activity of the Na-Cl cotransporter in the apical membrane of the early distal tubule also promotes kaliuresis and the development of hypokalemia due to downstream effects in the collecting duct.

Thiazide Diuretics

These agents promote volume loss (i.e., natriuresis and chloruresis) via inhibition of the Na-Cl cotransporter. Enhanced K^+ secretion occurs along the collecting duct due to (1) flow-dependent maxi-K channels in the apical membrane of α[alpha]-ICs, (2) secondary hyperaldosteronism, and (3) increased luminal [Na] in the presence of increased ENaC channel activity, which increases lumen electronegativity. The effect of thiazides to cause hypocalciuria, as opposed to the hypercalciuric effect of loop diuretics, may increase lumen electronegativity and explain, in part, why hypokalemia is more marked with thiazides.

Gitelman Syndrome

Genetic mutations that decrease the activity of the thiazide-sensitive cotransporter cause Gitelman syndrome, another inherited hypokalemic metabolic alkalosis [120]. Unlike Bartter syndrome, all individuals with Gitelman syndrome have a mutation in this single transport element. Affected individuals with this autosomal recessive disorder usually present later in life (i.e., the second or third decade) than those with Bartter syndrome, often with muscle weakness due to hypokalemia [139]. Also in contradistinction to Bartter syndrome, individuals with Gitelman syndrome have hypocalciuria and hypomagnesemia (which makes treatment of the hypokalemia more difficult).

Connecting Tubule and Collecting Duct

As discussed, the connecting tubule and collecting duct are the major sites of K^+ secretion so it is not surprising that any process affecting the collecting duct can produce a dyskalemia. Therefore, from a pathophysiological standpoint, it is convenient to divide the etiologies into those associated with elevated aldosterone levels and those with suppressed aldosterone levels. The main disorders are reviewed briefly here.

Classic Distal Renal Tubular Acidosis

Hypokalemia, which can be severe, is a nearly invariant finding in classical or Type I RTA, and results from renal K^+ wasting. The development of severe hypokalemia in the setting of distal RTA is puzzling [140], because metabolic acidosis tends to decrease the activity of the ROMK channel. Although simple leakage of K^+ across the apical membrane of the collecting duct could explain K^+ wasting in distal RTA due to amphotericin B, the "leakage" explanation does not hold for the other forms of distal RTA. The renal K^+ loss may result from secondary hyperaldosteronism due to concomitant renal Na^+ wasting [141]. Another hypothesis is defective H^+/K^+-ATPase pumps in the apical membrane of α[alpha]-ICs [140]. Primary dysfunction of this pump would simultaneously decrease H^+ secretion and K^+ reabsorption, promoting metabolic acidosis and hypokalemia, respectively.

Treatment

Experts have recommended that when hypokalemia is accompanied by acidosis, potassium should be repleted before correcting the acidosis to avoid exacerbation of hypokalemia. However, the availability of K^+ salts containing citrate, acetate, or gluconate (all organic anions that are converted to bicarbonate in the liver) allows both to be repleted simultaneously.

Toluene Intoxication

The "sniffing" of substances that contain toluene (e.g., airplane glue, spray paint, paint thinners, etc.) can produce a normal anion gap metabolic acidosis resembling type 1 (distal) renal tubular acidosis [142]. Many of these patients develop marked hypokalemia due to the overproduction of hippurate (a nonresorbable anion) resulting from the metabolism of toluene [143, 144]. The hypokalemia can be severe enough to cause muscle paralysis, so (repeated) episodes of paralysis due to "sniffing" can be confused with hypokalemic periodic paralysis, especially in young patients presenting to the emergency department. This is one setting where the urine [K^+] and TTKG is helpful, because it will be low (i.e., less than 3) in HypoPP and high (i.e., greater than 4) in those with toluene intoxication. Of course, patients with the latter will also have a metabolic acidosis.

States of High Renin and High Aldosterone

Primary increases in renin cause hyperaldosteronism and can lead to hypertension and hypokalemia. The differential diagnosis of primary hyperreninemia includes (1) renal artery stenosis, (2) malignant hypertension, (3) renin secreting tumors, and mostly in the past, (4) some formulations of oral contraceptives. The incidence of hypokalemia differs among these disorders.

Renal Artery Stenosis

In patients with renovascular disease, underperfusion of the affected kidney stimulates renin secretion from the JG cells. K^+ secretion in the collecting duct is stimulated by the secondary increase in aldosterone. For unclear reasons, hypokalemia only develops in about 15–20 % of adult patients.

Malignant Hypertension

Pressure-induced renal damage and ischemia can cause renin release from the JG cells, leading to "pressure natriuresis" and hypokalemia in up to 50 % of cases [145]. A similar pathogenesis has been reported in pheochromocytoma [146].

Renin Secreting Tumors

Neoplasms that secrete renin are quite rare. Most cases arise from benign tumors in the kidney and are due to transformation of pericytes of the juxtaglomerular apparatus (e.g., hemangiopericytomas or histiopericytomas). In contrast to renal reninomas, extrarenal renin secreting tumors tend to be malignant, including pancreatic malignancies, oat cell carcinoma and in children with Wilms' tumor. As expected, these patients develop hyperaldosteronism with hypertension and hypokalemia that normalizes following resection of the tumor. In a recent case report, a 22-year-old woman with a blood pressure of 160/110 and marked hypokalemia (serum [K^+] 2.7 mM) was found to have a 1.5 cm renin secreting tumor in one kidney [147]. Her hypertension, hypokalemia, and hyperreninemic hyperaldosteronism all resolved following tumor resection.

States of Low Renin and High Aldosterone

This group of disorders includes primary hyperaldosteronism due to adrenal adenoma (Conn syndrome), adrenal carcinoma, bilateral adrenal cortical hyperplasia, and glucocorticoid remediable hyperaldosteronism (GRA). Hypokalemia is a classical finding in primary hyperaldosteronism not only due to the effect of increased aldosterone on the collecting duct, but also because of the development of metabolic alkalosis and increased distal fluid and sodium delivery. Indeed, the latter may deserve special emphasis because patients with primary hyperaldosteronism who are not sodium overloaded (i.e., by dietary salt restriction and/or use of K^+-sparing diuretics) appear to have much less renal K^+ loss. This may explain, in part, why a significant subset of these patients is normokalemic [148]. Currently, aldosterone-producing adenomas (APAs) account for about one-third of the cases of primary aldosteronism, while the other two-thirds is due to idiopathic bilateral cortical hyperplasia (many of the latter are normokalemic) [149].

Adrenal Adenoma

The most common form of primary hyperaldosteronism with hypokalemia is due to an aldosterone-secreting adrenal cortical tumor. Although adrenal aldosteronomas are almost always benign, one of the original 18 patients did have an adrenal adenocarcinoma [150]. The most common symptoms, muscle weakness and polyuria in 75 % of the patients, are directly referable to hypokalemia. Hypokalemia impairs urinary concentration (i.e., produces a nephrogenic diabetes insipidus) and is associated with a decrease in aquaporin-2 water channels in the collecting duct [151].

Primary aldosteronism is the most common form of secondary hypertension (5–13 % of all patients with hypertension), so it is very important to maintain a high clinical suspicion for this disorder. Surgical resection of benign aldosteronomas should be curative. If surgery is not an option (as in bilateral adrenal cortical hyperplasia), medical management with aldosterone antagonists (e.g., spironolactone, eplerenone) is usually helpful, although K^+ supplementation and additional antihypertensive agents are often necessary.

Molecular Pathogenesis

A major advance in our understanding of the molecular pathophysiology of primary aldosteronism is the very recent discovery of mutations in a specific K^+ channel found in adrenal glomerulosa cells [152]. Aldosterone secretion in these cells is stimulated by membrane depolarization, which opens voltage-dependent calcium channels.

In this landmark study, the investigators analyzed APAs from 22 patients and identified a small number of somatic mutations in each tumor, and found one gene—*KCNJ5*—mutated in two tumors. The gene product of *KCNJ5* is Kir3.4, an inwardly rectifying K^+ channel. Among these tumors, two mutations in Kir3.4 were identified: G151R in 33 % of tumors and L168R in 29 % of tumors. Of great interest, both mutations are in or near the highly conserved selectivity filter that includes the GYG motif seen in every known K^+ channel. The G151R mutation changes the GYG motif to RYG, and the L168R mutation is adjacent to the tyrosine side chain of the GYG motif. As a result, both mutations convert the channel to a nonselective cation channel that allows Na^+ entry, which chronically depolarizes the adrenal glomerulosa cells. This results in chronic aldosterone secretion, and the constant elevation in cellular calcium promotes cellular proliferation. With regard to hypokalemia, the serum [K^+] in these 22 patients averaged 3.5±0.4 mM (range 2.5–4.5); 10 of the 22 had serum [K^+] less than 3.5 mM [152].

Glucocorticoid Remediable Aldosteronism

Also known as dexamethasone-suppressible hyperaldosteronism, glucocorticoid remediable aldosteronism (GRA) is a hereditary cause of human hypertension in which aldosterone secretion comes under the control of adrenocorticotropin (ACTH). The molecular mechanism of this autosomal dominant disorder is a crossover event resulting in a chimeric gene where sequences of the 11β[beta]-hydroxylase and aldosterone synthase genes fuse [153]. The presence of an ACTH response element with the coding region of aldosterone synthase allows ACTH to drive abnormal aldosterone synthesis from the zona fasciculata, which can produce hypokalemia, especially in patients taking loop or thiazide diuretics. The phenotype can be quite variable though, and many patients remain normokalemic. Glucocorticoids are a remedy for the disorder because they suppress ACTH secretion, so administration of dexamethasone is useful for both diagnosis and therapy.

States of Low Renin and Low Aldosterone

This group of disorders includes the so-called pseudohyperaldosterone states, due either to an increase (or apparent increase) in a mineralocorticoid other than aldosterone. Congenital or acquired disorders include (1) congenital adrenal hyperplasia, (2) Cushing syndrome, and (3) acquired inhibition of 11β[beta]-hydroxysteroid dehydrogenase type 2 (11β[beta]-HSD2) (AME). The major inherited disorders are (1) activating mutations of the mineralocorticoid receptor, (2) genetic inhibition of 11β[beta]-HSD2 (AME), and (3) Liddle syndrome.

Congenital Adrenal Hyperplasia

Two of the cytochrome P450 enzymes involved in the biosynthesis of adrenal corticosteroids are 11β[beta]-hydroxylase and 17α[alpha]-hydroxylase. Deficiency of either of these enzymes results in significant reductions in cortisol biosynthesis and a consequential increase in corticotrophin (ACTH). In fact, 11β[beta]-hydroxylase deficiency is the second most common form of congenital adrenal hyperplasia (steroid 21-hydroxylase deficiency is by far the most common cause). Persistently elevated secretion of ACTH stimulates adrenal production of 11-deoxycortisol, 11-deoxycorticosterone, and adrenal androgens. Excess adrenal androgens cause hypertension, hypokalemia, and virilization.

Treatment. Therapy for these disorders is aimed at administering glucocorticoids (e.g., dexamethasone) at doses sufficient to reduce ACTH secretion.

Cushing Syndrome

Hypokalemia can be seen in Cushing syndrome, particularly in those with the acute ectopic corticotrophin syndrome [154]. The latter is most often seen in patients with small cell lung carcinoma and consists of the rapid onset of hypertension, hypokalemia (may be mild), edema, and glucose intolerance. In a review of 58 patients with Cushing syndrome due to ectopic ACTH secretion [155], hypertension was seen in 78 % of the patients, while hypokalemia occurred in 57 %. The presence of hypokalemia was strongly correlated to urinary cortisol levels, suggesting that high plasma levels may allow cortisol access to the mineralocorticoid receptor.

Treatment. Obviously, the therapy of choice is to remove the ACTH-secreting tumor when possible. When not possible, adrenal enzyme inhibitors may control the hypercortisolism. Under some conditions (e.g., indolent nonresectable tumors), bilateral adrenalectomy may be necessary.

Activating Mutations of the Mineralocorticoid Receptor

In 2000, a novel activating mutation (S810L) in the mineralocorticoid receptor (MR) was discovered [156]. The associated syndrome is autosomal dominant and the mutation confers constitutive activation of the receptor and causes a conformational change that allows non-mineralocorticoids (e.g., progesterone) and even aldosterone antagonists (e.g., spironolactone) to act as potent agonists. Because progesterone will act as a potent mineralocorticoid in this disorder, female patients who become pregnant can develop severe hypertension with mild hypokalemic metabolic alkalosis.

Syndrome of Apparent Mineralocorticoid Excess

Aldosterone is not the only endogenous agonist that can bind to the MR. Cortisol can also bind to the MR, and because circulating levels of cortisol are much higher than aldosterone, mechanisms must be in place to prevent cortisol from binding to the MR. The major mechanism is the enzymatic conversion of cortisol to cortisone via 11β[beta]-HSD2, and cortisone does not activate the MR. Therefore, genetic or acquired defects in 11β[beta]-HSD2 that allow inappropriate binding of cortisol to the MR will result in AME often producing the classic triad of hypertension, hypokalemia, and metabolic alkalosis [157]. Genetic mutations in 11β[beta]-HSD2 cause a familial form of human hypertension [158], often with hypokalemia. Because plasma renin activity and aldosterone secretion are suppressed, the syndrome is also known as autosomal recessive pseudohyperaldosteronism.

The most common forms of acquired inhibition of 11β[beta]-HSD2 relates to ingestion of competitive inhibitors of the enzyme, including carbenoxolone, bioflavonoids, and most notably, licorice. Glycyrrhetinic acid (GA), found in the natural licorice root (*Glycyrrhiz glabra*) and used as a flavoring, contains ~2 mg of GA per gram on average, but the range of variability is huge (0.026–98 mg) [159]. Individuals ingesting enough licorice to develop clinical issues are almost always hypokalemic, sometimes markedly so. In a recent report, a 55-year-old man presented with a serum [K^+] of 1.7 mM and metabolic alkalosis (total CO_2 36 mM), although his blood pressure was only 125/85 mmHg [160]. On questioning, he admitted to consuming 25 g of licorice root per day after he quit smoking. His licorice root contained 23 mg of GA per gram, for a total of 525 mg of GA per day. Indeed, the hypokalemic effect of GA has been suggested as a potential therapy to control hyperkalemia in dialysis patients with anuria [161].

Treatment. Therapy for patients found to be ingesting GA is simply to discontinue the offending substance. Potassium supplementation is only necessary to replete the initial K^+ deficit (see estimating equation in the next section). Patients with the hereditary disorder often respond to treatment with aldosterone antagonists (i.e., spironolactone, eplerenone).

Liddle Syndrome

This rare autosomal dominant form of inherited human hypertension has led to an explosion of knowledge about the molecular and cell biology of the epithelial Na^+ channel (ENaC). The entry of Na^+ across the apical membrane of PCs via ENaC is the rate limiting step of sodium reabsorption along the collecting duct [162]. The basic molecular defect in Liddle syndrome involves mutations in the β[beta]-subunit (and rarely the γ[gamma]-subunit) of ENaC, which leads to a gain-of-function and hyper-reabsorption of Na^+ [60]. The cellular basis of the disorder primarily relates to abnormal trafficking due to decreased membrane retrieval of ENaC, resulting in an increase in the number of functional channels in the apical membrane [163].

These patients often present with the classic triad of hypertension, hypokalemia, and metabolic alkalosis [164]. In the original kindred, the proband was a 16-year-old girl with a blood pressure of 180/110 and a serum [K^+] of 2.8 mM. Her younger brother had a blood pressure of 200/110 and a serum [K^+] of 2.7 mM. The syndrome is also known as autosomal dominant pseudohyperaldosteronism because hyper-reabsorption of Na^+ via ENaC is independent of aldosterone, so plasma renin activity and aldosterone secretion are completely suppressed. As expected, the pathogenesis of the hypokalemia relates to an increase in the lumen electronegativity of the collecting duct and the development of metabolic alkalosis, both of which promote K^+ secretion via ROMK [165].

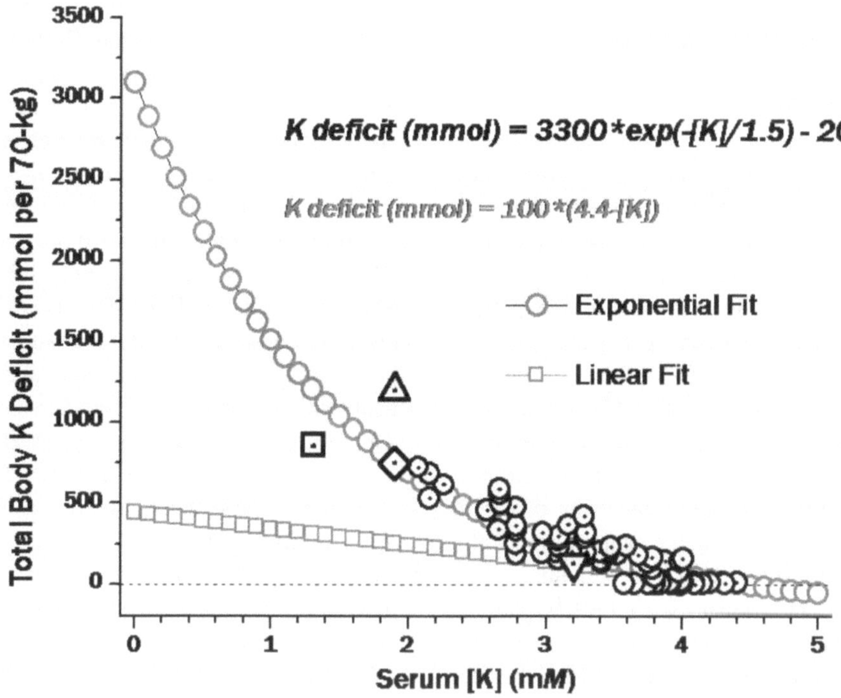

Fig. 3.5 Relationship of serum [K^+] and estimated total body K^+ deficit. The total body K^+ deficit has traditionally been estimated using a linear equation, as shown by the *squares*, for example. The exponential equation (*circles*) was derived by fitting data (*dotted circles*) obtained by Sterns et al. [166]. The estimated total body K^+ deficit (per 70-kg) in mmol is given by $3,300 \times exp(-[K^+]/1.5)-200$, where [$K^+$] is in mM. Other patients from the literature are also plotted, including the mean deficit from patients reported by Kassirer and Schwartz (*dotted inverted triangle*) [71], Murthy et al. (*dotted triangle*) [168], Murakami et al. (*dotted diamond*) [167], and Yasue et al. (*dotted square*) [169]

Treatment. The main goal of therapy is to control blood pressure, which is best accomplished with dietary sodium restriction combined with effective blockade of ENaC with amiloride or triamterene. Aldosterone antagonists are not effective.

Vomiting and Nasogastric Drainage

Loss of gastric fluid due to vomiting or NG drainage is the most common situation for upper GI processes associated with hypokalemia. Although some of the K^+ loss occurs from the gut because the [K^+] of gastric fluid is 10–15 mM, most of the K^+ loss (up to 200 mmol/day) occurs through urinary K^+ loss secondary to the effects of metabolic alkalosis with bicarbonaturia, ECF volume depletion with hyperaldosteronism, and chloride depletion [116]. Therefore, a high urine K^+ is usually a key laboratory finding in distinguishing upper GI losses from lower GI losses, where the urine K^+ will be low.

Treatment. Patients who have been vomiting or undergoing NG drainage develop hypokalemia in association with hypochloremic (saline-responsive) metabolic alkalosis and an element of ECF volume contraction. Therefore, the cornerstone of treatment is potassium in the form of KCl and volume repletion with NaCl, which will also relieve the secondary aldosteronism. The amount of isotonic NaCl infused should be based on an assessment of clinical volume status, and should be continued until the patient is euvolemic. The amount of K^+ needed will vary among patients, some of whom will require more than 250 mmol. An estimate of the amount of K^+ needed can be obtained from the graphical relationship and equation shown in Fig. 3.5.

Treatment of Hypokalemia

General Principles

Hypokalemia is usually not a medical emergency unless severe (serum [K^+] <2.5 mM) or symptomatic (e.g., disturbances in cardiac conduction, dysrhythmias, neuromuscular weakness, or paralysis). The therapeutic approach to the patient with hypokalemia consists of: (1) identification of the site and cause of K^+ loss; (2) therapy directed at the underlying cause; (3) estimation of the total body K^+ deficit; (4) choice of potassium-containing preparation, route, and rate of administration; and (5) adequate monitoring of serum [K^+] in order to modify therapy appropriately and prevent the development of hyperkalemia.

An important corollary is to identify patients at risk to develop hypokalemia and take preventative measures such as (1) using the lowest effective dose of loop and thiazide diuretics; (2) advising patients to avoid high salt and water intake to prevent increased distal delivery of Na^+ and high urine flow rates; (3) checking for hypomagnesemia and repleting magnesium prior to repleting K^+; and (4) preventing bicarbonaturia and mitigating against metabolic alkalosis.

Estimation of the Total Body K⁺ Deficit

Because more than 98 % of total body K^+ is intracellular, estimation of the K^+ deficit based on sampling the serum [K^+] is not simple or straightforward. A rough rule of thumb is the linear estimation that the serum [K^+] falls by ~0.3 mM for each loss of 100 mmol of total body K^+ [166]. Transforming and using these data, this writer derived the following exponential equation to provide a more accurate estimation of the total body K^+ deficit:

$$K^+ \text{ deficit (mmol)} = 3{,}300 \times \exp(-[K^+]/1.5) - 200$$

where [K^+] is the patient's serum [K^+]. Both the linear and exponential relationships between the serum [K^+] and the estimated K^+ deficit are plotted in Fig. 3.5. It is immediately apparent that the exponential is a much more realistic model, as might have been expected. For example, although both curves meet the boundary condition that the K^+ deficit is ~0 mmol at a serum [K^+] of 4.4 mM, extrapolation to the boundary condition of a serum [K^+] of 0 mM yields a realistic result only for the exponential. The linear relationship yields a total body K^+ deficit of only ~450 mmol, whereas the exponential predicts a total body K^+ deficit of 3,100 mmol, which is quite reasonable.

How well does the exponential relationship predict actual total body K^+ deficits in real life? A few cases taken from the literature shows that the exponential fits well with the empirical results for patients with moderate and severe hypokalemia.

- In subjects with an average serum [K^+] of 3.2 mM, the mean net K^+ loss was 128 mmol; the equations predict a K^+ deficit of 124 mmol [71].
- A single patient with severe hypokalemia ([K^+] = 1.9 mM) in association with metabolic acidosis due to an enterovesical fistula [167]. This patient required ~750 mmol of K^+ to correct her deficit, close to the 788 mmol value predicted by the exponential equation.
- A 22-year-old woman presented with a serum [K^+] of 1.9 mM in the setting of DKA and coma [168]. This patient would also be expected to have a total body K^+ deficit of ~800 mmol. In the actual case, she required 660 mmol of intravenous K^+ during the first 12 h of admission, and then required 40–80 mmol of oral K^+ per day for the next 8 days (320–640 mmol). Therefore, the total amount of K^+ she required was between 980 and 1,300 mmol K^+, more than predicted. However, this is not surprising because this patient also required an insulin drip, which would be expected to obligate additional K^+.
- A 93-year-old woman who presented with hypertension and paralysis and severe hypokalemia (serum [K^+] 1.3 mM) due to chronic ingestion of licorice [169]. The exponential equation estimates a total body K^+ deficit of 1,218 mmol for this patient. In actuality, she required 858 mmol of intravenous and oral K^+, but it is important to note that her management included a K^+-sparing diuretic (spironolactone), which would be predicted to decrease the amount of supplemental K^+ required for repletion.

Given the highly lopsided distribution between the amount of K^+ in the ICF and ECF, it stands to reason that any linear "rule of thumb" would be a small tail trying to wag a large dog. In contrast, the exponential equation is more analytically appealing and appears to provide a much more realistic model for estimating the total body K^+ deficit. Regardless of the method used, one must always be mindful of the limitations of estimating total body K^+ deficit and that there may be considerable variation among patients.

Choice of Potassium-Containing Preparation, Route, and Rate of Administration

Whenever possible, supplemental K^+ should be given orally (or enterally) to emulate the usual physiological and homeostatic mechanisms [101]. Under most conditions, potassium chloride (KCl) is the drug of choice for patients with hypokalemia, metabolic alkalosis, and/or volume depletion. Typically, patients with ongoing losses (e.g., those taking loop or thiazide diuretics) require 20–80 mmol of KCl per day. For hypokalemia developing in the setting of metabolic acidosis (e.g., with diarrhea or renal tubular acidosis), alkalinizing K^+ salts (acetate, citrate, gluconate, or bicarbonate) can be used.

Intravenous (IV) K^+ replacement should be reserved for symptomatic hypokalemia or situations with an element of time urgency (e.g., patients taking digoxin) or in which oral K^+ is not feasible (e.g., vomiting, nasogastric suction, ileus) or not tolerated due to gastrointestinal irritation. When K^+ must be given via the IV route, a "low and slow" approach should be taken [101]. That is, the bag should contain only a limited amount of K^+ (e.g., no more than 40 mM) and the infusion rate should not exceed 20 mmol/h. To minimize insulin-mediated cellular K^+ uptake, the K^+ salt should be dissolved in glucose-free solutions [170]. Infusion via peripheral IV lines is preferred, and to avoid pain and phlebitis, should not exceed 40 mM. Higher concentrations can be given via a central line [171]. For patients with symptomatic or severe hypokalemia (serum $[K^+]$ <2.0 mM) who may require more than 160 mmol over the first few hours of treatment, two peripheral IV lines are required. Such patients should be on a cardiac monitor in the intensive care unit, and serum $[K^+]$ should be measured every 2–4 h and carefully followed [172].

Reducing Renal K^+ Secretion

A therapeutic option in the treatment of hypokalemia is to interfere with K^+ secretion along the collecting duct. This can be achieved either by aldosterone antagonists (spironolactone or eplerenone) or by directly blocking ENaC (amiloride or triamterene). Present day management of hypertension often includes ACE inhibitors or ARBs, which also reduce renal K^+ secretion. Therefore, one way to mitigate the development of thiazide-induced hypokalemia is to combine HCTZ with these agents, and combination pills are now widely available.

Risk of Hyperkalemia

It is important to emphasize that there is always a risk of hyperkalemia when patients are receiving K^+ supplements and/or agents that reduce renal K^+ secretion. Indeed, supplemental K^+ is the most common cause of hyperkalemia in hospitalized patients [86], which can be serious and occasionally lethal. Similar caution is advised for patients who are oliguric or taking nonsteroidal anti-inflammatories, ACE inhibitors, ARBs, or aldosterone antagonists. The importance of careful and frequent monitoring of serum $[K^+]$ in these patients cannot be overstated.

Hyperkalemia: Specific Disorders

Pseudohyperkalemia

The possibility of pseudohyperkalemia should be considered whenever the *serum* $[K^+] \geq$ *plasma* $[K^+] + 0.5$ mM. Also known as factitious hyperkalemia, pseudohyperkalemia is due to an artifact occurring in vitro, and was first described in association with thrombocytosis. If present, it is important to make the diagnosis because pseudohyperkalemia requires no treatment. Indeed, the major hazard associated with pseudohyperkalemia is inadvertent treatment, which could lead to dangerous hypokalemia.

As is the case when RBCs lyze during or after a blood draw, it is the sample—not the individual—that is hyperkalemic. This artifactual increase due to excess K^+ leakage out of the blood cells in the sample can be caused by (1) severe thrombocytosis or leukocytosis; (2) mechanical trauma during venipuncture or fist clenching during phlebotomy, or (3) familial pseudohyperkalemia. In most of the hereditary forms, the pseudohyperkalemia is a result of temperature-sensitive leakage of K^+ out of cells kept below body temperature [173].

Transfer of K^+ from ICF to ECF

Transcellular shifts of K^+ from cells to the ECF occurs under a number of conditions related to *cell lysis* (e.g., rhabdomyolysis, tumor lysis syndrome, massive hemolysis, and ischemic tissue injury), *certain drugs and toxins* (e.g., succinylcholine, somatostatin, digoxin and digoxin-like substances, and barium and fluoride poisonings), or *hyperkalemic periodic paralysis*. It is important to note that in some of these conditions (e.g., digoxin toxicity), the "transcellular shift" may result more from impaired cellular uptake of K^+ (e.g., due to insulinopenia) rather than increased K^+ efflux. For example, the hyperkalemia associated with DKA is primarily due to insulin deficiency.

Cell Lysis

Injury that leads to cell lysis always increases the ECF K^+ load and causes transient hyperkalemia, which can be life threatening if the intensity of the lysis overwhelms internal and external homeostatic mechanisms. Usually, cell lysis does not result in significant hyperkalemia in the absence of other defects in K^+ disposal. However, it is not uncommon for the processes leading to cell lysis to be attended by hypovolemia and/or acute kidney injury (AKI).

Rhabdomyolysis, the breakdown of muscle tissue, has numerous causes both traumatic [174] and nontraumatic [175], and can lead to myoglobinuric AKI. Treatment is supportive, and hyperkalemia developing in normovolemic patients with AKI can be temporized with Kayexalate®, insulin (and glucose), and β_2[beta2]-agonists until dialysis treatment commences.

Tumor lysis syndrome most commonly occurs in hematological malignancies such as acute leukemia and Burkitt's lymphoma, and may be spontaneous or related to chemotherapy. The pathogenesis of hyperkalemia in acute tumor lysis syndrome is analogous to that in rhabdomyolysis, except the lyzed cells are tumor rather than muscle, and the cause of AKI relates to uric acid rather than myoglobin. Treatment for the hyperkalemia itself is as outlined for rhabdomyolysis. Allopurinol has long been the standard treatment to manage the hyperuricemia, although recombinant urate oxidase (rasburicase) is emerging as an effective alternative.

Ischemic tissue injury can occur in patients with severe vascular disease (particularly celiomesenteric) or those who develop arterial embolisms (e.g., lower extremity) or compartment syndromes. Such patients are at high risk to develop hyperkalemia due to ischemic or necrotic tissue. A typical situation is a patient with mesenteric insufficiency who develops hyperkalemia due to ischemic gut. Optimal treatment is surgical management of the underlying lesion when possible; otherwise, treatment is supportive and as outlined above.

Drugs and Toxins

Any drug or toxin that interferes with the action of the Na^+/K^+-ATPase pump (e.g., cardiac glycosides) will promote the development of hyperkalemia, primarily by interfering with cellular K^+ uptake. In addition to digitalis, substances with a ouabain-like effect include several traditional Chinese medicines (e.g., Chan Su, Lu-Shen-Wan, Dan Shen, and Asian ginseng), and herbal remedies prepared from foxglove, lily of the valley, oleander, yew berry, dogbane, red squill, and toad skin. Use of these agents can be tragic; recently, an otherwise healthy man died of severe hyperkalemia after ingestion of aphrodisiac pills containing toad venom [176].

Digoxin

Clinically, digoxin is by far most commonly encountered cardiac glycoside. Digoxin and K^+ both bind to the extracellular side of the Na^+/K^+-

ATPase, and are able to displace each other. This means not only that digoxin toxicity promotes hyperkalemia, but also that hypokalemia potentiates digoxin toxicity. Patients who develop hyperkalemia ([K^+] >5.5 mM) in the setting of digoxin toxicity are also considered to be at increased risk of death. Because calcium is thought to increase arrhythmogenicity in digoxin toxicity, it has long been recommended that calcium salts be given slowly and with caution if at all.

Succinylcholine

Significant hyperkalemia associated with succinylcholine was first reported to occur during anesthesia in patients with severe burns, but also occurs in debilitated patients with degenerative or inflammatory neuromuscular diseases. The pathophysiology appears to involve an increase the number of acetylcholine receptors (AChRs), which migrate out beyond the neuromuscular junction in these conditions and spread throughout the muscle [177]. It is thought that subsequent depolarization of these AChRs by succinylcholine and its metabolites causes K^+ efflux, presumably via voltage-gated K^+ channels. If it is not possible to avoid the use of succinylcholine to anesthetize patients at risk, the prepared anesthesiologist will monitor the EKG and plasma [K^+] carefully and be equipped to treat with insulin (and glucose), if necessary.

Hyperkalemic Periodic Paralysis

HyperPP is caused by hereditary (autosomal dominant) mutations in the α[alpha]-subunit of SCN4A, the voltage-gated Na^+ channel in skeletal muscle [178]. The disorder is characterized by episodic muscle weakness precipitated by exposure to cold, rest following exercise, K^+ ingestion, or glucocorticoids. There are at least four different mutations of SCN4A [179], and certain mutations are associated with fixed muscle weakness. The electrophysiological phenotype is impaired fast inactivation of the channel causing persistent Na^+ currents and prolonged depolarization of skeletal muscle fibers, producing membrane inexcitability and muscle paralysis. A similar disorder has been described in a subset of quarter horses [180] who are descendents of the sire Impressive. Indeed, the number of affected quarter horses has increased rapidly because the muscular phenotype has been a popular selection by show judges.

Treatment

Salbutamol, a β_2[beta]-adrenergic agonist, has been shown to be effective in treating and perhaps preventing attacks. Acetazolamide, which is effective in HypoPP, has also been effective in some patients with HyperPP.

Post-parathyroidectomy

Hyperkalemia develops in the majority of chronic dialysis patients who undergo parathyroidectomy [181]. Although the hyperkalemia is treated with dialysis, the underlying mechanism is uncertain. It is possible that hyperkalemia is a consequence of hypocalcemia, which could promote K^+ transfer out of muscle cells. There is evidence that voltage-gated sodium channels require calcium ions to close [182]. Incomplete closure of voltage-gated sodium channels would tend to depolarize muscle cells, which increases the electrochemical gradient for K^+ efflux.

Excess Potassium Intake

Under normal conditions, excessive K^+ intake should not result in clinically significant hyperkalemia. Indeed, as previously discussed, early human cultures consumed a diet that was much higher in K^+ (up to 400 mmol/day) than our present Western diet, and presumably people did not develop symptomatic hyperkalemia. Of course, it is likely that the steady-state ECF [K^+] was higher in those consuming a higher K^+ diet. On the other hand, reduction of K^+ intake remains a cornerstone in the therapeutic approach to any patient predisposed to hyperkalemia from other factors such as CK$^+$D, so a short discussion of K^+-rich substances is warranted.

Fruits and vegetables are rich in K^+: whereas a typical banana contains 12 mmol K^+, a half cup of raisins contains 15 mmol, a half cup of dried prunes contains 16 mmol, and a baked potato (with skin) contains over 18 mmol. K^+-containing salt substitutes are also a concern, especially in patients with decreased GFR who may also be taking ACEIs or ARBs [183]. There are also a number of herbal remedies that are very high in K^+ including alfalfa, dandelion, hawthorne berries, horsetail, milkweed, nettle, and noni juice. The latter, which has been touted to have a number of health benefits, has ~56 mM of K^+, about the same as in tomato and orange juice.

Finally, there are a few types of pica (pathological craving for substances not generally regarded as food) that harbor danger for high K^+ loads, including ingestion of riverbed clay (geophagia; this clay contains ~1 mmol/g) and ingestion of burnt match heads (cautopyreiophagia) [184]. A patient maintained on hemodialysis with hypogeusia due to zinc deficiency developed cautopyreiophagia and ate enough burnt match heads to add 80 mmol to his daily K^+ intake, and presented with an ECF [K^+] >8 mM [185]. Repletion of zinc reversed both his taste disorder and his cautopyreiophagia.

Decreased Potassium Excretion

Mineralocorticoid Deficiency

A complete description of the causes of primary mineralocorticoid deficiency and mineralocorticoid resistance is beyond the scope of this chapter. All of these etiologies (listed in Table 3.2) impair renal K^+ secretion and therefore predispose to hyperkalemia.

Heparin-Induced Aldosterone Suppression

Heparin and its congeners can decrease renal K^+ secretion because of interference with aldosterone biosynthesis [186, 187]. Heparin-induced hyperkalemia [188], appears to also involve a decrease in the number and affinity of Ang II receptors in the zona glomerulosa of the adrenal cortex, which inhibits Ang II-stimulation of aldosterone production.

Increases in ECF [K^+] occur in about 7–8 % of patients, although significant hyperkalemia is rare in the absence of additional factors that disrupt K^+ handling by the kidney [186]. Aldosterone suppression, which may be clinically heralded by a natriuresis reminiscent of the initial effect of spironolactone, is apparent within 72 h. The effect is reversible, and aldosterone synthesis returns to normal within a week after heparin is discontinued. Because heparin and low molecular weight heparin are so commonly used, heparin-induced aldosterone suppression should be suspected in the differential diagnosis of hyperkalemia in any patient receiving these anticoagulants.

Table 3.2 Mineralocorticoid deficiency (or resistance) predisposing to hyperkalemia

Primary mineralocorticoid deficiency (Addison disease)
1. Autoimmune adrenalitis
a. Isolated adrenal insufficiency
b. Polyglandular autoimmune syndrome
2. Infectious adrenalitis
a. HIV and AIDS
b. Tuberculosis (TB)
c. Disseminated fungal infection
d. Syphilis
3. Congenital adrenal hyperplasia (e.g., 21-hydroxylase deficiency)
4. Isolated aldosterone synthase deficiency
5. Heparin and low molecular weight heparin
6. Adrenal hemorrhage or infarction
7. Metastatic cancer
8. Congenital adrenal hypoplasia
9. Familial hypoaldosteronism
Hyporeninemic hypoaldosteronism
1. Kidney disease (most often diabetic nephropathy)
2. Nonsteroidal anti-inflammatory drugs (NSAIDS)
3. Angiotensin converting enzyme inhibitors (ACEIs)
4. Angiotensin receptor blockers (ARBs)
5. Cyclosporine
6. Obstructive uropathy
Mineralocorticoid resistance
1. Aldosterone antagonists
a. Spironolactone
b. Eplerenone
2. Epithelial Na^+ Channel (ENaC) blockers
a. Amiloride
b. Triamterene
c. Pentamidine
d. Trimethoprim
3. Tubulointerstitial disease
a. Acute kidney injury
Obstructive uropathy
Acute interstitial nephritis
Papillary necrosis
a. Chronic kidney disease
Sickle cell disease
Lupus nephritis
Amyloidosis
Post kidney transplant
4. Pseudohypoaldosteronism

Hyperkalemia Complicating Drug Therapy

Inhibition of the RAAS has become central in the pharmacological management of cardiovascular disease (hypertension and congestive heart failure) and CKD. Given the growing number of patients with diabetes and hypertension who also have nephropathy, hyperkalemia has become a constant concern and common complication in this patient population, especially those with reduced GFR [189]. Hyperkalemia is also a feature of Type 4 RTA, which is most often seen in association with diabetic nephropathy and CKD, but also occurs in the elderly and in patients with obstructive uropathy and sickle cell disease. Kidney transplant recipients may be at additional risk because calcineurin inhibitors (CNIs) such as cyclosporine A and tacrolimus inhibit renal K^+ secretion (see below). As outpatients, use of nonsteroidal anti-inflammatory drugs (NSAIDs) or coxibs will also impair renal K^+ secretion in these patient populations. Finally, when hospitalized for suspicion of an acute coronary syndrome, use of heparin can further reduce renal K^+ secretion in these patients (see section on heparin). Table 3.3 summarizes the clinical circumstances that predispose to hyperkalemia.

Table 3.3 Clinical circumstances predisposing to hyperkalemia

Disease states
1. Diabetes mellitus
2. Type 4 RTA
3. Hyporeninemic hypoaldosteronism
4. Congestive heart failure (CHF)
5. Hypertension
6. Renal hypoperfusion and/or oliguria
7. Chronic kidney disease (CKD)
8. Acute kidney injury (AKI)
Antihypertensives
2. Angiotensin converting enzyme inhibitors (ACEIs)
3. Angiotensin receptor blockers (ARBs)
4. Aldosterone antagonists
a. Spironolactone
b. Eplerenone
5. Epithelial Na^+ channel (ENaC) blockers
c. Amiloride
d. Triamterene
6. Nonspecific β-adrenergic (β_2) blockers
e. Propranolol
f. Labetolol
g. Carvedilol
Other drugs
1. K^+ supplements
2. Nonsteroidal anti-inflammatory drugs (NSAIDs)
3. Cyclooxygenase-2 (COX-2) inhibitors
4. Heparin and congeners
5. Digoxin
6. Calcineurin inhibitors (CNIs)
a. Cyclosporine A (CsA)
b. Tacrolimus (FK506)
7. ENaC blockers
a. Trimethoprim
b. Pentamidine

ACE Inhibitors and ARBs

Angiotensin converting enzyme inhibitors (ACEIs) inhibit the conversion of angiotensin I to Ang II, which leads to a decrease in adrenal aldosterone secretion. ARBs prevent Ang II from binding to the AT1 receptors in arterioles and in the adrenal gland and in arterioles. Both ACEIs and ARBs impair renal K^+ disposal by at least two mechanisms: (1) decreased GFR due to inhibition of Ang II-mediated constriction of the efferent arteriole and (2) decreased adrenal aldosterone secretion. Although hyperkalemia develops in only ~1.5 % of patients without the diseases listed in Table 3.2 [190], it occurs in ~10 % of outpatients treated with ACEIs [191], and ~10–40 % of inpatients receiving ACEIs [86, 90]. While some studies have suggested that ARBs cause less hyperkalemia than ACEIs (e.g., comparison of valsartan versus lisinopril [192]), no significant difference was seen in other studies (e.g., candesartan versus lisinopril [193]).

Aldosterone Antagonists

These K^+-sparing diuretics, spironolactone and eplerenone, bind to the mineralocorticoid receptor and directly interfere with the K^+ secretory effects of aldosterone along the distal nephron. The clinical use of these agents has increased enormously since 1999, after the RALES study suggested that spironolactone use significantly reduced morbidity and mortality in patients with moderate to severe CHF [91]. Although the incidence of hyperkalemia was low in this study (spironolactone was stopped in 8 % of patients), one must bear in mind that patients were excluded for baseline serum

$[K^+]$ >5 mM or serum [creatinine] >2.5 mg/dL, and patients in the study were carefully monitored. Analysis of the impact of the RALES study on spironolactone-associated hyperkalemia performed 5 years later showed a significant increase in both the rate of hospitalization for hyperkalemia (from 2.4 to 11.0 per 1,000 patients) and mortality related to hyperkalemia (from 0.3 to 2.0 per 100 patients) [92].

In one retrospective study [194], 125 consecutive patients referred to a heart failure clinic (mean left ventricular ejection fraction 29 %) were studied. The majority (90 %) had either New York Heart Association (NYHA) class II or III, the mean age was 72.9 years and the baseline serum $[K^+]$ was 4.2 ± 0.3 mM. Sixty of the patients were already on spironolactone, and the remaining 65 were placed on spironolactone. The majority of patients (86 %) were taking an ACEI or ARB and 76 % were initially taking K^+ supplements (presumably discontinued unless proven necessary). Over the 2-year study, 36 % of the patients developed serum $[K^+]$ >5 mM, with 17 % >5.5 mM and 10 % >6 mM. The authors conclude that the risk factors for hyperkalemia include age, NYHA functional class, and ejection fraction.

Other groups have demonstrated similar results, emphasizing that the conditions of the RALES study do not necessarily translate to the clinic, especially because of differences in patient comorbidities such as diabetes and medications, particularly beta-blockers.

ENaC Blockers

Blockade of the ENaC conductance in the apical membrane of PCs abrogates the membrane depolarization that drives K^+ secretion along the collecting duct. In addition to classical diuretics (amiloride and triamterene), the antimicrobials trimethoprim [195] and pentamidine have been shown to cause hyperkalemia by ENaC blockade.

Nonspecific β[beta]-Adrenergic (β_2) [beta2] Blockers

As mentioned, β_2[beta2]-adrenergic receptor agonists promote cellular uptake of K^+ by stimulating the Na^+/K^+-ATPase, such that nonspecific β[beta]-blockers can impair internal K^+ homeostasis. Because the sympathetic nervous system stimulates renin release, these agents can also impair external K^+ homeostasis. Although the use of first-generation nonspecific β[beta]-blockers (e.g., propanolol) has declined in recent years, the clinical utility of labetalol and especially carvedilol has led to a resurgence. Although hyperkalemia is rare when β[beta]-blockers are used alone, their use may predispose to a significant increase in serum $[K^+]$ when used in combination with ACEIs, ARBs, and/or aldosterone antagonists.

NSAIDs and Coxibs

By interfering with prostaglandin (especially PGE2 ad PGI2) biosynthesis, these agents impair renal K^+ disposal by lowering GFR by constriction of the afferent arteriole, and by decreasing renin release. The latter attenuates aldosterone-mediated effects on distal K^+ secretion. The risk of hyperkalemia is higher in patients with advanced age, CKD, and those taking ACEIs, ARBs, and/or aldosterone antagonists [90, 189].

Calcineurin Inhibitors

The ability of CNIs to impair renal K^+ secretion may be multifactorial, as studies have suggested that they inhibit renin secretion, decrease tubular sensitivity to aldosterone, inhibit the activity of the Na^+/K^+-ATPase pump, and suppress apical K^+ channels in (rabbit) collecting duct.

Clinical Approach to Hyperkalemia

The risk for the development of hyperkalemia should be assessed in all patients who have an underlying defect in renal K^+ excretion. Factors placing a patient at high risk include advanced age and any of the items listed in Tables 3.2 and 3.3. Steps to assess and minimize the development of hyperkalemia include:

1. *Restrict K^+ intake.* Take a complete dietary and medication history and eliminate any unnecessary K^+ intake. A list and/or picture menu of foods high in K^+ should be discussed and given

to every patient at risk. Many patients are not aware that some salt substitutes and many fruits, vegetables, and juices are rich in potassium.

2. *Minimize the use of NSAIDs and coxibs.* Discuss alternative methods to relieve chronic pain (e.g., exercise, physical therapy, acetaminophen, gabapentin, etc.). Attempt to discontinue any other nonessential substances that may interfere with K^+ excretion.
3. *Add a loop or thiazide diuretic.* Thiazides can promote K^+ excretion in patients with hypertension. Loop diuretics also increase K^+ excretion and should be used in patients with hypervolemic disorders and/or those with CKD (stage 4 or worse).
4. *Begin therapy with the minimally effective dose of ACEIs, ARBs, and aldosterone antagonists.* For example, although the typical dose of spironolactone is 25 mg daily, some patients may only require 12.5 mg daily.
5. *Measure serum [K^+] and [creatinine] within 10–14 days after adding or modifying ACEI, ARB, or aldosterone antagonist therapy.*
6. *Monitor serum [K^+] periodically.* Doses of these medications should be decreased if serum [K^+] rises to 5.6 mM; the drug should be stopped if serum [K^+] rises further.

Finally, careful attention should be paid to maintaining euvolemia because hypovolemia potentiates the development of hyperkalemia in patients on any of these medications.

Treatment of Hyperkalemia

Severe hyperkalemia is a medical emergency. Although there is some variation among institutions, hyperkalemia here is defined as serum [K^+] >5.0 mM. Grading the severity of hyperkalemia varies somewhat in the medical literature, but has been classified as mild (5.5–6.0 mM), moderate (6.1–6.9 mM), or severe (>7.0 mM) [4]. Once pseudohyperkalemia has been considered and excluded, the most important (and sometimes the most difficult) step is deciding who is in need of immediate therapy. Beyond the "snapshot" level of serum [K^+], other factors should be considered in making the decision to initiate therapy for hyperkalemia: (1) any effects on the cardiac conduction system, (2) the presence of muscle weakness, (3) the rate of change in serum [K^+], (4) other medications, particularly digoxin or drugs that impair K^+ excretion, (5) kidney function, (6) the degree to which adaptation to hyperkalemia can be expected to have occurred [19], and (7) the underlying cause, particularly if there is good reason to believe a further increase in ECF [K^+] is likely (e.g., rhabdomyolysis).

Hyperkalemia causes membrane depolarization that decreases cardiac cell conduction velocity and increases the rate of repolarization. In general, worsening hyperkalemia is associated with a progression in ECG abnormalities (see Fig. 3.6): (1) peaked or "tented" T waves, (2) prolonged PR interval, (3) widening of the QRS complex, (4) decrease or loss of P waves, (5) degeneration into a "sine-wave" pattern, and finally (6) asystole. Therefore, it is no surprise that many authorities consider the presence of any acute ECG abnormality to be a medical emergency that should be immediately antagonized with calcium salts.

On the other hand, it must be appreciated that the ECG is not reliable as a sensitive indicator of hyperkalemia; poor correlation between the two has been exemplified in cases where the ECG was largely unaffected despite severe hyperkalemia [196]. The correlation between hyperkalemia and ECG abnormalities tends to be tighter in animal studies, probably because the experimental protocols more closely simulate acute hyperkalemia, whereas human hyperkalemia often has a chronic component. In human studies where acute hyperkalemia was induced by ingestion of large boluses of potassium salts, most of the otherwise healthy volunteers exhibited the abnormalities expected on ECG [197, 198]. If enough potassium is ingested to cause the serum [K^+] to exceed 6.5 mM, essentially all volunteers will at least exhibit peaked T waves [198]. On the other hand, patients with CKD "adapt" to hyperkalemia (see [19] and section on potassium adaptation) and may not exhibit ECG abnormalities until hyperkalemia becomes severe (e.g., >7.5 mM) [199].

There is a four-pronged therapeutic approach for the patient with severe hyperkalemia (sum-

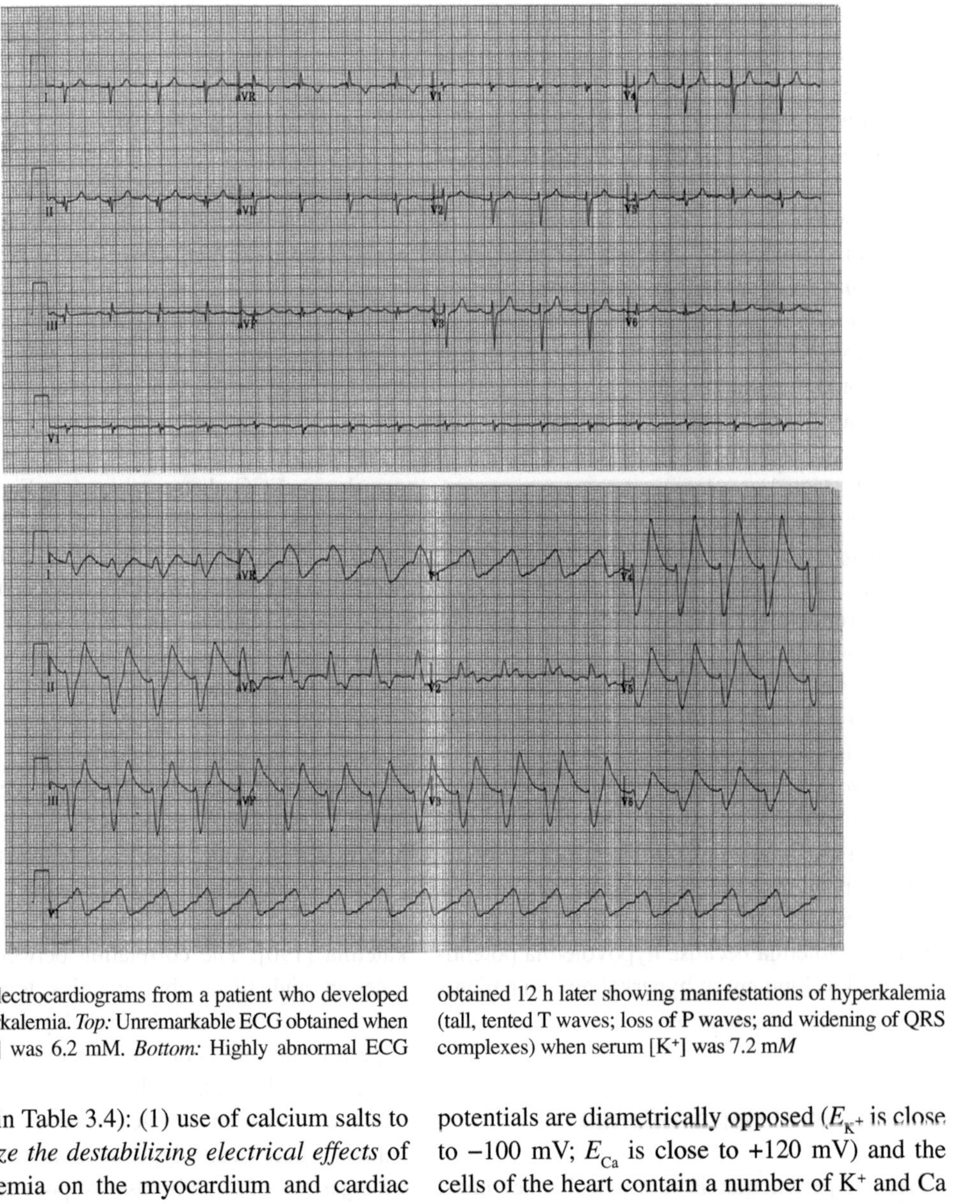

Fig. 3.6 Electrocardiograms from a patient who developed acute hyperkalemia. *Top:* Unremarkable ECG obtained when serum [K+] was 6.2 mM. *Bottom:* Highly abnormal ECG obtained 12 h later showing manifestations of hyperkalemia (tall, tented T waves; loss of P waves; and widening of QRS complexes) when serum [K+] was 7.2 m*M*

marized in Table 3.4): (1) use of calcium salts to *antagonize the destabilizing electrical effects* of hyperkalemia on the myocardium and cardiac conduction system, (2) use of insulin (with glucose), β_2[beta2]-agonists, and perhaps bicarbonate to *promote the cellular uptake of K+* from ECF to ICF, (3) *removal of K+* from the body, and (4) identification (and elimination) of the underlying cause(s) to plan *long-term management.*

Antagonize the Destabilizing Electrical Effects of Hyperkalemia on the Heart

The mutual antagonism between calcium and potassium salts lies in the fact that their Nernst potentials are diametrically opposed (E_{K^+} is close to −100 mV; E_{Ca} is close to +120 mV) and the cells of the heart contain a number of K^+ and Ca channels that are tightly regulated by voltage [200]. However, the precise molecular mechanisms underlying this mutual antagonism are not known with certainty. The "surface charge hypothesis" is a possible explanation [201]. According to this hypothesis, the deposition of divalent Ca^{2+} ions on the extracellular surface creates a microenvironment that tends to repolarize the myocardial membrane, which helps stabilize otherwise depolarized voltage-gated channels. If the "surface charge hypothesis" is correct, it should be possible to substitute another divalent cation (e.g., Mg^{2+}) with

Table 3.4 Treatment of hyperkalemia

1) Protect the heart a. *Calcium salts:* to antagonize the destabilizing electrical effects of hyperkalemia on the myocardium and cardiac conduction system i. Ampule (10 mL) of 10 % Ca-Gluconate pushed over 2–3 min (20–30 min if patient on cardiac glycosides) and repeated in 5 min if needed ii. Effect is short-lived, ~20 min
2) Reduce ECF [K^+] a. Replete ECF volume b. Promote transfer of K^+ from ECF→ICF i. *Insulin* 10 units IV followed by a 50-mL ampule of 50 % dextrose (in non-hyperglycemic patients) 1. Works by activating the Na^+/K^+-ATPase 2. Effect begins within 20 min, peaks at 30–60 min, and lasts 4–6 h 3. Follow fingerstick blood sugar ii. β_2(beta2)-adrenergic receptor agonists 1. Works via the cAMP second messenger system 2. Inhaled albuterol 10–20 mg by nebulizer 3. Effect begins within 30 min, peaks at 90–120 min, and lasts 4–6 h
3) Remove K^+ from the body a. Enhance renal K^+ excretion i. Stop ACEIs, ARBs, and spironolactone ii. Loop and/or thiazide diuretics iii. Fludrocortisone b. Promote enteral K^+ loss i. *Cation exchange resins* combined with an osmotic laxative 1. Sodium polystyrene sulfonate (Kayexalate®) 2. May give orally or as a high colonic 3. Risk of colonic necrosis c. Conventional hemodialysis i. Most efficient and reliable method for removing K^+ ii. Up to half of the K^+ removed from the ECF is "replaced" by transfer of K^+ from the ICF
4) Follow-up and long-term management a. Carefully monitor ECF [K^+] and watch for rebound b. Look for the presence of any dietary factors (e.g., fruits and vegetables high in K^+) or the use of salt substitutes containing K^+ c. Carefully review the medication list for any drugs that might impair K^+ excretion d. Caution patients who take combinations of diuretics, K^+ supplements, NSAIDs, ACE inhibitors, ARBs, and/or aldosterone antagonists to hold these medications if they develop acute volume losses (e.g., acute gastroenteritis)

equal efficacy, but this does not appear to be the case.

It is possible that Ca^{2+} effectively antagonizes hyperkalemic depolarization by allowing voltage-gated Na^+ channels to close. Experiments performed on squid axon strongly suggest that voltage-gated Na^+ channels must bind a Ca^{2+} ion in order to close [182, 202, 203]. If this requirement holds in hearts subjected to the depolarizing effect of hyperkalemia, then administration of Ca^{2+} would facilitate the closing of voltage-gated Na^+ channels, which would allow repolarization of the membrane potential. Perhaps this mechanism, in addition to possible surface charge effects, underlies the salutary action of calcium in stabilizing the cardiac membrane in hyperkalemia.

Administration of Calcium Salts in Hyperkalemia

Most authorities recommend that calcium be given to patients with severe hyperkalemia ([K^+] >7.0 mM) or those with moderate hyperkalemia who manifest acute abnormalities on ECG [204]. ECG changes (see Fig. 3.6) include tall or tented T waves larger than 5 mm ([K^+] 6–7 mM), small or absent P waves, widening of the QRS complex ([K^+] 7–8 mM), sinusoidal QRST waveform ([K^+] 8–9 mM), and A-V dissociation or ventricular tachycardia or fibrillation ([K^+] >9 mM). As mentioned however, there have been case reports of patients with [K^+] >8 mM without significant abnormalities on ECG [196].

Either calcium gluconate or calcium chloride can be administered intravenously, but calcium gluconate is preferred because it can be given through a peripheral line and is less irritating to the vasculature and to surrounding tissues in case of extravasation. A 10 mL ampule of 10 % calcium gluconate (93 mg of elemental calcium) can be given as an intravenous push over 2–5 min, and repeated in 5 min if there is no improvement or further deterioration. The onset of the effect is rapid, often within seconds and should clearly be apparent within several minutes. As expected however, the efficacy of an ampule only lasts on the order of minutes, from less than 20 min to up to 60 min.

Use of Calcium Salts in Hyperkalemic Patients Taking Cardiac Glycosides

Most authorities recommend that intravenous calcium salts be used with extreme caution (if at all) in hyperkalemic patients taking cardiac glycosides. Older studies supported the existence of a synergistic relationship between digitalis and calcium [205, 206], but controversy has developed over the years [206] as more carefully performed studies failed to demonstrate such synergism [207]. A study performed in dogs addressed the question directly, and the investigators concluded that a dangerous interaction only occurred with severe hypercalcemia (serum calcium >30 mg/dL) [208].

Finally, it is important to emphasize that patients with digoxin toxicity often present with hyperkalemia as a direct result of inhibition of the Na^+/K^+-ATPase. Optimal treatment under these conditions would include the use of digoxin-specific Fab fragments [209, 210]. In the first of these case reports [209], the digitoxic patient had a $[K^+]$ of 8.1 mM that worsened to 8.8 mM despite treatment with intravenous calcium, insulin and glucose, and bicarbonate. In the second report [210], the patient was severely digitoxic (8.4 ng/mL) and presented with a serum $[K^+]$ of 9.9 mM. Both patients were treated with hemodialysis and digoxin Fab fragments and recovered. Interestingly, both of these severely hyperkalemic and digitoxic patients were also treated with intravenous 10 % calcium chloride (two ampules in the first patient) without ill effects.

Reduce the Extracellular K^+

Of course, the administration of calcium salts does not affect the distribution or excretion of potassium so dangerously high ECF $[K^+]$ levels will persist unless other measures are taken. At this point, therapy is focused on maneuvers that reduce the extracellular K^+ load and promote the cellular uptake of K^+ and alter its distribution.

Replete ECF Volume

An often overlooked aspect in the treatment of hyperkalemia is awareness of the benefit of repleting ECF volume if a component of hypovolemia is present. Consider a 70-kg man who takes an ARB and normally has an ECF volume of 14 L and serum $[K^+]$ of 4.5 mM. The total amount of ECF K^+ is 63 mmol. Now imagine he becomes ill, loses 3 L of ECF volume, and is found to have a serum $[K^+]$ of 7.5 mM (total amount of ECF K^+ now 7.5 mmol/L × 11 L = 82.5 mmol). By simply giving the patient 3 L of isotonic saline, the ECF $[K^+]$ will decrease from a dangerous level of 7.5 mM to a much safer level of 5.9 mM, even in the absence of kidney function.

Promote the Cellular Uptake of K^+

A cornerstone of care in the acute management of hyperkalemia is to administer agents that transfer K^+ from ECF→ICF. Several classes of medications have been used over the decades, and some traditional agents (e.g., sodium bicarbonate, especially in dialysis patients [204]) have fallen out of favor due to lack of proven efficacy. Currently, the major drugs used to promote the cellular uptake of K^+ are *insulin* (usually given with glucose) and β_2[beta2]-*adrenergic receptor agonists.*

Insulin

Baseline insulin levels play a key role in extrarenal potassium homeostasis, and intravenous insulin is uniformly efficacious in promoting the cellular uptake of K^+. A simple, effective approach is to administer 10 units of regular insulin as an intravenous bolus, followed by a 25 g bolus of glucose (one 50 mL ampule of 50 % dextrose) in patients who are not hyperglycemic (i.e., blood glucose level <250 mg/dL). Although glucose should also stimulate endogenous insulin secretion in nondiabetics, the bolus of dextrose is primarily aimed at preventing hypoglycemia. The hypokalemic effect of insulin usually begins within 20 min, peaks between 30 and 60 min, and lasts for 4–6 h. To decrease the incidence of hypoglycemia, some have advocated giving the bolus of dextrose before the insulin. In addition to frequent measurements of serum $[K^+]$, patients should be monitored closely for signs of hypoglycemia and fingerstick blood glucose levels carefully followed.

β_2[beta2]-Adrenergic Receptor Agonists

Stimulation of the β_2[beta2]-adrenergic receptor promotes cellular uptake of K^+ via the cAMP second messenger system. The effect is independent of insulin, aldosterone, and kidney function. In the United States, intravenous administration of β_2[beta2]-agonists is not approved for the treatment of hyperkalemia, so inhaled albuterol is the current β_2[beta2]-adrenergic agonist of choice. The dose is 10–20 mg (5 mg/mL) conveniently delivered by nebulizer, which is five to ten times the dose used in the treatment of asthma. The onset of action is usually within 30 min, with peak effect occurring at 90–120 min. The main side effect is tachycardia. Responders experience a decrease in ECF [K^+] of 0.6–1 mM, but it is important to note that for unclear reasons, 40–50 % of patients on dialysis do not respond to this therapy [211]. Therefore, it is recommended that inhaled albuterol should not be used as monotherapy for hyperkalemia.

Sodium Bicarbonate

Bicarbonate therapy is no longer considered a first- or even second-line agent in the treatment of hyperkalemia. Although studies in the pre-dialysis era suggested a salutary effect, careful recent studies have failed to show bicarbonate has a role in the initial management (first hour) of hyperkalemia in patients without significant acidosis [212, 213]. In view of the other, more reliable agents discussed above and potential adverse side effects including volume overload, sodium bicarbonate use in hyperkalemia should be limited to those patients who also have severe metabolic acidosis.

Combination Therapy

Because insulin and β_2[beta2]-adrenergic agonists activate the Na^+/K^+-ATPase by independent mechanisms, these two treatments may be combined to achieve an additive hypokalemic effect [214]. Such an approach also has the advantages of reducing the chance of hypoglycemia and being effective in most dialysis patients [211].

Remove K^+ from the Body

Assuming hyperkalemia is due to total body K^+ overload, ultimate therapy of hyperkalemia requires maneuvers that remove K^+ from the body. There are three routes for elimination of K^+: (1) via the kidney using diuretics or mineralocorticoids, (2) via the lower GI tract using cation exchange resins, mineralocorticoids, and/or inducing diarrhea, and (3) via an extracorporeal circuit using dialysis.

Enhance Renal K^+ Excretion

The two main maneuvers involve certain diuretics and mineralocorticoids.

Diuretics

Patients with CKD often have comorbid conditions including hypertension and/or volume overload, and some may develop chronic hyperkalemia particularly if there management includes ACE inhibitors, ARBs, and/or aldosterone blockers. The kaliuretic effect of thiazide or loop diuretics in this setting can help potassium homeostasis is such patients. Of course, the efficacy of diuretics in this setting is limited by functioning nephron mass, and will be of minimal benefit to patients maintained on dialysis.

Mineralocorticoids

Theoretically, exogenous mineralocorticoids (e.g., fludrocortisone 0.1–0.2 mg/day) could be used to increase both colonic and renal K^+ secretion. Practically, however, this therapy directly conflicts with the benefits associated with ACE inhibitors, ARBs, and/or aldosterone blockers; and is limited by increased Na^+ reabsorption and exacerbation of hypertension and/or volume overload.

Promote Enteral K^+ Loss

In the absence of adequate kidney function, the only way to remove K^+ from the body without (or while arranging for) dialysis is to stimulate enteral K^+ secretion. GI losses of K^+ are enhanced by cation exchange resins and agents that induce osmotic diarrhea. Both modes of action are combined when a cathartic such as sorbitol is used with sodium polystyrene sulfonate (SPS, Kayexalate®) resin. A third way to promote colonic K^+ secretion is to activate the MR in these cells; either directly with an exogenous mineralocorticoid, or indirectly via inhibition of the enzyme (11β[beta]-HSD2) that converts cortisol to cortisone.

Cation Exchange Resin

Kayexalate® contains 4 mmol Na^+ per gram and binds secreted K^+ (in exchange for Na^+) primarily in the colon. Each gram of resin binds ~0.4–1.2 mmol of K^+ in exchange for ~2–3 mmol of Na^+; so 30-g of resin can be expected to remove ~12–36 mmol of K^+, but at the "cost" of an Na^+ load of ~60–90 mmol.

Originally, SPS resin was given as a powder in water, but more often a resin-laxative combination was given orally or as a (high colonic) enema. Patients have usually been given 15–60 g of the resin with 25 g of sorbitol. When given orally, it takes at least 2 h to get to the site of K^+ secretion, but most or all of the exchange sites in the resin will be utilized. The peak effect occurs after 4–6 h, and may continue for 24 h. For more urgent situations, a retention enema was recommended at a dose of 40–60 g of the resin with 25 g of sorbitol in 250 mL of water.

SPS resin in combination with sorbitol (33 or 70 %) was used for ten decades, but increasing reports of colonic necrosis in certain types of patients led the Food and Drug Administration (FDA) to recommend against their simultaneous use in September 2009. Colonic necrosis is the most serious adverse effect associated with resin-cathartic therapy, and appears to be more related to sorbitol than to the resin [215]. Patients at particular risk are those who are volume-depleted, have significant vascular or gastrointestinal disease, or are post-operative [216–218]. The incidence of this catastrophic complication has been estimated to be 1.8 % in post-operative patients [216].

Importantly, the FDA warning has been applied only to the use of SPS resin with 70 % sorbitol, and has not been expressly applied to the label of the premixed suspension of SPS resin in 33 % sorbitol still stocked by many hospitals. This is presumably because nearly all of the reports of colonic necrosis have been associated with the use of 70 % sorbitol. The following text is taken from the FDA Web site (accessed April 1, 2011) (http://www.fda.gov/Safety/MedWatch/SafetyInformation/ucm186845.htm)

> FDA September 2009: Colonic Necrosis
>
> Cases of colonic necrosis and other serious gastrointestinal adverse events (bleeding, ischemic colitis, perforation) have been reported in association with Kayexalate use. The majority of these cases reported the concomitant use of sorbitol. Risk factors for gastrointestinal adverse events were present in many of the cases including prematurity, history of intestinal disease or surgery hypovolemia, and renal insufficiency and failure. Concomitant administration of sorbitol is not recommended.
>
> FDA January 2011: Colonic Necrosis
>
> Cases of intestinal necrosis, which may be fatal, and other serious gastrointestinal adverse events (bleeding, ischemic colitis, perforation) have been reported in association with Kayexalate use.
>
> Do not use in patients who do not have normal bowel function. This includes postoperative patients who have not had a bowel movement post surgery.
>
> Do not use in patients who are at risk for developing constipation or impaction (including those with history of impaction, chronic constipation, inflammatory bowel disease, ischemic colitis, vascular intestinal atherosclerosis, previous bowel resection, or bowel obstruction)
>
> Discontinue use in patients who develop constipation. Do not administer repeated doses in patients who have not passed a bowel movement.
>
> Concomitant use of Sorbitol with Kayexalate has been implicated in cases of colonic intestinal necrosis, which may be fatal.

Recommendations for Using SPS

Although the overall efficacy and safety of SPS remains controversial [219, 220], we generally agree with the viewpoints expressed by Watson et al. [220] that—in the absence of dialysis—SPS is currently the only way to remove potassium from hyperkalemic patients who lack kidney function. In circumstances where hyperkalemia occurs in the setting of acute kidney failure (e.g., crush injury, earthquakes, etc.) or when chronic dialysis patients cannot get to a functional dialysis unit (e.g., during Hurricane Katrina), SPS may be the only treatment available. Keeping the FDA warnings in mind, we initially recommend the use of SPS powder in water whenever possible. If that is not effective, we would consider the use of premixed SPS in 33 % sorbitol orally as long as the patient is not in any of the categories specified in the FDA warning. High colonic retention enemas of SPS in aqueous solutions can be given when the oral route cannot be used, but SPS enemas in combination with sorbitol should not be used. Given the delay of several hours before SPS becomes effective, the risk probably outweigh the benefits in a chronic dialysis patient with access who can be placed on dialysis within 3–4 h.

Caveats on Using SPS

The use of SPS presents a dilemma. On the one hand, the temptation to administer SPS is almost irresistible when caring for a hyperkalemic patient with decreased kidney function and no established access for dialysis. On the other hand, there seems little doubt that a substantial percentage of SPS use is probably unnecessary and does expose the patient to small but real risks. Therefore, in addition to the recommendations above, the following caveats should be kept in mind:

- It is likely that SPS is overused in dialysis patients. As mentioned, the risk of SPS probably outweighs the benefits in chronic dialysis patients with a functional access who can be placed on dialysis within 4 h
- There is no guarantee that SPS is safe even in the absence of sorbitol. SPS crystals can often be detected adherent to the injured mucosa in human pathological specimens [221, 222]. For instance, a case of colonic necrosis following oral SPS without sorbitol directly implicates SPS [223].
- The risk of colonic necrosis exists even when patients at "high-risk" are avoided. The risk of intestinal necrosis is thought to be greatest when SPS is given with sorbitol within the first post-operative week. For example, when SPS with sorbitol was given to 117 patients within the first post-operative week, two patients (1.7 %) developed intestinal necrosis [216]. Notably, however, in a recent case series of patients given SPS in sorbitol, only 2 of the 11 confirmed cases of intestinal necrosis occurred in the post-operative setting [221].

Laxatives and Cathartics

Despite the FDA warnings regarding the combined use of SPS and cathartics, 70 % sorbitol alone is still available as an osmotic laxative. Even without a resin, stimulation of the bowel and a decrease in transit time enhances K^+ loss from the GI tract. In one study of healthy subjects, the effect of several laxatives with and without a resin was compared using 12 h stool collections [224]. The results showed that yellow phenolphthalein/docusate (Correctol®) caused more Na^+ and K^+ losses than either sorbitol or sodium sulfate, and that resin recovery in the stool was also higher with the phenolphthalein/docusate. Total fecal K^+ excretion was highest when phenolphthalein/docusate and resin were combined. Notably, sorbitol caused more adverse effects in these healthy subjects, which is significant because sorbitol use has been associated with colonic necrosis, as mentioned [225]. These results suggest that phenolphthalein/docusate is superior to sorbitol and that the most efficacious combination for K^+ loss from the GI tract is phenolphthalein/docusate and sodium polystyrene sulfonate.

Efficacy in End Stage Kidney Disease

Whether the resin itself is actually effective in dialysis patients is unclear. One study showed not only that adding resin to phenolphthalein/docusate did not increase the net fecal potassium, but also that none of four resin-cathartic combinations produced significant decreases in the serum $[K^+]$ [226]. Indeed, some authorities are not convinced that a resin removes more K^+ than the diarrhea induced by the cathartic alone, and they no longer use resins in the treatment of acute hyperkalemia [227].

Mineralocorticoid Receptor Activation

One study has shown that administration of GA for 2 weeks lowered the serum [K^+] of anuric dialysis patients without increasing blood pressure [161]. Recall that GA is the substance found in black licorice that inhibits 11β[beta]-HSD2, which then allows cortisol to access the MR. In a recent prospective, double-blind, placebo-controlled crossover study, chronic hemodialysis patients were given cookies or bread rolls containing 18-β-glycyrrhetinic acid (500 mg twice daily) or placebo [228]. The results of this 6-month study showed that average serum [K^+] was ~1 mM lower on GA, and the incidence of hyperkalemia ([K^+] ≥6 mM) decreased from 9 to 0.6 %. Although no toxic side effects were noted, chronic MR stimulation in the cardiovascular system is known to promote inflammation and fibrosis.

Extracorporeal Removal of K^+ from the Body

Conventional hemodialysis is the most efficient and reliable method for removing K^+ from the body. However, the problem in practice is the delay inherent in establishing access to the circulation (in non-dialysis patients) and assembling the dialysis team when patients with severe hyperkalemia present during off-hours.

The total amount of K^+ removed depends on physical factors such as the characteristics of the hemofilter (e.g., surface area), antiparallel flow rate between blood and dialysate, and the intensity of the treatment (e.g., duration, blood-dialysate K^+ gradient). Other important factors include the rate at which K^+ removed from the ECF is "replaced" by K^+ from the ICF for subsequent removal and the glucose level of the dialysate [229]. Glucose-free dialysates are associated with more efficient K^+ removal, probably because of lower intra-dialytic insulin release. In general, about 40 % of the total K^+ removed by hemodialysis comes from the ECF.

One study performed on stable dialysis patients showed that total K^+ removal over a 4 h dialysis session was ~50 mmol on a standard 2 mM K^+ bath, ~63 mmol on a 1 mM bath, and 78.5 mmol on a K^+-free bath [230]. Consider a 65-kg male dialysis patient with a pre-dialysis serum [K^+] of 6.0 mM. His total ECF K^+ is $13 \times 6 = 78$ mmol. If dialyzed for 4 h against a standard 2 mM bath and 50 mmol K^+ was removed exclusively from the ECF (with no change in volume), his post-dialysis serum [K^+] would be ~2.15 mM. However, it would more likely be ~4.0 mM, suggesting that about half the K^+ removed from the ECF is "replaced" by K^+ from the ICF. Extrapolating from this example, dialyzing him against a 1 mM bath would result in a post-dialysis [K^+] of ~3.6 mM; a K^+-free bath would remove the equivalent of all of his ECF K^+, but ~39 mmol would move out from the ICF, resulting in a post-dialysis [K^+] of about 3.0 mM.

Obviously, more K^+ will be removed from patients with hyperkalemia due to a higher blood-dialysate gradient. It follows that the highest rate of K^+ removal will occur during first hour of dialysis. However, rapid falls in serum [K^+]—which are more likely to occur with 0–1 mM K^+ dialysates—may be associated with problems such as rebound hypertension or arrhythmias [231]. Therefore, it may be prudent to minimize the use of very low K^+ dialysates, put patients at risk on a cardiac monitor, and perhaps use potassium profiling to remove K^+ steadily but gradually [232].

Follow-Up and Long-Term Management

The serum [K^+] may rebound after acute maneuvers to treat hyperkalemia (e.g., post-dialysis rebound), so it should be checked every 2–4 h until stable acceptable values are achieved. Once the acute episode is over, efforts must be made to determine the underlying causes leading to the development of hyperkalemia, and a plan should be made to avoid future difficulties with potassium homeostasis. As discussed, loop or thiazide diuretics may help certain patients who still have some functioning renal mass.

Table 3.5 Substances predisposing to hyperkalemia

Exogenous potassium
High K^+ foods
K^+-containing salt substitutes
K^+ supplements
K^+-containing medication (e.g., K^+ penicillin G)
Other sources of K^+ in hospitalized patients
Stored blood
Collins solution
Nutritional supplements
TPN
Herbal remedies
Alfalfa
Dandelion
Hawthorne berries
Horsetail
Milkweed
Nettle
Noni juice
Transcellular shift (ICF→ECF)
Herbal remedies that inhibit the Na^+/K^{++}-ATPase
Chan su
Dogbane
Foxglove
Lily of the valley
Oleander
Red squill
Siberian ginseng
Toad skin
Yew berry

Table 3.5 lists some usual and some unusual substances that can predispose to hyperkalemia, and a review of the following points with patients and their family is recommended:

- Look for the presence of any dietary factors, such as the ingestion of favorite fruits and vegetables that have come into season or the use of salt substitutes containing K^+.
- A list—or better yet, picture menus—of foods with acceptable levels of K^+ and foods high in K should be given to all patients at risk for hyperkalemia.
- Carefully review the medication list for any drugs that might impair K excretion.
- Caution patients who take combinations of diuretics, K supplements, NSAIDs, ACE inhibitors, ARBs, and/or aldosterone antagonists to hold these medications if they develop acute volume losses (e.g., acute gastroenteritis) and to call their physician immediately.

References

1. Fulop M. Hyperkalemia in diabetic ketoacidosis. Am J Med Sci. 1990;299:164–9.
2. Singhal PC, Venkatesan J, Gibbons N, Gibbons J. Prevalence and predictors of rhabdomyolysis in patients with hypokalemia. N Engl J Med. 1990;323:1488.
3. Helfant RH. Hypokalemia and arrhythmias. Am J Med. 1986;80:13–22.
4. Mandal AK. Hypokalemia and hyperkalemia. Med Clin North Am. 1997;81:611–39.
5. Schwartz WB, Relman AS. Effects of electrolyte disorders on renal structure and function. N Engl J Med. 1967;276:383–9. contd.
6. Montague BT, Ouellette JR, Buller GK. Retrospective review of the frequency of ECG changes in hyperkalemia. Clin J Am Soc Nephrol. 2008;3:324–30.
7. Littmann L, Monroe MH, Taylor 3rd L, Brearley Jr WD. The hyperkalemic Brugada sign. J Electrocardiol. 2007;40:53–9.
8. Tanawuttiwat T, Harindhanavudhi T, Bhan A, Dia M. Hyperkalemia-induced Brugada pattern: an unusual manifestation. J Cardiovasc Med (Hagerstown). 2010;11:285–7.
9. Mason B. Principles of geochemistry. 3rd ed. New York: Wiley; 1966.
10. Hardison R. Hemoglobins from bacteria to man: evolution of different patterns of gene expression. J Exp Biol. 1998;201:1099–117.
11. Clausen T. Na^+-K^+ pump regulation and skeletal muscle contractility. Physiol Rev. 2003;83:1269–324.
12. Stein WD. The sodium pump in the evolution of animal cells. Philos Trans R Soc Lond B Biol Sci. 1995;349:263–9.
13. Hebert SC, Desir G, Giebisch G, Wang W. Molecular diversity and regulation of renal potassium channels. Physiol Rev. 2005;85:319–71.
14. Bygrave FL. The ionic environment and metabolic control. Nature. 1967;214:667–71.
15. Giebisch GH. A trail of research on potassium. Kidney Int. 2002;62:1498–512.
16. Mills B, Tupper JT. Cell cycle dependent changes in potassium transport. J Cell Physiol. 1976;89: 123–32.
17. Davy H. 1807 Bakerian Lecture: on some new phenomena of chemical changes produced by electricity, particularly the decomposition of fixed alkalies, and the exhibition of the new substances which constitute their bases: and on the general nature of alkaline bodies. Philos Trans R Soc. 1808;98:1–44.
18. Skou JC. The influence of some cations on an adenosine triphosphatase from peripheral nerves. Biochim Biophys Acta. 1957;23:394–401.
19. Gennari FJ, Segal AS. Hyperkalemia: an adaptive response in chronic renal insufficiency. Kidney Int. 2002;62:1–9.
20. Dluhy RG, Axelrod L, Williams GH. Serum immunoreactive insulin and growth hormone response to

potassium infusion in normal man. J Appl Physiol. 1972;33:22–6.
21. Rosa RM, Silva P, Young JB, et al. Adrenergic modulation of extrarenal potassium disposal. N Engl J Med. 1980;302:431–4.
22. Brown RS. Extrarenal potassium homeostasis. Kidney Int. 1986;30:116–27.
23. Bia MJ, Lu D, Tyler K, De Fronzo RA. Beta adrenergic control of extrarenal potassium disposal. A beta-2 mediated phenomenon. Nephron. 1986;43:117–22.
24. Akaike N. Sodium pump in skeletal muscle: central nervous system-induced suppression by alpha-adrenoreceptors. Science (New York, NY). 1981;213:1252–4.
25. Williams ME, Rosa RM, Silva P, Brown RS, Epstein FH. Impairment of extrarenal potassium disposal by alpha-adrenergic stimulation. N Engl J Med. 1984;311:145–9.
26. Clausen T. Hormonal and pharmacological modification of plasma potassium homeostasis. Fundam Clin Pharmacol. 2010;24:595–605.
27. Rigato I, Blarasin L, Kette F. Severe hypokalemia in 2 young bicycle riders due to massive caffeine intake. Clin J Sport Med. 2010;20:128–30.
28. Passmore AP, Kondowe GB, Johnston GD. Caffeine and hypokalemia. Ann Intern Med. 1986;105:468.
29. Mudge DW, Johnson DW. Coca-Cola and kangaroos. Lancet. 2004;364:1190.
30. Fredholm BB, Battig K, Holmen J, Nehlig A, Zvartau EE. Actions of caffeine in the brain with special reference to factors that contribute to its widespread use. Pharmacol Rev. 1999;51:83–133.
31. Moreno M, Murphy C, Goldsmith C. Increase in serum potassium resulting from the administration of hypertonic mannitol and other solutions. J Lab Clin Med. 1969;73:291–8.
32. Sirken G, Raja R, Garces J, Bloom E, Fumo P. Contrast-induced translocational hyponatremia and hyperkalemia in advanced kidney disease. Am J Kidney Dis. 2004;43:e31–5.
33. Goldfarb S, Cox M, Singer I, Goldberg M. Acute hyperkalemia induced by hyperglycemia: hormonal mechanisms. Ann Intern Med. 1976;84:426–32.
34. Viberti GC. Glucose-induced hyperkalaemia: a hazard for diabetics? Lancet. 1978;1:690–1.
35. Conte G, Dal Canton A, Imperatore P, et al. Acute increase in plasma osmolality as a cause of hyperkalemia in patients with renal failure. Kidney Int. 1990;38:301–7.
36. Adrogue HJ, Madias NE. PCO_2 and [K+]p in metabolic acidosis: certainty for the first and uncertainty for the other. J Am Soc Nephrol. 2004;15:1667–8.
37. Adrogue HJ, Madias NE. Changes in plasma potassium concentration during acute acid-base disturbances. Am J Med. 1981;71:456–67.
38. Krapf R, Caduff P, Wagdi P, Staubli M, Hulter HN. Plasma potassium response to acute respiratory alkalosis. Kidney Int. 1995;47:217–24.
39. Jones JW, Sebastian A, Hulter HN, Schambelan M, Sutton JM, Biglieri EG. Systemic and renal acid-base effects of chronic dietary potassium depletion in humans. Kidney Int. 1982;21:402–10.
40. Rector Jr FC, Bloomer HA, Seldin DW. Effect of potassium deficiency on the reabsorption of bicarbonate in the proximal tubule of the rat kidney. J Clin Invest. 1964;43:1976–82.
41. Soleimani M, Burnham CE. Physiologic and molecular aspects of the Na^+:HCO_3^- cotransporter in health and disease processes. Kidney Int. 2000;57:371–84.
42. Fulop M. Serum potassium in lactic acidosis and ketoacidosis. N Engl J Med. 1979;300:1087–9.
43. Wiederseiner JM, Muser J, Lutz T, Hulter HN, Krapf R. Acute metabolic acidosis: characterization and diagnosis of the disorder and the plasma potassium response. J Am Soc Nephrol. 2004;15:1589–96.
44. Berliner RW, Kennedy Jr TJ, Hilton JG. Renal mechanisms for excretion of potassium. Am J Physiol. 1950;162:348–67.
45. Giebisch G, Stanton B. Potassium transport in the nephron. Annu Rev Physiol. 1979;41:241–56.
46. O'Neil RG, Hayhurst RA. Functional differentiation of cell types of cortical collecting duct. Am J Physiol. 1985;248:F449–53.
47. Madsen KM, Tisher CC. Structural-functional relationships along the distal nephron. Am J Physiol. 1986;250:F1–15.
48. Woda CB, Leite Jr M, Rohatgi R, Satlin LM. Effects of luminal flow and nucleotides on [Ca^{2+}]i in rabbit cortical collecting duct. Am J Physiol Renal Physiol. 2002;283:F437–46.
49. Palmer LG, Frindt G. High-conductance K channels in intercalated cells of the rat distal nephron. Am J Physiol Renal Physiol. 2007;292:F966–73.
50. Holtzclaw JD, Grimm PR, Sansom SC. Intercalated cell BK-alpha/beta4 channels modulate sodium and potassium handling during potassium adaptation. J Am Soc Nephrol. 2010;21:634–45.
51. Grimm PR, Irsik DL, Liu L, Holtzclaw JD, Sansom SC. Role of BKbeta1 in Na^+ reabsorption by cortical collecting ducts of Na^+-deprived mice. Am J Physiol Renal Physiol. 2009;297:F420–8.
52. Giebisch G, Krapf R, Wagner C. Renal and extrarenal regulation of potassium. Kidney Int. 2007;72:397–410.
53. DuBose Jr TD, Gitomer J, Codina J. H^+, K^+-ATPase. Curr Opin Nephrol Hypertens. 1999;8:597–602.
54. Field MJ, Stanton BA, Giebisch GH. Differential acute effects of aldosterone, dexamethasone, and hyperkalemia on distal tubular potassium secretion in the rat kidney. J Clin Invest. 1984;74:1792–802.
55. Muto S. Potassium transport in the mammalian collecting duct. Physiol Rev. 2001;81:85–116.
56. Alvarez de la Rosa D, Gimenez I, Forbush B, Canessa CM. SGK1 activates Na^+-K^+-ATPase in amphibian renal epithelial cells. Am J Physiol Cell Physiol. 2006;290:C492–8.
57. Alvarez de la Rosa D, Zhang P, Naray-Fejes-Toth A, Fejes-Toth G, Canessa CM. The serum and gluco-

corticoid kinase sgk increases the abundance of epithelial sodium channels in the plasma membrane of Xenopus oocytes. J Biol Chem. 1999;274:37834–9.

58. Pearce D, Kleyman TR. Salt, sodium channels, and SGK1. J Clin Invest. 2007;117:592–5.
59. Ring AM, Leng Q, Rinehart J, et al. An SGK1 site in WNK4 regulates Na^+ channel and K^+ channel activity and has implications for aldosterone signaling and K^+ homeostasis. Proc Natl Acad Sci U S A. 2007;104:4025–9.
60. Shimkets RA, Warnock DG, Bositis CM, et al. Liddle's syndrome: heritable human hypertension caused by mutations in the beta subunit of the epithelial sodium channel. Cell. 1994;79:407–14.
61. Wilson FH, Disse-Nicodeme S, Choate KA, et al. Human hypertension caused by mutations in WNK kinases. Science (New York, NY). 2001;293:1107–12.
62. Kahle KT, Wilson FH, Leng Q, et al. WNK4 regulates the balance between renal NaCl reabsorption and K^+ secretion. Nat Genet. 2003;35:372–6.
63. Ring AM, Cheng SX, Leng Q, et al. WNK4 regulates activity of the epithelial Na^+ channel in vitro and in vivo. Proc Natl Acad Sci U S A. 2007;104:4020–4.
64. Rastegar A, Biemesderfer D, Kashgarian M, Hayslett JP. Changes in membrane surfaces of collecting duct cells in potassium adaptation. Kidney Int. 1980;18:293–301.
65. Good DW, Wright FS. Luminal influences on potassium secretion: sodium concentration and fluid flow rate. Am J Physiol. 1979;236:F192–205.
66. Good DW, Velazquez H, Wright FS. Luminal influences on potassium secretion: low sodium concentration. Am J Physiol. 1984;246:F609–19.
67. Woda CB, Bragin A, Kleyman TR, Satlin LM. Flow-dependent K^+ secretion in the cortical collecting duct is mediated by a maxi-K channel. Am J Physiol Renal Physiol. 2001;280:F786–93.
68. Taniguchi J, Imai M. Flow-dependent activation of maxi K^+ channels in apical membrane of rabbit connecting tubule. J Membr Biol. 1998;164:35–45.
69. Satlin LM, Sheng S, Woda CB, Kleyman TR. Epithelial Na^+ channels are regulated by flow. Am J Physiol Renal Physiol. 2001;280:F1010–8.
70. Gennari FJ, Goldstein MB, Schwartz WB. The nature of the renal adaptation to chronic hypocapnia. J Clin Invest. 1972;51:1722–30.
71. Kassirer JP, Schwartz WB. The response of normal man to selective depletion of hydrochloric acid. Factors in the genesis of persistent gastric alkalosis. Am J Med. 1966;40:10–8.
72. Klastersky J, Vanderklen B, Daneau D, Mathiew M. Carbenicillin and hypokalemia. Ann Intern Med. 1973;78:774–5.
73. Ellison DH, Velazquez H, Wright FS. Stimulation of distal potassium secretion by low lumen chloride in the presence of barium. Am J Physiol. 1985;248: F638–49.
74. Amorim JB, Bailey MA, Musa-Aziz R, Giebisch G, Malnic G. Role of luminal anion and pH in distal tubule potassium secretion. Am J Physiol Renal Physiol. 2003;284:F381–8.
75. Welt LG. Experimental magnesium depletion. Yale J Biol Med. 1964;36:325–49.
76. Whang R, Welt LG. Observations in experimental magnesium depletion. J Clin Invest. 1963;42:305–13.
77. Altura BM, Altura BT. Interactions of Mg and K on blood vessels—aspects in view of hypertension. Review of present status and new findings. Magnesium. 1984;3:175–94.
78. Matsuda H, Saigusa A, Irisawa H. Ohmic conductance through the inwardly rectifying K channel and blocking by internal Mg^{2+}. Nature. 1987;325:156–9.
79. Lu Z, MacKinnon R. Electrostatic tuning of Mg^{2+} affinity in an inward-rectifier K^+ channel. Nature. 1994;371:243–6.
80. Yang L, Frindt G, Palmer LG. Magnesium modulates ROMK channel-mediated potassium secretion. J Am Soc Nephrol. 2010;21:2109–16.
81. Huang CL, Kuo E. Mechanism of hypokalemia in magnesium deficiency. J Am Soc Nephrol. 2007;18:2649–52.
82. Wei Y, Zavilowitz B, Satlin LM, Wang WH. Angiotensin II inhibits the ROMK-like small conductance K channel in renal cortical collecting duct during dietary potassium restriction. J Biol Chem. 2007;282:6455–62.
83. Yue P, Sun P, Lin DH, Pan C, Xing W, Wang W. Angiotensin II diminishes the effect of SGK1 on the WNK4-mediated inhibition of ROMK1 channels. Kidney Int. 2011;79:423–31.
84. Schnermann J, Homer W. Smith Award lecture. The juxtaglomerular apparatus: from anatomical peculiarity to physiological relevance. J Am Soc Nephrol. 2003;14:1681–94.
85. Adrogue HJ, Madias NE. Sodium and potassium in the pathogenesis of hypertension. N Engl J Med. 2007;356:1966–78.
86. Rimmer JM, Horn JF, Gennari FJ. Hyperkalemia as a complication of drug therapy. Arch Intern Med. 1987;147:867–9.
87. Satlin LM, Carattino MD, Liu W, Kleyman TR. Regulation of cation transport in the distal nephron by mechanical forces. Am J Physiol Renal Physiol. 2006;291:F923–31.
88. Field MJ, Stanton BA, Giebisch GH. Influence of ADH on renal potassium handling: a micropuncture and microperfusion study. Kidney Int. 1984;25:502–11.
89. Greenberg A. Diuretic complications. Am J Med Sci. 2000;319:10–24.
90. Perazella MA. Drug-induced hyperkalemia: old culprits and new offenders. Am J Med. 2000;109:307–14.
91. Pitt B, Zannad F, Remme WJ, et al. The effect of spironolactone on morbidity and mortality in patients with severe heart failure. Randomized aldactone evaluation study investigators. N Engl J Med. 1999;341:709–17.
92. Juurlink DN, Mamdani MM, Lee DS, et al. Rates of hyperkalemia after publication of the randomized

aldactone evaluation study. N Engl J Med. 2004;351:543–51.
93. Loughlin J, Seeger JD, Eng PM, et al. Risk of hyperkalemia in women taking ethinylestradiol/drospirenone and other oral contraceptives. Contraception. 2008;78:377–83.
94. Genazzani AR, Mannella P, Simoncini T. Drospirenone and its antialdosterone properties. Climacteric. 2007;10 Suppl 1:11–8.
95. Hajjar IM, Grim CE, George V, Kotchen TA. Impact of diet on blood pressure and age-related changes in blood pressure in the US population: analysis of NHANES III. Arch Intern Med. 2001;161:589–93.
96. Institute of Medicine. Dietary reference intakes for water, potassium, sodium, chloride, and sulfate. In: Food and Nutrition Board. Washington, DC: National Academies Press; 2004. p. 173–246.
97. Rabinowitz L, Green DM, Sarason RL, Yamauchi H. Homeostatic potassium excretion in fed and fasted sheep. Am J Physiol. 1988;254:R357–80.
98. Lee FN, Oh G, McDonough AA, Youn JH. Evidence for gut factor in K^+ homeostasis. Am J Physiol Renal Physiol. 2007;293:F541–7.
99. Greenfeld D, Mickley D, Quinlan DM, Roloff P. Hypokalemia in outpatients with eating disorders. Am J Psychiatry. 1995;152:60–3.
100. Elisaf M, Liberopoulos E, Bairaktari E, Siamopoulos K. Hypokalaemia in alcoholic patients. Drug Alcohol Rev. 2002;21:73–6.
101. Gennari FJ. Hypokalemia. N Engl J Med. 1998;339:451–8.
102. Lin SH. Thyrotoxic periodic paralysis. Mayo Clin Proc. 2005;80:99–105.
103. Cannon SC. Pathomechanisms in channelopathies of skeletal muscle and brain. Annu Rev Neurosci. 2006;29:387–415.
104. Jurkat-Rott K, Mitrovic N, Hang C, et al. Voltage-sensor sodium channel mutations cause hypokalemic periodic paralysis type 2 by enhanced inactivation and reduced current. Proc Natl Acad Sci U S A. 2000;97:9549–54.
105. Manoukian MA, Foote JA, Crapo LM. Clinical and metabolic features of thyrotoxic periodic paralysis in 24 episodes. Arch Intern Med. 1999;159:601–6.
106. Ryan DP, da Silva MR, Soong TW, et al. Mutations in potassium channel Kir2.6 cause susceptibility to thyrotoxic hypokalemic periodic paralysis. Cell. 2010;140:88–98.
107. Lin SH, Lin YF, Chen DT, Chu P, Hsu CW, Halperin ML. Laboratory tests to determine the cause of hypokalemia and paralysis. Arch Intern Med. 2004;164:1561–6.
108. Lin SH, Chu P, Cheng CJ, Chu SJ, Hung YJ, Lin YF. Early diagnosis of thyrotoxic periodic paralysis: spot urine calcium to phosphate ratio. Crit Care Med. 2006;34:2984–9.
109. Ko GT, Chow CC, Yeung VT, Chan HH, Li JK, Cockram CS. Thyrotoxic periodic paralysis in a Chinese population. QJM. 1996;89:463–8.
110. Lin SH, Lin YF. Propranolol rapidly reverses paralysis, hypokalemia, and hypophosphatemia in thyrotoxic periodic paralysis. Am J Kidney Dis. 2001;37:620–3.
111. Huang TY, Lin SH. Thyrotoxic hypokalemic periodic paralysis reversed by propranolol without rebound hyperkalemia. Ann Emerg Med. 2001;37:415–6.
112. Brambilla G, Cenci T, Franconi F, et al. Clinical and pharmacological profile in a clenbuterol epidemic poisoning of contaminated beef meat in Italy. Toxicol Lett. 2000;114:47–53.
113. Bahlmann H, Lindwall R, Persson H. Acute barium nitrate intoxication treated by hemodialysis. Acta Anaesthesiol Scand. 2005;49:110–2.
114. Brown RS. Potassium homeostasis and clinical implications. Am J Med. 1984;77:3–10.
115. Knochel JP, Dotin LN, Hamburger RJ. Pathophysiology of intense physical conditioning in a hot climate. I. Mechanisms of potassium depletion. J Clin Invest. 1972;51:242–55.
116. Schwartz WB, Kassirer JP. Medical management of chronic renal failure. Am J Med. 1968;44:786–802.
117. Solomon R. The relationship between disorders of K^+ and Mg^{2+} homeostasis. Semin Nephrol. 1987;7:253–62.
118. Gill Jr JR, Frolich JC, Bowden RE, et al. Bartter's syndrome: a disorder characterized by high urinary prostaglandins and a dependence of hyperreninemia on prostaglandin synthesis. Am J Med. 1976;61:43–51.
119. Stein JH. The pathogenetic spectrum of Bartter's syndrome. Kidney Int. 1985;28:85–93.
120. Simon DB, Lifton RP. The molecular basis of inherited hypokalemic alkalosis: Bartter's and Gitelman's syndromes. Am J Physiol. 1996;271:F961–6.
121. Simon DB, Karet FE, Hamdan JM, DiPietro A, Sanjad SA, Lifton RP. Bartter's syndrome, hypokalaemic alkalosis with hypercalciuria, is caused by mutations in the Na-K-2Cl cotransporter NKCC2. Nat Genet. 1996;13:183–8.
122. Rodriguez-Soriano J. Bartter and related syndromes: the puzzle is almost solved. Pediatr Nephrol (Berlin, Germany). 1998;12:315–27.
123. Wrong O, Metcalfe-Gibson A, Morrison RB, Ng ST, Howard AV. In vivo dialysis of faeces as a method of stool analysis. I. Technique and results in normal subjects. Clin Sci. 1965;28:357–75.
124. Kavic SM, Frehm EJ, Segal AS. Case studies in cholera: lessons in medical history and science. Yale J Biol Med. 1999;72:393–408.
125. Oster JR, Materson BJ, Rogers AI. Laxative abuse syndrome. Am J Gastroenterol. 1980;74:451–8.
126. de Wolff FA, de Haas EJ, Verweij M. A screening method for establishing laxative abuse. Clin Chem. 1981;27:914–7.
127. Shelton JH, Santa Ana CA, Thompson DR, Emmett M, Fordtran JS. Factitious diarrhea induced by stimulant laxatives: accuracy of diagnosis by a clinical reference laboratory using thin layer chromatography. Clin Chem. 2007;53:85–90.
128. Holmberg C. Congenital chloride diarrhoea. Clin Gastroenterol. 1986;15:583–602.

129. Blondon H, Bechade D, Desrame J, Algayres JP. Secretory diarrhoea with high faecal potassium concentrations: a new mechanism of diarrhoea associated with colonic pseudo-obstruction? Report of five patients. Gastroenterol Clin Biol. 2008;32:401–4.
130. Simon M, Duong JP, Mallet V, et al. Over-expression of colonic K^+ channels associated with severe potassium secretory diarrhoea after haemorrhagic shock. Nephrol Dial Transplant. 2008;23:3350–2.
131. Van Dinter Jr TG, Fuerst FC, Richardson CT, et al. Stimulated active potassium secretion in a patient with colonic pseudo-obstruction: a new mechanism of secretory diarrhea. Gastroenterology. 2005;129: 1268–73.
132. Sandle GI, Hunter M. Apical potassium (BK) channels and enhanced potassium secretion in human colon. QJM. 2010;103:85–9.
133. Sebastian A, McSherry E, Morris Jr RC. On the mechanism of renal potassium wasting in renal tubular acidosis associated with the Fanconi syndrome (type 2 RTA). J Clin Invest. 1971;50:231–43.
134. Messiaen T, Deret S, Mougenot B, et al. Adult Fanconi syndrome secondary to light chain gammopathy. Clinicopathologic heterogeneity and unusual features in 11 patients. Medicine. 2000;79:135–54.
135. Estevez R, Boettger T, Stein V, et al. Barttin is a Cl^- channel beta-subunit crucial for renal Cl^- reabsorption and inner ear K^+ secretion. Nature. 2001;414: 558–61.
136. Miyamura N, Matsumoto K, Taguchi T, et al. Atypical Bartter syndrome with sensorineural deafness with G47R mutation of the beta-subunit for ClC-Ka and ClC-Kb chloride channels, barttin. J Clin Endocrinol Metabol. 2003;88:781–6.
137. Schlingmann KP, Konrad M, Jeck N, et al. Salt wasting and deafness resulting from mutations in two chloride channels. N Engl J Med. 2004;350:1314–9.
138. Vargas-Poussou R, Huang C, Hulin P, et al. Functional characterization of a calcium-sensing receptor mutation in severe autosomal dominant hypocalcemia with a Bartter-like syndrome. J Am Soc Nephrol. 2002;13:2259–66.
139. Cruz DN, Shaer AJ, Bia MJ, Lifton RP, Simon DB. Gitelman's syndrome revisited: an evaluation of symptoms and health-related quality of life. Kidney Int. 2001;59:710–7.
140. Batlle D, Moorthi KM, Schlueter W, Kurtzman N. Distal renal tubular acidosis and the potassium enigma. Semin Nephrol. 2006;26:471–8.
141. Sebastian A, McSherry E, Morris Jr RC. Impaired renal conservation of sodium and chloride during sustained correction of systemic acidosis in patients with type 1, classic renal tubular acidosis. J Clin Invest. 1976;58:454–69.
142. Taher SM, Anderson RJ, McCartney R, Popovtzer MM, Schrier RW. Renal tubular acidosis associated with toluene "sniffing". N Engl J Med. 1974;290: 765–8.
143. Streicher HZ, Gabow PA, Moss AH, Kono D, Kaehny WD. Syndromes of toluene sniffing in adults. Ann Intern Med. 1981;94:758–62.
144. Carlisle EJ, Donnelly SM, Vasuvattakul S, Kamel KS, Tobe S, Halperin ML. Glue-sniffing and distal renal tubular acidosis: sticking to the facts. J Am Soc Nephrol. 1991;1:1019–27.
145. Gill Jr JR, George JM, Solomon A, Bartter FC. Hyperaldosteronism and renal sodium loss reversed by drug treatment for malignant hypertension. N Engl J Med. 1964;270:1088–92.
146. Lenz T, Thiede HM, Nussberger J, Atlas SA, Distler A, Schulte KL. Hyperreninemia and secondary hyperaldosteronism in a patient with pheochromocytoma and von Hippel-Lindau disease. Nephron. 1992;62:345–50.
147. Leogite J, Schillo F, Viennet G, et al. Reninoma: a rare but curable cause of high blood pressure, a case report. Ann Endocrinol. 2003;64:198–201.
148. Conn JW, Cohen EL, Rovner DR, Nesbit RM. Normokalemic primary aldosteronism. A detectable cause of curable "essential" hypertension. JAMA. 1965;193:200–6.
149. Schirpenbach C, Reincke M. Primary aldosteronism: current knowledge and controversies in Conn's syndrome. Nat Clin Pract. 2007;3:220–7.
150. Conn JW, Knopf RF, Nesbit RM. Clinical characteristics of primary aldosteronism from an analysis of 145 cases. Am J Surg. 1964;107:159–72.
151. Marples D, Frokiaer J, Dorup J, Knepper MA, Nielsen S. Hypokalemia-induced downregulation of aquaporin-2 water channel expression in rat kidney medulla and cortex. J Clin Invest. 1996;97: 1960–8.
152. Choi M, Scholl UI, Yue P, et al. K^+ channel mutations in adrenal aldosterone-producing adenomas and hereditary hypertension. Science. 2011;331: 768–72.
153. Lifton RP, Dluhy RG, Powers M, et al. A chimaeric 11 beta-hydroxylase/aldosterone synthase gene causes glucocorticoid-remediable aldosteronism and human hypertension. Nature. 1992;355:262–5.
154. Orth DN. Cushing's syndrome. N Engl J Med. 1995;332:791–803.
155. Torpy DJ, Mullen N, Ilias I, Nieman LK. Association of hypertension and hypokalemia with Cushing's syndrome caused by ectopic ACTH secretion: a series of 58 cases. Ann N Y Acad Sci. 2002;970: 134–44.
156. Geller DS, Farhi A, Pinkerton N, et al. Activating mineralocorticoid receptor mutation in hypertension exacerbated by pregnancy. Science (New York, NY). 2000;289:119–23.
157. Morineau G, Sulmont V, Salomon R, et al. Apparent mineralocorticoid excess: report of six new cases and extensive personal experience. J Am Soc Nephrol. 2006;17:3176–84.
158. Mune T, Rogerson FM, Nikkila H, Agarwal AK, White PC. Human hypertension caused by mutations in the kidney isozyme of 11 beta-hydroxysteroid dehydrogenase. Nat Genet. 1995;10:394–9.
159. van Uum SH. Liquorice and hypertension. Neth J Med. 2005;63:119–20.
160. Mumoli N, Cei M. Licorice-induced hypokalemia. Int J Cardiol. 2008;124:e42–4.

161. Serra A, Uehlinger DE, Ferrari P, et al. Glycyrrhetinic acid decreases plasma potassium concentrations in patients with anuria. J Am Soc Nephrol. 2002;13:191–6.
162. Rossier BC. 1996 Homer Smith Award Lecture. Cum grano salis: the epithelial sodium channel and the control of blood pressure. J Am Soc Nephrol. 1997;8:980–92.
163. Snyder PM. Minireview: regulation of epithelial Na^+ channel trafficking. Endocrinology. 2005;146:5079–85.
164. Liddle GW, Bledsoe T, Coppage WS. A familial renal disorder simulating primary aldosteronism but with negligible aldosterone secretion. Trans Assoc Am Physicians. 1963;76:99–213.
165. Gennari FJ, Hussain-Khan S, Segal A. An unusual case of metabolic alkalosis: a window into the pathophysiology and diagnosis of this common acid-base disturbance. Am J Kidney Dis. 2010;55:1130–5.
166. Sterns RH, Cox M, Feig PU, Singer I. Internal potassium balance and the control of the plasma potassium concentration. Medicine. 1981;60:339–54.
167. Murakami K, Tomita M, Kawamura N, et al. Severe metabolic acidosis and hypokalemia in a patient with enterovesical fistula. Clin Exp Nephrol. 2007;11:225–9.
168. Murthy K, Harrington JT, Siegel RD. Profound hypokalemia in diabetic ketoacidosis: a therapeutic challenge. Endocr Pract. 2005;11:331–4.
169. Yasue H, Itoh T, Mizuno Y, Harada E. Severe hypokalemia, rhabdomyolysis, muscle paralysis, and respiratory impairment in a hypertensive patient taking herbal medicines containing licorice. Intern Med. 2007;46:575–8.
170. Kunin AS, Surawicz B, Sims EA. Decrease in serum potassium concentrations and appearance of cardiac arrhythmias during infusion of potassium with glucose in potassium-depleted patients. N Engl J Med. 1962;266:228–33.
171. Kruse JA, Carlson RW. Rapid correction of hypokalemia using concentrated intravenous potassium chloride infusions. Arch Intern Med. 1990;150:613–7.
172. Hamill RJ, Robinson LM, Wexler HR, Moote C. Efficacy and safety of potassium infusion therapy in hypokalemic critically ill patients. Crit Care Med. 1991;19:694–9.
173. Sugimoto T, Kume S, Osawa N, Nakazawa J, Koya D, Kashiwagi A. Familial pseudohyperkalemia: a rare cause of hyperkalemia. Intern Med. 2005;44:875–8.
174. Bywaters EGL, Beall D. Crush injuries with impairment of renal function. Br Med J. 1941;1:427.
175. Grossman RA, Hamilton RW, Morse BM, Penn AS, Goldberg M. Nontraumatic rhabdomyolysis and acute renal failure. N Engl J Med. 1974;291:807–11.
176. Gowda RM, Cohen RA, Khan IA. Toad venom poisoning: resemblance to digoxin toxicity and therapeutic implications. Heart (British Cardiac Society). 2003;89:e14.
177. Martyn JA, Richtsfeld M. Succinylcholine-induced hyperkalemia in acquired pathologic states: etiologic factors and molecular mechanisms. Anesthesiology. 2006;104:158–69.
178. Lehmann-Horn F, Jurkat-Rott K. Voltage-gated ion channels and hereditary disease. Physiol Rev. 1999;79:1317–72.
179. Ptacek LJ, Johnson KJ, Griggs RC. Genetics and physiology of the myotonic muscle disorders. N Engl J Med. 1993;328:482–9.
180. Pickar JG, Spier SJ, Snyder JR, Carlsen RC. Altered ionic permeability in skeletal muscle from horses with hyperkalemic periodic paralysis. Am J Physiol. 1991;260:C926–33.
181. Cruz DN, Perazella MA. Biochemical aberrations in a dialysis patient following parathyroidectomy. Am J Kidney Dis. 1997;29:759–62.
182. Armstrong CM. Distinguishing surface effects of calcium ion from pore-occupancy effects in Na^+ channels. Proc Natl Acad Sci U S A. 1999;96:4158–63.
183. Ponce SP, Jennings AE, Madias NE, Harrington JT. Drug-induced hyperkalemia. Medicine. 1985;64:357–70.
184. Perry MC. Cautopyreiophagia. N Engl J Med. 1977;296:824.
185. Abu-Hamdan DK, Sondheimer JH, Mahajan SK. Cautopyreiophagia. Cause of life-threatening hyperkalemia in a patient undergoing hemodialysis. Am J Med. 1985;79:517–9.
186. Oster JR, Singer I, Fishman LM. Heparin-induced aldosterone suppression and hyperkalemia. Am J Med. 1995;98:575–86.
187. Conn JW, Rovner DR, Cohen EL, Anderson Jr JE. Inhibition by heparinoid of aldosterone biosynthesis in man. J Clin Endocrinol Metabol. 1966;26:527–32.
188. Wilson ID, Goetz FC. Selective hypoaldosteronism after prolonged heparin administration. A case report, with postmortem findings. Am J Med. 1964;36:635–40.
189. Palmer BF. Managing hyperkalemia caused by inhibitors of the renin-angiotensin-aldosterone system. N Engl J Med. 2004;351:585–92.
190. Goldberg AI, Dunlay MC, Sweet CS. Safety and tolerability of losartan potassium, an angiotensin II receptor antagonist, compared with hydrochlorothiazide, atenolol, felodipine ER, and angiotensin-converting enzyme inhibitors for the treatment of systemic hypertension. Am J Cardiol. 1995;75:793–5.
191. Reardon LC, Macpherson DS. Hyperkalemia in outpatients using angiotensin-converting enzyme inhibitors. How much should we worry? Arch Intern Med. 1998;158:26–32.
192. Bakris GL, Siomos M, Richardson D, et al. ACE inhibition or angiotensin receptor blockade: impact on potassium in renal failure. VAL-K Study Group. Kidney Int. 2000;58:2084–92.

193. Preston RA, Baltodano NM, Alonso AB, Epstein M. Comparative effects on dynamic renal potassium excretion of ACE inhibition versus angiotensin receptor blockade in hypertensive patients with type II diabetes mellitus. J Clin Pharmacol. 2002;42:754–61.
194. Svensson M, Gustafsson F, Galatius S, Hildebrandt PR, Atar D. Hyperkalaemia and impaired renal function in patients taking spironolactone for congestive heart failure: retrospective study. BMJ (Clinical research ed). 2003;327:1141–2.
195. Velazquez H, Perazella MA, Wright FS, Ellison DH. Renal mechanism of trimethoprim-induced hyperkalemia. Ann Intern Med. 1993;119: 296–301.
196. Szerlip HM, Weiss J, Singer I. Profound hyperkalemia without electrocardiographic manifestations. Am J Kidney Dis. 1986;7:461–5.
197. Keith NM, Osterberg AE, Burchell HB. Some effects of potassium salts in man. Ann Intern Med. 1942;16:879–92.
198. Thomson WAR. The effect of potassium on the heart in man. Br Heart J. 1939;1:269–82.
199. Tarail R. Relationship of abnormalities in concentration of serum potassium to electrocardiographic disturbances. Am J Med. 1948;5:828–37.
200. Nerbonne JM, Kass RS. Molecular physiology of cardiac repolarization. Physiol Rev. 2005;85:1205–53.
201. Frankenhaeuser B, Hodgkin AL. The action of calcium on the electrical properties of squid axons. J Physiol. 1957;137:218–44.
202. Armstrong CM, Cota G. Calcium ion as a cofactor in Na channel gating. Proc Natl Acad Sci U S A. 1991;88:6528–31.
203. Armstrong CM, Cota G. Calcium block of Na^+ channels and its effect on closing rate. Proc Natl Acad Sci U S A. 1999;96:4154–7.
204. Allon M. Hyperkalemia in end-stage renal disease: mechanisms and management. J Am Soc Nephrol. 1995;6:1134–42.
205. Gold H, Kwit N. Digitalis and calcium synergism. Science (New York, NY). 1937;86:330–1.
206. Smith PK, Winkler AW, Hoff HE. Calcium and digitalis synergism: the toxicity of calcium salts injected intravenously into digitalized animals. Arch Int Med. 1939;64:322–8.
207. Lown B, Black H, Moore FD. Digitalis, electrolytes and the surgical patient. Am J Cardiol. 1960;6:309–37.
208. Nola GT, Pope S, Harrison DC. Assessment of the synergistic relationship between serum calcium and digitalis. Am Heart J. 1970;79:499–507.
209. Fenton F, Smally AJ, Laut J. Hyperkalemia and digoxin toxicity in a patient with kidney failure. Ann Emerg Med. 1996;28:440–1.
210. Van Deusen SK, Birkhahn RH, Gaeta TJ. Treatment of hyperkalemia in a patient with unrecognized digitalis toxicity. J Toxicol. 2003;41:373–6.
211. Allon M, Dunlay R, Copkney C. Nebulized albuterol for acute hyperkalemia in patients on hemodialysis. Ann Intern Med. 1989;110:426–9.
212. Blumberg A, Weidmann P, Shaw S, Gnadinger M. Effect of various therapeutic approaches on plasma potassium and major regulating factors in terminal renal failure. Am J Med. 1988;85:507–12.
213. Blumberg A, Weidmann P, Ferrari P. Effect of prolonged bicarbonate administration on plasma potassium in terminal renal failure. Kidney Int. 1992;41:369–74.
214. Flatman JA, Clausen T. Combined effects of adrenaline and insulin on active electrogenic Na^+-K^+ transport in rat soleus muscle. Nature. 1979;281: 580–1.
215. Lillemoe KD, Romolo JL, Hamilton SR, Pennington LR, Burdick JF, Williams GM. Intestinal necrosis due to sodium polystyrene (kayexalate) in sorbitol enemas: clinical and experimental support for the hypothesis. Surgery. 1987;101:267–72.
216. Gerstman BB, Kirkman R, Platt R. Intestinal necrosis associated with postoperative orally administered sodium polystyrene sulfonate in sorbitol. Am J Kidney Dis. 1992;20:159–61.
217. Rogers FB, Li SC. Acute colonic necrosis associated with sodium polystyrene sulfonate (Kayexalate) enemas in a critically ill patient: case report and review of the literature. J Trauma. 2001;51:395–7.
218. Kelsey PB, Chen S, Lauwers GY. Case records of the Massachusetts General Hospital. Weekly clinicopathological exercises. Case 37–2003. A 79-year-old man with coronary artery disease, peripheral vascular disease, end-stage renal disease, and abdominal pain and distention. N Engl J Med. 2003;349: 2147–55.
219. Sterns RH, Rojas M, Bernstein P, Chennupati S. Ion-exchange resins for the treatment of hyperkalemia: are they safe and effective? J Am Soc Nephrol. 2010;21:733–5.
220. Watson M, Abbott KC, Yuan CM. Damned if you do, damned if you don't: potassium binding resins in hyperkalemia. Clin J Am Soc Nephrol. 2010;5:1723–6.
221. McGowan CE, Saha S, Chu G, Resnick MB, Moss SF. Intestinal necrosis due to sodium polystyrene sulfonate (Kayexalate) in sorbitol. South Med J. 2009;102:493–7.
222. Rashid A, Hamilton SR. Necrosis of the gastrointestinal tract in uremic patients as a result of sodium polystyrene sulfonate (Kayexalate) in sorbitol: an underrecognized condition. Am J Surg Pathol. 1997;21:60–9.
223. Cheng ES, Stringer KM, Pegg SP. Colonic necrosis and perforation following oral sodium polystyrene sulfonate (Resonium A/Kayexalate) in a burn patient. Burns. 2002;28:189–90.
224. Emmett M, Hootkins RE, Fine KD, Santa Ana CA, Porter JL, Fordtran JS. Effect of three laxatives and a cation exchange resin on fecal sodium and

potassium excretion. Gastroenterology. 1995;108: 752–60.
225. Dardik A, Moesinger RC, Efron G, Barbul A, Harrison MG. Acute abdomen with colonic necrosis induced by Kayexalate-sorbitol. South Med J. 2000;93:511–3.
226. Gruy-Kapral C, Emmett M, Santa Ana CA, Porter JL, Fordtran JS, Fine KD. Effect of single dose resin-cathartic therapy on serum potassium concentration in patients with end-stage renal disease. J Am Soc Nephrol. 1998;9:1924–30.
227. Kamel KS, Wei C. Controversial issues in the treatment of hyperkalaemia. Nephrol Dial Transplant. 2003;18:2215–8.
228. Farese S, Kruse A, Pasch A, et al. Glycyrrhetinic acid food supplementation lowers serum potassium concentration in chronic hemodialysis patients. Kidney Int. 2009;76:877–84.
229. Sherman RA, Hwang ER, Bernholc AS, Eisinger RP. Variability in potassium removal by hemodialysis. Am J Nephrol. 1986;6:284–8.
230. Hou S, McElroy PA, Nootens J, Beach M. Safety and efficacy of low-potassium diasylate. Am J Kidney Dis. 1989;13:137–43.
231. Karnik JA, Young BS, Lew NL, et al. Cardiac arrest and sudden death in dialysis units. Kidney Int. 2001;60:350–7.
232. Lameire N, Van Biesen W, Vanholder R. Did 20 years of technological innovations in hemodialysis contribute to better patient outcomes? Clin J Am Soc Nephrol. 2009;4 Suppl 1:S30–40.

4 Disorders of Calcium, Phosphate, and Magnesium Metabolism

Ali Hariri, David B. Mount, and Ashghar Rastegar

Disorders of Calcium Metabolism

General Considerations

Serum calcium concentration plays a major role in many biologic processes including skeletal mineralization, neuromuscular excitability, and blood clotting. Intracellular calcium, which is maintained at a 1,000-fold lower concentration than serum calcium, plays a vital role in most physiological processes, including muscular contraction, hormone secretion, nerve conduction, cell proliferation, differentiation, and motility. Skeleton contains approximately 99 % of total body calcium, but only 1 % is freely available for exchange with extracellular calcium. Serum calcium is present in two fractions as bound and free calcium. Calcium binds tightly to albumin at a ratio of approximately 0.8 mg per gram of albumin. Free or ionized calcium is the active component of extracellular calcium pool and accounts for 47 % of total calcium.

A. Hariri, M.D. • A. Rastegar, M.D.
Section of Nephrology, Department of Medicine, Yale School of Medicine, 333 Cedar St., New Haven, CT 06520, USA

D.B. Mount, M.D. (✉)
Renal Division, VA Boston Healthcare System, and, Brigham and Women's Hospital, Harvard Medical School, Boston, MA, USA
e-mail: dmount@rics.bwh.harvard.edu; david.mount2@va.gov

Calcium Homeostasis

Calcium homeostasis reflects the interaction between gut, bone, and kidney. This interaction is orchestrated by several hormones, including parathyroid hormone (PTH), vitamin D, and calcitonin, and involves several organs, including gut, bone, kidney, and parathyroid gland (Fig. 4.1). Regulation of serum calcium is unique among all ions due to the presence of a negative feedback loop that allows minute-to-minute regulation of its concentration. This loop is activated by interaction between ionized calcium and a unique receptor, calcium-sensing receptor (CaR), present on parathyroid, specialized thyroid, and renal epithelial cells. CaR is a G-protein-coupled receptor with an extracellular cation-binding site that responds to ambient concentration of calcium and to a lesser extent magnesium [1]. This receptor was first discovered on parathyroid cells, where it plays a major role in synthesis and secretion of PTH. A minor decrease in serum calcium concentration is sensed by the CaR, resulting in rapid stimulation of the parathyroid gland and secretion of PTH. Within the kidney CaR is present in virtually all tubular segments, expressed at the including luminal membrane of proximal tubules, at the basolateral membrane of medullary thick ascending limb (MTAL), cortical thick ascending limb (CTAL), distal convoluted tubule (DCT), and at the apical surface of medullary collecting duct (MCD). In the kidney CaR is able to respond to both plasma and interstitial calcium

D.B. Mount et al. (eds.), *Core Concepts in the Disorders of Fluid, Electrolytes and Acid-Base Balance*, DOI 10.1007/978-1-4614-3770-3_4, © Springer Science+Business Media New York 2013

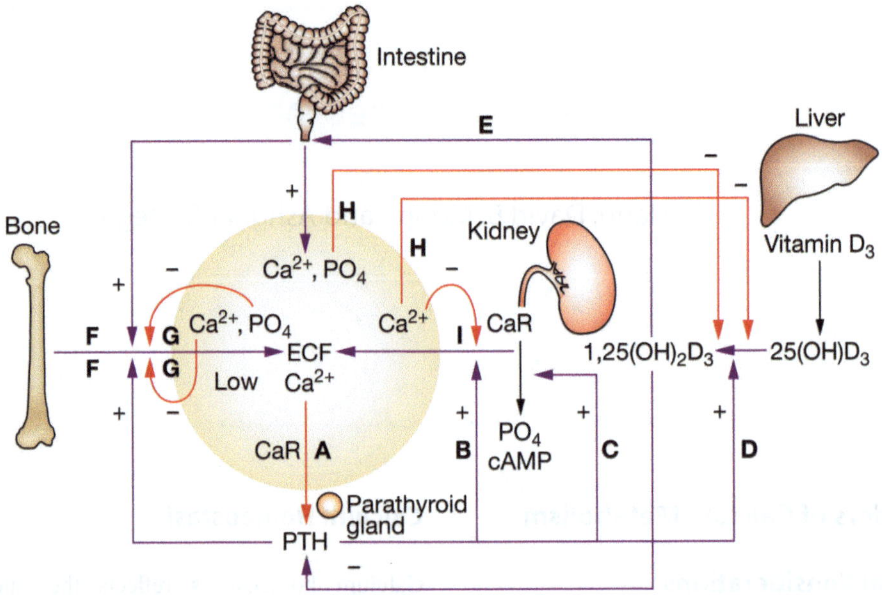

Fig. 4.1 Schematic diagram to illustrate the principal elements of extracellular calcium homeostasis. Actions that increase extracellular calcium levels are denoted by *purple arrows*; actions that decrease levels are shown by *red arrows*. *Abbreviations*: *1,25(OH)$_2$D$_3$* 1,25-dihydroxyvitamin D_3, *25(OH)D$_3$* 25-hydroxyvitamin D_3; *Ca^2* calcium ions; *cAMP* cyclic AMP; *CaR* extracellular calcium-ion-sensing receptor; *ECF* extracellular fluid; *PO^4* phosphate ions; *PTH* parathyroid hormone. From Brown EM [1]; used with permission

concentration as well as tubular fluid concentration, modulating both the amount as well as concentration of calcium in urine and pH of the urine. Calcitonin-secreting cells of thyroid gland also express CaR, which, in presence of high ambient calcium, stimulate these cells to release calcitonin. For more detailed discussion please see review by Brown [1].

PTH, an 84-amino-acid peptide, is the master hormone orchestrating overall regulation of ionized calcium concentration. It is synthesized in chief cells of parathyroid gland in response to ionized calcium level. Intact PTH level is cleared by the kidney and liver with a half-life of 4 min. In liver, it is metabolized by the Kupffer cells into multiple fragments. The C-terminal fragment is renally excreted and therefore has a longer half-life in renal failure [2]. The PTH N-terminal fragment binds to PTH receptor, a G-protein coupled receptor, and exerts its well-known biologic activity which includes the following: (1) Stimulation of 1-α(alpha)-hydroxylase enzyme and production of active vitamin D by proximal renal tubular cells, (2) Activation of osteoclasts resulting in bony resorption and release of calcium and phosphate, and (3) Stimulation of calcium and inhibition of phosphate reabsorption by the kidney.

Calcitonin, a 32-amino-acid peptide, is synthesized by the C-cells of thyroid gland. Calcitonin secretion is modulated by changes in serum calcium. Calcitonin rapidly inhibits osteoclastic bone resorption, but the effect is short-lived [3]. The overall role of calcitonin in calcium homeostasis in man is not clear. For example, patients who lack a thyroid gland and patients with calcitonin-producing tumors of the thyroid gland have normal serum calcium.

Calcium homeostasis is also regulated by fibroblast growth factor 23 (FGF23), which was initially identified as the disease gene for autosomal dominant hypophosphatemic rickets (ADHR—OMIM 193100) [4]. Increases in FGF23 activity, as seen in ADHR, X-linked hypophosphatemic rickets, and tumor-induced osteomalacia, cause hypophosphatemia and osteomalacia. FGF23 is a phosphaturic factor secreted by bone cells [5]. This novel hormone has several evolving roles in calcium

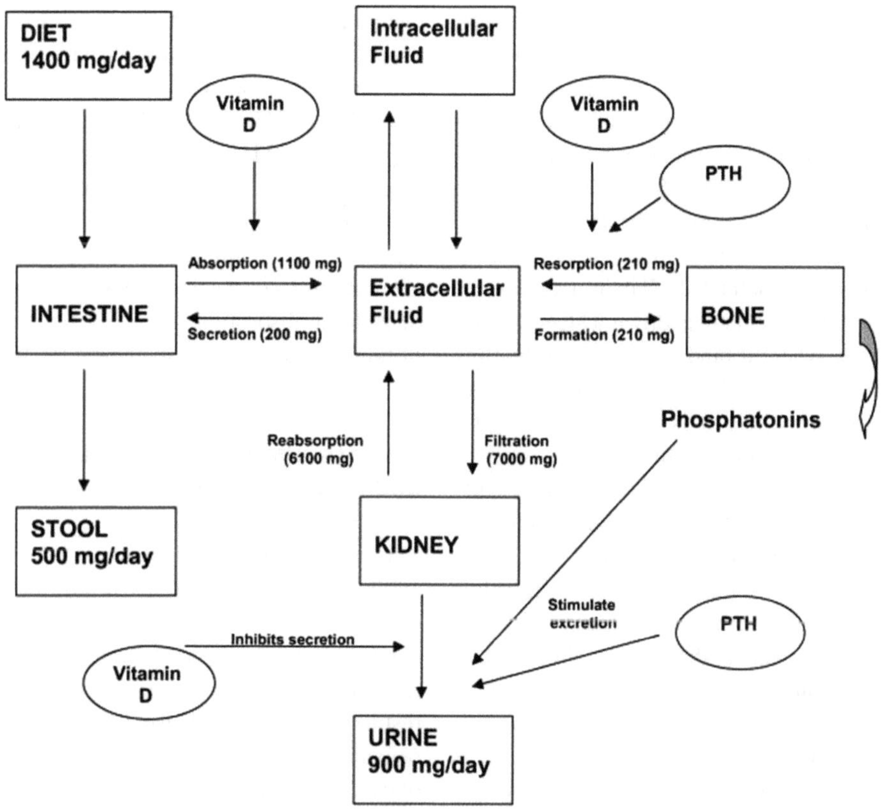

Fig. 4.2 Summary of the phosphate metabolism for a normal adult in neutral phosphate balance. PTH = parathyroid hormone. From Gaasbeek et al. [88]; used with permission

and phosphate homeostasis. Perhaps the most prominent effect of FGF23 on calcium homeostasis is due to inhibition of the renal 1-α-hydroxylase enzyme that generates the active form of vitamin D, 1,25-dihydroxyvitamin D_3 (calcitriol). Reduced activity of FGF23 thus causes familial tumoral calcinosis, characterized by hyperphosphatemia and elevated calcitriol, with progressive deposition of calcium phosphate crystals in periarticular spaces, soft tissues, and bone [5].

Regulation of Calcium Absorption by Intestine

Normal daily calcium content of a Western diet is about 1.0 g, 30 % of which (300 mg) is normally absorbed in upper small intestine with a small amount absorbed in colon [6]. Secretion of calcium by the gut is fixed at 150 mg/day, resulting in a net absorption of 150 mg, which is matched by renal excretion. In adults in zero calcium balance bony remodeling does not impact on overall calcium homeostasis (Fig. 4.2).

Calcium absorption in the intestine is regulated by the level of 1,25-dihydroxyvitamin D_3. Vitamin D is either ingested in diet or synthesized in the skin by ultraviolet light. This is hydroxylated at 25 position in the liver and then further hydroxylated at C-1 position by the enzyme, 1-α-hydroxylase, in the proximal tubule of the kidney. This enzyme, which controls the level of this active hormone, is regulated by PTH, phosphate, calcium as well as its own product, 1,25-dihydroxyvitamin D_3. 1,25-dihydroxyvitamin D_3 also increases phosphate absorption by the intestine. Calcium absorption occurs primarily in duodenum with minor reabsorption in jejunum [7]. Active calcium absorption involves specific channels and intracellular calcium-binding protein. Briefly both intestinal mucosal cells in duodenum as well as renal epithelial cells in distal convoluted tubules (DCT) and connecting tubules (CNT) have calcium-transporting channels in their luminal membranes. These channels are members of a large cation-transporting channel family, i.e., transient receptor potential (TRP) family [8]; TRPV5 and TRPV6 are the major absorptive calcium channels in the intestine, duodenum, kidney, and other vitamin D-responsive epithelia [8]. Calcium enters the cell through these channels down a steep chemical gradient, where it binds to a calcium-binding protein (calbindin). It then diffuses to the basolateral membrane where it is extruded through a calcium-sodium counter-transporter as well as the calcium-ATPase pump. This process is highly regulated by the calcitropic hormones including vitamin D, PTH as well as "Klotho," novel vitamin-D controlled signaling protein [8]. While vitamin D and PTH seem to increases the abundance of TRP channels through regulation of its transcription and translation, Klotho, through its enzymatic activity, traps the channel in the plasma cell membrane. This highly controlled process ensures that intracellular as well as plasma calcium is tightly regulated during calcium abundance as well as deprivation (for detailed discussion please see [8]). Calcium is primarily secreted in ileum where it binds to free fatty acids resulting in their saponification. The CaR is present in small and large intestine; however, its physiologic role is not yet well defined.

Renal Handling of Calcium

Ionized calcium is freely filtered and then reabsorbed along the nephron, resulting in a fractional excretion of approximately 2–3 %. In the proximal tubule two-third of filtered calcium is reabsorbed along with sodium and water. In the thick ascending limb of the Loop of Henle, the intraluminal positive charge created by sodium absorption and potassium recycling results in calcium and magnesium absorption through the paracellular pathway [9, 10]. The CaR is heavily expressed at the basolateral membrane of thick ascending limb cells; activation of this basolateral receptor inhibits transepithelial Na^+-Cl^- and K^+ transport, thus reducing the lumen-positive potential difference and inhibiting transepithelial calcium and magnesium transport by the thick ascending limb [9]. Finally urinary excretion of calcium is fine-tuned in distal convoluted tubule through TRPV5 and TRPV6, calcium channels regulated by PTH and vitamin D [8]. In summary, calcium absorption in the proximal tubule is regulated by factors regulating sodium absorption. However, in the more distal nephron, calcium absorption is regulated increasingly independent of sodium absorption, allowing tight regulation of final urinary calcium excretion [8, 10].

Defense Against Hypocalcemia and Hypercalcemia

The complex interplay between several organs and hormones described above allows tight control of serum calcium concentration within a very narrow range. A fall in serum calcium is sensed rapidly by CaR in the parathyroid gland cells resulting in rapid release of PTH to increase osteoclastic bone resorption, renal reabsorption of calcium and activation of vitamin D to increase intestinal calcium and phosphate absorption. This series of events restores calcium concentration to normal levels. The converse occurs when serum calcium increases for any reason. In addition CaR has a role, independent of PTH, in defense against hypercalcemia by increasing urinary calcium [11]. The overall response is more effective in mitigating hypocalcemia than hypercalcemia. There is, however, a limit to the effectiveness of these defense mechanisms, such that hypercalcemia or hypocalcemia can occur despite maximum activation of these mechanisms or due to failure of one or more of its components.

Disorders of Calcium Concentration

Serum calcium concentration is made up of three distinct fractions; 47 % as ionized or free calcium, 47 % bound to serum albumin and globulin, and 6 % complexed with several anions, including citrate, acetate, phosphate, and sulfate. At pH of 7.4 each gram of albumin binds 0.8 mg (0.2 mmol) of calcium, and therefore, total calcium concentration should always be corrected for increases or decreases in serum albumin. Acute acidemia increases and alkalemia decreases ionized calcium without changing total calcium. Hypercalcemia is defined as total calcium level corrected for albumin concentration above 10.2 mg/dL (2.55 mmol/L) and ionized calcium above 5.6 mg/dL (1.4 mmol/L). Hypocalcemia is defined as total calcium corrected for albumin of less than 8.5 mg/dL (<2.1 mmol/L) and ionized calcium of less than 4.5 mg/dL (<1.1 mmol/L).

Hypercalcemia

Clinical Presentation

Symptoms of hypercalcemia depend on its severity and duration. Mild hypercalcemia is often asymptomatic, but severe hypercalcemia presents with renal, GI, and neurological symptoms including polyuria, polydipsia, constipation, nausea, vomiting, drowsiness, lethargy, stupor, and coma. Long-standing hypercalcemia could present with sign and symptoms of nephrolithiasis, nephrocalcinosis, renal failure, and rarely uremia. Bony symptoms may be present if hypercalcemia is associated with calcium mobilization from the bone, such as in hyperparathyroidism or in malignancy-associated hypercalcemia.

Causes of Hypercalcemia

The most common causes of hypercalcemia are listed in Table 4.1. These are discussed briefly below.

Table 4.1 Causes of hypercalcemia

Primary hyperparathyroidism
Malignancy-associated hypercalcemia
PTH-rP-associated hypercalcemia
Hypercalcemia secondary to bony metastasis
Activation of vitamin D
PTH-associated hypercalcemia
Milk–alkali syndrome (MAS)
Granulomatous disease
Sarcoidosis
Tuberculosis
Silicone-induced
Candidiasis
Leprosy
Inactivation of CaR
Familial hypocalciuric hypercalcemia
Neonatal severe hyperparathyroidism
Endocrine-associated hypercalcemia
Adrenal insufficiency
Hyperthyroidism
Immobilization
Drugs
Thiazide diuretics
Lithium
Vitamin D
Vitamin A
Estrogen/antiestrogen
Theophylline

Primary Hyperparathyroidism

Primary hyperparathyroidism (PHPT) is a relatively common disease with approximately 100,000 new cases annually diagnosed in the United States. It occurs most commonly in older patients with peak incidence in the sixth decade and a female to male ratio of 3:2. The incidence of PHPT is highest in postmenopausal women, estimated at 1:1,000 [12, 13]. Primary hyperparathyroidism is most often due to a single adenoma, accounting for 85 % of all cases. In 15 % of patients PHPT is due to parathyroid hyperplasia and could be familial in nature or in association with MEN syndromes. In MEN I hyperparathyroidism [HPT] is the most common endocrine presentation, with a penetrance approaching 100 % by 50 years of age. Less commonly HPT is seen as part of MEN II syndrome [14]. Finally, parathyroid carcinoma, which can present with biochemical parameters similar to PHPT, accounts for less than 1 % of the cases of HPT [15].

Clinical presentation of PHPT. With the advent of automated multiphasic screening tests, the clinical presentation of primary hyperparathyroidism in Western countries has changed dramatically [12, 13]. Most patients are now diagnosed because of abnormal biochemical tests rather than specific symptoms. The classical presentation of bone pain, kidney stone, and change in mental state is now rare [13]. It is not clear if this change is due to earlier diagnosis of a slowly progressive disease or due to a change in the nature of the disease (see below). Renal presentation of hyperparathyroidism can include polyuria, hypercalciuria, nephrolithiasis, nephrocalcinosis, and renal failure; however, these are typically late manifestations of the disease and are less commonly seen today. Nephrolithiasis, the most common renal manifestation, is reported in up to 20 % of these patients [12, 13]; however, this is probably an overestimation and reflects the estimate in more severe cases. Another renal manifestation is mild proximal renal tubular acidosis secondary to PTH-induced inhibition of bicarbonate (and phosphate) reabsorption by the proximal tubule. Symptomatic bone disease is now reported in less than 15 % of patients. Nonspecific neuropsychiatric symptoms are common, encompassing weakness, fatigue, depression, cognitive impairment, anxiety, and sleep disturbance; some but not all studies suggest improvement in these symptoms with surgery [16]. Less common manifestations include chondrocalcinosis presenting as pseudogout. Gastrointestinal manifestation includes peptic ulcer disease and pancreatitis.

The natural history of asymptomatic hyperparathyroidism was studied in a group of 121 patients, 101 of whom were totally asymptomatic; during the 10-year follow-up 50 % underwent surgical parathyroidectomy. Interestingly of 52 asymptomatic patients, 27 % became symptomatic and the remainder had no changes in their biochemical and clinical presentation during this time. The latter group, which would have gone undiagnosed before advent of routine screening, has significantly impacted on our understanding of the natural history of HPT [17].

Diagnosis of PHPT. PHPT should be considered when hypercalcemia is associated with elevated or "normal" levels of PTH. Serum calcium is often only mildly elevated with concomitant mild depression in serum phosphorous and increase in urinary calcium. PTH level is either frankly elevated or elevated relative to concentration of serum calcium. In some patients serum calcium is only intermittently elevated and in a rare patient, it is always normal. In the latter group PHPT is suspected because of elevated serum PTH level often obtained to evaluate bone disease. In these patients, secondary causes of hyperparathyroidism, especially vitamin D deficiency, should be strongly considered and ruled out, before a diagnosis of PHPT is made [18].

Routine bone studies in patients with PHPT are usually normal; however, bone densitometry often shows decreased density at radial head with minimal changes in the spine and intermediate changes in hip region. This variation reflects the effect of PTH on cortical vs. cancellous bone. The incidence of bone fracture in patients with PHPT is conflicting and reflects the severity of the underlying disease. Fracture rates are increased in cortical but not vertebral bones (reviewed in [12]). The classical finding of osteitis fibrosa cystica, subperiosteal bone resorption involving the phalanges, and "salt and pepper" appearance of the skull are now very uncommon in Western countries.

Pathophysiology of HPT. In PHPT, due to a single adenoma, the normal relationship between calcium and PTH secretion is altered resulting in a shift of the "set point" of the calcium receptor response [19]. There is, however, wide variation in the set point in different adenomas [20]. In PHPT due to hyperplasia, while each cell responds normally to the negative feedback mechanism, PTH secretion is increased due to the overall size of the gland. The cellular and molecular events leading to formation of parathyroid adenoma remains elusive. In rare cases such as HPT-Jaw tumor syndrome or in some patients with MEN 1 and 2, a genetic abnormality is now recognized. The clonal origin of most cases of PHPT suggests a defect at the level of parathyroid cell proliferation [21]. In some patients overexpression of cyclin D1, a cell-cycle regulator, is implicated in the development of parathyroid adenoma.

Management of patients with PHPT. In symptomatic patients surgery is recommended and is very effective in normalizing biochemical findings and reversing most clinical symptoms. In asymptomatic patients, a recent consensus report (2008 Third International Workshop on the Management of Asymptomatic Primary Hyperparathyroidism) recommends surgery for patients with (a) calcium that is 1 mg/dL greater than the upper limits of normal, (b) an estimated GFR that is <60 mL/min, (c) markedly reduced bone density (*t*-score of <2.5) at any sites, and/or previous fracture fragility, and (d) age <50 [18]. Hypercalciuria in the absence of nephrolithiasis is no longer regarded as an indication for surgery, since hypercalciuria is but one of several factors contributing to the risk of renal stones [18].

Surgery should be carried out by a surgeon experienced in the removal of parathyroid adenoma, using minimally invasive techniques and intraoperative PTH assays for more "focused" surgery [22]. This procedure utilizes intraoperative PTH assay to ensure that only a single adenoma is present. The reported success rate is as high as 98 % with very low complication rates [18]. Before surgery, the adenoma should be localized by imaging studies. The most common imaging procedure, T99 sistamibi SPECT, has a sensitivity of up to 90 % for single adenomas; however, such parathyroid scans can miss 27 % of double adenomas and 57 % of hyperplastic glands [22]. The sensitivity of preoperative imaging can be increased by addition of other modalities, including neck ultrasound. In patients who are not considered to be a candidate for surgery because they do not meet the above criteria, regular follow-up is recommended, with measurement of serum calcium and creatinine every 6 months and bone densitometry biannually [18]. It is particularly important to note that patients may start to lose bone density after 8–10 years, such that monitoring should continue long term [18].

Medical therapy of PHPT is not considered equivalent to surgery [18] but is appropriate for patients who refuse surgery, are not appropriate surgical candidates, or have failed a parathyroidectomy (with residual hyperparathyroidism) [18, 23, 24]. There are four classes of medical therapies for primary hyperparathyroidism: calcimetics (cinacalcet), bisphosphonates, estrogen, and selective estrogen modulators (SERMs) [23]. The calcimimetic cinacalcet, by activating the parathyroid CaR, inhibits PTH secretion in patients with hyperparathyroidism [23]. Cinacalcet has been shown to be highly effective in reducing both PTH and calcium in patients with a broad range of disease severity [24]. However, it has little effect on bone density [24]. Bisphosphonates, in contrast, have little effect on PTH levels yet improve bone density. Estrogen and the SERM raloxifene have similar positive effects on bone; however, the adverse nonskeletal effects of estrogen replacement tend to limit its use for this purpose [23].

Malignancy-Associated Hypercalcemia

Malignancy-associated hypercalcemia (MAHC) is the most common cause of hypercalcemia in hospitalized patients, usually occurring in patients with advanced disease. MAHC is most commonly secondary to lung, breast, and hematological malignancies but can be seen in other tumors [25]. The most common cause of MAHC is due to presence of a circulating factor secreted by the tumor, the so-called humoral hypercalcemia of malignancy (HHM). This accounts for 80 % of MAHC. In 20 % of patients, hypercalcemia is due to local factors secreted by tumor invading the bone directly and stimulating osteolytic bony resorption. In rare patients hypercalcemia is due to activation of vitamin D or secretion of PTH by the tumor (Table 4.2) [25].

MAHC was first noted in 1920s; as early as the 1940s, it was suggested to be due to a circulating factor, possibly PTH. The discovery of a peptide, PTH-related protein (PTHrP), in 1987 was a seminal event expanding our understanding of HHM. This hormone, with a 70 % homology to the first 13 amino acids of the N-terminal of PTH, binds to PTH receptors, mimicking the biologic activities of PTH [26]. PTHrP is found in normal tissues and has many important physiologic effects, including regulation of placental calcium transport, mammary gland development, cell proliferation, and apoptosis [27, 28]. Hypercalcemia from PTHrP is due to stimulation of adenylate cyclase in target tissues, resulting in an increase in intestinal calcium absorption, osteoclastic bony resorption, and renal calcium reabsorption [29].

Table 4.2 Subtypes of hypercalcemia associated with cancer

Cancer type	Frequency	Bone metastases	Causative mediator	Typical tumors
Local osteolytic hypercalcemia	20 %	Common and extensive	Cytokines, chemokines, PTHrP	Breast cancer, myeloma, lymphoma
Humoral hypercalcemia	80 %	Minimal or absent	PTHrP	Squamous cell cancer; renal, ovarian, or endometrial cancer; HTLV-associated lymphoma; breast cancer
Calcitriol-secreting	<1 %	Variable	1,25-$(OH)_2D_3$ (calcitriol)	Lymphoma
Ectopic hyperparathyroidism	<1 %	Variable	PTH	Variable

PTH parathyroid hormone; *PTHrP* PTH-related protein; *1,25*$(OH)_2D$ 1,25-dihydroxyvitamin D; *HTLV* human T-cell lymphotrophic virus

The most common tumors associated with PTHrP-mediated hypercalcemia include squamous cell carcinomas of the lung, head and neck, as well as renal cell, prostate, breast, pancreas, and liver cancers and, on rare occasions, pheochromocytoma. PTHrP determination, measured by immunoradiometric assay (IRMA), is highly sensitive and specific and does not cross react with PTH or its fragments [30]. Interestingly, MAHC may on occasion be due to PTH secretion by the tumor [31] or transactivation of the parathyroid gene by a tumor gene product; this mechanism, however, is extremely rare.

Clinical features of MAHC. The clinical presentation of patients with PTHrp-induced hypercalcemia is a combination of the signs and symptoms of underlying cancer, in addition to the effects of hypercalcemia. The tumor is often far advanced, but in rare cases hypercalcemia can be the first presenting sign of malignancy. The biochemical profile is similar to patients with PHPT, with low serum phosphate, high fractional excretion of phosphate, and hypercalciuria. However, the serum level of 1,25 vitamin D is low in these patients; this may be due to the severity of hypercalcemia, overriding the stimulatory effect of PTH on the 1-α-hydroxylase enzyme [32]. Workup in these patients should include imaging studies to evaluate bony metastasis as well as measurement of PTH, PTHrP, and 1,25 vitamin D levels.

Hypercalcemia due to bony metastasis accounts for up to 35 % of MAHC and is most commonly seen in breast cancer and multiple myeloma. It is postulated that these tumors secrete a local osteoclast-activating factor (OAF) resulting in bony resorption. Among local osteolytic factors postulated are several lymphokines and chemokines including interleukin 1 α(alpha) and 1 β(beta), TNF, TGF β(beta)α(alpha). In addition PTHrP acting through paracrine mechanism can induce local bone resorption around the area of metastasis [33].

Another cause of HHM is activation of vitamin D by 1-α-hydroxylase enzyme present in macrophages. This is seen primarily in patients with Hodgkin's and non-Hodgkin's lymphomas, although it has also been reported in other tumors [34]. In these patients PTH and PTHrp levels are low to normal and 1,25 vitamin D level is elevated.

Treatment of MAHC. Management of these patients should include treatment of underlying tumor, as well as treatment of hypercalcemia. As noted above these tumors may be in advanced stages, and therefore, treatment is often very difficult. Hypercalcemia is often severe and needs to be treated promptly by increasing renal excretion of calcium by volume expansion while inhibiting bony resorption with calcitonin and bisphosphonates. This is discussed in detail later in this section. In hypercalcemia secondary to activation of vitamin D, glucocorticoids are the drug of choice. Glucocorticoids are also effective in hematological malignancy complicated by hypercalcemia.

Hypercalcemia Due to Milk–Alkali Syndrome

Milk–alkali syndrome (MAS) was a common problem in first half of the previous century, when peptic ulcer disease was routinely treated with milk and absorbable alkali [35]. The syndrome typically encompassed hypercalcemia, hyperphosphatemia, renal failure and metabolic alkalosis. MAS essentially disappeared with the use of new drugs for peptic ulcers, including nonabsorbable alkali, H2-blockers, and hydrogen pump inhibitors. More recently with the extensive use of calcium containing salts for prevention and treatment of osteoporosis, a new form of MAS or more appropriately alkali-associated hypercalcemia (AAH) or calcium–alkali syndrome, has appeared [36, 37]. In a recent review Beall and colleagues summarized the clinical and laboratory presentation of this new syndrome in 54 patients, with mean age of 50.3 and equal gender distribution. Hypercalcemia was due to the use of calcium carbonate in all, supplemented with milk and dairy food in some. The mean serum calcium was 15.1 mg/dL (range 11.1–27.5 mg/dL). Irreversible renal failure developed in 20 % of these patients [35]. In a recent report of 125 patients with hypercalcemia by Picolos and colleagues, AAH was the third most common cause of hypercalcemia in hospitalized patients and the second most common cause of severe hypercalcemia (>3.5 mmol/L), accounting for 8.8 and 25.7 % of cases respectively [36]. Interestingly in contrast to classical MAS, in more recent case series the serum phosphate is normal to low in the majority of patients [35, 37]. This is due to binding of dietary phosphate in GI tract by calcium carbonate. AAH is also reported in post-heart and heart and lung transplants treated with high dose calcium-containing antacids; in one report, 65/297 (22 %) of these patients developed significant hypercalcemia [38]. Other biochemical findings in this group included metabolic alkalosis in 31 % and renal failure in 37 %. Treatment of AAH includes discontinuation of absorbable antacids and standard treatment of acute hypercalcemia, as discussed later in this section.

Hypercalcemia Due to Granulomatous Diseases

Hypercalcemia is common in granulomatous disease such as sarcoidosis, tuberculosis, leprosy, and foreign body-associated granuloma (Reviewed in ref. [39]); although sarcoidosis is the most common cause in the developed world, more than 20 granulomatous disorders have been reported to cause calcitriol-mediated hypercalcemia [40]. In sarcoidosis hypercalcemia occurs in 10–20 % and hypercalciuria in up to 50 % of patients (reviewed in [41]). Hypercalcemia is a manifestation of multiple opportunistic infections in patients with AIDS including disseminated candidiasis and CMV and pneumocystis carinii [39, 40]. More recently hypercalcemia has been reported in AIDS patients with immune reconstitution syndrome and disseminated mycobacterium tuberculosis [42]. Hypercalcemia in these granulomatous disorders is due to activation of vitamin D by macrophage 1-α-hydroxylase enzyme [43]. The overactive extrarenal 1-α-hydroxylase enzyme is highly substrate-dependent, such that these patients are very sensitive to sunshine and seasonal variation in sunshine [44], in addition to calcium and vitamin D intake. Patients with sarcoidosis may also demonstrate normal serum calcium and high calcitriol levels, with suppressed PTH levels due to the direct inhibitory effect of calcitriol on PTH expression [45]. Normocalcemic hypercalciuria is also common, attributed to enhanced intestinal absorption of calcium (due to increased calcitriol) with reduced renal tubular calcium reabsorption due to suppressed PTH [45].

Hypercalcemia in sarcoidosis and other granulomatous disorders responds quickly to glucocorticoids, which reduce calcitriol synthesis by macrophages [46] and also reduce intestinal calcium absorption [47]. Low-dose prednisone (10–20 mg/day) is typically sufficient in sarcoidosis for long-term control of hypercalcemia; however, calcitriol-mediated hypercalcemia in lymphomas may require higher doses. Alternatives to prednisone include bisphosphonates [48], choroquine [43], hydroxychloroquine [49], and ketoconazole [50]. Treatment should also include a decrease in calcium and vitamin D intake, in addition to specific treatment of the underlying disease.

Hypercalcemia Due to Inactivation of Calcium-Sensing Receptor

Discovery of calcium-sensing receptor (CaR) has allowed better understanding of several genetic and acquired disorders presenting with hypercalcemia. One such disorder is an inactivating mutation of this receptor, decreasing its sensitivity to ambient calcium. The biochemical features of this syndrome include hypercalcemia, elevated PTH level, and hypocalciuria [51]. Familial hypocalciuric hypercalcemia (FHH—OMIM 145980) is due to heterozygous loss-of-function mutations, while neonatal severe primary hyperparathyroidism (NSHPT—OMIM 239200) is caused by homozygous loss-of-function mutations [52]. Patients with FHH are usually asymptomatic despite variable elevation in serum calcium. The PTH level is usually within normal range but elevated for the level of serum calcium. Serum magnesium is also elevated, reflecting the role of this receptor in regulating this cation. The urinary calcium is very low, a feature often used to distinguish this disorder from PHPT. This is likely due to the reduction in CaR-mediated inhibition of Na^+-Cl^- and K^+ transport by the thick ascending limb, resulting in reduced transcellular calcium transport by this nephron segment. In NSHPT calcium level can be as high as 7.5 mmol/L (30 mg/dL). In contrast to FHH these patients are often very symptomatic, presenting with weakness, hypotonia, and fractures, at times requiring urgent parathyroidectomy [52, 53]. Over 100 inactivating mutations are now recognized, with each family expressing a specific mutation. Phenotype–genotype correlations have shown that both these disorders are quite heterogeneous, with significant clinical variability among different kindred. A definitive diagnosis may therefore require genetic analysis [1, 54], which is clinically available in the United States.

Miscellaneous Causes of Hypercalcemia

Endocrine. Mild hypercalcemia is seen in 15–50 % of patients with thyrotoxicosis [55]. This is attributed to activation of osteoclasts by thyroid hormone [55, 56]. Treatment should be directed toward management of the hyperthyroidism; beta-blockers have been reported to partially ameliorate hypercalcemia in this disorder. Mild hypercalcemia has also been reported in Addison disease, secondary to both bone resorption and a decrease in urinary calcium. The latter is resolved quickly with volume expansion. However, physiologic doses of glucocorticoids are necessary to normalize skeletal calcium homeostasis [57].

Immobilization. Prolonged immobilization results in hypercalciuria in all patients; hypercalcemia in this context occurs primarily in patients with high bone turnover such as adolescents and those with Paget disease, thyrotoxicosis, hyperparathyroidism, and malignancy. This is due to an increase in osteoclastic activity and a concomitant decrease in osteoblastic [58]. Prolonged immobilization is associated with osteopenia and nephrolithiasis. Biochemical studies show suppressed PTH and calcitriol levels. Treatment includes weight-bearing exercises when possible; if this is not possible, treatment with volume expansion, loop diuretics, bisphosphonates, and calcitonin should be considered. For example, the prophylactic use of intermittent bisphosphonates in hemiplegic patients is associated with lower serum calcium and better preservation of bone density on the hemiplegic side [59].

Drugs. In addition to vitamin D and calcium supplements, which were discussed above, thiazides as well as Lithium are important causes of drug-induced hypercalcemia. Thiazides induce hypocalciuria via proximal tubular hyperabsorption of calcium, leading to hypercalcemia [60]. This is more commonly seen in patients with mild asymptomatic hyperparathyroidism [61]. Hypercalcemia is seen in up to 10 % of patients on Lithium and is usually mild. This is due to a change in calcium-PTH set point, presumably due to the interaction between lithium and the CaR [62, 63]. This is supported by recent reports of favorable response to Cinacalcet in two patients with Li-induced hypercalcemia [64].

Approach to the Patient with Hypercalcemia

History and physical examination often offer the strongest clues to the final diagnosis in these patients. Most patients with mild chronic asymptomatic hypercalcemia have PHPT, whereas most patients with severe hypercalcemia have MAH. PHPT may present with history of renal and bone disease while patients with MAH often present with a known malignancy. A careful medication history, including over-the-counter antacids or other calcium-containing medications, is very helpful in patients with hypercalcemia of unknown etiology. Diagnosis of hypercalcemia secondary to granulomatous and other endocrine disorders is often challenging and requires careful attention to diagnostic tests such as serum cortisol, thyroid, and vitamin D metabolites. Diagnosis of hypercalcemia is greatly aided by the availability of sensitive tests to measure PTH, PTHrP as well as vitamin D metabolites. These tests, however, should be interpreted in the light of other clinical data. Finally, multiple myeloma should be ruled out with the appropriate tests, including serum and urine immunoelectrophoresis and serum free light chain levels.

Treatment of Hypercalcemia

Treatment of mild hypercalcemia (calcium <11.9 mg/dL) should focus on the diagnosis and treatment of the underlying disorder. In patients with PHPT, the definitive treatment is ultimately a parathyroidectomy; however, therapy with cinacalcet can rapidly normalize serum calcium [24]. In patients with malignancy-associated hypercalcemia, treatment of the underlying malignancy is often ineffective; it also does not change the ultimate outcome in these patients. In moderate and severe hypercalcemia, defined as calcium level above 12 and 14 mg % respectively [25], it is critical to treat hypercalcemia rapidly while searching for the underlying etiology. This is because severe hypercalcemia creates a vicious cycle due to its renal, CNS and GI effects. Hypercalcemia decreases GFR by afferent arteriolar vasoconstriction as well as polyuria-induced volume depletion. This results in a decrease in the filtered load of calcium and a reduced ability of the kidney to excrete calcium. Hypercalcemia also results in nausea, vomiting decreasing fluid intake and worsening volume depletion. The CNS effects of hypercalcemia include lethargy, headache, decreased cognitive function, and finally stupor and coma; again these neuropsychiatric symptoms, by decreasing food and fluid intake, worsen volume depletion and hypercalcemia. These multiple effects thus create a vicious cycle, leading to hypercalcemic crisis.

Treatment of hypercalcemia should initially include supportive therapy including decreasing oral or enteral calcium intake, discontinuation of drugs that result in hypercalcemia and treatment of hypophosphatemia [25]. If this fails or hypercalcemia is severe, treatment should include maneuvers to increase calcium excretion and when indicated, decrease calcium resorption from bone and/or absorption from the gut (Table 4.3). Increase in calcium excretion is achieved initially by infusion of large amount of normal (0.9 %) saline to replete the extracellular fluid volume and increase GFR; this will lead to an initial drop in serum calcium. This initial calciuresis can then be augmented by the use of loop diuretics such as furosemide to inhibit calcium reabsorption by the thick ascending limb [65]. In patients with relatively normal renal function this maneuver is often highly successful in decreasing serum calcium rapidly. Major side effects include hypokalemia, hypomagnesemia, and

Table 4.3 Causes of hypocalcemia

1. Hypoparathyroidism a. Developmental: branchial dysembryogenesis (DiGeorge's syndrome) b. Autoimmune: polyglandular autoimmune disorders (APECD) c. Idiopathic: isolated late-onset d. Postsurgical e. Infiltrative diseases f. Irradiation g. Hypomagnesemia
2. PTH resistance: pseudohypoparathyroidism
3. Activating mutation of Car
4. Vitamin D deficiency a. Nutritional deficiency b. Malabsorption c. Anticonvulsant therapy d. Liver disease
5. 1-α-hydroxylase deficiency (vitamin D-dependent rickets, Type I)
6. Vitamin D resistance (vitamin D-dependent rickets, Type II)
7. Medications: bisphosphonates, phosphate, anticonvulsants, calcitonin
8. Malignancy a. Osteoblastic metastases b. Tumor-lysis syndrome
9. Acute pancreatitis
10. Sepsis

occasionally volume overload. The furosemide dose and frequency should be adjusted to generate urine volumes in excess of 4–6 L/day. This volume should be replaced by fluid containing both sodium as well as potassium chloride. It is important to initiate forced diuresis with furosemide only *after* correction of volume deficit commonly present in these patients. In patients with irreversible severe renal failure and patients on dialysis, treatment with dialysis using low calcium bath is essential. Oral phosphate is occasionally used if serum phosphate is low (<3.0 mg/dL) but this is rarely effective.

In patients with primary hyperparathyroidism and malignancy where bone resorption plays an important role in the development of hypercalcemia, inhibition of bone resorption has an important role in controlling hypercalcemia. Bisphosphonates acting through inhibition of osteoclastic activity and induction of osteoclast apoptosis are effective antiresorptive agents (for details refer to ref. [25]). These drugs are poorly absorbed orally and therefore must be given intravenously. Table 4.3 summarizes the dose and mode of administration of the most commonly used bisphosphonates. Three drugs, pamidronate, zoledronate, and ibandronate, have been approved by the Food and Drug Administration (FDA) for use in the United States while in Europe an additional drug, clodronate, is also available. The initial response to bisphosphonates requires 2–4 days, with the greatest drop in serum calcium seen between days 4 and 7. Response rate varies from 60 to 90 % with the effect lasting for several weeks (for a detailed discussion refer to refs. [25] and [66]). Although zoledronate is simpler to administer and has a slightly greater efficacy, it is more expensive than pamidronate. The major side effects of these drugs include flu-like symptoms, fatigue, nausea, dyspnea, and edema. The most important but fortunately uncommon side effect is acute kidney injury, with acute tubular necrosis [66]. This is most common with zolendronate and least common with ibandronate [66]. Pamidronate but not other bisphosphonates has also been reported to cause nephrotic syndrome secondary to FSGS [66]. These drugs should therefore be used cautiously in patients with acute kidney injury and/or chronic kidney disease. Initial emphasis in these patients should be on aggressive volume repletion with normal saline. Bisphosphonates should only be utilized if subsequent therapy with furosemide and saline is not successful, and/or if definitive management of the underlying disorder is not feasible. Options include IV ibandronate, which may have less nephrotoxicity [66], or renally adjusted dosing with IV pamidronate over several hours.

Recently gallium nitrate has become available for treatment of MAH. In a double-blind study, gallium nitrate was at least as effective as pamidronate in normalizing of serum calcium. This drug was well tolerated with minimal side effects [67]. Calcitonin is occasionally used acutely; however, its effect is short-lived and needs to be followed by a more definitive therapy. Mithramycin, once the drug of choice in MAH, is now rarely used. Dose and route of administration of these drugs are summarized in Table 4.3. High dose glucocorticoids are effective in patients with vitamin-D dependent hypercalcemia such as in sarcoidosis or T-cell lymphomas; it has also been used successfully in certain hematological malignancies such as multiple myeloma. In patients with severe renal failure or on dialysis, hypercalcemia should be treated with low calcium dialysis.

Hypocalcemia

Hypocalcemia is defined as total serum calcium, corrected for albumin, of less than 8.4 mg/dL (2.1 mmol/L) or ionized calcium of less than 4.48 mg/dL (1.12 mmol/L). Hypocalcemia seen in acutely ill patients is often secondary to hypoalbuminemia. It is therefore essential that calcium level is corrected for albumin concentration, and if needed hypocalcemia is verified by measurement of ionized calcium.

Clinical Presentation of Hypocalcemia

Clinical features of hypocalcemia are a function of severity, the rate of decrease in serum calcium, and the presence or absence of other electrolyte abnormalities such as hypomagnesemia or hypokalemia. The primary clinical features of hypocalcemia are neuromuscular and cardiovascular in nature. Some of these signs and symptoms, such as irritability and weakness, are nonspecific in nature; however, other manifestations, such as tetany, laryngospasm, seizure, and/or a positive Trousseau or Chvostek sign, should strongly suggest this diagnosis.

Hypocalcemia increases neuronal excitability, presenting clinically as paresthesia, tetany, laryngospasm, bronchospasm, and muscle cramps. Centrally hypocalcemia can cause a change in mental status, resulting in stupor and seizure. Long-standing hypocalcemia can result in CNS calcification as well as papilledema. Chvostek and Trousseau signs both reflect increased excitability of neuronal tissue. The Chvostek sign is elicited by a sharp tap over the facial nerve, resulting in twitching of facial and upper lip muscles. The Trousseau sign is elicited by inflation of the sphygmomanometer cuff to 10 mm above the systolic pressure for 3 min; the resultant carpopedal spasm is due to increased sensitivity of peripheral nerves to hypoxia. In general, the Trousseau sign is more specific than that of Chvostek, which is seen in 10 % of normal individuals. It is important to note that similar signs and symptoms can be elicited in patients with hypomagnesemia as well as severe respiratory alkalosis.

Calcium level is critical for both myocardial contractility as well as electrical conduction. Cardiovascular presentation therefore includes arrhythmias, bradycardia, abnormal EKG with prolonged QT, congestive heart failure, and hypotension [68]. Other clinical findings include cataract, coarse brittle hair, and dry skin, primarily seen in chronic hypocalcemia.

Causes of Hypocalcemia

Hypocalcemia is primarily due to decrease in parathyroid secretion or resistance to PTH, or due to vitamin D deficiency. Table 4.3 summarizes the major causes of hypocalcemia.

Hypoparathyroidism

Hypoparathyroidism is the most important cause of chronic hypocalcemia. Hypoparathyroidism can be developmental, often presenting in the neonatal period, or autoimmune, presenting in childhood. Acquired hypoparathyroidism, primarily postsurgical, can occur at any age, but often presents in adulthood.

Developmental hypoparathyroidism is seen primarily in patients with chromosome 21q11.2 deletion presenting with a variety of phenotypic expression, including DiGeorge and its closely related velocardiofacial syndrome [69]. These syndromes are due to incomplete development of brachial arch resulting in variety of defects including agenesis or hypogenesis of parathyroid and thymus glands, as well as facial and cardiac abnormalities. Hypoparathyroidism develops in 17–60 % of patients, typically improving over time with subsequent hypertrophy of the remnant gland. Thymal hypogenesis results in a T-cell defect in about 80 % of patients. Antibody production is, however, normal, but these patients are prone to viral and superimposed bacterial infections. Cardiac anomalies included interrupted aortic arch, isolated ventricular septal defect and Tetralogy of Fallot. Other anomalies include delay in speech development as well as anatomic defects in genitourinary and ophthalmic systems. The specific gene(s) involved in this heterogeneous syndrome remains unknown [69].

Autoimmune hypoparathyroidism is seen as a component of autoimmune polyendocrinopathy–candidiasis–ectodermal dystrophy (APECED) syndrome. It is a rare monogenic autosomal recessive disorder due to mutation in autoimmune regulatory gene (AIRE) on chromosome 21q22.3. Although mutation in AIRE gene causes loss of self-tolerance, its specific function is not fully known [70]. The majority of patients develop the classical triad of hypoparathyroidism, hypoadrenalism, and mucocutaneous candidiasis; other findings can include hypothyroidism, hepatitis, keratoconjunctivitis, and other endocrinopathies. Hypoparathyroidism is the most common endocrine disorder and develops in 2/3 of the patients as the first endocrine deficiency [71]. Adrenal insufficiency develops later, often during adolescence. Diabetes mellitus, testicular failure, and hypothyroidism develop in middle age. Interstitial nephritis is reported in 9 % of patients reported from Finland [72]. Clinical presentations vary greatly in the same family, with final diagnosis made anywhere from infancy to middle age [72].

Sporadic hypoparathyroidism is a rare disease presenting with clinical and biochemical signs of hypoparathyroidism, cataract, basal ganglia calcification, and seizure. The etiology is thought to be autoimmune in origin, presenting in the third and fourth decades of life. Recently autoantibody to the CaR has been documented in 49 % of patients versus 13.3 % of a control group. The etiologic roles of these antibodies need further studies [73].

Postsurgical hypoparathyroidism is seen in patients with extensive surgery for thyroid cancer, Grave's disease, head and neck cancer, or parathyroid hyperplasia. With the increase in popularity of radiation therapy in the treatment of Grave's disease, the incidence of postsurgical hypoparathyroidism has decreased. Postsurgical hypoparathyroidism can be permanent, often becoming apparent few hours after surgery, or transient. The latter is due to ischemia of normal parathyroid glands or due to chronic suppression of normal glands by a hyperfunctioning adenoma. In patients with long-standing hyperparathyroidism, removal of the adenoma is often followed by hungry bone syndrome, presenting as severe hypocalcemia and hyperphosphatemia, in the immediate postoperative period. This is more common in patients with more severe hyperparathyroidism presenting with higher serum calcium, higher PTH, larger adenomas [74], and preoperative vitamin D deficiency [75].

Hypomagnesemia is associated with a decrease in PTH secretion as well as end organ resistance to the action of PTH. These patients often do not respond to calcium or vitamin D supplementation until hypomagnesemia is corrected [76]. Hypoparathyroidism is occasionally seen in patients treated with external radiation to the neck as well as radioactive iodine treatment for Grave's disease [77]. Hypoparathyroidism has also been reported in infiltrative diseases such as Wilson disease, hemochromatosis, and metastatic cancer.

Pseudohypoparathyroidism

Albright and colleagues in 1942 reported a group of patients with skeletal and developmental defects who presented with biochemical features of hypoparathyroidism. These patients were, however, resistant to bovine PTH infusion. This disorder called pseudohypoparathyroidism (PsHPT) includes a heterogeneous group with different biochemical and clinical features. PsHPT is now classified as type 1a, 1b, type II as well as pseudopseudohypoparathyroidism (PsPsHPT) [78]. Patients with type 1a PsHPT have developmental and skeletal defects including brachydactyly, short stature, mental retardation, hypocalcemia, hyperphosphatemia, and resistance to the action of many hormones. Patients with type 1b have resistance to renal effect of PTH but present with normal appearance. Patients with PsPsHPT present with skeletal abnormalities of PsHPT type 1a, but with normal biochemical features and normal hormonal responsiveness. This group can be seen in the same family as type 1a. The genetic defect in these patients is in the alpha subunit of GTP-binding protein. This explains the associated resistance to several hormones in this type of PsHPT [78]. The heterogeneity reflects type of mutation as well as mode of inheritance in affected patients [78].

PsHPT type II present with normal developmental features but are hypocalcemic. Nephrogenous CAMP generation is normal; however, the phosphaturic effect is blunted, resulting in hyperphosphatemia. It is postulated that these patients have normal G-protein coupled response with a defect in renal response to C-AMP. The genetic abnormality in type II remains unknown at this time [78].

Diagnosis of hypoparathyroidism. Hypoparathyroidism should be considered in any patient with hypocalcemia, especially in association with hyperphosphatemia. In patients with normal renal function the differential diagnosis includes severe vitamin D deficiency and pseudohypoparathyroidism. In patients with mucocutaneous candidiasis or other endocrine deficiencies, diagnosis of polyglandular endocrinopathy should be entertained. Diagnosis should be confirmed with measurement of PTH as well as vitamin D level. Patients with pseudohypoparathyroidism have biochemical abnormalities similar to hypoparathyroidism but with normal to elevated PTH level. As noted

Table 4.4 Biochemical findings in hypocalcemic states

Diagnosis	Phosphate	PTH	25(OH)D	$1,25(OH)_2D_3$
Hypoparathyroidism	↑	↓	N	↓
Pseudohypoparathyroidism	↑	↑	N	↓
Vitamin D deficiency	↓	↑	↓	↓, N, ↑
Renal failure	↑	↑	N	↓
Severe liver disease	↓	↑	↓	↓, N
Nephrotic syndrome	↓	↑	↓	↓, N
Hypomagnesemia	↓, N	↓	N	↓, N
Vitamin D-dependent rickets, type I	↓	↑	N, ↑	↓
Vitamin D-dependent rickets, type II	↓	↑	N, ↑	↑

Table 4.5 Oral calcium preparations

Salt	Tablet size (mg)	Elemental calcium (mg) (%)	Tablets/day to provide 1.0 g of elemental calcium
Calcium gluconate	500	45 (9 %)	22
Calcium lactate	650	84 (13 %)	12
Calcium carbonate	1,250	500 (40 %)	2
Calcium citrate	950	200 (24 %)	5

Table 4.6 Vitamin D preparations

Nonproprietary name	Abbreviation	Commercial name	Effective dose
Cholecalciferol	Vitamin D_3		400–1,000 U/day
Ergocalciferol	Vitamin D_2	Calciferol	25,000–100,000 U 3×/week
Calcifediol	$25(OH)D_3$	Calderol	20–50 μ9(mu)g 3×/week–once/day
Dihydrotachysterol	DHT	Dihydrotachysterol	0.1–1 mg/day
Calcitriol	$1,25(OH)_2D_3$	Rocaltrol	0.25–1 μ(mu)g 1–2×/day
Paricalcitol	19-nor-1α(alpha),25 $(OH)_2D_3$	Zemplar	1.0–2.0 μ(mu)g/day or 2.0–4.0 μ(mu)g 3×/week
Doxecalciferol	1α(alpha),OHD_3	Hectorol	1.0–3.5 μ(mu)g/day

above skeletal abnormalities are seen in some but not all patients with PsHPTH. Biochemical findings in hypocalcemic states are summarized in Table 4.4 [78].

Treatment of hypoparathyroidism. The standard treatment of hypoparathyroidism and PsHPT is use of one of the many vitamin D and calcium preparations with the goal of raising serum calcium level to low normal level (Tables 4.5 and 4.6). Vitamin D increases calcium absorption by the gut; however, in the absence of PTH, this can result in hypercalciuria, nephrocalcinosis, nephrolithiasis, and renal failure [79]. In addition, dose titration is often difficult and should be done with close monitoring of serum as well as urinary calcium, with the goal of maintaining low normal calcium levels. Recently recombinant human (1–34) PTH has become available for the treatment of osteoporosis. In a randomized parallel group open labeled study of 20 patients with hypoparathyroidism of different etiologies, patients were treated with either PTH sc or oral cholecalciferol on twice daily basis for 3 years. Serum calcium was similar in both groups but urinary calcium was higher in cholecalciferol group. Markers of bone remodeling were similar in both groups. PTH injection was well tolerated [80]. The experience with this drug is, however, limited and further studies are required before this logical therapy replaces conventional therapy with vitamin D.

Hypocalcemia Secondary to Activating Mutation Of CaR

Autosomal dominant hypercalciuric hypocalcemia is a rare disease due to an activating mutation of CaR. This mutation induces excessive calcium-induced inhibition of the parathyroid gland, resulting in hypocalcemia and hypercalciuria. Hypocalcemia is often mild and asymptomatic. Some patients may present as Bartter's syndrome [81], consistent with dysfunction of the thick ascending limb nephron segment. The CaR is heavily expressed at the basolateral membrane of thick ascending limb cells; genetic activation of CaR inhibits transepithelial Na^+-Cl^- and K^+ transport, thus producing a Bartter's syndrome phenotype [9, 81]. Attempts at normalization of serum calcium will aggravate hypercalciuria and result in nephrolithiasis and nephrocalcinosis. Recently exogenous PTH hormone has been shown to be effective in a single patient with this disorder [82].

Vitamin D Deficiency

Vitamin D deficiency, when mild or moderate, is typically associated with normal serum calcium and high PTH level. However, if severe or if associated with calcium malabsorption, it will present with hypocalcemia and osteomalacia. Vitamin D deficiency can be dietary in nature or due to a defect in the activation of vitamin D. Dietary-induced vitamin D deficiency is less common in western countries, where milk and certain other foods are fortified with this vitamin. Mild vitamin D deficiency is, however, relatively common, primarily in elderly and alcoholics with marginal food intake and low exposure to sunshine. Vitamin D deficiency is also seen in patients with malabsorption due to pancreatitis, celiac disease, cystic fibrosis, primary biliary cirrhosis, and short bowel syndrome. Vitamin D deficiency seen in patients on long-term phenobarbitol is due to enhanced metabolism of this vitamin resulting from the induction of hepatic microsomal enzymes by this drug. Hypocalcemia is also occasionally seen in patients on phenytoins; this is due to a decrease in intestinal calcium absorption, as well as calcium release by bone [83].

Vitamin D-dependent rickets refers to patients presenting in childhood with hypocalcemia, severe osteomalacia, high PTH level, and hypophosphatemia, who are responsive to 1,25 vitamin D, but not to the parent compounds [84]. This disorder is due to a deficiency in 1-α-hydroxylase enzyme required for activation of vitamin D. If hypocalcemia is prolonged these patients will develop secondary hyperparathyroidism with its classical bony abnormalities. Hereditary vitamin D-resistant rickets refers to patients who do not respond to 1,25 vitamin D (type II); this disorder is caused by loss-of-function defects in the vitamin D receptor.

Treatment of vitamin D deficiency is primarily through the provision of a physiologic amount of vitamin D with or without calcium supplementation, in food or as an oral medication (Table 4.6). Treatment of the vitamin D-dependent group involves provision of physiologic dose of 1,25 cholecalciferol; treatment of vitamin D resistant rickets is very difficult and may require prolonged calcium infusion.

Hypocalcemia Secondary to Magnesium Deficiency

This is discussed under the section on "Hypomagnesemia" in this chapter.

Acute Reversible Hypocalcemia

This is seen primarily in patients with acute pancreatitis as well as sepsis. The mechanism of hypocalcemia in acute pancreatitis is due to (a) release of pancreatic lipases resulting in deposition of calcium in area of fat necrosis and (b) release of calcitonin and glucagons [85]. Hypocalcemia seen in septic patients is secondary to release of inflammatory mediators and is not seen in postsurgical patients in intensive care unit who are not septic [86].

Diagnostic Evaluation of Hypocalcemia

This should always begin by correction of total calcium for changes in serum albumin and if needed, by measurement of ionized calcium. In patients with true hypocalcemia careful history with special attention to the time of onset, severity of symptoms, surgical, dietary, medication and family history. On physical examination attention should be paid to presence or absence of developmental or acquired skeletal abnormalities, bony fracture and mucocutaneous candidiasis. The biochemical profile of patients with hypocalcemia is summarized in Table 4.4. Workup should therefore include evaluation of serum magnesium, PTH as well as vitamin D metabolites. Presence of other endocrine abnormalities should raise the possibility of polyglandular syndromes associated with hypoparathyroidism. Further workup should be dictated by the initial findings and may include imaging as well as genetic testing.

Most adult patients presenting with hypocalcemia, often associated with hyperphosphatemia, have primary hypoparathyroidism. In infants and young children less common syndromes such as pseudohypoparathyroidism or APECD syndrome should also be considered.

Treatment of Hypocalcemia

Treatment of hypocalcemic syndrome depends greatly on the final diagnosis and is discussed under specific diseases above. In this section we only discuss the acute treatment of hypocalcemia. Hypocalcemia should be treated if patients have any symptoms or signs referable to this abnormality including tetany, seizure, papilledema, hypotension, arrhythmia, positive Chvostek or Trousseau signs, or prolonged QT interval. Acute hypocalcemia often occurs in patients with extensive neck surgery or after removal of large parathyroid adenomas presenting as hungry bone syndrome. In addition patients with nutritional deficiency complicated by magnesium deficiency or with acute pancreatitis could present with acute rapidly declining serum calcium. In patients with severe or life-threatening hypocalcemia 10–20 mL of calcium gluconate containing 90–180 mg of elemental calcium should be given intravenously while monitoring the patient [87]. This can be repeated as needed. If hypocalcemia persists an infusion of calcium gluconate should be initiated to provide 10–15 mg/kg of elemental calcium over 6–8 h. Calcium chloride can also be used but it is more irritating at the site of infusion. If hypocalcemia is expected to persist, treatment should include oral calcium supplement providing 1–2 g of elemental calcium and vitamin D. Table 4.5 summarizes amount of calcium in popular calcium preparations. Table 4.6 summarized the vitamin D preparation available and effective dose.

Disorders of Phosphate Metabolism

General Considerations

Phosphorous, present in the body primarily as inorganic phosphate, plays a major role in many biologic systems including membrane function, energy metabolism, cell signaling, oxygen transport, and skeletal muscle metabolism [88]. Total body phosphorous pool is 99 % intracellular, of which 85 % is bound to skeleton as hydroxyapatite and remainder in the soft tissues. The extracellular pool of phosphorous is approximately 600 mg. Given a pKa of 6.8, the plasma inorganic phosphate exists primarily as $H2PO_4^{2-}$; HPO_4^- with a ratio of 4 divalent to 1 monovalent molecule. The concentration of plasma inorganic phosphate is reported as the concentration of elemental phosphorous in the plasma and is between 2.5 and 4.5 mg/dL or 0.81 and 1.4 mmol/L. Plasma phosphate is 10 % protein bound. There is a diurnal variation in the concentration of plasma phosphorous of about 0.2 mmol with nadir at 11:00 a.m. and peak between midnight and 3:00 a.m. The extent and timing of the diurnal variation is dependent on dietary phosphate intake [89]. Given the 99:1 ratio of intra- to extracellular phosphate, serum phosphorous may not be a good indicator of total body phosphate. In addition the ratio between intracellular and extracellular phosphate is affected by multiple factors, including acid–base status, glucose metabolism, as well as several hormones, in particular insulin and catecholamines. These are discussed further under specific disorders.

Phosphate intake in Western diet is about 20 mg/kg/day or 1,400 mg in a 70 kg man. Approximately 1,100 mg is absorbed in the upper intestine, primarily in the proximal jejunum, while 200 mg is secreted in bile and salivary juices resulting in a net absorption of 900 mg and loss of 500 mg in stool. In adults bone resorption and formation is equal and this therefore has no impact on overall phosphate homeostasis. Finally renal excretion of phosphorous equals the net phosphorous absorption (Fig. 4.2).

Phosphate Homeostasis

Intestinal Absorption of Phosphate

Intestinal phosphate absorption is both active through sodium-phosphate cotransporter, as well as passive by diffusion. Sodium phosphate cotransport is accomplished by a family of Na^+-P type II cotransporters (NaPi-II), with type IIa and IIc located in the luminal membrane of renal proximal tubule and IIb in the luminal membrane of intestine of man [90]. Phosphate absorption is increased by an increase in the number of transporters shuffled to the membrane and decreased when these transporters are shifted internally and degraded.

At low phosphate intake most intestinal phosphate absorption occurs through active pathway; however, on high phosphate intake, passive absorption plays a more major role. Phosphate absorption is regulated through an interaction between serum phosphorous, PTH, and 1,25 vitamin D [91]. 1,25 vitamin D directly stimulates phosphate absorption while PTH and serum phosphorous, through regulation of vitamin D activation to 1,25 vitamin D, indirectly control net phosphate absorption. The final pathway for 1,25 vitamin D modulation of phosphate absorption is through the regulation of the number of sodium-phosphate cotransporters in the luminal membrane of enterocytes, primarily in early jejunum.

Renal Regulation of Phosphate

Although plasma phosphate is 10–15 % protein bound, the filtered load can be calculated as if it is freely filtered. This is partly due to the effect of Gibbs–Donnan equilibrium on distribution of anion across a semi-permeable membrane and partly due to the need to correct plasma volume for space occupied by plasma protein. Most filtered phosphate is reabsorbed, resulting in a fractional excretion of about 10–15 %. Phosphate is actively reabsorbed in the proximal tubule primarily through Na^+-Pi-IIa and to a lesser extent, Na^+-P-IIc cotransporters. By the end of the accessible proximal tubule less than 30 % of filtered phosphate remains in the tubular fluid. The remainder of filtered phosphate is reabsorbed in the distal portion of proximal tubule with a small amount reabsorbed in distal nephron. Phosphate is not secreted by any segment of the nephron.

Renal phosphate handling is regulated by PTH, dietary phosphate and to a lesser extent vitamin D. PTH is the major regulator of phosphate handling by the kidney. The PTH effect is primarily in the proximal tubule, where it binds to its receptor on the apical and basolateral membranes, downregulating Na^+-Pi-IIa and Na^+-Pi-IIc abundance in apical brush border membrane. Acute changes in phosphate absorption involve movement of Na^+-Pi from an intracellular pool to brush border membrane and vice versa. Long-term regulation depends on production or destruction of Na^+-Pi transporters through transcription or degradation pathways. The transporter(s) in basolateral membrane responsible for phosphate exit is still unknown. The effect of PTH is dependent on the activation of both phospholipase C and protein kinase C, as well as protein kinase A-dependent pathways [91, 92]. Dietary phosphate also rapidly modulates phosphate reabsorption in proximal tubules through similar mechanism [91]; this effect is, however, independent of PTH level. In addition the phosphaturic response to PTH is markedly blunted in phosphate-deprived states. The effects of vitamin D metabolites are complex and depend partly on direct effects on the tubule, in addition to effects on total body phosphate homeostasis. Short-term administration of vitamin D metabolites is phosphaturic in phosphate-replete and antiphosphaturic in phosphate-depleted individuals. Chronic administration of vitamin D increases gut absorption of phosphate and secondarily increases urinary phosphate excretion [93]. Growth hormone, insulin, and thyroid hormone increase and calcitonin, glucocorticoids, and atrial natriuretic factor decrease phosphate reabsorption (reviewed in ref. [91]).

In 1994 Kumar et al. documented the presence of inhibitor(s) of phosphate transport in the serum of a patient with tumor-induced osteomalacia (TIO) who presented with hypophosphatemia, phosphaturia, low 1,25 vitamin D, and rickets

Table 4.7 Factors affecting phosphate handling by the kidney

Factors that increase Pi reabsorption	*Factors that decrease Pi reabsorption*
• Phosphate depletion	• Phosphate loading
• Hypocalcemia	• Hypercalcemia
• Parathyroidectomy	• PTH, PTHrP, and cyclic AMP
• 1-α 25(OH)$_2$ D$_3$	• Phosphatonins: (FGF-23, SFRP-4, MEPE, FGF7)
• Volume contraction	• Volume expansion
• Hypocapnia	• Acid–base disturbance
• Hormones: growth hormone, thyroid hormone, insulin	• Calcitonin, glucocorticoids, atrial naturetic peptide
	• Miscellaneous (Carbonic anhydrase inhibitors, dopamine, glucose, and alanine)

[94]. These inhibitors, collectively called phosphatonins, are only discussed briefly here; readers are referred to several excellent reviews for more in-depth discussions [5, 95]. The major known phosphatonin is fibroblast growth factor 23 (FGF23) [5]. This peptide inhibits renal and intestinal absorption of phosphate directly by inhibition of the Na^+-P-IIa cotransporter. It also inhibits activation of vitamin D to 1,25 vitamin D through inhibition of 1-α-hydroxylase enzyme [5]. The biochemical findings in patients with TIO are similar to the phenotype of two genetic syndromes, autosomal dominant hypophosphatemic rickets (ADHR—OMIM 193100) and X-linked hypophosphatemic rickets (XHR—OMIM 307800). In patients with ADHR, a mutated form of FGF23 with a prolonged half-life induces severe phosphaturia, hypophosphatemia, and rickets [5]. In XHR mutations in a gene, "phosphate-regulating gene with homology to endopeptidases on X-chromosome" (PHEX), are involved [5]; this enzyme regulates degradation of FGF23 and other phosphatonins. The physiological role of this peptide in normal man is still a rapidly evolving area of investigation. However, oral phosphate loading and calcitriol stimulate FGF23 secretion, whereas dietary phosphate restriction inhibits [96]. FGF23 levels increase progressively in chronic kidney disease (CKD), suggesting that FGF23 excess plays an important role in the CKD-associated inhibition of the 1-α-hydroxylase enzyme that generates active calcitriol [96]. These findings support important physiologic roles for FGF23 in the regulation of phosphate and calcium; however, further studies are needed to fully evaluate its role in heath and disease. Several other phosphatonins, including matrix extracellular phosphoglycoprotein (MEPE), frizzle-related protein 4 (s-FRP4), and FGF7, have also been implicated in TIO. However, their role in phosphate homeostasis in man is still speculative. Table 4.7 summarizes factors involved in the regulation of serum phosphorous by the kidney.

Hypophosphatemia

Hypophosphatemia is defined by a decrease in serum phosphorous concentration below lower limits of normal of <2.5 mg/dL. Mild to moderate hypophosphatemia is defined as values between 1.0 and 2.5 mg/dL and severe hypophosphatemia as phosphorous level below 1.0 mg/dL. Phosphate deprivation refers to deficiency in dietary phosphate intake, and phosphate depletion to abnormally low total body phosphate. Given the fact that 99 % of total body phosphate is intracellular, phosphate deprivation and/or depletion may or may not be associated with hypophosphatemia. Hypophosphatemia could also occur without phosphate depletion by intracellular shift of phosphate, as seen in acute respiratory alkalosis.

Hypophosphatemia is relatively common in the hospital population. The incidence is reportedly from 0.4 to 2 %, depending on the definition of hypophosphatemia and the patient population included in the study. In certain populations, such as alcoholics or patients with sepsis, it can reach as high as 23 % [97]and as high as 75 % and 80 % in patients with burn and sepsis respectively (reviewed in ref. [88]). Severe hypophosphatemia is, however, much less common and estimated at 0.1 % [98]. Notably, however, in a retrospective study severe hypophosphatemia was associated with fourfold increases in mortality [99].

Signs and Symptoms of Hypophosphatemia

Signs and symptoms of hypophosphatemia depend on the severity, associated deficiencies and underlying illness. Mild to moderate hypophosphatemia is often asymptomatic while severe hypophosphatemia can result in multiple clinical manifestations including:

- Musculoskeletal: Musculoskeletal symptoms include weakness, muscle pain and frank rhabdomyolysis. Although these symptoms are commonly attributed to hypophosphatemia, they are often seen in patients, such as alcoholics, who have multiple comorbidities including other electrolyte and acid–base abnormalities. It is therefore difficult to document an independent role for hypophosphatemia alone. Rhabdomyolysis defined as CK >1.5 upper limits of normal was reported in 36 % of 129 hypophosphatemic patients with mean phosphate of 1.5 mg/dL. These patients had multiple other electrolyte abnormalities and none had signs and symptoms referable to elevation in CK [100]. Animals deprived of phosphate for several weeks develop only mild muscle abnormalities including subclinical myopathy (reviewed in ref. [101]). A more severe form of proximal muscle weakness is seen in patients with hypophosphatemia rickets. Pathological finding includes nonspecific atrophy probably from disuse and nutritional deficiency common in these patients [102].
- Cardiovascular: Reversible myocardial depression in human has been reported in severe but not mild to moderate hypophosphatemia. In one study of seven patients with severe hypophosphatemia (mean serum phosphorous of 0.97 mg/dL), normalization of serum phosphorous was associated with increase in left ventricular stroke work by 44 % [103]. In contrast in another study with mean serum phosphorous of 1.88 mg/dL reversal of hypophosphatemia had no effect on cardiac function [104]. These finding were validated in another study comparing baseline serum phosphorous of 0.90 with 1.40 mg/dL [105]. Chronic moderate hypophosphatemia in patients with hypophosphatemic rickets with mean serum phosphorous concentration of 2.6 mg/dL was not associated with measurable depression of myocardial function or clinical CHF [106]. Hypophosphatemia is associated with cardiac arrhythmia, which improves with phosphate repletion [107].
- Respiratory failure: The clinical impact of hypophosphatemia is perhaps the most apparent in patients with respiratory failure. Gravelyn et al. documented significant improvement in maximal inspiratory and expiratory pressure in 16 of 23 patients with moderate hypophosphatemia with mean phosphate of 1.9 mg/dL [108]. Aubier et al. studied the effect of phosphate repletion in eight patients with acute respiratory failure and moderate hypophosphatemia (mean serum phosphorous 1.2 mg/dL) and documented doubling of trans-diaphragmatic pressure after phosphate repletion [109]. Hypophosphatemia is common in patients hospitalized with respiratory illnesses including COPD [110]. In one series 21 % of patients with COPD had phosphorous <2.5 mg/dL. This did not correlate with phosphate intake but patients with hypophosphatemia had lower renal phosphate threshold and were on drugs, which are known to enhance renal phosphate excretion [110]. In intubated patients hypophosphatemia may delay successful intubation. Although well-documented cases remain rare, given the well-known effect of hypophosphatemia on diaphragmatic muscle, it should be treated aggressively in patients with respiratory failure.
- Neurologic: Severe neurological symptoms, including central pontine mylinolysis, peripheral neuropathy, paresthesia, weakness, and coma, have been reported in patients with very severe hypophosphatemia [111, 112]. It is important to note that these patients have multiple nutritional and electrolyte disturbances, making it difficult to assign an independent role for hypophosphatemia.
- Hematologic: Phosphate depletion decreases 2,3 DPG as well as ATP concentration increasing hemoglobin affinity for oxygen and decreasing release of oxygen at tissue level Hemolysis is thought to be secondary to ATP depletion resulting in deformity of RBC membrane and RBC breakdown. This event,

however, is very rare in human and is only reported in patients with severe hypophosphatemia, especially when serum phosphate decreases rapidly [113]. Although hypophosphatemia also reduces ATP content of leukocytes and may decrease oxygen consumption and generation of superoxide critical for intracellular killing, there is little evidence that this is associated with increased risk of infection (reviewed in ref. [101]).

- Miscellaneous effect: Phosphate depletion increases calcium absorption from the intestine secondary to activation of vitamin D to 1,25 vitamin D. It also increases release of calcium from the skeleton. The well-known hypercalciuria associated with phosphate depletion is partly due to the above events and partly due to a defect in calcium absorption in proximal tubule [114]. In addition hypophosphatemia not only decreases PTH level but also causes resistance to renal effect of PTH resulting in increased renal calcium excretion [115].

Table 4.8 Causes of hypophosphatemia

1. Decreased intestinal absorption
a. Decrease in phosphate intake
b. Phosphate binding antacids
c. Vitamin-D deficiency/resistance
d. Malabsorption
2. Redistribution hypophosphatemia
a. Respiratory alkalosis
b. Refeeding hypophosphatemia
c. Hormonal-induced
d. Rapid cell proliferation
3. Renal hypophosphatemia
a. Primary tubular damage
i. Hereditary
ii. Acquired
b. Circulating factors
i. Hyperparathyroidism
ii. PTHrp
iii. Phosphatonins
1. Tumor-induced osteomalacia
2. ADHR
3. XLH
c. Volume expansion
d. Diuretics
e. Liver resection
4. Multiple factors
a. DKA
b. Alcoholism

Causes of Hypophosphatemia

Hypophosphatemia can be due to decreased intake and/or absorption of phosphate, cellular shift, renal loss, or to a combination of these factors. The approach to patients with hypophosphatemia should always begin with careful history and physical examination followed by evaluation of selected laboratory studies. The latter should include serum electrolytes, calcium, magnesium, and arterial blood gases. When appropriate, more selective studies such as measurement of PTH, vitamin D metabolites, fractional excretion of phosphate, or tubular threshold corrected for GFR (Tm/GFR), as well as imaging studies will be very helpful in establishing specific diagnosis. Classification of hypophosphatemia is summarized in Table 4.8.

Hypophosphatemia Due to Decreased Intake and/or Intestinal Absorption

This alone rarely causes hypophosphatemia; however, hypophosphatemia can be seen in the setting of decreased absorption secondary to malabsorption or aggressive use of phosphate binders. This is commonly seen in patient with poor nutrition and now accounts for the majority of patients in this category. Vitamin D deficiency could result in a decrease in intestinal phosphate absorption; however, hypophosphatemia in this setting is partly due renal loss due to secondary hyperparathyroidism PTH level. Steatorrhea could result in hypophosphatemia partly as a result of vitamin D deficiency and partly to decreased absorption of phosphate independent of vitamin D. Hypophosphatemia is occasionally seen in patients with prolonged starvation such as in Kwashiorkor; this is, however, very uncommon.

Hypophosphatemia Due to Intracellular Shift

Redistribution hypophosphatemia is the most common cause of this disorder, and can be seen with normal or low total body phosphate (Table 4.8). Intracellular phosphate shifts can occur under the influence of insulin and catecholamines, or can be secondary to respiratory alkalosis or rapid cell proliferation. Infusion of glucose or oral intake of carbohydrate stimulates insulin secretion and results in increased cellular uptake of glucose and phosphate [116]. Catecholamine-mediated phosphate shift is seen in sepsis, myocardial infarction, burn, and thyrotoxicosis [117]. This is also seen in patients receiving sympathomimetics, such as nebulized salbutamol. This response is blunted by the administration of propanolol, suggesting a role for beta-adrenergic stimulation [118].

The most common cause of redistribution hypophosphatemia with normal total body phosphate is acute respiratory alkalosis. In this disorder the lowering of the pCO_2 is rapidly reflected intracellularly, resulting in intracellular alkalosis. The alkaline pH stimulates phosphofructokinase, the rate-limiting enzyme in glycolysis, resulting in rapid metabolism of glucose and utilization of phosphate [119]. This is quickly reversible with resolution of hyperventilation. In metabolic alkalosis, the intracellular pH changes more slowly and hypophosphatemia is therefore milder in nature [120]. Hypophosphatemia seen in liver disease, sepsis, heat stroke, CNS catastrophy, and neuroleptic-malignant syndrome is attributed to the respiratory alkalosis associated with these disorders.

Treatment of redistribution hypophosphatemia without phosphate depletion should focus on the treatment of the underlying disorder(s). If serum phosphate is less than 1 mg % (especially if it is less than 0.5 mg %) or if it is associated with clinical symptoms, phosphate repletion should be initiated, with the goal of raising serum phosphate to about 1 mg %. Redistribution hypophosphatemia is also reported in patients with rapid cell growth, such as patients with pernicious anemia treated with B12.

Starvation results in total body phosphate, potassium, magnesium as well as mineral and vitamin depletion. On presentation serum concentration of these ions is often within normal range, which decreases rapidly with refeeding [121]. During starvation most of the caloric needs are generated through fat metabolism; however, during refeeding the body switches to carbohydrate metabolism, resulting in stimulation of a series of hormones, most importantly insulin. This response is enhanced after a period of starvation. The intracellular shift of glucose is accompanied with a shift of phosphate and potassium resulting in hypophosphatemia and hypokalemia. This effect is most pronounced in patients who are started on high caloric intake [121]. Refeeding hypophosphatemia can be severe enough to result in respiratory failure, cardiac arrhythmia, heart failure, muscle paralysis, coma, and death. Treatment of refeeding hypophosphatemia should begin by identifying patients that are prone to develop this complication; these include patients with severe weight loss, hypophosphatemia, and hypokalemia on admission as well as sign and symptoms of vitamin deficiency. In addition the high-risk patients include patients with anorexia nervosa, classical Marasmus/Kwashiorkor, chronic alcoholics, and patients with underlying chronic diseases [121]. In these patients preventive measures include initiation of treatment for phosphate depletion before development of hypophosphatemia [122]. Refeeding should be started with low caloric intake (no more than 25 % of caloric need), increased slowly over 3–5 day period. These patients should be followed closely and if signs and symptoms of severe hypophosphatemia develop, aggressive phosphate repletion should be initiated (see below in treatment of hypophosphatemia).

Hypophosphatemia Due to Renal Loss

Renal hypophosphatemia could be due to (a) renal tubular damage or (b) inhibition of phosphate reabsorption by specific circulating factor(s).

Renal hypophosphatemia due to tubular damage can be isolated in nature or be part of a more generalized proximal tubular damage such as Fanconi syndrome. Fanconi syndrome can be due to an inborn error of metabolism such as cystinosis or be acquired in nature due to tubular injury from paraproteins or drug toxicity [123]. Ifosfamide, used primarily in children, can result in Fanconi syndrome in up to 4–25 % of children; adult cases have also been described [123]. It is often subclinical but may result in hypophosphatemic rickets [124]. Hypophosphatemia is the second most common (after hyperuricemia) electrolyte disorder in patients with HIV disease, often due to drug-associated Fanconi syndrome. It is particularly common in patients treated with the acyclic nucleoside phosphonates antiviral drugs, i.e., adefovir, cidofovir, and tenofivir [123]. Renal hypophosphatemia due to circulating factors: The most common cause of renal hypophosphatemia secondary to circulating factors is primary or secondary hyperparathyroidism. Primary hyperparathyroidism is a relatively common disease, presenting primarily in older women. Phosphaturia is often mild with serum phosphate rarely below 2.0 mg/dL. The mild nature of hypophosphatemia may be secondary to activation of vitamin D by PTH as well as low phosphate resulting in an increase in increase intestinal phosphate absorption. (For more detailed discussion refer to discussion under "Hyperparathyroidism" in this chapter). A less common cause of renal hypophosphatemia is due to presence of circulating phosphatonin(s), particularly FGF23 [5]. Patients with tumor-induced osteomalacia (TIO) develop severe renal hypophosphatemia and osteomalacia, which is reversed by the removal of the tumor [125].This is a rare disease associated with benign soft tissue and bony tumors; renal hypophosphatemia is due to over-expression of FGF23 (see section on "Phosphate Homeostasis" for more in-depth discussion). In these patients PTH level is normal and 1,25 vitamin D level is low. FGF23 is elevated in X-Linked Hypophosphatemic rickets, in association with loss of function mutations in an endopeptidase (PHEX) that has been implicated in FGF23 homeostasis [5].

Acute hypophosphatemia is reported in up to 100 % of patients undergoing partial liver resection as live liver donors or for treatment of liver metastasis [126, 127]. Severe hypophosphatemia was seen in 70 % of 18 live liver donors [126] despite phosphate repletion. In another study of 21 patients undergoing liver resection for cancer all developed hypophosphatemia with the nadir occurring on the second postoperative day. Mean serum phosphate nadir was 1.86 mg/dL with a range of 1.0–2.2 mg/dL, despite aggressive phosphate repletion. Urinary fractional excretion of phosphate increased to 45 % by day 2 and decreased to 13 % by day 4. PTH and 1,25 vitamin D level were normal. FGF23 measured in four patients did not show any specific pattern [127]. The pathogenesis of this interesting phenomenon may involve a circulating factor, but this remains speculative.

A more common cause of acute hypophosphatemia is rapid volume expansion. The mechanism is secondary to decrease in proximal tubular reabsorption of sodium, calcium as well as phosphate and an acute increase in PTH level secondary to the associated decrease in ionized calcium [128].

Hypophosphatemia Due to Multiple Causes

Alcoholism. Hypophosphatemia is uncommon with acute alcohol intoxication, reported in less than 5 % of patients, but very common in chronic alcoholics admitted for inpatient treatment [129]. De Marchi et al. studied 61 patients over a 4-week period and documented presence of hypophosphatemia in 30 %, often associated with hypomagnesaemia and hypocalcemia [97]. Causes of hypophosphatemia in these patients include (a) decrease intestinal absorption due to poor nutrition, malabsorption and use of phosphate-binding antacids, (b) cellular shift of phosphate due to respiratory alkalosis, refeeding hyperinsulinemia and high catecholamine level and (c) decrease threshold for phosphate reabsorption observed in 78 % of patients with hypophosphatemia. Hypophosphatemia was part of a generalized proximal tubular defect that included hypouricemia, glycosuria, and aminoaciduria and is considered to be due to renal tubular toxicity of alcohol. This improved during the 4-week of abstinence [97].

Diabetic ketoacidosis (DKA). Serum phosphate in DKA is often normal despite marked phosphaturia, caused by the release of intracellular phosphate and subsequent phosphaturia, accentuated by glycosuria and metabolic acidosis hypophosphatemia, due to intracellular shift of phosphate by administered insulin, develops within 12–24 h, and can be very severe [130].

Hypophosphatemia is common after renal transplantation [131]. This is partly due to post-operative fluid expansion as well as persistent hyperparathyroidism in the face of more normal renal function [132]. Although serum phosphate often normalizes after several months, patients continue to have mild phosphaturia. The pathogenesis of persistent phosphaturia is not clear and in some patients is independent of PTH level. This syndrome has recently been linked to persistent "tertiary" FGF23, resulting in phosphaturia and suppressed calcitriol generation [96].

Treatment of Hypophosphatemia

The correlation between hypophosphatemia and true phosphate depletion is poor at best. It is therefore important to distinguish between hypophosphatemia associated with low or normal total body phosphate (see under classification of hypophosphatemia) before treatment is initiated. In rare cases where the patient is either symptomatic or has very severe hypophosphatemia (<0.5 mg/dL), emergent treatment should be considered before etiology of hypophosphatemia is elucidated.

In hypophosphatemia secondary to phosphate shift, treatment should focus on the reversal of the underlying disorder. This is particularly true when the shift is due to acute respiratory alkalosis, often associated with life-threatening disorders such as sepsis, hepatic failure or CNS bleed. In refeeding hypophosphatemia, as discussed above, the focus should be on prevention, by identifying high-risk patients and increasing caloric intake in a stepwise fashion. In hypophosphatemia due to true phosphate depletion, treatment would depend on the severity, presence or absence of signs and symptoms, and reversibility. Treatment should only be considered if hypophosphatemia is severe (less than 1.0 mg/dL), if the patient is symptomatic or if hypophosphatemia is predicted to persist for a prolonged time. For example in patients with DKA or alcoholism who are able to eat, hypophosphatemia often reverses with increase dietary intake and no supplemental replacement is needed. However, in patients with ongoing phosphate loss due to persistent renal leakage or ongoing malabsorption, phosphate replacement may be initiated with moderate hypophosphatemia. The replacement dose should always be expressed in millimole of elemental phosphate (and not mEq which would vary with pH of the solution) or mg of phosphate. The conversion factor is 31 (1 mmol of phosphate being equivalent to 31 mg of elemental phosphorous). Therefore, 1 L of 9-mM phosphate contains 279 mg of elemental phosphorous. The standard dose is between 0.08 and 0.16 mmol/kg given over 6 h; if the patient is symptomatic the dose could be increased with maximum dose of 0.25 mol/kg.

To achieve a more rapid normalization, doses as high as 0.6 mmol/kg has been used safely in the ICU setting. In one study [133] the administration of 2 mg/kg of elemental phosphorous as 9-mM potassium phosphate every 6 h resulted in elevation of serum phosphorous from a baseline of 0.81–1.67 mg/dL in 24 h and 2.8 mg/dL in 48 h. It is, however, not clear if such an aggressive treatment of hypophosphatemia in asymptomatic patients has significant clinical impact. We therefore would recommend more cautious replacement in these patients. The intravenous treatment should be switched to oral treatment as soon as a level above 1.5 mg/dL has been reached and patient is able to tolerate oral intake.

In patients with mild to moderate long-standing hypophosphatemia oral treatment is preferred. There are several oral preparations, as either sodium and/or potassium salt (Table 4.9). The usual dosage is 1–2 g of elemental phosphorous per day. Milk contains approximately 1 g of elemental phosphorous per quart; in patients that can tolerate milk, low fat or skim milk should be considered as a means to treat moderate hypophosphatemia. This dose of 1–2 g would replenish total body phosphate in approximately 7–10 days. We should also remember that major side effect or oral phosphorous is diarrhea. This is dose related and resolves with a decrease in dosage or by giving the medication in divided dose. Oral phosphorous in high dosage, especially in children and elderly patients with renal failure, can cause severe hyperphosphatemia (see below under hyperphosphatemia); phosphate replacement should always be performed cautiously in patients with renal failure. Intravenous phosphate replacement can result in hypocalcemia, hypomagnesemia, soft tissue calcification, hyperkalemia (with potassium

Table 4.9 Commonly available phosphate preparations

	pH	Phosphorus (mg)	Sodium (mEq)	Potassium (mEq)
Oral preparations				
K-phos neutral tablets	7.4	250/tab	12/tab	2/tab
Neutraphos capsules	7.3	250/cap	7.1/cap	7.1/cap
Neutraphos K capsules	7.3	250/cap	–	14.2/cap
Fleet's phosphosoda	4.8	128.6/mL	4.8/mL	–
Parenteral preparations				
Potassium phosphate	6.6	93.1/mL	–	4.3/mL
Sodium phosphate	5.7	93.0/mL	4.0/mL	–
Neutral sodium phosphate	7.35	2.8/mL	0.16/mL	–
Neutral sodium, potassium phosphate	7.4	3.1/mL	0.16/mL	0.02/mL

preparation) and volume overload (with sodium preparation). If calcium supplementation is considered, it should be administered in a separate line to prevent precipitation. Finally, some of the phosphate preparations are acidic and can result in metabolic acidosis.

Hyperphosphatemia

Hyperphosphatemia, defined as phosphate level of 5.0 mg/dL in adult and 6 mg % in children, is due to increased exogenous load, decreased renal output, increased endogenous release or a combination of these factors (Table 4.10). A decrease in renal output is due to renal failure and is only dealt with briefly in this chapter.

Table 4.10 Causes of hyperphosphatemia

Increased exogenous load
Oral supplement with decreased GFR
Defects in bowel mucose
Vitamin D intoxication
Intravenous infusion of phosphate-containing solution
Decreased urinary excretion
Reduced GFR
Hypoparathyroidism (congenital, acquired)
Pseudohypoparathyroidism (Type I, II)
Acromegaly
Thyrotoxicosis
Sickle cell anemia
Etidronate disodium
Increased endogenous load
Acute respiratory acidosis
Metabolic acidosis
Tumor lysis syndrome
Rhabdomyolysis

Increase Exogenous Load

Hyperphosphatemia occasionally occurs due to an increase oral or IV phosphate intake. An increase in oral intake above 2 g/day is often associated with diarrhea, limiting the intestinal absorption of phosphate. However, in patients with decreased gut motility, such as children with Hirschsprung's disease, older patients with chronic constipation, or patients with mucosal inflammation, phosphate is absorbed by the colon, resulting in hyperphosphatemia. This is potentiated by any decrease in GFR, common in older patients.

Fleet phosphosoda is routinely used for the treatment of constipation and preparation for colonoscopy. The routine dose is 90 mL, containing 11.5 g of elemental phosphorous, given in two equal doses. In a study of 70 patients with mean age of 47 years and measured creatinine clearance of >70 mL/min, serum phosphate rose to above 8 mg/dL in 36.7 % of patients and to above 10 mg/dL in seven patients. The elevation is serum phosphate correlated closely with age but not creatinine clearance [134]. Phosphate-based colonoscopy preparations have been linked to acute phosphate nephropathy, leading to significant restrictions in use. Markowitz et al. have reported renal biopsy and clinical findings in 21 patients with ARF following intake of oral phosphate for colonoscopy. These 21 patients

(17 women and 4 men, with a mean age of 64) were identified from 31 biopsies with diagnosis of nephrocalcinosis who had no known etiology for this finding except for exposure to oral phosphate purgatives. ARF was discovered from 1 day to several months after exposure. The mean serum creatinine before exposure was 1.1 mg/dL and rose to a mean of 3.9 mg/dL. Five patients developed ESRD (mean follow-up 16.7 months) and the remainder developed chronic renal insufficiency. The pathologic findings included extensive tubular calcium phosphate deposition with variable degree of chronic tubulointerstitial fibrosis and tubular atrophy; in patients with an acute presentation, signs of tubular injury and interstitial edema predominated [135]. Risk factors for acute phosphate nephropathy include advanced age, preexisting CKD, hypertension, volume depletion, female gender, and use of angiotensin-converting enzyme inhibitors or angiotensin receptor blockers [136].

Vitamin D toxicity is still seen especially in older patients on vitamin D supplementation. This is associated with mild to moderate hyperphosphatemia due to vitamin D-induced increase in intestinal absorption, coupled with a decrease in renal excretion due to low PTH level. This is almost always associated with hypercalcemia.

Decreased Renal Excretion of Phosphate

Serum phosphate is maintained in the normal range by the ability of the kidney to match phosphate excretion to intake. The filtered load of phosphate in an adult individual with GFR of 100 mL/min is approximately 5.5 g/day. To maintain homeostasis, the kidney must excrete 20 % of the filtered load, an amount equal to the net gut absorption of approximately 1.0 g/day. As GFR decreases, serum phosphate concentration is maintained within normal range by an increase in fractional excretion of phosphate. This is due to an increase in PTH level, triggered by hypocalcemia, calcitriol deficiency, as well as hyperphosphatemia; "secondary" increases in FGF23 are thought to play an important role in the associated calcitriol deficiency [96]. As the GFR drops to approximately 20 % of normal, the increase in fractional excretion of phosphate will not suffice, resulting in hyperphosphatemia; this is a predictable complication of advanced CKD.

Hyperphosphatemia associated with hypoparathyroidism or pseudohypoparathyroidism is due to an increase in phosphate absorption by the kidney. This is partly mitigated by a decrease in intestinal absorption of phosphate due to a decrease in 1,25 vitamin D level. Patients with hypoparathyroidism present with hypocalcemia, tetany, cataract, and basal ganglia calcification and decreased bony mineralization. Serum phosphate can be as high as 8–9 mg/dL in patients with severe, hypoparathyroidism. Hypoparathyroidism can be due to congenital causes, autoimmune disease, surgical removal, radiation, or hemochromatosis. Pseudohypoparathyroidism presents with similar biochemical findings but with high PTH level. This is due to skeletal and renal resistance to PTH; this syndrome is more fully discussed in the section on "Hypocalcemia" in this chapter.

Mild hyperphosphatemia is also seen in acromegaly, hyperthyroidism and occasionally patients with Paget's disease. Mild hyperphosphatemia secondary to increased tubular absorption of phosphate is seen in acromegaly and is thought to be due to the effect of increased level of insulin-like growth factor. The hyperphosphatemia seen in thyrotoxicosis is due to an increase release of phosphate from muscle, coupled with an increase in tubular absorption of phosphate. Similar mechanisms exist in sickle cell anemia, where hyperphosphatemia is due to increased phosphate release from red cells as well as an increase in tubular absorption.

Increase in Endogenous Load

This subtype of hyperphosphatemia is due to either shift or release of phosphate from intracellular compartments. Phosphate shift occurs primarily due to the inhibitory effect of acidemic pH on phosphofructokinase, the rate-limiting enzyme in glycolysis, resulting in a decrease in intracellular utilization of phosphate [120] This is more pronounced with respiratory acidosis where a rise in pCO_2 results in rapid drop in intracellular pH. In metabolic acidosis, hyperphosphatemia is more common in organic acidosis such as DKA or lactic acidosis.

Hyperphosphatemia due to release of intracellular phosphate occurs in tumor lysis syndrome and rhabdomyolysis. Tumor lysis syndrome (TLS) occurs when the release of intracellular material is greater than body's excretory ability. This syndrome usually presents with hyperuricemia, hyperphosphatemia, hyperkalemia and hypocalcemia [137]. Acute renal failure secondary to urate nephropathy and/or calcium phosphate deposition is a common finding in TLS. Although spontaneous TLS has been reported, TLS is almost always due to rapid cell lysis secondary to treatment of aggressive tumors such as acute leukemias and lymphomas. Tumors that are associated with TLS have rapid growth rate, involve abdominal organs, are in highly advanced stages and are sensitive to chemotherapy. Risk factors for TLS include elevated LDH, leukocytosis, spontaneous hyperuricemia, and a decrease in GFR. In the largest series of 46 episodes of TLS in 37 patients with Burkitt's lymphoma, hyperphosphatemia occurred in 31 % of patients with normal GFR and in all patients with reduced GFR before chemotherapy [138]. Rhabdomyolysis presents in similar fashion to TLS although acute renal failure is a more predictable complication of this disorder. In these patients hyperuricemia, hyperphosphatemia, hyperkalemia, and hypocalcemia occur out of proportion to the degree of renal failure.

Clinical Consequences of Hyperphosphatemia

Mild hyperphosphatemia is often asymptomatic; however, severe hyperphosphatemia, especially when acute, can cause severe hypocalcemia with its associated symptoms of tetany, seizure, and hypotension. Severe hyperphosphatemia due to cell lysis is often associated with renal failure and its clinical consequences. As discussed above, acute hyperphosphatemia in the setting of cell lysis is associated with multiple other electrolyte abnormalities and therefore presents with signs and symptoms related to other electrolyte disorders. Chronic hypophosphatemia is frequent in chronic renal failure and is associated with hypocalcemia, secondary hyperparathyroidism, and renal osteodystrophy.

Treatment of Hyperphosphatemia

Treatment of hyperphosphatemia depends on its severity, duration, and on the presence or absence of renal failure. Mild hyperphosphatemia does not require any treatment; however, severe hyperphosphatemia, especially when acute, must be dealt with promptly. If renal function is normal or near normal, then maneuvers to increase renal excretion of phosphate, such as volume expansion and administration of acetazolamide, should be used. In patients with significant renal failure and severe hyperphosphatemia, insulin and glucose can be used to shift phosphate intracellularly. This should always be followed with dialysis to help with phosphate removal. Phosphate removal in patients with TLS syndrome is quite challenging. Intermittent hemodialysis with high flow is effective but often needs to be repeated every 12–24 h. Continuous venovenous hemofiltration with dialysis (CVVHD) is also effective and should be considered in patients with a rapid rise in serum phosphate (reviewed in ref. [137]). Treatment of severe hyperphosphatemia, especially when acute, is a difficult challenge. It is therefore important to prevent its development as much as possible. Oral phosphate should not be used as purgative in older patients and patients with underlying renal disease. Patients with aggressive tumors who are at risk for TLS should be volume expanded before any treatment is given. Use of alkali, recommended for prevention and treatment of urate nephropathy, could result in the precipitation of calcium phosphate crystals in soft tissue, including kidneys, resulting in acute renal failure and therefore should be used cautiously. In these patients, it is therefore imperative to prevent development of hyperuricemia with the use of allopurinol or recombinant uric acid oxidase. Chronic hyperphosphatemia is almost always associated with severe renal failure and is not discussed in this chapter.

Disorders of Magnesium Homeostasis

General Considerations

Magnesium, with a molecular weight of 24.3, is predominantly an intracellular divalent cation. It is critical for many metabolic processes, including the production and utilization of energy. This cation activates many enzymes, including several involved in key steps of intermediary metabolism. These enzymes are important in regulating various processes in the cell and cell membrane. Magnesium is essential for the function of several critical transporters such as the Na^+-K^+-ATpase, H-ATPase, and Ca-ATPase holoenzymes. Magnesium is also critical in the synthesis of protein and DNA, in the transcription of DNA and RNA, and in the translation of messenger RNA. In addition, magnesium may play an important role in the regulation of mitochondrial function.

Normal Magnesium Homeostasis

Body Mg^{2+} Pools

In a normal adult, the total body magnesium (Mg^{2+}) content is approximately 1,000 mmol (24,000 mg). This is present in bone, muscle, and intracellular and extracellular space. More than 60 % of total body Mg^{2+} is present in bone, with about one third of the bone Mg^{2+} adsorbed to the surface of bone crystals. The latter form is relatively readily exchangeable with serum magnesium. The Mg^{2+} content of muscle is approximately 17 % of the total body content. While the intracellular Mg^{2+} concentration is greater than the extracellular concentrations, the latter more accurately reflect the total body Mg^{2+} content. There are, however, practical problems in measuring the intracellular concentrations. The majority of intracellular pool of Mg^{2+} is thus bound to various proteins, ATP, RNA and less than 3 % is in free (ionized) form. In addition, Mg^{2+} is compartmentalized in different organelles within the cell. The extracellular pool of magnesium is in dynamic relationship with the intracellular pool. This relationship is affected by several factors including catecholamines, alkalosis (or rapid correction of acidosis), refeeding, among others. Serum magnesium therefore may or may not reflect the state of total body magnesium (Fig. 4.3).

Intestinal Absorption of Magnesium

The recommended daily intake of magnesium, in a Western diet, is 10–15 mmol. The bioavailability of Mg^{2+} varies based on the specific salt content of magnesium. Only 30–60 % of dietary magnesium is absorbed which, in normal individual, is matched by renal loss, thus maintaining overall homeostasis (Fig. 4.2).

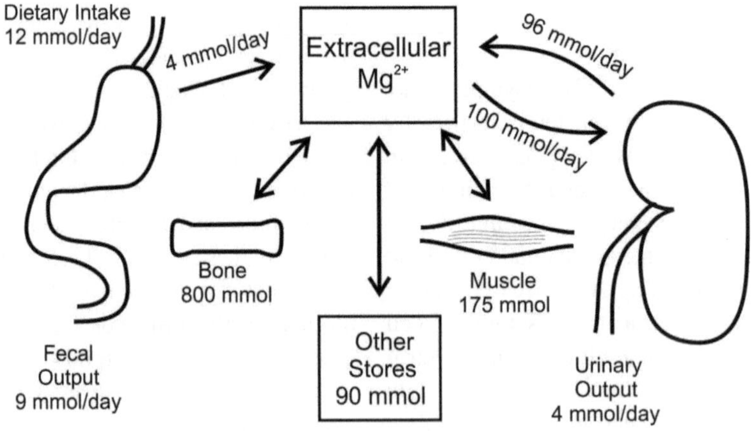

Fig. 4.3 The distribution of magnesium between the various body pools, including the intestine, extracellular space, the intracellular space, bone, and the kidney

Mg^{2+} absorption in the intestine has saturable (transcellular) and nonsaturable (paracellular) components. The primary site of Mg^{2+} absorption in humans appears to be the distal small intestine, with some absorption taking place in the colon. Specifically, triple lumen perfusion studies in humans indicate that Mg^{2+} absorption occurs in the ileum and proximal jejunum [139]. The exact mechanisms involved in absorption of Mg^{2+} are not well understood. However, two members of the transient receptor potential (TRP) cation channel, subfamily M, TRPM6 and TRPM7, are involved in these processes. These two form a dimer and TRPM7 is known to be a functional channel for Mg^{2+}. *TRPM6* mRNA is expressed in the surface and crypt epithelial cells of the colon and in villous epithelial cells of the duodenum and plays a major role in magnesium absorption. This gene is mutated in the syndrome of hypomagnesemia with secondary hypocalcemia (HSH) [140]. In animal models, an increase in dietary Mg^{2+} causes an increase in TRPM6 gene expression.

The role of vitamin D in the GI absorption of the Mg^{2+} remains controversial. Studies in vitamin D-deficient animals indicate that vitamin D acts to increase Mg^{2+} absorption. Perfusion studies of the jejunum in patients with renal failure also show that 1,25 dihydroxyvitamin D (calcitriol) stimulates Mg^{2+} absorption. Metabolic balance studies in humans, however, indicate that active vitamin D only minimally affects the net absorption of Mg^{2+} [141]. In contrast to calcium absorption, there is no relation between the steady-state plasma levels of calcitriol and the net absorption of Mg^{2+} [142]. These conflicting data remain unexplained and may reflect the variable effect of calcitriol in vitamin D deficient vs. vitamin D replete states.

Renal Handling of Magnesium

Magnesium is partially bound to protein, and approximately 70–75 % of plasma magnesium is ultrafilterable. The majority of filtered Mg^{2+} is reabsorbed by the renal tubules, resulting in fractional excretion of 3–5 %. Approximately 15–25 % of the filtered Mg^{2+} is reabsorbed in the proximal tubule, 65–75 % in the thick ascending limb (TAL), and 5–10 % in the distal convoluted tubule (DCT), where the final fine-tuning takes place. Studies of the rare diseases presenting with hypomagnesemia have shown that Paracelin-1 (PCNLN-1, Claudin 16) and Claudin 19, coexpressed in the tight junctions in the TAL, are responsible for the paracellular reabsorption of Mg^{2+} in TAL [143, 144]. Claudin-16 and Claudin-19 interact to confer the cation-selectivity of tight junctions in the TAL, contributing significantly to the transepithelial absorption of magnesium and other cations by this nephron segment [144]. In DCT Mg^{2+} is absorbed through TRPM6-channels; mutations in this gene results in the syndrome of hypomagnesemia with secondary hypocalcemia [145].

With respect to control of renal magnesium absorption, Mg^{2+} and Ca are both ligands for CaR expressed primarily in TAL, however; the affinity of this receptor is four to five times less for Mg^{2+} [146]. Notably, however, the concentration of Mg^{2+} in the tubules is high enough to react with the CaR. Epidermal growth factor (EGF) has recently emerged as a novel "magnesiotropic" hormone. This role was discovered via characterization of point-mutations in the EGF gene, in patients with isolated autosomal recessive hypomagnesemia [147] (OMIM 611718). These mutations impair basolateral sorting of a transmembrane precursor form of (pro-EGF) expressed in DCT cells. Wild-type pro-EGF is thought to undergo cleavage at the basolateral membrane, with autocrine stimulation of apical TRPM6 channels via the basolateral EGF receptor [147, 148].

Disorders of Magnesium Homeostasis

The normal range for serum Mg^{2+} is 0.75–0.98 mmol/L (1.5–2.0 mEq/L or 1.8–2.4 mg/dL); the normal range is slightly higher in children younger than 5 years of age. There are also differences based on race and sex, with blacks having slightly lower concentrations than whites and males having higher concentrations than females [149]. Mg^{2+} is approximately 30 % protein-bound, 55–60 % in free (ionized) form, and the remainder chelated to phosphate, citrate, and other anions. Since Mg^{2+} is predominantly intracellular, an individual with hypomagnesemia might have normal intracellular Mg^{2+}. However, in most cases, by the time the serum Mg^{2+} has declined below normal level, the total body Mg^{2+} is severely depleted. Similarly, an individual with normal serum Mg^{2+} may have low total body Mg^{2+}.

Hypomagnesemia

The reported incidence or prevalence of hypomagnesemia should be evaluated in the light of the fact that magnesium is predominantly intracellular and serum Mg^{2+} therefore may or may not reflect total body Mg^{2+}. Hypomagnesemia, defined as Mg^{2+} concentration below 1.8 mg/dL, is present in 14.5 % of the general population [150]. The incidence of hypomagnesemia has been reported to be approximately 65 % in patients admitted to a medical intensive care unit, 4.0 % in outpatients with hypertension, and 7.0 % in hospitalized patients not in an intensive care setting [151]. Hypomagnesemia is more prevalent among hypertensive patients [152]; however, Mg^{2+} therapy in these patients has not been shown to be helpful in control of hypertension. It is possible that a single common mutation or group of common mutations predispose these patients to both hypomagnesemia and hypertension.

Signs and Symptoms of Hypomagnesemia

Patients with severe hypomagnesemia, defined as serum Mg^{2+} below 0.5 mmol/L (1.2 mg/dL), are often symptomatic. The major manifestations of hypomagnesemia are cardiac and neuromuscular in nature. This is not surprising, as Mg^{2+} is a cofactor in regulating various ionic channels and pumps and is critical for the function of excitable tissue. In addition, these tissues are heavily ATP dependent, and Mg^{2+} is required for ATP generation in these tissues.

Neuromuscular abnormalities are nonspecific (Table 4.11) and include tremor, fasciculation, positive Chvostek and Trousseau signs, and tetany. Severe hypomagnesemia may also be manifested as generalized convulsions, which is only responsive to Mg^{2+} replacement.

Hypomagnesemia has been purported to contribute to an increased morbidity and mortality in various cardiac disorders. Lewis et al. [151] found that in patients with mild to moderate hypomagnesemia, Mg^{2+} repletion was associated with a reduction in the incidence of ventricular ectopia. Mg^{2+} supplementation has also been shown to decrease the frequency of ventricular ectopic beats following acute myocardial infarction [153].

Furthermore, a diet rich in Mg^{2+} may reduce the morbidity and mortality of subjects with a high risk for coronary artery disease. In addition Mg^{2+} therapy may have a role in controlling the ventricular rate in atrial fibrillation [154]. Patients with severe hypomagnesemia have a higher mortality rate despite a similar APACHE score [155]. These observations suggest that severe hypomagnesemia should be treated aggressively.

Associated Electrolyte Abnormalities

Hypomagnesemia is frequently seen in association with certain other electrolyte abnormalities, particularly hypokalemia and hypocalcemia. Approximately 40–60 % of the patients with hypokalemia have concomitant hypomagnesemia. This co-occurrence of hypokalemia and hypomagnesemia is at least partially due to inappropriate renal coexcretion of both cations, due for example to cisplatin-associated tubular necrosis. However, Mg^{2+} depletion also has effects on potassium homeostasis. Magnesium deficiency thus results in refractory hypokalemia, particularly if the plasma Mg^{2+} is less than 0.5 mmol/L [156]; hypomagnesemic patients are refractory to K^+ replacement in the absence of Mg^{2+} repletion [157, 158].

Several mechanisms appear to contribute to the effect of magnesium depletion on potassium homeostasis. Magnesium depletion has inhibitory effects on muscle Na^+/K^+-ATPase activity, resulting in significant efflux from muscle and a secondary kaliuresis. Distal tubular potassium secretion also appears to be enhanced, due to a reduction in the normal physiological inward rectification of ROMK (Renal Outer Medullar K^+ channel) secretory K^+ channels in principal cells, with a subsequent increase in outward conductance [159, 160]. ROMK and structurally related potassium channels are inward rectifying, i.e., K^+

Table 4.11 Signs and symptoms associated with hypomagnesemia

Cardiovascular	Arrhythmias	Ventricular ectopic beats
		Tachycardia and fibrillation ventricular
		Fibrillation multifocal atrial tachycardia atrial
		Torsades des pointes treatment
		Refractory arrhythmias
	EKG changes	Prolonged QT intervals
		Inverted T waves
		ST segment depression
		Wide QRS complexes
		Prolonged PR interval
	Others	Essential hypertension
		Pregnancy-induced hypertension
		Increased sensitivity to digitalis glycosides
Neuromuscular	Acute	Parasomnias
		Confusion, coma, psychosis, agitation, delirium, depression, weakness, tremors, tetany, spasticity, seizures, increased deep tendon reflexes, paresthesias
	Chronic	Alzheimer's
		Amyotrophic lateral sclerosis and Parkinson–dementia complex of Guam Stroke
Electrolytes		Hypocalcemia
		Hypokalemia
		Hypophosphatemia
Miscellaneous		Preterm labor
		Fetal PTH suppression
		Serum calcitriol decreased

flows inward more readily than outward; even though outward conductance is usually less than inward conductance, K^+ efflux predominates in principal cells since the membrane potential is more positive than the equilibrium potential for K^+. Intracellular Mg^{2+} plays a key role in inward rectification, binding and blocking the pore of the channel from the cytoplasmic side [159, 160]. The hypomagnesemia-associated reduction in cytoplasmic Mg^{2+} in principal cells reduces inward rectification of ROMK, increasing outward conductance by as much as 30 % [160] and increasing K^+ secretion. In addition, it has been suggested that the repletion of intracellular K^+ is impaired in hypomagnesemia, even in normokalemic patients [161]. Decreased intracellular Mg^{2+} enhances K^+ efflux from the cytoplasm of cardiac and perhaps skeletal myocytes, likely due to reduced intracellular blockade of inward rectifying K^+ channels (increased efflux) and inhibition of the Na^+/K^+-ATPase (decreased influx); plasma K^+ levels thus remain normal at the expense of intracellular K^+ [161, 162].

Hypocalcemia is another electrolyte abnormality commonly associated with hypomagnesemia. Mild hypomagnesemia may stimulate PTH secretion, while more severe hypomagnesemia suppresses the secretion of PTH and produces resistance to actions of PTH on both bone and the kidney. In addition, the serum levels of calcitriol are low in hypomagnesemic patients [163]. Therefore, serum Mg^{2+} should be routinely measured in all patients with hypokalemia and/or hypocalcemia.

Approach to Patient with Hypomagnesemia

Evaluating Serum Magnesium

Diagnosis of hypomagnesemia is often a reflection of the frequency of measurement of this cation as part of routine laboratory evaluation. Whang et al. documented that 47 % of patients seen in an urban primary care hospital, had Mg^{2+} concentrations of less than 0.74 mmol (<1.70 mg/dL). Interestingly in 90 % of these patients the measurement of serum Mg^{2+} was not requested (and therefore would have gone undetected) by the primary physician [164]. The incidence of hypomagnesemia is also affected by the fact that the normal value varies significantly in different medical centers and outpatient laboratories.

The symptoms of Mg^{2+} depletion may not appear until the serum levels fall below the normal range by 0.25–0.35 mmol/L (0.60–0.85 mg/dL) [149]. As a result, it is not surprising that many hypomagnesemic patients are not recognized [164]. As emphasized before, since Mg^{2+} is primarily intracellular, Mg^{2+} depletion can be present with normal serum Mg^{2+} levels. Low serum Mg^{2+} could occur due to low serum albumin; however, most labs do not measure ionized Mg^{2+}. A reduction in albumin results in reduction of total serum Mg^{2+} without affecting the ionized fraction. The following formula is recommended to correct the serum Mg^{2+} for the contribution of hypoalbuminemia:

Corrected serum Mg^{2+} (mmol/L) = measured total serum Mg^{2+} + [0.005 × (40 − serum albumin {g/L})

Intracellular Mg^{2+} can be measured by several different methods developed in a variety of cells including red cells, lymphocytes and muscle. However, these methods are not available for routine clinical use and remain as research tools. In addition none of these specialized tests have been shown to be reliable clinically as a predictor of Mg^{2+} content of the body. The measurement of Mg^{2+} in erythrocytes, lymphocytes, rectal mucosa, and hair follicle are offered through many laboratories; however, these are not standardized. While NMR studies in the muscle are very informative, NMR technique is not readily available and is very expensive.

Evaluating Urinary Magnesium

After determination of hypomagnesemia, urinary magnesium expressed as fractional excretion of Mg^{2+} (FEMg) should be measured to differentiate GI from renal loss of magnesium. If hypomagnesemia is of extrarenal origin, FEMg should be less than <1 % (<1 mmol/24 h). Although $FEMg^{2+}$ is dependent on the magnesium intake, in a hypomagnesemic patient, FEMg >15 % is consistent with the TAL as the site of Mg^{2+} loss; in contrast, a value of 5–15 % is more consistent with the DCT as the site of Mg^{2+} loss. Standardized Mg^{2+} loading test could be also helpful in evaluating the state of total body Mg^{2+} content; however, this test is rarely indicated in a clinical setting.

Classification of Hypomagnesemia

Hypomagnesemia could be due to a decrease in GI absorption or to a decrease in renal reabsorption. While chelation and intracellular shift of Mg^{2+} could lead to hypomagnesemia, these are very uncommon. In this chapter we only briefly discuss hypomagnesemia due to GI loss and focus primarily on renal causes of hypomagnesemia.

Intestinal Losses and Reduced Intestinal Absorption of Magnesium

Mg^{2+} intake is markedly reduced in patients with prolonged nasogastric suction, starvation, parenteral fluid administration, or enteral tube feeding. Other conditions including various malabsorption syndromes, intestinal bypass surgery, enteric fistulas may substantially reduce intestinal Mg^{2+} absorption. Laxative abuse may produce a pseudo-Bartter's syndrome with hypomagnesemia, hypocalcemia, hypokalemia, and hypophosphatemia.

Proton-pump inhibitors (PPIs—omeprazole, esomeprazole, pantoprazole, and rabeprazole) have emerged as a reasonably common cause of hypomagnesemia, due to reduced intestinal absorption [165]. It seems that passive absorption of magnesium is intact in these patients, with presumed inhibition of TPPM6/7-mediated absorption by these drugs, via an unknown mechanism. Intestinal calcium absorption is also reduced in PPI-associated hypomagnesemia, with concomitant hypocalcemia and hypokalemia.

Renal Losses of Magnesium

Familial Disorders of Renal Magnesium Loss

Despite the importance of Mg^{2+} in biological process, most of our information regarding Mg^{2+} homeostasis comes from the studies of rare genetic diseases presenting with hypomagnesemia. A summary of all the familial causes of hypomagnesemia is shown in Table 4.12.

Table 4.12 Inherited disorders of hypomagnesemia

Disorder	Mode of inheritance	Gene	Urinary calcium	Other lab findings
Gitelman	AR	NCCT	Low	Alkalosis, hypokalemia, salt wasting, high bone density
Bartter	AR	CLCB	High/NRL/Low	Alkalosis, hypokalemia, salt wasting
SeSAME syndrome	AR	KIR4.1		Epilepsy, metabolic alkalosis
Hypomagnesemia/ hypercalciuria syndrome	AR	CLD-16/19	High	Nephrocalcinosis
Hypomagnesemia	AR	EGF	Low	
Isolated hypomagnesemia	AD	FXYD2	Low	
Hypomagnesemia and hypocalciuria	AR	TRPM6	Low	Low PTH
Autosomal dominant hypoparathyroidism	AD	CASR	High	Hyperphosphatemia
Metabolic hypomagnesemia	Maternal	tRNAIe	Low	Hypertension, hypercholesterolemia

Both Bartter's syndrome and Gitelman's syndrome (OMIM 263800) can present with hypomagnesemia, hypokalemia and alkalosis. Bartter's syndrome is secondary to defects in a variety of transport and regulatory genes expressed in the TAL, while Gitelman's syndrome is due to loss-of-function mutations in the thiazide-sensitive sodium chloride cotransporter of the distal convoluted tubule (DCT). Although the majority of patients with Bartter's syndrome have normal serum magnesium, approximately 20 % are hypomagnesemic due to renal Mg^{2+} wasting [166]. The majority of the latter group has abnormalities in the chloride B channel (ClCB) located in basolateral membrane of TAL cells. These patients, in contrast to other patients with Bartter's syndrome, are not typically hypercalciuric. The age of onset of hypomagnesemia is higher among the patients with Gitelman's syndrome. These patients also have low urinary calcium. Although the specific genes involved in the pathogenesis of Gitelman's and Bartter's syndromes are well characterized, the mechanism(s) of hypomagnesemia are not clear. It is, however, known that TRPM6 expression is reduced after thiazide treatment and in an animal model of Gitelman's syndrome [60].

Familial renal Mg^{2+} wasting with hypomagnesemia has also been reported in association with hypercalciuria (OMIM 248250). These patients have a mutation in Paracellin-1 (claudin-16) or Claudin 19 [143, 144]. Since these patients have hypomagnesemia, with FEMg as high 15–50 %, and hypercalciuria, it is not surprising that the defect is in the TAL. Patients with this genetic disorder suffer from ocular abnormalities and gouty arthritis. Other biochemical abnormalities include elevated levels of PTH and high uric acid levels. These patients develop nephrocalcinosis and renal failure, which can progress to end-stage renal disease. Hypermagnesuria and hypercalciuria does not reoccur when these patients received a functioning renal transplant, indications that the defect is specific to the renal tubule. Family members have a 42 % incidence of hypercalciuria and an increased incidence of medullary sponge kidneys. These patients also have an increased risk of urinary tract infection.

Autosomal recessive hypomagnesemia and hypocalcemia (OMIM 602014) is known to be caused by a mutation in TRPM6 [145]. These patients have decreased absorption of Mg^{2+} in the intestine with decreased renal Mg^{2+} reabsorption in the DCT; FEMg is between 5 and 15 %. They also have hypocalciuria and hypocalcemia; the hypocalcemia is probably secondary to hypomagnesium-induced hypoparathyroidism and PTH resistance. As indicated previously the presence of TRPM6 in the GI tract and the kidney suggests that this protein is a major regulator of Mg^{2+} homeostasis.

Patients with loss-of-function mutations in the KCNJ10 gene that encodes the KIR4.1 potassium channel develop a syndrome encompassing epilepsy, ataxia, sensorineural deafness, and tubulopathy (EAST or SeSAME syndrome—OMIM 612780) [167, 168]. The associated tubulopathy encompasses hypokalemia, metabolic alkalosis, hypocalciuria, and hypomagnesemia [167, 168]; KIR4.1 knockout mice demonstrate a greater natriuresis than littermate controls, in addition to hypocalciuria [167]. The KIR4.1/KIR5.1 and KIR4.2/KIR5.1 channels at the basolateral membrane of DCT cells are hypothesized to function in basolateral K^+ recycling, maintaining adequate Na^+/K^+-ATPase activity for Na^+-Cl^- absorption and other aspects of DCT function.

Autosomal dominant hypomagnesemia (OMIM 154020) is reported in two Dutch families with identity by descent (IBD). These patients demonstrate hypomagnesemia with hypocalciuria. The genetic defect is due to a mutation in Na^+/K^+ ATPase gamma subunit expressed in the DCT [169]. Activating mutations of CASR could lead to autosomal dominant hypoparathyroidism characterized by hypocalcemia and hypercalciuria with occasional hypomagnesemia. For further details refer to the section on calcium disorders in this chapter. More recently, a loss-of-function mutation in the Kv1.1 potassium channel has been described in a family with autosomal dominant hypomagnesemia [170]. The Kv1.1 protein is coexpressed with TRPM6 at the apical membrane of DCT cells, where it is postulated to generate a favorable luminal membrane potential for TRPM6-mediated Mg^{2+} reabsorption.

Finally, there are many reports of hypomagnesemia in patients with mitochondrial disorders, especially Kearns–Sayre syndrome. These patients typically have large deletions in the mitochondrial genome. One kindred presented with hypomagnesemia, hypertension and hypercholesterolemia (OMIM 500005). These patients also had hypocalciuria consistent with other magnesium abnormalities, due to a defect in the DCT. The pattern of inheritance in this kindred is through the maternal lineage. These patients show a point mutation in the mitochondrial tRNAIle [171]. This position is conserved through the evolution in all the tRNAs. In addition, these patients show reduced ATP production as measured by NMR in vivo.

Table 4.13 Medications causing hypomagnesemia

Class	Names
Diuretics	Loop, thiazide, mannitol
Antibiotics	Amphotericin, pentamidine, aminoglycoside, tetracycline, foscarnet, carbenicillin, ticracillin
Oncologic	GMCSF, cisplatin, cetuximab
Immunosuppressant	Cyclosporine, FK 506
Endocrine	Corticosteroid, estrogen

Drugs Affecting Renal Handling of Magnesium

Various drugs can increase urinary magnesium and lead to Mg^{2+} depletion (Table 4.13).

Diuretics

As discussed before most Mg^{2+} is reabsorbed in the TAL via paracellular tight junctions, driven by the lumen-positive potential difference generated by combined apical Na^+-K^+-$2Cl^-$ transport and apical K^+ channel activity. The loop diuretics, which block the TAL Na^+-K-$2Cl^-$ transporter, augment urinary magnesium acutely and cause Mg^{2+} depletion. Thiazide diuretics have minimal acute effect on Mg^{2+} excretion; however, when given over the long term, they may induce urinary Mg^{2+} losses and hypomagnesemia [172], attributed to a reduction in TRPM6 expression in the DCT [60]. In reality hypomagnesemia is more common in patients on long-term thiazide than on furosemide. This is very similar to the observation in Gitelman's and Bartter's syndromes, as discussed before. This apparent paradox as well as the exact mechanism resulting in magnesium wasting remains unexplained.

In contrast, the potassium-sparing diuretics, (amiloride or triamterene), *reduce* urinary Mg^{2+} excretion and are not associated with hypomagnesemia [173].

Aminoglycosides

Hypomagnesemia alone or in combination with hypocalcemia, hypokalemia, and metabolic alkalosis, has been reported in nearly 5 % of patients receiving aminoglycoside antibiotics [174]. The risk is greater with an increase in the dose and the duration of therapy. The elderly are more prone to develop hypomagnesemia, perhaps since they often get a higher dose than appropriate to their level of kidney function. Although specific mechanisms remain elusive, the clinical picture is compatible with distal tubular toxicity.

Calcineurin Inhibitors

The immunosuppressive drug cyclosporine A (CSA) and FK506 (Prograf) may lead to renal wasting of Mg^{2+} and hypomagnesemia. Hypomagnesemia following renal transplantation was rare prior to the introduction of CSA. Furthermore, hypomagnesemia has now been described during treatment with CSA and Fk506 in liver transplant recipients [175]. There was no correlation between the serum Mg^{2+} levels and the blood calcineurin inhibitor levels. CSA has been shown to downregulate the expression of Claudin-14 and as a result causes an increase in FEMg [176]; it also appears to inhibit TRPM6 [177]. In addition CSA reduces the rate of replication of mitochondria in different tissues, resulting in a decrease in energetics and Mg^{2+} wasting.

Cisplatin

Renal Mg^{2+} wasting also occurs with cisplatin; this may be severe and can persist for years after cessation of therapy [178]. Brock et al. [178] studied 40 children treated with cisplatin for solid tumors; the follow-up ranged from 1.5 to 7 years. Among the 21 children with serum Mg^{2+} measurements, six had low values at follow-up. Hypomagnesemia may also persist in patients treated with cisplatin for ovarian cancer [179]. Hypocalciuria, hypokalemic metabolic alkalosis, and evidence of renal Mg^{2+} wasting are seen, consistent with a "pseudo-Gitelman's" syndrome [180].

Cardiac Glycosides

Digoxin, and other cardiac glycosides, may produce hypomagnesemia due to renal Mg^{2+} wasting. Hypomagnesemia increases the sensitivity of the Na^+ pump to digitalis glycosides; thus increasing the likelihood of overt digitalis toxicity.

Foscarnet

Foscarnet toxicity includes hypomagnesemia and hypocalcemia is common in foscarnet treated patients. This is most commonly seen in AIDS patients treated for CMV retinitis, in approximately 70 % of these patients [181]. Hypomagnesemia occurs acutely after an intravenous dose of foscarnet and is often self-limited but can also be severe. The exact mechanism of foscarnet-induced hypomagnesemia is still unclear, but presumably relates to tubular toxicity given the propensity of this drug to cause tubular necrosis.

EGF Inhibitors

Epidermal growth factor (EGF) functions as an autocrine stimulant of apical TRPM6 channels in DCT cells, via the basolateral EGF receptor [147, 148] (see above). In consequence, inhibition of the EGF receptor kinase with the recombinant inhibitor cetuximab, utilized in oncology, is associated with hypomagnesemia and hypokalemia [147].

Other Causes of Hypomagnesemia

Phosphate Depletion

Phosphate deprivation can lead to hypercalciuria and hypermagnesuria, with resultant hypomagnesemia. Phosphate depletion reduces Mg^{2+} transport as well as that of calcium in the TAL and in the distal convoluted tubule [149]. This is not surprising, as phosphate depletion leads to ATP depletion and resultant energy deprivation necessary for reabsorptive function.

Hypercalcemia

Hypercalcemia, independent of etiology, often results in renal Mg^{2+} wasting. The mechanism is probably secondary to activation of CaR in the basolateral membrane of cells in the TAL. This would then result in inhibition of apical $Na\text{-}K^+\text{-}2Cl^-$ cotransport and apical K^+ channel activity, with a secondary decrease in paracellular Mg^{2+} and Ca reabsorption [9] (see section under "Calcium Homeostasis" in this chapter). In primary hyperparathyroidism, this effect of hypercalcemia to induce Mg^{2+} wasting may be offset by the ability of PTH to enhance the tubular reabsorption of Mg^{2+}; hence the serum Mg^{2+} in hyperparathyroidism may be normal, low, or high.

Hungry Bone Syndrome

Hypomagnesemia may arise due to the rapid deposition of Mg^{2+} into the bone matrix after parathyroidectomy or osteoblastic metastasis.

This is discussed fully in this chapter under hypocalcemia.

Administration of Nutrients

Magnesium is shifted intracellularly during rapid infusion of nutrients, such as glucose or amino acids, or insulin administration. This shift is probably in response to increased intracellular enzymatic activities and the need for increased ATP production.

Transfusion or Plasmapheresis

The administration of citrate for blood transfusion or plasmapheresis can lead to Mg^{2+} chelation, with an approximately 30 % decrease in serum values [182].

Cardiopulmonary Bypass

Hypomagnesemia, probably secondary to intracellular Mg^{2+} shift, occurs commonly in coronary artery bypass surgery [183]. In a prospective study by Aglio et al. [183] approximately 18 % of patients had hypomagnesemia prior to surgery. This increased to 71 % after termination of the cardiopulmonary bypass. Robertie et al. [184] noted that both $[Ca^{2+}]i$ and $[Mg^{2+}]i$ fell on initiation of cardiopulmonary bypass. This was associated with a paradoxical suppression of PTH level that did not respond to Mg^{2+} administration [184].

Pregnancy

Serum Mg^{2+} is commonly low in pregnancy [185], particularly during the last trimester. The hypomagnesemia of pregnancy is partly due to a shift of Mg^{2+} into the fetus or other developing tissues, such as the uterus and/or placenta. Furthermore, the marked increase in GFR during pregnancy would result in an increase in filter load of Mg^{2+} and an increase in urinary Mg^{2+}.

Alcoholism

Hypomagnesemia as well as other electrolyte abnormalities are common in chronic alcoholics (also see under "Hypophosphatemia" in this chapter). Hypomagnesemia and Mg^{2+} depletion in these patients is due to several additive factors, including protein-calorie malnutrition, diarrhea, and increased urinary excretion of Mg^{2+}. Renal loss of Mg^{2+} in the alcoholic is probably related to direct toxicity of alcohol reducing the renal tubular reabsorption of Mg^{2+}, with nearly a threefold increase of urinary Mg^{2+}. Alcoholic ketoacidosis and phosphate depletion with hypophosphatemia may also contribute to renal Mg^{2+} losses. De Marchi et al. reported a reversible tubular defect in approximately 20 % of alcoholics; this defect encompassed aminoaciduria, glycosuria, a reduced renal threshold for phosphate excretion, renal magnesium wasting, and impaired urinary acidification following an acid load. These abnormalities are very similar to Fanconi's syndrome with disorders in ATP production in the proximal tubules. These abnormalities were reversed after abstinence for 4 weeks [97].

Diabetes Mellitus

Hypomagnesemia is common in patients with diabetes mellitus, reported in 40 % of these patients. Hypermagnesuria is reported in up to 55 % of insulin-dependent diabetics [186]. The increase in urinary Mg^{2+} is partly due to hyperglycemia-induced glycosuria. Hypomagnesemia may also be due to an intracellular shift of Mg^{2+}.

Treatment of Hypomagnesemia

Treatment of hypomagnesemia should begin by treating the underlying causative disorder or disorders. This includes discontinuation of drugs such as cisplatin and toxins such as alcohol, treatment of diarrhea and other GI disorders, as well as correction of malnutrition. Magnesium supplementation should, however, be used if hypomagnesemia is clinically significant and/or the underlying disorder is not rapidly reversible. Mg^{2+} replacement can be accomplished through IV, oral and peritoneal routes. Typically a symptomatic patient or a patient refractory to oral magnesium therapy should receive IV magnesium treatment. Oral replacement is usually given to asymptomatic patients as well as patients with chronic persistent hypomagnesemia. Finally, in a patient who fails chronic IV and oral magnesium supplementation, peritoneal treatment may need to be considered.

Intravenous Magnesium

Although magnesium can be administered intramuscularly, this route of administration is very painful. The magnesium preparation for intravenous use is Magnesium sulfate ($MgSO_4$ $7H_2O$)

Table 4.14 Partial list of magnesium preparations for oral and parenteral use

Salt	Formula	Percent	Form	Mg, mmol[a] preparation	Diarrhea
Sulfalc	$MgSO_4$□$7H_2O$	10	Injection (2 mL)	4.0	N/A
Sulfate	$MgSO_4$□$7H_2O$	10	Powder (15 g)[b]	61.2	++
Oxide	MgO	60	Tablet (140 mg)[c]	3.5	++
Hydroxide[d]	$Mg(OH)_2$	42	Suspension (10 mL)	14.5	++
Hydroxide	$Mg(OH)_2$	42	Tablet (400 mg)[c]	3.5	++
Citrate[d]	$C_{12}H_{22}MgO_{14}$	16	Solution (10 mL)	4.2	++
Lactate	$C_6H_{10}MgO_6$	10	Tablet[f]	3.5	+
Chloride	$MgCl_2$□$6H_2O$	12	Solution[g] (10 mL)	2.5	+
Gluconate	$C_{12}H_{22}MgO_{14}$	5.8	Tablet (500 mg)	1.2	±
Proteinate	(Soy protein)		Tablet	5.5	±

[a]Content per dosage unit
[b]Usual cathartic dose (Epsom salts)
[c]Marketed as a magnesium supplement (Uro-Mag)
[d]Marketed as a laxative (milk of magnesia) but sometimes prescribed for its magnesium content
[e]A proprietary mixture of 200 mg each of magnesium and aluminum hydroxide (Maalox), widely used as an antacid
[f]Marketed as sustained release magnesium supplement (Mag-Tab-SR)
[g]Compounded with syrup

with, MW 246.5, containing 9.7 % elemental magnesium. The drug is available in 2 mL vials containing 1 g (4 mmol) of magnesium sulfate or 97 mg of elemental Mg^{2+}. In life-threatening situations 4–8 mmol is diluted in 250–500 cm^3 of dextrose and water and given over a 10–15 min period while monitoring patient for any arrhythmias. In severe but not life-threatening hypomagnesemia, 40 mmol (1,000 mg), or as much as 125–200 mmol (3,000–4,800 mg is given intravenously over 24 h. The rate of administration should be slow to allow equilibration of the extracellular and intracellular Mg^{2+} levels. If magnesium sulfate is infused rapidly, it is renally excreted. When patients are severely Mg^{2+}-depleted it is therefore best to infuse Mg^{2+}-containing solutions over a long period of time. However, the total amount given over 24 h should not exceed 125–200 mmol (3,000–4,800 mg). In severely depleted patients, several days are required to achieve near total repletion.

Oral Magnesium Replacement Therapy

Many laxatives and antacids contain Mg^{2+} salts. Most Mg^{2+} supplements are available over the counter (Table 4.14). Several oral compounds, such as magnesium citrate, magnesium hydroxide, and magnesium sulfate, have a major effect on intestinal motility and are primarily used as laxatives. Others, such as magaldrate, magnesium carbonate, magnesium trisilicate, and magnesium oxide, are primarily used as antacids. Although these compounds enhance intestinal motility, net absorption of Mg^{2+} is also increased. Magnesium chloride, magnesium gluconate, magnesium proteinate, and magnesium lactate have an even lesser tendency to cause diarrhea. The sustained release preparations (Slow Mg^{2+} or mag-tab SR) provide 2.5–3.5 mmol of Mg^{2+} per tablet. To enhance its absorption it is best if these drugs are given in divided doses.

Intraperitoneal

Intraperitoneal administration has been shown to be effective. While high concentration of magnesium in the IP fluid leads to severe lower abdominal pain, this pain is dose dependent. In a single patient administration of 1 g of magnesium sulfate in 500 mL of DW 5 % at twice daily rate was effective to maintain a normal magnesium level.

Potassium-Sparing Diuretics

Administration of the potassium-sparing diuretics triamterene or amiloride can reduce the urinary excretion of magnesium [172, 173]. In 6-day clinical trials in patients with congestive heart failure who had been receiving furosemide followed by furosemide plus amiloride, the addition of amiloride resulted in a significant reduction of both urinary magnesium and potassium, while the lymphocyte content of both magnesium and potassium rose significantly [187]. In a recent study of 116 consecutive patients with CHF treated with placebo or spironolactone 20 mg daily in addition to conventional therapy for 6 months, the latter group had significantly higher Plasma Mg^{2+} concentration, erythrocyte Mg^{2+} concentration, and lower erythrocyte Mg^{2+} efflux. Patients on spironolactone therapy also had a marked decrease of 24-h mean heart rate, ventricular and atrial premature beats, and the risk of atrial fibrillation/flutter [188]. Potassium sparing diuretics are also partially effective in patients with Gitelman's syndrome, [189].

Other Treatments

There is limited evidence in support of other modes of treatment of hypomagnesemia including calcitriol. In rare cases of renal hypomagnesemia unresponsive to aggressive medical therapy, renal transplantation has been considered. Administration of theophylline has been suggested as a mode of increasing ATP/cAMP. The risks of theophylline treatment are, however, substantial, due to the increased risk of cardiac arrhythmia in patients who are already susceptible due to underlying hypomagnesemia.

Hypermagnesemia

Hypermagnesemia is only observed in the patients with decreased GFR and/or markedly increased Mg^{2+} intake. Surprisingly most patients with stage-4 and even stage-5 chronic kidney disease (CKD)havenormalmagnesium.Hypermagnesemia would, however, occur in these patients if they ingest magnesium-containing antacid or enema.

Mild hypermagnesemia seen in association with severe volume depletion, such as in patients with adrenal insufficiency; this is thought to be secondary to increased tubular reabsorption of Mg^{2+}. Autosomal dominant hypocalciuric hypercalcemia is associated with hypermagnesemia; this is due to loss of function of CaR. Hypermagnesemia is more common in the homozygous cases, neonatal severe hyperparathyroidism (for more detailed discussion please refer to the section on "Hypercalcemia" in this chapter).

Sign and Symptoms of Hypermagnesemia

Moderate hypermagnesemia due to infusion of Mg^{2+} containing solutions commonly causes vasodilatation, resulting in a feeling of warmth with flushing. Severe hypermagnesemia also causes hypotension. A further increase in serum Mg^{2+} may result in impaired motor function, muscular weakness, impaired ventilation due to paralysis of the respiratory muscles, loss of deep tendon reflexes, bradycardia, prolongation of the PR interval, and cardiac arrhythmias (specially with serum Mg^{2+} levels above 10 mg/dL). Further increase in Mg^{2+} will lead to alterations in consciousness. In a patient with CKD, the hypermagnesemia could be chronic in nature and result in minimal clinical signs and symptoms. In addition sign and symptoms of hypermagnesemia could be masked by uremia.

Management of Hypermagnesemia

In a patient with normal renal function and Mg^{2+} overload, discontinuation of exogenous Mg^{2+} is often effective in reversing hypermagnesemia. The administration of intravenous calcium in doses of 100–200 mg of elemental calcium may aid in reversal of symptoms of hypermagnesemia. In ESRD patients with symptomatic and marked hypermagnesemia, dialysis may be needed to lower the magnesium level. If magnesium-free dialysate solution is not available, the use of a standard dialysate solution with a magnesium concentration of 0.5 mEq/L will remove adequate amounts of Mg^{2+} and lower the serum Mg^{2+} level over time.

References

1. Brown EM. Clinical lessons from the calcium-sensing receptor. Nat Clin Pract Endocrinol Metab. 2007;3:122–33.
2. Hruska KA, Korkor A, Martin K, Slatopolsky E. Peripheral metabolism of intact parathyroid hormone. Role of liver and kidney and the effect of chronic renal failure. J Clin Invest. 1981;67:885–92.
3. Deftos LJ. Calcitonin. In: Favus M et al., editors. Primer on the metabolic bone diseases and disorders of mineral metabolism. 2nd ed. New York: Raven; 1993. p. 70–6.

4. The ADHR Consortium. Autosomal dominant hypophosphataemic rickets is associated with mutations in FGF23. Nat Genet. 2000;26:345–8.
5. Alon US. Clinical practice: fibroblast growth factor (FGF)23: a new hormone. Eur J Pediatr. 2010; 170(5):545–54.
6. Barger-Lux MJ, Heaney RP, Recker RR. Time course of calcium absorption in humans: evidence for a colonic component. Calcif Tissue Int. 1989;44:308–11.
7. Bell NH. Vitamin D-endocrine system. J Clin Invest. 1985;76:1–6.
8. Dimke H, Hoenderop JG, Bindels RJ. Molecular basis of epithelial Ca^{2+} and Mg^{2+} transport: insights from the TRP channel family. J Physiol. 2010;589 (Pt 7):1535–42.
9. Hebert SC. Calcium and salinity sensing by the thick ascending limb: a journey from mammals to fish and back again. Kidney Int Suppl. 2004;91:S28–33.
10. Bindels RJ. Homer W. Smith Award: Minerals in motion: from new ion transporters to new concepts. J Am Soc Nephrol. 2010;21:1263–9.
11. Kantham L, Quinn SJ, Egbuna OI, et al. The calcium-sensing receptor (CaSR) defends against hypercalcemia independently of its regulation of parathyroid hormone secretion. Am J Physiol Endocrinol Metab. 2009;297:E915–23.
12. Silverberg SJ, Bilezikian JP. The diagnosis and management of asymptomatic primary hyperparathyroidism. Nat Clin Pract Endocrinol Metab. 2006;2: 494–503.
13. Silverberg SJ, Bilezikian JP. Clinical presentation of primary hyperparathyroidism in the United States. In: Bilezikian JP, editor. The parathyroids. 2nd ed. New York: Academic; 2001. p. 349–60.
14. Brandi ML, Gagel RF, Angeli A, et al. Guidelines for diagnosis and therapy of MEN type 1 and type 2. J Clin Endocrinol Metab. 2001;86:5658–71.
15. Shane E, Bilezikian JP. Parathyroid carcinoma: a review of 62 patients. Endocr Rev. 1982;3:218–26.
16. Silverberg SJ, Lewiecki EM, Mosekilde L, Peacock M, Rubin MR. Presentation of asymptomatic primary hyperparathyroidism: proceedings of the third international workshop. J Clin Endocrinol Metab. 2009;94:351–65.
17. Silverberg SJ, Shane E, Jacobs TP, Siris E, Bilezikian JP. A 10-year prospective study of primary hyperparathyroidism with or without parathyroid surgery. N Engl J Med. 1999;341:1249–55.
18. Bilezikian JP, Khan AA, Potts Jr JT. Guidelines for the management of asymptomatic primary hyperparathyroidism: summary statement from the third international workshop. J Clin Endocrinol Metab. 2009;94:335–9.
19. Khosla S, Ebeling PR, Firek AF, Burritt MM, Kao PC, Heath 3rd H. Calcium infusion suggests a "set-point" abnormality of parathyroid gland function in familial benign hypercalcemia and more complex disturbances in primary hyperparathyroidism. J Clin Endocrinol Metab. 1993;76:715–20.
20. Brown EM. Four-parameter model of the sigmoidal relationship between parathyroid hormone release and extracellular calcium concentration in normal and abnormal parathyroid tissue. J Clin Endocrinol Metab. 1983;56:572–81.
21. Simonds WF, James-Newton LA, Agarwal SK, et al. Familial isolated hyperparathyroidism: clinical and genetic characteristics of 36 kindreds. Medicine (Baltimore). 2002;81:1–26.
22. Udelsman R, Pasieka JL, Sturgeon C, Young JE, Clark OH. Surgery for asymptomatic primary hyperparathyroidism: proceedings of the third international workshop. J Clin Endocrinol Metab. 2009;94:366–72.
23. Khan A, Grey A, Shoback D. Medical management of asymptomatic primary hyperparathyroidism: proceedings of the third international workshop. J Clin Endocrinol Metab. 2009;94:373–81.
24. Peacock M, Bilezikian JP, Bolognese MA, et al. Cinacalcet HCl reduces hypercalcemia in primary hyperparathyroidism across a wide spectrum of disease severity. J Clin Endocrinol Metab. 2011;96:E9–18.
25. Stewart AF. Clinical practice. Hypercalcemia associated with cancer. N Engl J Med. 2005;352:373–9.
26. Abou-Samra AB, Juppner H, Force T, et al. Expression cloning of a common receptor for parathyroid hormone and parathyroid hormone-related peptide from rat osteoblast-like cells: a single receptor stimulates intracellular accumulation of both cAMP and inositol trisphosphates and increases intracellular free calcium. Proc Natl Acad Sci U S A. 1992;89:2732–6.
27. Wysolmerski JJ, Stewart AF. The physiology of parathyroid hormone-related protein: an emerging role as a developmental factor. Annu Rev Physiol. 1998;60:431–60.
28. Asa SL, Henderson J, Goltzman D, Drucker DJ. Parathyroid hormone-like peptide in normal and neoplastic human endocrine tissues. J Clin Endocrinol Metab. 1990;71:1112–8.
29. Yates AJ, Gutierrez GE, Smolens P, et al. Effects of a synthetic peptide of a parathyroid hormone-related protein on calcium homeostasis, renal tubular calcium reabsorption, and bone metabolism in vivo and in vitro in rodents. J Clin Invest. 1988;81:932–8.
30. Pandian MR, Morgan CH, Carlton E, Segre GV. Modified immunoradiometric assay of parathyroid hormone-related protein: clinical application in the differential diagnosis of hypercalcemia. Clin Chem. 1992;38:282–8.
31. Nussbaum SR, Gaz RD, Arnold A. Hypercalcemia and ectopic secretion of parathyroid hormone by an ovarian carcinoma with rearrangement of the gene for parathyroid hormone. N Engl J Med. 1990;323: 1324–8.
32. Shaker JL, Krawczyk KW, Findling JW. Primary hyperparathyroidism and severe hypercalcemia with low circulating 1,25-dihydroxyvitamin D. J Clin Endocrinol Metab. 1990;71:1305–9.

33. Guise TA, Mundy GR. Cancer and bone. Endocr Rev. 1998;19:18–54.
34. Seymour JF, Gagel RF. Calcitriol: the major humoral mediator of hypercalcemia in Hodgkin's disease and non-Hodgkin's lymphomas. Blood. 1993;82:1383–94.
35. Beall DP, Henslee HB, Webb HR, Scofield RH. Milk-alkali syndrome: a historical review and description of the modern version of the syndrome. Am J Med Sci. 2006;331:233–42.
36. Picolos MK, Lavis VR, Orlander PR. Milk-alkali syndrome is a major cause of hypercalcaemia among non-end-stage renal disease (non-ESRD) inpatients. Clin Endocrinol (Oxf). 2005;63:566–76.
37. Patel AM, Goldfarb S. Got calcium? Welcome to the calcium-alkali syndrome. J Am Soc Nephrol. 2010;21:1440–3.
38. Kapsner P, Langsdorf L, Marcus R, Kraemer FB, Hoffman AR. Milk-alkali syndrome in patients treated with calcium carbonate after cardiac transplantation. Arch Intern Med. 1986;146:1965–8.
39. Sharma OP. Hypercalcemia in granulomatous disorders: a clinical review. Curr Opin Pulm Med. 2000;6:442–7.
40. Kallas M, Green F, Hewison M, White C, Kline G. Rare causes of calcitriol-mediated hypercalcemia: a case report and literature review. J Clin Endocrinol Metab. 2010;95:3111–7.
41. Berliner AR, Haas M, Choi MJ. Sarcoidosis: the nephrologist's perspective. Am J Kidney Dis. 2006;48:856–70.
42. Ferrand RA, Elgalib A, Newsholme W, Childerhouse A, Edwards SG, Miller RF. Hypercalcaemia complicating immune reconstitution in an HIV-infected patient with disseminated tuberculosis. Int J STD AIDS. 2006;17:349–50.
43. Adams JS, Diz MM, Sharma OP. Effective reduction in the serum 1,25-dihydroxyvitamin D and calcium concentration in sarcoidosis-associated hypercalcemia with short-course chloroquine therapy. Ann Intern Med. 1989;111:437–8.
44. Taylor RL, Lynch Jr HJ, Wysor Jr WG. Seasonal influence of sunlight on the hypercalcemia of sarcoidosis. Am J Med. 1963;34:221–7.
45. Subramanian P, Chinthalapalli H, Krishnan M, et al. Pregnancy and sarcoidosis: an insight into the pathogenesis of hypercalciuria. Chest. 2004;126: 995–8.
46. Sandler LM, Winearls CG, Fraher LJ, Clemens TL, Smith R, O'Riordan JL. Studies of the hypercalcaemia of sarcoidosis: effect of steroids and exogenous vitamin D3 on the circulating concentrations of 1,25-dihydroxy vitamin D3. Q J Med. 1984;53: 165–80.
47. Kimberg DV, Baerg RD, Gershon E, Graudusius RT. Effect of cortisone treatment on the active transport of calcium by the small intestine. J Clin Invest. 1971;50:1309–21.
48. Gibbs CJ, Peacock M. Hypercalcaemia due to sarcoidosis corrects with bisphosphonate treatment. Postgrad Med J. 1986;62:937–8.
49. Barre PE, Gascon-Barre M, Meakins JL, Goltzman D. Hydroxychloroquine treatment of hypercalcemia in a patient with sarcoidosis undergoing hemodialysis. Am J Med. 1987;82:1259–62.
50. Adams JS, Sharma OP, Diz MM, Endres DB. Ketoconazole decreases the serum 1,25-dihydroxyvitamin D and calcium concentration in sarcoidosis-associated hypercalcemia. J Clin Endocrinol Metab. 1990;70:1090–5.
51. Marx SJ, Attie MF, Levine MA, Spiegel AM, Downs Jr RW, Lasker RD. The hypocalciuric or benign variant of familial hypercalcemia: clinical and biochemical features in fifteen kindreds. Medicine (Baltimore). 1981;60:397–412.
52. Pollak MR, Brown EM, Chou YH, et al. Mutations in the human Ca(2+)-sensing receptor gene cause familial hypocalciuric hypercalcemia and neonatal severe hyperparathyroidism. Cell. 1993;75:1297–303.
53. Pollak MR, Brown EM, Estep HL, et al. Autosomal dominant hypocalcaemia caused by a Ca(2+)-sensing receptor gene mutation. Nat Genet. 1994;8:303–7.
54. Guarnieri V, Canaff L, Yun FH, et al. Calcium-sensing receptor (CASR) mutations in hypercalcemic states: studies from a single endocrine clinic over three years. J Clin Endocrinol Metab. 2010;95:1819–29.
55. Mosekilde L, Eriksen EF, Charles P. Effects of thyroid hormones on bone and mineral metabolism. Endocrinol Metab Clin North Am. 1990;19:35–63.
56. Mundy GR, Shapiro JL, Bandelin JG, Canalis EM, Raisz LG. Direct stimulation of bone resorption by thyroid hormones. J Clin Invest. 1976;58:529–34.
57. Montoli A, Colussi G, Minetti L. Hypercalcaemia in Addison's disease: calciotropic hormone profile and bone histology. J Intern Med. 1992;232:535–40.
58. Stewart AF, Adler M, Byers CM, Segre GV, Broadus AE. Calcium homeostasis in immobilization: an example of resorptive hypercalciuria. N Engl J Med. 1982;306:1136–40.
59. Kim GH, Martin SW, Fernandez-Llama P, Masilamani S, Packer RK, Knepper MA. Long-term regulation of renal Na-dependent cotransporters and ENaC: response to altered acid-base intake. Am J Physiol Renal Physiol. 2000;279:F459–67.
60. Nijenhuis T, Vallon V, van der Kemp AW, Loffing J, Hoenderop JG, Bindels RJ. Enhanced passive Ca^{2+} reabsorption and reduced Mg^{2+} channel abundance explains thiazide-induced hypocalciuria and hypomagnesemia. J Clin Invest. 2005;115:1651–8.
61. Christensson T, Hellstrom K, Wengle B. Hypercalcemia and primary hyperparathyroidism. Prevalence in patients receiving thiazides as detected in a health screen. Arch Intern Med. 1977;137: 1138–42.
62. Mallette LE, Eichhorn E. Effects of lithium carbonate on human calcium metabolism. Arch Intern Med. 1986;146:770–6.
63. Spiegel AM, Rudorfer MV, Marx SJ, Linnoila M. The effect of short term lithium administration on suppressibility of parathyroid hormone secretion by calcium in vivo. J Clin Endocrinol Metab. 1984;59: 354–7.

64. Sloand JA, Shelly MA. Normalization of lithium-induced hypercalcemia and hyperparathyroidism with cinacalcet hydrochloride. Am J Kidney Dis. 2006;48:832–7.
65. Suki WN, Yium JJ, Von Minden M, Saller-Hebert C, Eknoyan G, Martinez-Maldonado M. Acute treatment of hypercalcemia with furosemide. N Engl J Med. 1970;283:836–40.
66. Perazella MA, Markowitz GS. Bisphosphonate nephrotoxicity. Kidney Int. 2008;74:1385–93.
67. Cvitkovic F, Armand JP, Tubiana-Hulin M, Rossi JF, Warrell Jr RP. Randomized, double-blind, phase II trial of gallium nitrate compared with pamidronate for acute control of cancer-related hypercalcemia. Cancer J. 2006;12:47–53.
68. Suzuki T, Ikeda U, Fujikawa H, Saito K, Shimada K. Hypocalcemic heart failure: a reversible form of heart muscle disease. Clin Cardiol. 1998;21:227–8.
69. Brunet A, Gabau E, Perich RM, et al. Microdeletion and microduplication 22q11.2 screening in 295 patients with clinical features of DiGeorge/velocardiofacial syndrome. Am J Med Genet A. 2006;140:2426–32.
70. Rizzi M, Ferrera F, Filaci G, Indiveri F. Disruption of immunological tolerance: role of AIRE gene in autoimmunity. Autoimmun Rev. 2006;5:145–7.
71. Ahonen P, Myllarniemi S, Sipila I, Perheentupa J. Clinical variation of autoimmune polyendocrinopathy-candidiasis-ectodermal dystrophy (APECED) in a series of 68 patients. N Engl J Med. 1990;322: 1829–36.
72. Perheentupa J. Autoimmune polyendocrinopathy-candidiasis-ectodermal dystrophy. J Clin Endocrinol Metab. 2006;91:2843–50.
73. Goswami R, Brown EM, Kochupillai N, et al. Prevalence of calcium sensing receptor autoantibodies in patients with sporadic idiopathic hypoparathyroidism. Eur J Endocrinol. 2004;150:9–18.
74. Brasier AR, Nussbaum SR. Hungry bone syndrome: clinical and biochemical predictors of its occurrence after parathyroid surgery. Am J Med. 1988;84:654–60.
75. Stewart ZA, Blackford A, Somervell H, et al. 25-Hydroxyvitamin D deficiency is a risk factor for symptoms of postoperative hypocalcemia and secondary hyperparathyroidism after minimally invasive parathyroidectomy. Surgery. 2005;138:1018–25. discussion 25–6.
76. Cholst IN, Steinberg SF, Tropper PJ, Fox HE, Segre GV, Bilezikian JP. The influence of hypermagnesemia on serum calcium and parathyroid hormone levels in human subjects. N Engl J Med. 1984;310:1221–5.
77. Burch WM, Posillico JT. Hypoparathyroidism after I-131 therapy with subsequent return of parathyroid function. J Clin Endocrinol Metab. 1983;57: 398–401.
78. Levine MA. Clinical spectrum and pathogenesis of pseudohypoparathyroidism. Rev Endocr Metab Disord. 2000;1:265–74.
79. Quack I, Zwernemann C, Weiner SM, et al. Dihydrotachysterol therapy for hypoparathyroidism: consequences of inadequate monitoring. Five cases and a review. Exp Clin Endocrinol Diabetes. 2005;113:376–80.
80. Winer KK, Ko CW, Reynolds JC, et al. Long-term treatment of hypoparathyroidism: a randomized controlled study comparing parathyroid hormone-(1–34) versus calcitriol and calcium. J Clin Endocrinol Metab. 2003;88:4214–20.
81. Watanabe S, Fukumoto S, Chang H, et al. Association between activating mutations of calcium-sensing receptor and Bartter's syndrome. Lancet. 2002;360: 692–4.
82. Shiohara M, Shiozawa R, Kurata K, et al. Effect of parathyroid hormone administration in a patient with severe hypoparathyroidism caused by gain-of-function mutation of calcium-sensing receptor. Endocr J. 2006;53:797–802.
83. Pack AM, Morrell MJ. Adverse effects of antiepileptic drugs on bone structure: epidemiology, mechanisms and therapeutic implications. CNS Drugs. 2001;15:633–42.
84. Fraser D, Kooh SW, Kind HP, Holick MF, Tanaka Y, DeLuca HF. Pathogenesis of hereditary vitamin-D-dependent rickets. An inborn error of vitamin D metabolism involving defective conversion of 25-hydroxyvitamin D to 1 alpha,25-dihydroxyvitamin D. N Engl J Med. 1973;289:817–22.
85. Stewart AF, Longo W, Kreutter D, Jacob R, Burtis WJ. Hypocalcemia associated with calcium-soap formation in a patient with a pancreatic fistula. N Engl J Med. 1986;315:496–8.
86. Lind L, Carlstedt F, Rastad J, et al. Hypocalcemia and parathyroid hormone secretion in critically ill patients. Crit Care Med. 2000;28:93–9.
87. Tohme JF, Bilezikian JP. Hypocalcemic emergencies. Endocrinol Metab Clin North Am. 1993;22:363–75.
88. Gaasbeek A, Meinders AE. Hypophosphatemia: an update on its etiology and treatment. Am J Med. 2005;118:1094–101.
89. Portale AA, Halloran BP, Morris Jr RC. Dietary intake of phosphorus modulates the circadian rhythm in serum concentration of phosphorus. Implications for the renal production of 1,25-dihydroxyvitamin D. J Clin Invest. 1987;80:1147–54.
90. Murer H, Forster I, Biber J. The sodium phosphate cotransporter family SLC34. Pflugers Arch. 2004;447:763–7.
91. Murer H, Hernando N, Forster I, Biber J. Proximal tubular phosphate reabsorption: molecular mechanisms. Physiol Rev. 2000;80:1373–409.
92. Bacic D, Lehir M, Biber J, Kaissling B, Murer H, Wagner CA. The renal Na+/phosphate cotransporter NaPi-IIa is internalized via the receptor-mediated endocytic route in response to parathyroid hormone. Kidney Int. 2006;69:495–503.
93. Gloor HJ, Bonjour JP, Caverzasio J, Fleisch H. Resistance to the phosphaturic and calcemic actions of parathyroid hormone during phosphate depletion. Prevention by 1,25-dihydroxyvitamin D3. J Clin Invest. 1979;63:371–7.

94. Cai Q, Hodgson SF, Kao PC, et al. Brief report: inhibition of renal phosphate transport by a tumor product in a patient with oncogenic osteomalacia. N Engl J Med. 1994;330:1645–9.
95. Berndt T, Kumar R. Novel mechanisms in the regulation of phosphorus homeostasis. Physiology (Bethesda). 2009;24:17–25.
96. Wolf M. Forging forward with 10 burning questions on FGF23 in kidney disease. J Am Soc Nephrol. 2010;21:1427–35.
97. De Marchi S, Cecchin E, Basile A, Bertotti A, Nardini R, Bartoli E. Renal tubular dysfunction in chronic alcohol abuse—effects of abstinence. N Engl J Med. 1993;329:1927–34.
98. Larsson L, Rebel K, Sorbo B. Severe hypophosphatemia—a hospital survey. Acta Med Scand. 1983;214:221–3.
99. Camp MA, Allon M. Severe hypophosphatemia in hospitalized patients. Miner Electrolyte Metab. 1990;16:365–8.
100. Singhal PC, Kumar A, Desroches L, Gibbons N, Mattana J. Prevalence and predictors of rhabdomyolysis in patients with hypophosphatemia. Am J Med. 1992;92:458–64.
101. Amanzadeh J, Reilly Jr RF. Hypophosphatemia: an evidence-based approach to its clinical consequences and management. Nat Clin Pract Nephrol. 2006;2:136–48.
102. Dastur DK, Gagrat BM, Wadia NH, Desai M, Bharucha EP. Nature of muscular change in osteomalacia: light- and electron-microscope observations. J Pathol. 1975;117:211–28.
103. O'Connor LR, Wheeler WS, Bethune JE. Effect of hypophosphatemia on myocardial performance in man. N Engl J Med. 1977;297:901–3.
104. Vered Z, Battler A, Motro M, Frank M, Inbar R, Neufeld HN. Left ventricular function in patients with chronic hypophosphatemia. Am Heart J. 1984;107:796–8.
105. Davis SV, Olichwier KK, Chakko SC. Reversible depression of myocardial performance in hypophosphatemia. Am J Med Sci. 1988;295:183–7.
106. Vered I, Vered Z, Perez JE, Jaffe AS, Whyte MP. Normal left ventricular performance in children with X-linked hypophosphatemic rickets: a Doppler echocardiography study. J Bone Miner Res. 1990;5:469–74.
107. Venditti FJ, Marotta C, Panezai FR, Oldewurtel HA, Regan TJ. Hypophosphatemia and cardiac arrhythmias. Miner Electrolyte Metab. 1987;13:19–25.
108. Gravelyn TR, Brophy N, Siegert C, Peters-Golden M. Hypophosphatemia-associated respiratory muscle weakness in a general inpatient population. Am J Med. 1988;84:870–6.
109. Aubier M, Murciano D, Lecocguic Y, et al. Effect of hypophosphatemia on diaphragmatic contractility in patients with acute respiratory failure. N Engl J Med. 1985;313:420–4.
110. Fiaccadori E, Coffrini E, Ronda N, et al. Hypophosphatemia in course of chronic obstructive pulmonary disease. Prevalence, mechanisms, and relationships with skeletal muscle phosphorus content. Chest. 1990;97:857–68.
111. Michell AW, Burn DJ, Reading PJ. Central pontine myelinolysis temporally related to hypophosphataemia. J Neurol Neurosurg Psychiatry. 2003;74:820.
112. Yagnik P, Singh N, Burns R. Peripheral neuropathy with hypophosphatemia in a patient receiving intravenous hyperalimentation. South Med J. 1985;78:1381–4.
113. Jacob HS, Amsden T. Acute hemolytic anemia with rigid red cells in hypophosphatemia. N Engl J Med. 1971;285:1446–50.
114. Lau K, Agus ZS, Goldberg M, Goldfarb S. Renal tubular sites of altered calcium transport in phosphate-depleted rats. J Clin Invest. 1979;64:1681–7.
115. Steele TH, Stromberg BA, Underwood JL, Larmore CA. Renal resistance to parathyroid hormone during phosphorus deprivation. J Clin Invest. 1976;58:1461–4.
116. Annino JS, Relman AS. The effect of eating on some of the clinically important chemical constituents of the blood. Am J Clin Pathol. 1959;31:155–9.
117. Body JJ, Cryer PE, Offord KP, Heath 3rd H. Epinephrine is a hypophosphatemic hormone in man. Physiological effects of circulating epinephrine on plasma calcium, magnesium, phosphorus, parathyroid hormone, and calcitonin. J Clin Invest. 1983;71:572–8.
118. Ljunghall S, Joborn H, Rastad J, Akerstrom G. Plasma potassium and phosphate concentrations—influence by adrenaline infusion, beta-blockade and physical exercise. Acta Med Scand. 1987;221:83–93.
119. Trivedi B, Danforth WH. Effect of pH on the kinetics of frog muscle phosphofructokinase. J Biol Chem. 1966;241:4110–2.
120. Mostellar ME, Tuttle Jr EP. Effects of alkalosis on plasma concentration and urinary excretion of inorganic phosphate in man. J Clin Invest. 1964;43:138–49.
121. Kraft MD, Btaiche IF, Sacks GS. Review of the refeeding syndrome. Nutr Clin Pract. 2005;20:625–33.
122. De Cock A, Mana F, Velkeniers B, Urbain D. Hypophosphatemia and refeeding: a corrective or a preventive attitude? Acta Clin Belg. 2006;61:134–7.
123. Izzedine H, Launay-Vacher V, Isnard-Bagnis C, Deray G. Drug-induced Fanconi's syndrome. Am J Kidney Dis. 2003;41:292–309.
124. Skinner R, Pearson AD, English MW, et al. Risk factors for ifosfamide nephrotoxicity in children. Lancet. 1996;348:578–80.
125. Jonsson KB, Zahradnik R, Larsson T, et al. Fibroblast growth factor 23 in oncogenic osteomalacia and X-linked hypophosphatemia. N Engl J Med. 2003;348:1656–63.
126. Pomposelli JJ, Pomfret EA, Burns DL, et al. Life-threatening hypophosphatemia after right hepatic lobectomy for live donor adult liver transplantation. Liver Transpl. 2001;7:637–42.

127. Salem RR, Tray K. Hepatic resection-related hypophosphatemia is of renal origin as manifested by isolated hyperphosphaturia. Ann Surg. 2005;241:343–8.
128. Suki WN, Martinez-Maldonado M, Rouse D, Terry A. Effect of expansion of extracellular fluid volume on renal phosphate handling. J Clin Invest. 1969;48:1888–94.
129. Rauchenzauner M, Kountchev J, Ulmer H, et al. Disturbances of electrolytes and blood chemistry in acute alcohol intoxication. Wien Klin Wochenschr. 2005;117:83–91.
130. Kebler R, McDonald FD, Cadnapaphornchai P. Dynamic changes in serum phosphorus levels in diabetic ketoacidosis. Am J Med. 1985;79:571–6.
131. Moorhead JF, Wills MR, Ahmed KY, Baillod RA, Varghese Z, Tatler GL. Hypophosphataemic osteomalacia after cadaveric renal transplantation. Lancet. 1974;1:694–7.
132. Ward HN, Pabico RC, McKenna BA, Freeman RB. The renal handling of phosphate by renal transplant patients: correlation with serum parathyroid hormone (SPTH), cyclic 3′,5′-adenosine monophosphate (cAMP) urinary excretion, and allograft function. Adv Exp Med Biol. 1977;81:173–81.
133. Vannatta JB, Whang R, Papper S. Efficacy of intravenous phosphorus therapy in the severely hypophosphatemic patient. Arch Intern Med. 1981;141:885–7.
134. Gumurdulu Y, Serin E, Ozer B, Gokcel A, Boyacioglu S. Age as a predictor of hyperphosphatemia after oral phosphosoda administration for colon preparation. J Gastroenterol Hepatol. 2004;19:68–72.
135. Markowitz GS, Stokes MB, Radhakrishnan J, D'Agati VD. Acute phosphate nephropathy following oral sodium phosphate bowel purgative: an underrecognized cause of chronic renal failure. J Am Soc Nephrol. 2005;16:3389–96.
136. Heher EC, Thier SO, Rennke H, Humphreys BD. Adverse renal and metabolic effects associated with oral sodium phosphate bowel preparation. Clin J Am Soc Nephrol. 2008;3:1494–503.
137. Davidson MB, Thakkar S, Hix JK, Bhandarkar ND, Wong A, Schreiber MJ. Pathophysiology, clinical consequences, and treatment of tumor lysis syndrome. Am J Med. 2004;116:546–54.
138. Cohen LF, Balow JE, Magrath IT, Poplack DG, Ziegler JL. Acute tumor lysis syndrome. A review of 37 patients with Burkitt's lymphoma. Am J Med. 1980;68:486–91.
139. Brannan PG, Vergne-Marini P, Pak CY, Hull AR, Fordtran JS. Magnesium absorption in the human small intestine. Results in normal subjects, patients with chronic renal disease, and patients with absorptive hypercalciuria. J Clin Invest. 1976;57:1412–8.
140. Voets T, Nilius B, Hoefs S, et al. TRPM6 forms the Mg^{2+} influx channel involved in intestinal and renal Mg^{2+} absorption. J Biol Chem. 2004;279:19–25.
141. Hodgkinson A, Marshall DH, Nordin BE. Vitamin D and magnesium absorption in man. Clin Sci (Lond). 1979;57:121–3.
142. Wilz DR, Gray RW, Dominguez JH, Lemann Jr J. Plasma 1,25-(OH)2-vitamin D concentrations and net intestinal calcium, phosphate, and magnesium absorption in humans. Am J Clin Nutr. 1979;32:2052–60.
143. Simon DB, Lu Y, Choate KA, et al. Paracellin-1, a renal tight junction protein required for paracellular Mg^{2+} resorption. Science. 1999;285:103–6.
144. Hou J, Renigunta A, Konrad M, et al. Claudin-16 and claudin-19 interact and form a cation-selective tight junction complex. J Clin Invest. 2008;118:619–28.
145. Schlingmann KP, Weber S, Peters M, et al. Hypomagnesemia with secondary hypocalcemia is caused by mutations in TRPM6, a new member of the TRPM gene family. Nat Genet. 2002;31:166–70.
146. Pearce SH, Williamson C, Kifor O, et al. A familial syndrome of hypocalcemia with hypercalciuria due to mutations in the calcium-sensing receptor. N Engl J Med. 1996;335:1115–22.
147. Groenestege WM, Thebault S, van der Wijst J, et al. Impaired basolateral sorting of pro-EGF causes isolated recessive renal hypomagnesemia. J Clin Invest. 2007;117:2260–7.
148. Thebault S, Alexander RT, Tiel Groenestege WM, Hoenderop JG, Bindels RJ. EGF increases TRPM6 activity and surface expression. J Am Soc Nephrol. 2009;20:78–85.
149. Kobrin SM, Goldfarb S. Magnesium deficiency. Semin Nephrol. 1990;10:525–35.
150. Schimatschek HF, Rempis R. Prevalence of hypomagnesemia in an unselected German population of 16,000 individuals. Magnes Res. 2001;14: 283–90.
151. Lewis RV, Tregaskis B, McLay J, Service E, McDevitt DG. Oral magnesium reduces ventricular ectopy in digitalised patients with chronic atrial fibrillation. Eur J Clin Pharmacol. 1990;38:107–10.
152. Ma J, Folsom AR, Melnick SL, et al. Associations of serum and dietary magnesium with cardiovascular disease, hypertension, diabetes, insulin, and carotid arterial wall thickness: the ARIC study. Atherosclerosis risk in communities study. J Clin Epidemiol. 1995;48:927–40.
153. Dyckner T. Relation of cardiovascular disease to potassium and magnesium deficiencies. Am J Cardiol. 1990;65:44K–6.
154. Brodsky MA, Orlov MV, Capparelli EV, et al. Magnesium therapy in new-onset atrial fibrillation. Am J Cardiol. 1994;73:1227–9.
155. Rubeiz GJ, Thill-Baharozian M, Hardie D, Carlson RW. Association of hypomagnesemia and mortality in acutely ill medical patients. Crit Care Med. 1993;21:203–9.
156. Gennari FJ. Hypokalemia. N Engl J Med. 1998;339:451–8.
157. Rodriguez M, Solanki DL, Whang R. Refractory potassium repletion due to cisplatin-induced magnesium depletion. Arch Intern Med. 1989;149:2592–4.

158. Whang R, Flink EB, Dyckner T, Wester PO, Aikawa JK, Ryan MP. Magnesium depletion as a cause of refractory potassium repletion. Arch Intern Med. 1985;145:1686–9.
159. Huang CL, Kuo E. Mechanism of hypokalemia in magnesium deficiency. J Am Soc Nephrol. 2007;18:2649–52.
160. Yang L, Frindt G, Palmer LG. Magnesium modulates ROMK channel-mediated potassium secretion. J Am Soc Nephrol. 2010;21:2109–16.
161. Whang R, Whang DD, Ryan MP. Refractory potassium repletion. A consequence of magnesium deficiency. Arch Intern Med. 1992;152:40–5.
162. Vandenberg CA. Inward rectification of a potassium channel in cardiac ventricular cells depends on internal magnesium ions. Proc Natl Acad Sci U S A. 1987;84:2560–4.
163. Abbott LG, Rude RK. Clinical manifestations of magnesium deficiency. Miner Electrolyte Metab. 1993;19:314–22.
164. Whang R, Ryder KW. Frequency of hypomagnesemia and hypermagnesemia. Requested vs routine. JAMA. 1990;263:3063–4.
165. Hoorn EJ, van der Hoek J, de Man RA, Kuipers EJ, Bolwerk C, Zietse R. A case series of proton pump inhibitor-induced hypomagnesemia. Am J Kidney Dis. 2010;56:112–6.
166. Scoble JE, Screaton GR, Havard CW. Renal magnesium wasting in Bartter's syndrome. Nephrol Dial Transplant. 1990;5:388–90.
167. Bockenhauer D, Feather S, Stanescu HC, et al. Epilepsy, ataxia, sensorineural deafness, tubulopathy, and KCNJ10 mutations. N Engl J Med. 2009;360:1960–70.
168. Scholl UI, Choi M, Liu T, et al. Seizures, sensorineural deafness, ataxia, mental retardation, and electrolyte imbalance (SeSAME syndrome) caused by mutations in KCNJ10. Proc Natl Acad Sci U S A. 2009;106:5842–7.
169. Meij IC, Koenderink JB, van Bokhoven H, et al. Dominant isolated renal magnesium loss is caused by misrouting of the Na(+), K(+)-ATPase gamma-subunit. Nat Genet. 2000;26:265–6.
170. Glaudemans B, van der Wijst J, Scola RH, et al. A missense mutation in the Kv1.1 voltage-gated potassium channel-encoding gene KCNA1 is linked to human autosomal dominant hypomagnesemia. J Clin Invest. 2009;119:936–42.
171. Wilson FH, Hariri A, Farhi A, et al. A cluster of metabolic defects caused by mutation in a mitochondrial tRNA. Science. 2004;306:1190–4.
172. Ryan MP. Diuretics and potassium/magnesium depletion. Directions for treatment. Am J Med. 1987;82:38–47.
173. Ryan MP. Magnesium and potassium-sparing diuretics. Magnesium. 1986;5:282–92.
174. Shah GM, Kirschenbaum MA. Renal magnesium wasting associated with therapeutic agents. Miner Electrolyte Metab. 1991;17:58–64.
175. Craven JL. Cyclosporine-associated organic mental disorders in liver transplant recipients. Psychosomatics. 1991;32:94–102.
176. Chang CT, Hung CC, Tian YC, Yang CW, Wu MS. Cyclosporin reduces paracellin-1 expression and magnesium transport in thick ascending limb cells. Nephrol Dial Transplant. 2007;22:1033–40.
177. Ikari A, Okude C, Sawada H, Takahashi T, Sugatani J, Miwa M. Down-regulation of TRPM6-mediated magnesium influx by cyclosporin A. Naunyn Schmiedebergs Arch Pharmacol. 2008;377:333–43.
178. Brock PR, Koliouskas DE, Barratt TM, Yeomans E, Pritchard J. Partial reversibility of cisplatin nephrotoxicity in children. J Pediatr. 1991;118:531–4.
179. Markmann M, Rothman R, Reichman B, et al. Persistent hypomagnesemia following cisplatin chemotherapy in patients with ovarian cancer. J Cancer Res Clin Oncol. 1991;117:89–90.
180. Panichpisal K, Angulo-Pernett F, Selhi S, Nugent KM. Gitelman-like syndrome after cisplatin therapy: a case report and literature review. BMC Nephrol. 2006;7:10.
181. Palestine AG, Polis MA, De Smet MD, et al. A randomized, controlled trial of foscarnet in the treatment of cytomegalovirus retinitis in patients with AIDS. Ann Intern Med. 1991;115:665–73.
182. Mercan D, Bastin G, Lambermont M, Dupont E. Importance of ionized magnesium measurement for monitoring of citrate-anticoagulated plateletpheresis. Transfusion. 1997;37:418–22.
183. Aglio LS, Stanford GG, Maddi R, Boyd 3rd JL, Nussbaum S, Chernow B. Hypomagnesemia is common following cardiac surgery. J Cardiothorac Vasc Anesth. 1991;5:201–8.
184. Robertie PG, Butterworth 4th JF, Royster RL, et al. Normal parathyroid hormone responses to hypocalcemia during cardiopulmonary bypass. Anesthesiology. 1991;75:43–8.
185. Mimouni F, Miodovnik M, Tsang RC, Holroyde J, Dignan PS, Siddiqi TA. Decreased maternal serum magnesium concentration and adverse fetal outcome in insulin-dependent diabetic women. Obstet Gynecol. 1987;70:85–8.
186. McNair P, Christensen MS, Christiansen C, Madsbad S, Transbol I. Renal hypomagnesaemia in human diabetes mellitus: its relation to glucose homeostasis. Eur J Clin Invest. 1982;12:81–5.
187. Ryan MP, Ryan MF, Counihan TB. The effect of diuretics on lymphocyte magnesium and potassium. Acta Med Scand Suppl. 1981;647:153–61.
188. Gao X, Peng L, Adhikari CM, Lin J, Zuo Z. Spironolactone reduced arrhythmia and maintained magnesium homeostasis in patients with congestive heart failure. J Card Fail. 2007;13:170–7.
189. Colussi G, Rombola G, De Ferrari ME, Macaluso M, Minetti L. Correction of hypokalemia with antialdosterone therapy in Gitelman's syndrome. Am J Nephrol. 1994;14:127–35.

Management of Fluid and Electrolyte Abnormalities in Children

5

John T. Herrin

Correction of fluid and electrolyte abnormalities is based on the anatomy of fluid spaces, rate of water turnover, and a knowledge of the composition of common losses. In childhood, fluid spaces as a proportion of body weight, water turnover rates, surface area–mass ratio, renal function, and "skin physiology" (water loss varies with thickness and the nature of skin) differ as a function of age [1]. Integration of growth rate with continuing maturation in renal, hormonal, and gastrointestinal function allows homeostasis to be maintained as children develop. GFR is 15 ml/min/1.73m^2 at birth and reaches 120 ml/min/1.73 m^2 by age 2 years, a time when growth rate falls significantly. Concentrating ability is limited in the younger infant at a time when growth is most rapid and sodium, potassium, and phosphate are being included in new cells so that surfeit requiring excretion is limited. Concentrating ability subsequently increases with exposure to higher solute as growth rate decreases.

The aim of fluid therapy is to maintain normal volume and composition of body fluids and correct existing abnormalities. Repletion therapy replaces current existing water electrolyte deficits, to return the patient to normal volume electrolyte status. The tradition of fluid therapy in pediatrics has been based on a deficit therapy approach, administering maintenance needs plus past and ongoing losses, this "Holliday–Segar" regime [2] has for many years been the standard to minimize complications and improve clinical outcome. Recent reassessment [3] has come to appreciate these elaborate guidelines are often unnecessary and may be counterproductive [4]. Rapid ECF volume repletion in shock improves patient outcomes [3, 5, 6]. Such a scheme sets priority for restoration of circulation and reestablishing ECF to establish urine flow.

Rapid IV rehydration and the use of the standard oral replacement solutions (ORT) for rehydration and maintenance hydration fluids is a simple, safe and efficacious alternative route for most children in the setting of a dehydrating gastroenteritis [3]. The need for more precise assessment in the prescription of fluid and electrolyte therapy is necessary especially in children with nondiarrheal illness, with more complex disorders of fluid and electrolyte pathophysiology, e.g., perioperatively, in critically ill children with sepsis, burns, trauma, or in the malnourished child where an understanding of the distribution of body fluids, usual fluid and electrolyte requirements and homeostatic balance secondary to decreased effect of circulation, renal and hormonal response remains vital to the fluid prescription in the initial therapy and proper assessment of clinical response [5, 6]. This is particularly important in the child with endocrine or renal disease where normal renal homeostatic

J.T. Herrin, M.B.B.S., F.R.A.C.P. (✉)
Division of Nephrology, Department of Medicine,
Children's Hospital, 300 Longwood Avenue,
Boston, MA 02115, USA
e-mail: john.herrin@childrens.harvard.edu

D.B. Mount et al. (eds.), *Core Concepts in the Disorders of Fluid, Electrolytes and Acid-Base Balance*,
DOI 10.1007/978-1-4614-3770-3_5, © Springer Science+Business Media New York 2013

mechanisms, volume, and electrolyte regulation are already deranged.

The following discussion addresses hydration and maintenance fluid therapy, and an approach to common electrolyte abnormalities in childhood. Safe correction of such abnormalities requires adequate circulation and appropriate monitoring of blood pressure, pulse, respiration, weight change, urinary flow, and evaluation of blood and urinary chemistry profiles to evaluate response.

In order to initiate prompt management in severe depletion or shock central access is important, to allow volume replacement and obtain blood samples for appropriate laboratory studies. Two IV lines or one large IV line and an intraosseus line may be necessary in younger children [7]. Screening tests include electrolyte profile, glucose, ketones, blood urea nitrogen, creatinine, pH, pCO_2, bicarbonate, calcium, complete blood count, with differential white blood cell count. Ammonia and lactate levels should also be obtained if the etiology is not clear in the young infant or neonate where inborn errors of metabolism require consideration. Blood culture and other cultures are obtained as indicated.

Volume depletion sufficient to reduce effective circulating blood volume will lead to decreased tissue and organ perfusion and shock [7]. Shock may follow as a result of acute blood loss (hemorrhagic hypovolemic shock) [7]; gastroenteral losses from diarrhea, vomiting, or intestinal obstruction; renal losses such as sodium wasting disorders, diuretic therapy, or tubular diseases; from skin or respiratory losses in hyperthermia, hyperventilation, excess sweating, or skin damage such as burns [8, 9]; and in the extreme premature infant or from sequestration of fluid in "third space" losses [8]. Symptoms vary with the degree and type of volume depletion and the electrolyte and acid–base disorders produced. Rapid volume repletion is indicated in all patients with severe hypovolemia or hypovolemic shock and leads to improved outcome [3].

Nonhemorrhagic hypovolemic shock is the leading cause of morbidity and mortality in children who present in shock [7]. Rapid volume expansion along with supportive care including airway management and administration of 100 % oxygen and endotracheal intubation and assisted ventilation if necessary is the most appropriate initial therapy in all patients. Vasopressor medications do not have a place in the initial treatment of nonhemorrhagic hypovolemic shock; however, pressor dopamine, dobutamine, or epinephrine may be helpful in rare cases where response to large volume resuscitation is inadequate or decompensated shock ensues. An approach to acute resuscitation is outlined in Table 5.1.

Fluid and electrolyte therapy may be administered by intravenous infusion, nasogastric or jejunal tube, or provided orally in liquid or solid form. The route is determined by the size of the deficit, the status of circulation, urinary flow, gastrointestinal absorption capacity and renal function.

Table 5.1 Acute fluid management and resuscitation

1. If possible weigh the patient on admission prior to repletion.
2. If shock is present or if no urine is produced in the first 30 min: (a) Administer lactated Ringer solution, normal saline or 5 % albumin IV as a bolus. (b) Repeat bolus if adequate circulation is not established. (c) Some children require 60–100 ml/kg restore circulation. (d) Central venous monitoring may be required if circulation is not reestablished.
3. After the first 1 h continue isotonic crystalloid solution until: (a) Circulation and urine flow are established. (b) Calculate actual fluid and electrolyte deficits and rate.
4. If the patient is asymptomatic and/or dehydration is hyponatremic or isotonic: (a) Administer 50 % of the fluids calculated for 24 h over 8 h. (b) Administer remaining 50 % in next 16 h.
5. Hypertonic dehydration with shock: (a) Reestablish circulation and urine flow. (b) Next correct the remaining deficit slowly and evenly over 48 h.
6. Symptomatic Hyponatremia is an emergency: (a) Use 3 % saline until symptoms controlled.
7. Adequacy of therapy is indicated by: (a) Increase urine output (b) Normal circulation (c) Restoration of weight

Table 5.2 Fluid and electrolyte conditions in childhood

(A) Fluid imbalance	
Dehydration	Hyperosmolar states
Water intoxication	Hyposmolar states
(B) Electrolyte abnormalities	
Hyponatremia	Hypocalcemia
Hypernatremia	Hypercalcemia
Hypokalemia	Hypomagnesemia
Hyperkalemia	Hypermagnesemia
(C) Acid–base abnormalities	
(D) Metabolic disorders/inborn errors	
Disorders carbohydrate	Disorders of amino acid
Hyperglycemia	metabolism
Hypoglycemia	Urea cycle
Diabetic ketoacidosis	Abnormalities
Galactosemia	
(E) Emergencies	
Hypernatremia	Refeeding syndromes
Symptomatic	Drug effects
hyponatremia	Iatrogenic

In intravenous administration consideration must be given to osmolality of the solution, solute load, and rate of administration [10]. Although there are theoretical advantages to the use of colloid there is little objective evidence from trials or meta-analysis in adults to demonstrate these theoretical benefits in fact occur [11, 12]. Trial data in high-risk neonates suggest a probable benefit in high-risk neonates [13]. The pediatric task force on shock recommends the use of crystalloid for expansion [13]. Intravenous fluids are preferred in patients with unstable circulation, moderate hypovolemia, or patients who have hypo- or hypernatremia [13] or are unable to tolerate oral replacement therapy. The choice of peripheral versus central administration and calculation of an appropriate rate is based on the rate and type of solution required. Oral administration acceptance depends on taste and palatability, gastrointestinal absorption capacity, and the availability of a capable caretaker, since this is labor-intensive.

A classification of fluid and electrolyte abnormalities is outlined in Table 5.2 to demonstrate the range of common fluid and electrolyte abnormalities in children. A short review of physiology of normal fluid and electrolyte balance in childhood is provided to assist in understanding the differences in the therapy between childhood and adult [2, 10].

Maintenance Fluid Requirements

Fluid is continually lost from the body through the skin, lungs (insensible), feces, and urine, producing a constant "maintenance fluid" requirement equal to the amount of fluid of these losses and in childhood to provide water for growth. Actual maintenance requirements may vary considerably from the usual estimations (Table 5.3). Standard calculation assumes that the patient has a normal urinary output and renal function, and that the body temperature is within the range of 98–99 °F, with at least basal calorie food intake at environmental temperature and humidity are within temperate range. A number of methods for estimating average maintenance fluid requirements exist:

- Maintenance calculation fluid based on surface area: in infants weighing >10 kg renal function and body fluid requirements correlate best with body surface area (BSA). ECF volume is proportional to BSA in square meter (m^2), and water needs are expressed as ml/m^2/24 h. This system has the advantage that a single formula can be used for all ages. The normal water requirement is approximately 1,500 ml/m^2/24 h [2, 14].
- Maintenance fluid requirement calculated on the basis of calories expended. 100–150 ml fluid/100 cal metabolized is provided. This calculation is best suited to situations where caloric intake is limited.
- A common pediatric method which is simple to remember and calculate is based on body weight providing 100 ml/kg for the first 10 kg body weight; 50 ml/kg for the next 10 kg body weight; and 20 ml/kg for the weights above 20 kg [2, 14].

Maintenance fluid in the neonatal period is adjusted for gestational age, and the expected physiological contraction of extracellular fluid which occurs over the first few days before homeostasis becomes established (see *Neonatal Period in Special Conditions in Childhood*) [15–18]. Term infants lose approximately 5–10 % of birth weight, and premature infants as much as 15–20 % of birth weight (additional losses from

Table 5.3 Maintenance requirement and adjustments

Maintenance requirement	Increased requirement	Decreased requirement
Water		
Normal losses ml/m^2/24 h	Increased metabolic rate	Decreased metabolic rate
Respiratory and skin 775	Fever	Antidiuresis
(Insensible)	Tachypnea	Postoperative
Gastrointestinal 100	Increased solute loads	Nausea and vomiting
Urine 875	Glycosuria, ketoacidosis	Head injury
Water gained	Protein from catabolism	SIADH
Water oxidation 250	Trauma/burns	Positive pressure respiration
Net 1,500 ml/m^2/24 h	Increased water loss	Renal failure
	Diabetes insipidus	Oligoanuria
	Renal concentrating defect	Humidified air
	Skin—premature infant	
	Nursed on warming table	
Sodium		
Calculation based on:	Increased losses	Cardiac failure
BSA 20–50 mEq/m^2/24 h	Gastrointestinal loss	Renal failure
Body Wt 2–4 mEq/100 ml	Renal sodium wasting	
Calorie Provided 2–4 mEq/100 cal	Skin immaturity/damage	
Potassium		
Calculation based on:	Increased losses	Postoperative
BSA 20–50 mEq/m^2/24 h	Gastrointestinal	Catabolic states
Body Wt 2–3 mEq/100 m	Renal—tubulopathies	Prematurity day 2–3
Calorie provided 2–4 mEq/100 cal	Diuretic therapy	Renal failure
Calories for maintenance		
<10 kg 100 cal/kg	Fever	Environmental
10–20 kg 75–100 cal/kg	Stress	
>20 kg 65–75 cal/kg	Environmental	

Data from [10]

the skin 150—200 ml/kg/day in infants less than 28 weeks gestation, mainly with skin loss inversely proportional to gestational age) [15, 17, 18]. Neonates excrete less urine in the first 24–48 h of life [16, 18]. An output of less than 0.5 ml/kg/h suggests oliguria and requires assessment of urine SG, or Osm together with concurrent solute load, adequacy of hydration, and effective circulating volume. Although variation in urine flow rate (output) reflects both circulatory status and adequacy of hydration, urine output cannot be used to estimate renal function. Urine volume varies with intake, approximately 50 ml/kg/24 h is typical for the normal child [16]. Continuation of urinary output with isotonic or dilute urine in the presence of severe diarrhea suggests a polyuric state associated with intrinsic renal disease or hormonal abnormality (e.g., diabetes insipidus) [10, 16].

In younger infants it is important to consider the potential contribution of the renal solute load of the intake as well as loss from diarrhea or vomiting in producing a negative fluid balance [19]. Increased renal solute load may aggravate dehydration by causing obligatory urinary free-water loss in the infant who is already struggling to excrete an ingested solute load. The renal solute load (electrolyte and nitrogen for excretion) of a given feeding is different from the formula's measured osmotic load (which includes sugar and fat that are metabolized to CO_2 and water, in addition to electrolyte and nitrogen which require excretion) [19]. A clinical estimate of renal solute load of a formula may be based on nitrogen, sodium, potassium and chloride (1 g protein yields 4 mOsm, while sodium, potassium, and chloride yield 1 mOsm/1 mEq) [19, 20]. This calculation is appropriate if renal solute load is relatively high. In the presence of fever increased extrarenal water loss or increasing concentration of feedings to greater than 100 kcal/100 ml leads to a risk for negative fluid balance [19]. Infants cannot effectively concentrate urine much beyond 600 mOsm/kg [19, 20], so that cow's milk causes free-water losses three times greater than those of human milk, while boiled skim milk imposes a fourfold free-water loss. To avoid hypertonic dehydration, renal solute load should be minimized in infants with fluid losses and low solute feeding used in infants with a renal concentrating defect [19, 20].

Assessment of the Dehydrated Child

Initial Assessment

In the dehydrated child the initial assessment should include the following:

- History of urine output, weight change, infectious disease contacts, and an estimate of frequency of stooling or vomiting.
- Clinical and laboratory assessment of urine output, skin turgor, state of mucous membrane moisture, eye turgor, fullness of fontanel, and mental state; measurement of weight, complete blood count (CBC), serum and urine Na^+, K^+, Cl^-, pH, TCO_2, blood urea nitrogen (BUN), creatinine, osmolality, glucose, and calcium; urinalysis and appropriate cultures.

The urinary SG in dehydrated patients will be above 1.015 unless intrinsic renal disease is present. Ketonuria often accompanies dehydration without diabetes and trace or 1+ protein can be present, along with cellular debris and a few hyaline casts. A more active urine sediment signals underlying primary renal disease. Alkaline urine or with an increased urinary anion gap during dehydration should raise the question of renal tubular acidosis.

Estimates of deficits of water, sodium, and potassium in moderate to severe dehydration are available [10], and a recently developed clinical dehydration scale [21] for use in children less than 3 years of age allows clinical correlations between dehydration and general appearance, appearance based on the eyes, mucous membranes, and presence/absence of tears. This assessment is outlined in Table 5.4.

Assessment of Sodium and Potassium Losses

There is no practical means of assessing true K^+ loss; serum K^+ does not accurately reflect total body K^+ stores [10, 22]. However, one can assume in most instances that K^+ losses are equivalent to Na^+ losses [22, 23]. Estimation of Na^+ and K^+ deficits in a child with severe dehydration and in whom the serum Na^+ is known can be calculated from Na^+ deficit based on the current serum Na^+ concentration (dehydrated), the desired "normal" serum Na^+ concentration (usually 135 mEq/l), and the volume of distribution of Na^+, in total body water (TBW). The total body Na^+ deficit ($TBNa_d^+$) is the difference between the normal total body Na^+ ($TBNa_n^+$) and the current (dehydrated) total body Na^+ ($TBNa_c^+$), $TBNa_d^+ = TBNa_n^+ - TBNa_c^+$ [10]. The assumption on which the calculations are based is that Na^+ is the sole cation used for rehydration. This is a reasonable assumption, since rehydration preferentially should preserve the ECF (and thus the vascular space) over the ICF. In practice, the calculations actually provide for the deficit of total cations (Na^+ and K^+), which should be remembered when both Na^+ and K^+ are provided in the solutions used for rehydration.

Ongoing Losses

Loss of fluids and/or electrolytes while the patient is under observation may be continuous or sporadic. Although variation in renal output can accommodate small ongoing losses, optimal management dictates that larger losses be replaced in an orderly fashion.

Estimation of Ongoing Losses

Abnormal losses (nasogastric suction, surgical drainage, fistula drainage, vomitus) can be measured directly and may need sequential replacement each 1–6 h, particularly if there are

Table 5.4 Clinical estimates of dehydration

Clinical	Mild	Moderate	Severe	Special features
WT loss	3–5 %	6–9 %	10–15 %	
General appearance	N	Sunken eyes	Drawn with sunken eyes	Anxiety—restless
Behavior	N	Irritable	Lethargic Hyperirritable	Hyponatremia lethargic Seizures if extreme Hypernatremia shrill Mewling cry
Eyes tears Tension	N or decreased	Decreased	Absent	
Mucus membranes	N	Dry	Parched	Exaggerated appearance in hyponatremia
Thirst	Low	Moderate	Intense	Hyponatremia Intense early
Skin turgor Touch	N N	Tenting Dry	Absent Clammy or cold	Hyponatremia obvious decrease Doughy hypernatremia
Pulse	Regular	Increased	Very rapid	Thready or difficult to assess before shock
Urine flow	N	Reduced	Oliguria	Sg >1,015 unless concentrating defect
Anterior fontanelle Baby	Flat	Decreased	Sunken	

Data from [3, 10, 17]

Table 5.5 Composition of common body fluid for replacement

Fluid source	Na	K	Cl	HCO_3	pH	Osm
Gastric	50	10–15	150	O	1	300
Ileostomy	130	15–20	120	25–30	8	300
Diarrhea	50	35	40	50	7+	
Sweat	50	5	55	0		
Blood	140	4–5	100	25	7.4	285–290
Urine	0–100	20–100	70–100	0–5	4.5–8.5	50–1200

Electrolyte content expressed in mmol/l and osmolality as mOsm/l

significant volume losses or the losses from multiple sites with differing composition (urine, gastric, intestinal fistulae). In the absence of direct measurement, change in body weight can be used as a surrogate for the volume of fluid losses and estimates of electrolyte loss made from standard tables of concentration of common losses [10], replaced evenly over an equivalent period of time (Table 5.5). Large ongoing losses may require more frequent replacement (each 0.5–1 h), while smaller volume losses may be replaced daily. When providing replacement for large or unusual ongoing losses, periodic monitoring and reassessment of the patient's condition is necessary. Daily changes in weight are the best indicator of short-term (24–48 h) quantitative fluid loss and reflect changes in water and salt balance rather than caloric balance. Patients receiving maintenance fluids and calories should remain at a constant weight while insufficient calories are associated with loss of approximately 0.5 % body weight per day from loss of body fat stores metabolized to H_2O and other by-products.

General Principles of Repletion Therapy in Childhood

General principles have been outlined in numerous reviews [10, 14, 24]. Because loss is mainly

ECF, replacement therapy can advance rapidly, with volume and Na^+ restored by the end of 24–36 h. Estimates of losses developing in less than 3 days are 75–100 % from the ECF; if losses occur over a longer duration, combination losses are more frequent; losses 3–7 days are approx. 60–75 % ECF, and by 1 week ECF and ICF losses are approximately equal. Calculated or estimated total deficits of fluid and electrolytes are added to the maintenance requirement, after subtracting the amount provided during the initial resuscitation period from the total estimate. The remaining deficit and maintenance volume is provided over the first day. Deficit therapy is less effective than rapid rehydration [3, 4]; patients with gastroenteritis should receive rapid rehydration and ORT. If the patient is asymptomatic and dehydration is hypotonic or isotonic, one half of the remaining deficit together with maintenance fluids and electrolytes should be administered in the next 8 h and the remainder over the subsequent 16 h.

The strategy for replacing ongoing losses differs depending upon whether there is a deficit present at the initiation of therapy and the volume of ongoing loss. Patients without deficits at the initiation of therapy should be provided with maintenance fluid plus fluid and electrolytes and electrolytes and to replace the ongoing losses. If there are unusual urine losses or erratic urine output, therapy is designed to provide maintenance fluid equal to insensible fluid losses plus replacement of measured urine output and ongoing losses (400 $ml/m^2/24$ h plus measured urine output) [10]. Patients who are dehydrated at the initiation of therapy (as a result of vomiting or diarrhea) should have the measured or estimated volume of ongoing losses added to the calculated replacement fluid for maintenance and deficit. Adjustments to estimated losses should be made frequently, as more accurate data becomes available from actual measurement. Urine volume output is omitted from this calculation, since it is accounted for in the maintenance calculation. It is also important not to recalculate the overall deficits once rehydration of a dehydrated patient with ongoing losses has commenced, as this leads to an underestimation of true deficits.

Monitoring Fluid and Electrolyte Therapy

Periodic assessment is required, since the fluid and electrolytes provided to cover maintenance needs together with replacement of prior deficits and ongoing losses is based on a series of estimates and calculations. Adjustment to therapy is made based on response measured by monitoring circulation, urine flow, and chemical profile.

Clinical Assessment of Adequate Expansion

Expansion and stabilization of extracellular fluid (and vascular volume) results in increasing or stable weight, improvement in vital signs, increased blood pressure and central venous pressure, decreased pulse rate and respiratory rate, increased urinary output with decreasing urine specific gravity and osmolality, and increased sodium excretion [10]. Laboratory profile shows a decreasing hematocrit (in the absence of blood loss) together with a parallel fall in serum total protein concentration, and improvement in degree of metabolic acidosis with improved peripheral perfusion, decreasing BUN, creatinine, serum osmolality, and serum potassium.

Principles of acute fluid resuscitation as outlined in Table 5.1 are modified in the patient with diabetic ketoacidosis, where K^+ can be added to the initial solution (with careful monitoring), since rapid correction of dehydration, acidosis, and hyperglycemia may precipitate severe hypoglycemia and hypokalemia.

Correction of Abnormalities of Hydration

Gastroenteritis is the commonest cause of dehydration in childhood. Compared to adults, the greater insensible loss and increased daily water turnover decreases fluid reserve, such that reduced intake or mild increases in loss alone will lead to dehydration. In gastroenteritis rapid rehydration leads to increased gut perfusion and allows earlier return to feeding and increase in renal perfusion, with correction of fluid, electrolyte, and acid–base abnormalities (often without need for more specific therapy) with decreasing morbidity and mortality [24]. The intestine has a remarkable capacity to secrete or absorb water passively. The normal osmotic gradient is dictated by sodium transport via a sodium/hydrogen exchange, electrochemical gradient, and sodium coupled transport with glucose allowing potential for correction with ORT.

Rapid Rehydration Therapy

ECF restoration plays a major role in the therapy of most patients with dehydration. "Rapid rehydration" of ECF followed by maintenance treatment is safe and effective, and now considered the most appropriate treatment [24, 25]. Oral rehydration therapy may be initiated as soon as tolerated. For patients with mild dehydration, oral rehydration therapy (ORT) solution is administered to provide up to 5 ml/kg/h, containing 45–60 mEq/l of sodium over 12–24 h. In patients with moderate dehydration, oral rehydration therapy of 25–50 ml/kg is provided over 6–12 h. If IV rehydration is necessary for patients with severe dehydration (weight loss 10 % or greater), impaired circulation, evidence of interstitial fluid loss, 40 ml/kg lactated Ringer's solution or normal saline is given over 1–2 h, followed by ORT. If skin turgor, alertness, and pulse do not return to normal by the end of this infusion, one should infuse an additional bolus of 20–40 ml/kg over 1–2 h [25].

Rehydration Phase

Qualitatively, it is useful to separate dehydration states based on sodium and potassium loss in relation to the amount of water loss. The pathogenesis of abnormal plasma sodium concentrations allows rational diagnosis and treatment. Abnormal plasma sodium concentration results from abnormal water intake or output. In most cases hyponatremia is caused by inappropriate concentration of urine [26]. Determination of appropriateness of ADH secretion requires assessment of effective arterial volume and changing body weight. Hypernatremia follows impaired water intake or abnormal water loss, the site of which can be determined from urine osmolality. Hypernatremia is best treated by water replacement and measures to reduce abnormal water loss. The most appropriate route of delivery, oral or intravenous, and the type of replacement fluid depend on sodium status [13, 26].

In hypotonic dehydration fluid loss is from intravascular space and ECF compartments rather than the intracellular reservoir. Fall in ECF tonicity results in osmotic shifts to ICF which further depletes ECF leading to poor renal perfusion, oliguria, and decrease in renal regulation. Metabolic acidosis follows poor tissue perfusion, bicarbonate loss in the stool and with oliguria—renal retention of organic acids, chloride, sulfate, and phosphate anions. Circulatory compromise appears early, and dehydration is characterized by marked loss of skin turgor.

Causes of Hyponatremia

Hyponatremia is a result of differential sodium and water losses and is seen clinically with sodium loss in excess of water loss. Symptoms in hypopnatremia are nonspecific, and the rate of fall in serum sodium is as important as the absolute level of serum sodium in producing symptoms [10, 26]. Infants usually present soon after the onset of illness, since for a given weight loss, the clinical signs of dehydration are more marked in hypotonic dehydration than in isotonic or hypertonic dehydration [10]. Seizures occur infrequently, even with marked hyponatremia; however, generalized lethargy is common, and vascular collapse can occur early. Estimates of weight for mild, moderate, and severe dehydration from clinical signs are outlined in Table 5.4.

Therapy in Hyponatremia

The approach differs in hyponatremia depending on the following:

1. Volume status
   (a) Decreased extracellular fluid volume (ECF)
   (b) Increased ECF volume
   (c) Normal ECF volume [10, 13, 26]
2. The time hyponatremia has been present [26]

Factitious Causes

Pseudohyponatremia may occur with the following:

- Hyperlipidemia (if measured by flame photometer)
- Hyperosmolar hyponatremia secondary to hyperglycemia
- Use of osmotic agent, e.g., mannitol, must be distinguished from hypoosmolar hyponatremia and should be excluded

Hyponatremia with ECF Volume Depletion

This requires repletion with 0.9 % saline. Serum sodium less than 130 mmol/l follows net loss of salt from the following:

- Intestine (infantile diarrhea or intestinal obstruction)
- Urine (salt-losing renal disease, adrenal failure, or diabetic ketoacidosis)
- Sweat (hyperthermia or cystic fibrosis) particularly if the fluid loss is replaced with high volumes of low-solute fluids (e.g., fruit juice, "cola" soft drinks)

Very premature infants cannot conserve sodium, even if sodium balance is negative; hence, premature infants (<34 weeks gestation) receiving formula or breast milk without sodium supplementation can develop hyponatremia with minimal or no losses [27]. After 34 weeks gestation, renal sodium reabsorption becomes more efficient, and full-term neonates can retain sodium in the face of negative sodium balance. However, like premature infants they still exhibit limited ability to excrete sodium loads because of low GFR [27]. In addition to sodium loss from intestine, renal, or skin as in older children, specific predisposing factors in neonates include diuretic use, osmotic diuresis, and third space losses of extracellular fluid from skin damage, or necrotizing enterocolitis [16, 17]. Clinical signs in the neonate are similar to older children and adults with decrease in weight, poor skin turgor, tachycardia, and rising BUN and creatinine. Metabolic acidosis may occur if circulation is poor, with continuing diarrhea or renal bicarbonate loss; however, hypochloremic metabolic alkalosis may follow prolonged vomiting (pyloric stenosis, intestinal obstruction) or chronic diuretic use. Therapy in the newborn includes replacement of deficits and adjustment to match maintenance fluid plus ongoing losses. The type of fluid is dependent on the site of losses.

Hyponatremia with Normal Extracellular Volume

Hyponatremia with normal extracellular fluid volume occurs with excess fluid administration in the presence of inappropriate antidiuresis [26, 28] which may in childhood be associated with malignancy (lymphoma or cerebral), pulmonary disease (pneumonia, asthma, cystic fibrosis, positive pressure respiration), CNS disease such as infection or intracranial bleeding or drugs (anticonvulsants—carbamazepine; narcotics; vincristine; cyclophosphamide; NSAID; AVP analogs—desmopressin; "Ecstasy" 3, 4 methylenedioxy methamphetamine), gastrointestinal losses in inflammatory bowel disease, persistent nausea or vomiting or in neonates following intraventricular hemorrhage, and anoxia, sepsis, meningitis, pneumothorax, or positive pressure respiration [17, 26].

The diagnosis of SIADH rests on stable or increased weight with hyponatremia, euvolemia, a decreased serum Osm, and sometimes edema in younger infants or neonates. Oliguria is present with urine osmolality greater than 100 Osm/l; UNa>40 mEq/l (20 mEq/l in a neonate). Supplementary laboratory information includes a decreased BUN, creatinine, uric acid, with an increased urinary fractional excretion of sodium greater than 1 % and fractional excretion of urea greater than 55 % [23]. Low fractional excretion of sodium is more often present in infants with mature renal function than in adults [27]. The differential diagnosis includes cerebral salt wasting, a condition in which brain naturetic peptide is in excess and leads to proximal tubular sodium wasting [29]. The major differential feature is the fall weight in infants with cerebral salt wasting versus stable or gain in weight in SIADH. Clinical signs in cerebral salt wasting include evidence of decreased ECF volume. The therapeutic approach in SIADH is to treat the underlying disorder and restrict water intake to alleviate hypotonicity, while in patients with cerebral salt wasting salt repletion is required.

Therapy in Hyponatremia with Normal ECF Volume

In the child with asymptomatic hyponatremia there is no need to administer hypertonic saline based on laboratory anomalies alone. Rather free water should be restricted and maintenance sodium 2–3 mEq/kg/day plus replacement of ongoing sodium losses in addition to isotonic losses (135 mEq/l) calculated from present dehydration. If water restriction is not effective in correcting the defect or serum sodium concentration is below 120 mEq/l or neurological signs (lethargy or obtundation) are present, treatment should follow guidelines for furosemide administration and sodium replacement [30]. Sodium administration is discontinued if serum sodium rises at a greater rate than 10 mEq/24 h. Fluid restriction alone is preferred, once serum sodium concentration exceeds 120 mEq/l and neurological signs have cleared.

Hyponatremia with Extracellular Volume Excess

Hyponatremia due to extracellular fluid volume excess occurs in neonates and premature infants in the face of sepsis, decreased cardiac output, cardiac failure, necrotizing enterocolitis (NEC), or with fluid sequestration in areas of abnormal lymphatic drainage or neuromuscular paralysis. Decreased glomerular filtration and decreased tubular delivery of sodium and water follows the decreased effective circulating blood volume. Therapy includes sodium restriction together with measures to improve cardiac output in cardiac failure [10].

Hospital acquired hyponatremia is common, particularly if hypotonic fluid is used based on calculations for weight rather than energy expenditures. Most of the patients in reported series have had concurrent acute medical or surgical conditions, severe diarrhea, or elective surgery, and many had replacement with hypotonic fluid based on calculations for weight rather than for energy expenditure [3, 14]. An estimated 1.5 ml of water is generated for each 1 cal consumed. This generation of free water must also be considered in fluid balance and the variations in the expected maintenance (Table 5.3). It is necessary to reduced maintenance fluid appropriate to only cover the ongoing insensible loss and decreased urine volume loss. Delivery of otherwise hypotonic maintenance fluids indexed to body weight and not metabolic rate is an erroneous prescription delivering excess fluid [3, 14]. The average prescription under these circumstances should be reduced to approximately one half to one third volume "maintenance fluid" calculated under basal conditions. Other authors have argued for isotonic rather than hypotonic fluids should be given to children after surgery [31, 32]. Water restriction is still necessary to maintain balance particularly in the smaller infant; assessment of physiological need is the most important step in prevention of hyponatremia [14].

Treatment of Symptomatic Hyponatremia

Symptomatic hyponatremia is an emergency [30, 32]. Usually, the serum sodium must drop below 125 mmol/l to produce neurologic signs and symptoms, and serum sodium <115 mmol/l is associated with a substantial chance of grand mal seizures [30]. Symptomatic hyponatremia may be seen with a serum Na^+ concentration of 130 mEq/l or even above this level if the change in concentration has been sudden (e.g., ADH or

DDAVP treatment in a patient with diabetes insipidus). The patient's symptoms, the rate of development of symptoms, and the presence of volume deficit versus volume excess must be taken into account to determine the rate of correction of the serum Na^+ concentration [22, 30]. Regardless of the cause initial therapy is directed at raising the Na^+ concentration quickly, to control symptoms and then more slowly, correcting the remaining Na^+ deficit (correcting osmolar abnormalities). The primary problem in patients with symptomatic hyponatremia is cerebral edema; however, the risk of delayed therapy is greater than the risk of too rapid correction and osmotic demyelination [32, 33]. The rate of rise during the initial aggressive correction should not exceed a rise in serum sodium greater than 2 mEq/l/h in the first 3–4 h or until symptoms resolve. The initial goal is to raise serum sodium by 5 mEq/l over several hours [30]. In symptomatic patients 3 % NaCl (0.5 mEq/ml) prevents or terminates seizures with a usual initial dose of 5 ml/kg of 3 % NaCl given over 30 min to control seizures acutely.

Pontine myelinolysis is less of a risk in patients with hypotonic dehydration, where restoration of volume deficit leads to restoration of ECF and corrects the hyponatremia by inhibiting secretion of antidiuretic hormone. Patients who are in a state of hypotonic volume expansion, rather than volume depletion are at greater risk of pontine myelinolysis with correction of the serum sodium [3, 23].

In patients with serum sodium below 125 mEq/l, the aim is to avert vascular compromise and central nervous system damage. If the fall in serum sodium has been acute, hypertonic saline 3 % is administered, since it allows delivery of sodium with limited water. If the child with a known rapid measured fall is asymptomatic calculate the Na^+ deficit and provide hypertonic saline at a rate to deliver approximately 5 mEq/kg/h. However, if the duration or rate of fall in serum sodium is unknown and the patient is asymptomatic 3 % saline is not required and fluid restriction should be the initial therapy. If the patient is volume depleted 0.9 % saline expansion should be the first step. Otherwise, 0.9 % saline is given in place of (hypotonic) maintenance fluid and furosemide and given if the serum sodium does not rise steadily by 0.5–2 mEq/l/h. Total correction is not necessary and may induce symptomatic circulatory overload. Much of the sodium administered as 3 % saline is rapidly excreted in the urine so that the beneficial effect may be transient and hence the need for monitoring.

The therapy of asymptomatic hyponatremia should include testing to define etiology after gradual correction of the Na^+ deficit in increments of 10 mEq/l has commenced [32, 33]. Calculation of the sodium deficit is based on total body Na^+, e.g., $TBNa_d^+ = TBNa_n^+ - TBNa_c^+ = (Na_n^+ \times TBW) - [(TBW - FL) \times Na_c^+]$ where Na_d^+ = sodium deficit, Na_n^+ = normal sodium concentration, Na_c^+ = present measured sodium concentration, TBW equals total body water, FL equal fluid losses (weight change). Alternative approaches include calculation based on response to sodium chloride therapy which, although more accurate, adds a significant degree of complexity [26, 30].

Maintenance Na^+ is required in addition to the calculated sodium deficit. The volume and type of solution is then determined to deliver the calculated sodium load. It is important to note that K^+ deficit and acidosis both require specific therapy to allow for correction of the hyponatremia [10]. Hemoconcentration and prerenal azotemia will resolve with restoration of fluid status.

Isotonic Dehydration

Children with enteric losses, taking an intermediate solute load (e.g., breast milk, formula), arrive at a balanced dehydration where the net fluid loss is isotonic thus the deficit is represented by ECF loss. For a given weight loss, symptoms will be less dramatic clinically than in hypotonic dehydration. One can assume a weight loss of 5, 10, or 15 % for clinical estimation of mild, moderate, and severe dehydration, respectively (see Table 5.4).

Acute therapy in isotonic dehydration may be either rapid rehydration followed by ORT or deficit therapy. However, rapid rehydration therapy is the treatment of choice [3].

Hypertonic Dehydration

Hypertonic dehydration results from inappropriately high solute loads given as replacement fluid, or in the presence of a renal concentrating defect producing a large free-water loss. In infants this may follow treatment with a high solute load fluid (boiled skim milk or chicken broth) to replace bowel losses [19]. Although hypernatremia is the commonest hypertonic state, solutes such as glucose, urea, and mannitol can also produce a similar hypertonic disturbance clinically [34]. Even some children receiving low solute fluid replacement Pedialyte(R) may become hypertonic; the reason for this apparent paradox is unclear, although it is most likely related to the relative solute load and obligatory water loss producing a relative disparity between water loss and sodium loss.

Increasing ECF tonicity resulting from a hypertonic state produces movement of water out of the cell to the vascular space preserving circulation despite advancing dehydration [10, 35]. Intracellular dehydration of the brain can lead to permanent damage from cell volume changes [35], cerebral sinus thrombosis or hemorrhage from tearing of intracranial bridging vessels [36]. These children present with a clinical picture of neuromuscular and central nervous symptoms with substantial mortality [36]. Clinical signs of dehydration in infants with hypertonic dehydration can be deceptive. Skin turgor does not exhibit the usual tenting of advanced dehydration, but has a thick "doughy" consistency. Eyeball turgor, however, is decreased as in other dehydration states. Other findings include a shrill cry, or "mewling" sound, muscle weakness, tachypnea, and intense thirst in toddlers [36], and in infants hyperglycemia is present in 50 % of the patients, and calcium deficiency has been noted in 10 % with hypertonic dehydration [36].

Therapy of Hypernatremic Disorders

Therapy of hypernatremic disorders is best based on volume status—normal, decreased, or excess extracellular fluid volume [31, 32].

Hypernatremia with Decreased ECF Volume

Causes of this combination include the following:

- Increased insensible water loss from skin in very low birthweight infants
- ADH deficiency secondary to intraventricular hemorrhage
- Renal tubular insensitivity, e.g., nephrogenetic diabetes insipidus, hypercalcemia, or hypokalemia; renal immaturity, renal dysplasia, or after relief of obstruction may lead to water loss greater than sodium loss with consequent hypernatremia

Despite clinical dehydration the urine remains dilute in immature neonates [15–17]. Treatment aims at restoring circulation and subsequently increasing free water administration, effecting a slow but steady decrease in serum sodium. A more rapid rate of decrease in serum sodium approximately 1 mEq/kg/h in the small neonate is tolerated since hypernatremia results from water loss in excess of sodium loss, rather than excess total body sodium. The frequent monitoring in neonates allows early diagnosis so that the time that hypertonicity is present is short [15, 18, 37].

Hypernatremia with ECF Volume Excess

Causes of this combination include the following:

- Excess isotonic or hypertonic fluid administration in the presence of reduced cardiac output
- Excessive delivery of sodium as hypertonic sodium bicarbonate therapy for correction of acidosis or
- Errors in formula preparation in the neonatal period

Diagnostic features include weight gain with the edema. The infant may show significant neurological abnormalities including marked irritability, seizures, or coma, in addition to signs of fluid overload or edema. Therapy in this group includes correction of causative factors and sodium restriction. If the serum sodium levels are very high, furosemide 1 mg/kg may be the used and water losses replaced to produce a total body sodium deficit [34]. Dialysis may be necessary in cases of marked sodium overload with hypernatremia (salt poisoning), and sodium modeling may be helpful in controlling the rate of correction [38, 39]

General Principles of Treatment for Hypernatremia

The total fluid deficit should be replaced slowly over 48 h or more, aiming at a decrease in serum sodium by 10 mmol/l/day (<0.5 mmol/l/h) [10, 34]. Rapid correction may lead to cerebral (and sometimes pulmonary) edema. Excretion of sodium may be enhanced using a loop diuretic to augment urine sodium losses, with concurrent replacement of all the volume of urine output as free water.

If the patient has significant renal or cardiac compromise because of electrolyte imbalance, dialysis and ultrafiltration may be necessary [38, 39].

Guidelines to Therapy in Hypernatremia

- In the first 1 h: If shock is present restore circulation (Table 5.1). When circulation and urine flow has been reestablished this allows steady and controlled correction of the fluid deficit to be repleted at a slower, steady rate. In the initial phase lactated Ringer solution may be advantageous in reducing the chloride load in favor of lactate.
- Over the next 4 h aim at steadily reducing the serum Na^+ and serum osmolality. There is no universally accepted best regime. The rate and route of IV infusion is determined by the tonicity of the solution. Continue to infuse 10 ml/kg/h of 5 % dextrose in Ringer's lactate, Ringer's lactate, or a mixture of 2.5 % dextrose and 0.45 % saline to which is added 40 mEq/l. sodium bicarbonate of this time depending on the degree of acidosis and hyperglycemia. Adjust for measured rate of change in sodium to maintain a decrease at approximately 0.5 mEq/l/h.
- Potassium is added to the infusion as soon as there is an established urine flow.
- The next 48 h are utilized to replenish the fluid deficit (based on calculation) together with measured ongoing losses at a steady rate to minimize acute osmotic shifts [10, 35]. Should the serum sodium level fall at more than 0.5 mEq/l/h the intravenous infusion rate should be decreased. Should the serum sodium not continue to decrease at a steady rate ongoing losses are reviewed to be sure that replacement is adequate, and consideration of treatment with furosemide/free water replacement is given to produce an appropriate sodium deficit [34].
- Calculation of water deficit: provides a guide for necessary free water replacement Water deficit (liters) = usual body water − current body water. Unlike adults, children with hypernatremic dehydration are usually not significantly deficient in Na^+ but rather water depleted. Correction of the water deficit using sodium containing solutions may lead to severe Na^+ overload and possibly to an increased serum Na^+ concentration. It is unwise to attempt rapid control of hyperglycemia is present, as slower glucose metabolism provides a continuous source of free water delivered at a relatively constant rate and allows necessary ion shifts to occur as reequilibration proceeds.

Treatment of Acute Salt Excess with Hypernatremia

Patients presenting with serum $Na^+ \geq 160$ mEq/l and urine $Na^+ \geq 100$ mEq/l, after restoration of circulation, require consideration of dialysis or furosemide diuresis (1 mg/kg) with urine volume output replaced using 10 % dextrose in water solution each hour, monitoring Na^+ values every 4 h and repeating the administration of furosemide if urine output is not sustained [34, 40]. If the serum Na^+ concentration remains >180 mEq/l after circulation is reestablished, dialysis is usually necessary for correction [39]. In this case, peritoneal dialysis for slow correction using sodium modified dialysis fluid or hemodialysis with sodium modeling to control the rate of change in serum sodium and osmolality is necessary [38, 39].

Electrolyte Disturbances

Potassium Disturbances

Disorders of serum potassium are particularly important, since potassium ions have a significant effect on transmembrane potential and cell volume (related to the ratio of ICK^+/ECK^+).

Hypokalemia

Hypokalemia may result from renal tubular defects, including RTA [41], Bartter's syndrome and Gitelman's syndrome, from starvation [42], chronic diarrhea, or vomiting. Hypokalemia may also occur with diabetic ketoacidosis, hyperaldosteronism, chloride losing diarrhea, and/or chronic use of diuretics. Inadequate long-term replacement is usually accompanied by chloride depletion with metabolic alkalosis [42, 43]. Acid urine in the presence of metabolic alkalosis (paradoxical aciduria) indicates significant K^+ depletion. Hypokalemic metabolic alkalosis is usually accompanied by a K^+ deficit of at least 4–5 mEq/kg [10, 43].

Symptoms of hypokalemia can include muscle weakness, cramps, paralytic ileus, decreased reflexes, lethargy, and confusion. Chronic exposure to low serum potassium results in a decrease in renal concentrating ability, producing a vasopressin-resistant diabetes insipidus.

Cardiac effects of hypokalemia are reflected by changes in the electrocardiogram (ECG), which include a low-voltage T wave, the presence of a U wave, and a prolonged Q-T interval or arrhythmia [44] and indicate the need for immediate therapy.

Therapy for Hypokalemia

- If asymptomatic, oral replacement is preferred, particularly if hypokalemia is secondary to chronic and nonreversible causes such as congenital chloride diarrhea, renal tubulopathies, renal tubular acidosis [42, 43]. Supplements with 1–4 mEq/kg/day of potassium are usually required and should be distributed in doses evenly throughout the day, and titrated to correct the serum potassium. Potassium chloride is the desirable replacement in most tubulopathies and gastrointestinal losses [43]; however, potassium citrate is necessary in patients with renal tubular acidosis, where potassium chloride supplementation increases degree of acidosis [41, 43]. Patients with severe depression of serum potassium level, especially if acute and patients on digitalis may require intravenous treatment [43].
- If potassium level is <2.5 mEq/l and patient is symptomatic, slowly administer KCl 1–2 mEq/kg intravenously restricting the rate to 0.5–0.9 mEq/kg/h for 1–2 h while carefully monitoring cardiac status [42, 43, 45]. The maximal intravenous dose of K^+ is 1 mEq/kg/h, preferably administered into a large vein via intravenous pump. Replacement should not exceed these limits except in extreme circumstance, e.g., the serum potassium is less than 1.0 mEq/l, and/or arrhythmia is present and then only in the presence of a physician experienced in dealing with this problem and under continuous ECG monitoring in the Intensive Care Unit [45].

Hyperkalemia

Most commonly, a rapidly rising serum potassium is a component of acute renal compromise. Extracellular potassium concentration correlates with onset and degree of cardiotoxicity. Accompanying metabolic derangements such as acidosis or hypocalcemia may precipitate ECG changes [46].

In children hyperkalemia occurs in the setting of increased tissue breakdown and release such as hemolysis (either intravascular or extravascular, e.g., hemolytic uremic syndrome) or myoglobin release with muscle damage. This produces an increased risk of cardiac arrhythmia even with mild renal insufficiency, mineralocorticoid deficiency, Addison's disease, congenital adrenal cortical hyperplasia, overuse of potassium sparing diuretics, ACE inhibitor therapy, calcineurin inhibitor therapy, excess use of K^+ supplements, or inappropriate use of salt substitutes [10, 18, 46].

In the neonate potassium release from tissue destruction can occur in the context of birth trauma, cephalhematoma, intraventricular hemorrhage, hypothermia, bleeding disorders, intravascular or extravascular hemodialysis, asphyxia, or ischemia [18]. Decreased potassium clearance in neonates occurs with renal failure, oliguria, hyponatremia, or congenital adrenal hyperplasia.

False elevations of potassium may occur with heel-stick blood samples, thrombocytosis, or marked leukocytosis, as well as from hemolysis. These factitious causes should be considered particularly if the ECG is normal. Repeat serum potassium as a plasma or whole blood sample will avoid problems with hemolysis.

General Principles of Treatment in Hyperkalemia

Prevention is the best treatment for hyperkalemia [10, 18, 45, 46]. For established elevated potassium levels:

Discontinue all sources of exogenous potassium intake (IV solution, medication formula feedings). Review the medication list for potassium supplements or agents which prevent either intracellular potassium uptake (such as Beta-blockers) or decrease potassium excretion (ACE inhibitors, ARB, aldosterone antagonists, or calcineurin inhibitors). Review the composition and rate of parenteral nutrition solutions. Check the dose of potassium supplements and adjust if necessary. In the neonate medication error is the commonest cause of sudden unexpected hyperkalemia.

Identify the cause and any exacerbating factors—hypocalcemia, hyponatremia, acidosis, insulin deficiency and beta-blocker therapy. This step is performed while assessing the risk by ECG [46]. The toxic effects of hyperkalemia are mainly cardiac and generally develop when the serum potassium rises above 7 mEq/l [44, 46]. Plasma K^+ above this level interferes with normal nodal and bundle conduction producing ECG changes which include peaked T waves, increased P-R interval and widened QRS, depressed S-T segment, and atrioventricular or intraventricular heart block. The presence of such ECG changes in hyperkalemia signals the need for specific therapy. As serum K^+ rises above levels of 7.5 mEq/l, there is significant danger of heart block, ventricular tachycardia, and ventricular fibrillation [46].

If symptomatic from muscle weakness or ECG changes emergent therapy is required to stabilize cardiac cell membranes. This is achieved by giving calcium gluconate 10 %, 0.5 ml/kg intravenously under ECG monitoring. One should expect a response in ECG pattern within 2–3 min. Extra caution must be used if the patient is digitalized or receiving pressor therapy.

For longer-term control promote potassium shift into cells and into glycogen using sodium bicarbonate, insulin/glucose or, beta-2 agonists

Sodium Bicarbonate to Promote Potassium Shift into Cells

Controversy exists as to the role of treatment of hyperkalemia with sodium bicarbonate. Studies in adults show that sodium bicarbonate in the absence of metabolic acidosis is relatively ineffective in producing a intracellular potassium shift. However, in infants and children particularly immature infants, hyperkalemia is almost always associated with acidosis making sodium bicarbonate therapy reasonable [42, 43]. In addition sodium bicarbonate in patients with renal insufficiency, but sustained urine output leads to increased distal sodium delivery with increased potassium excretion in addition to intracellular shift associated with correction of acidosis [42, 43]. Since the protection offered by intracellular shift potassium is transient, there is a need for concurrent measures of potassium removal either diuretic therapy, Kayexalate (R) or dialysis. There a significant risks to therapy in the neonate and smaller infant with either the insulin/glucose (hypoglycemia, hypotension), bowel complications from Kayexalate(R) usage, and in premature infants (less than 34 weeks gestation) sodium bicarbonate may produce hypernatremia or intracranial hemorrhage [47]. Diluted sodium bicarbonate given slowly over 30 min for marked elevation in potassium with acidosis or as an infusion over 2–24 h if practical [47]. Diluted sodium bicarbonate may also be given with diuretic therapy in this younger age group. Sodium bicarbonate 1–2.5 mmol/kg is administered in older children to treat acidosis, and to shift potassium into cells. Response is expected over 30–60 min. Correction of acidosis produces a fall of potassium by 1 mEq/l for each 0.1 pH unit rise. Insulin increases cellular potassium uptake, leading to a shift of potassium from the extracellular space. This should usually be administered with glucose (4 g/1 unit regular insulin) to prevent hypoglycemia. Neonates are particularly sensitive to hypoglycemia, if there is not a balance between insulin and glucose both hypotension and hypoglycemia will occur [17]. Administration of glucose alone will usually stimulate sufficient endogenous insulin in most infants to produce the desired potassium shift to be used alone initially. If insulin is required use 0.05 units/kg insulin with 2 ml/kg of dextrose 10 % in water (0.2 g dextrose) given as a bolus and followed by a continuous infusion of 10 % dextrose in water at 2–4 ml/kg/h with regular insulin [17, 47].

Albuterol by nebulization may be helpful temporarily, and hyperventilation may be helpful particularly in an intubated neonate.

Eventual removal of K^+ from the body by increasing excretion will be required:

- Cation exchange resins: Sodium polystyrene sulfonate 1 g/kg by mouth should lower potassium by 1 mEq/l. Excessive or recurrent use of Kayexalate(R) may, however, produce hypocalcemia. In neonates, Kayexalate(R)—if absolutely necessary—should be administered in water or 5 % glucose solution rather than sorbitol, which can be toxic to the colon and lead to necrotizing enterocolitis. It should not be given orally or by nasogastric tube in preterm infants because of the risk of bowel hypomotility and may produce bezoar or plug formation, with intestinal obstruction.
- Furosemide 1 mg/kg/dose intravenously may be helpful in promoting potassium excretion if urine output is sustained [16–18].
- Hemodialysis or peritoneal dialysis should be initiated promptly if significant elevation of serum potassium persists despite therapy or if a potential further rise can be predicted from the underlying condition producing the hyperkalemia, e.g., hemolysis, tumor lysis syndrome.

Calcium Disturbances

Ionized Ca^{2+} constitutes about 47 % of total serum calcium and is involved in enzyme regulation, stabilization of neuromuscular membranes, coagulation processes, and bone formation [48]. Metabolic acidosis increases ionized Ca^{2+}, whereas metabolic alkalosis may decrease it, even to the point of symptomatic tetany.

Hypocalcemia

Hypocalcemia is most commonly seen in rickets, renal insufficiency, hypoalbuminemic states (liver disease or nephrosis), and in the neonate fed cow's milk or soy based formulae with increased phosphate loads [16, 18, 47, 48]. Drugs that cause hypocalcemia include furosemide, glucagon, calcitonin, mithramycin, bicarbonate, and corticosteroids [47] and in neonates exchange transfusion with acid citrate-preserved blood can cause hypocalcemia [17].

Depressed ionized Ca^{2+} is associated with Chvostek's and Trousseau's signs, carpopedal spasm, and, occasionally, mental confusion or seizures. Neonates commonly become "jittery" and may have seizures with tetany particularly after stimulation such as handling. The ECG shows prolongation of the Q-T interval relative to the rate.

Treatment of hypocalcemia should include IV and PO administration of Ca^{2+}. An IV bolus of Ca^{2+} 10 mg/kg over 10–20 min will transiently (for about 1 h) raise the serum Ca^{2+} level and provide symptomatic relief. Supplemental Ca^{2+} 20–40 mg/kg/day IV or oral supplements

60–100 mg/kg/day of elemental Ca^{2+} should be provided commencing under IV cover. Continuous IV administration is hazardous producing cardiac arrhythmias, phlebitis, subcutaneous calcification and tissues necrosis. Continuous IV replacement should be reserved for critical situations.

Hypercalcemia

Hypercalcemia can be produced by vitamin D intoxication, sarcoidosis, cancer, immobilization, thyrotoxicosis, Addison's disease, hypophosphatasia, hyperparathyroidism, and the "milk-alkali" syndrome in patients on calcium compounds as antacid or phosphate binders. In neonates, hypercalcemia may follow prolonged furosemide therapy, which produces secondary hyperparathyroidism.

Symptoms of increased Ca^{2+} include nausea, anorexia, vomiting, constipation, polyuria, dehydration, mental confusion, and eventually coma. Chronic elevation of Ca^{2+} can lead to nephrocalcinosis, extraskeletal calcification, and renal calculi.

Treatment in hypercalcemia is aimed at symptomatic control followed by investigation and treatment of the underlying disorder. The initial step is to provide hydration with normal saline to increase urinary excretion of calcium. If this is not sufficient to produce control, induce diuresis with furosemide 1 mg/kg and replacement of urine volume loss with saline to prevent dehydration; if normal serum calcium is not achieved, consider using calcitonin or bisphosphonate. Dialysis has a limited place in treatment of severe acute hypercalcemia seen in some patients with malignancy—the aim of dialysis is to produce symptomatic control while more chronic therapy and if possible specific treatment of the malignancy is instituted.

Magnesium Disturbances

Hypomagnesemia

Muscular twitching, disorientation, latent tetany, movement disorders, and seizures have been observed in hypomagnesemia, together with hyperreactivity to mechanical and auditory stimulation. Lowered serum concentrations and whole body deficits are found in patients with chronic diarrhea, vomiting, celiac disease, prolonged parenteral fluid therapy, hyperaldosteronism, renal tubular abnormalities, chronic diuretic therapy and in association with certain antibiotic therapies (aminoglycosides and amphotericin B). Monitoring and prophylactic oral administration should be undertaken in these situations [49].

If symptomatic, intramuscular injection of 0.1 ml of 24 % $MgSO_4 \cdot 7H_2O$ (0.2 mEq/kg) repeated each 6 h for 3–4 doses usually produces symptomatic and biochemical improvement. Magnesium can then be added to maintenance fluids or provided orally for patients requiring long-term therapy.

Hypermagnesemia

Hypermagnesemia results early in drowsiness, decreased deep tendon reflexes and later in respiratory depression, disturbances in atrioventricular and intraventricular conduction (at levels of approximately 5 mEq/l) [49]. Acute renal failure and Addison's disease are accompanied by significantly elevated serum magnesium levels, particularly if magnesium enema or cathartics are used.

Prophylactic restriction of magnesium intake in patients with adrenal or renal disease is warranted. In the symptomatic patient intravenous calcium gluconate rapidly reverses depressant effects and the associated cardiac abnormalities.

Specific Conditions in Childhood

This section describes a group of specialized conditions where the development or treatment of the fluid or electrolyte abnormality differs from adolescent or adult patients. The following clinical conditions and situations are briefly reviewed:

- The neonatal period
- Oligoanuria in the nursery
- Burns in childhood
- Pyloric stenosis

Table 5.6 Special conditions in prematurity

Condition	Potential problems	Monitoring	Treatment
1. Very low birth weight			
Day 1	Prediuretic	Weight q 12 h	Adjust fluid rate
Day 2–3	Diuresis 15–20 % wt loss	Check electrolytes q 6–8 h	Adjust electrolyte
	Hypernatremia	Check electrolyte	Avoid fluid excess
	Lung disease if no diuresis	Check glucose level	Adjust electrolytes
	Or excess fluid administration	Administration rate	Adjust glucose
Day 4–5	Homeostasis		
	Glucose intolerance		
2. Nonoliguric hyperkalemia 24–72 h			
From K shift	K>6 mEq/l	Serum K q 12 h on day 1–4	Avoid postnatal glucocorticoid dose
Occurs 25 % infants	Shift ICF—ECF varies prematurity		Withhold K administration
Wt<1,000 kg	Potential decrease Na-K ATPase		
3. Late hyponatremia of prematurity			
Occurs at 6–8 weeks	Rapid growth	Electrolytes twice	Na supplements
Low sodium intake—breast milk	Immature tubules	Weekly	
4. Chronic lung disease			
If diuretic therapy	Excess Na/water overload	Weight gain	Avoid Na/water overload
Furosemide	Nephrocalcinosis	Electrolytes if diuretics	
		Renal U/S	
5. Acute asphyxia			
Hypoxia/ischemic	Cerebral edema	Electrolytes	Restrict fluid
	Stress hyperglycemia	Weight	Prevent excess fluid and salt
	SIADH		
6. Premature fluid excess	RDS	Electrolytes	Avoid excess fluid
	NEC	Weight	
	PDA		
	Chronic lung disease		

Data from [17, 18]

- Congenital chloride diarrhea and pseudo obstruction syndromes
- Perioperative fluid therapy
- Homeostasis in the malnourished infant
- Special conditions related to premature infants (Table 5.6)

Neonatal Conditions

Major differences are present in the Neonate when compared to Adult physiology. Before birth water and electrolyte homeostasis in the fetus is controlled by maternal and placental homeostatic mechanisms. After birth there is an initial phase of readjustment before homeostasis occurs.

Major differences include anatomy of relative size of compartments for total body water, ICF, ECF space, and perinatal changes in total body water. The ECF in the newborn is approximately equal in size to ICF (and exceeds the size of the intracellular fluid space in premature infants) [1, 50]. The goal of fluid and electrolyte therapy in the immediate postnatal period is to allow expected physiological changes to occur without dangerous perturbation in fluid and electrolyte status rather than maintain external fluid and electrolyte balance [17, 18, 51]. Normally a phased contraction of the ECF space occurs over the first 1 week. In term infants, after 24 h of low urinary output, a "physiologic" diuresis leads to a deficit of total body water mainly from the extracellular fluid compartment occurring over the next 3–4 days in term infants. More marked weight loss, as much as 15–20 %, may occur in premature infants where increased surface area–body weight ratio and immaturity of skin function allows increased losses. Water loss from the skin is inversely proportional to gestational age [17, 18]. Fluid and electrolyte therapy needs to be individualized with requirements based on careful assessment of clinical and laboratory status plus an additional supplement of water and electrolyte needs to be provided for growth. Sodium supplementation is usually not required in the first 24–36 h except in small for gestational age term infants extracellular fluid expansion is necessary to maintain volume status [17].

Renal and hormonal maturation occur with increasing gestational age [51]. GFR is lower in preterm infant than in full-term infants; it is lowest in the prediuretic phase in day 1, and less well autoregulated in the neonate. Na^+ and volume regulatory mechanisms are qualitatively similar to adults, but functionally limited by low GFR, until maturation increases in response to solute load. The lower rate of GFR limits excretion of water, sodium, and potassium. The ability to conserve sodium with a normal extracellular fluid volume is limited by decreased sodium reabsorptive capacity of the proximal nephron in the preterm infant. Although preterm and full-term infants can dilute their urine nearly as well as adults they cannot concentrate to the same degree (maximal urine osmolality is approximately 600–700 mOsm/kg in a term infant, and 400–500 mOsm/l in premature infants) [51]. Obligate solute loads generated from that intravenous solutions, parenteral nutrition, or concentrated feedings require extra free water for their elimination [17–19]. Since infants cannot control their own fluid intake, sufficient fluid must be provided to balance need for solute excretion. Increased skin losses in the face of fever and illness add an additional risk in these infants. Nursing on a radiant warming table is often necessary to attend to the rapidly changing clinical status of the young infant, but stresses the infant, leading to increased fluid and electrolyte loss [17]. Early use of an incubator will significantly reduce insensible fluid loss. Bicarbonate and glucose thresholds are lower in infants less than 34 weeks gestation than in the term infant and the bicarbonate threshold remains lower in the term infant than an adult [16]. Acid excretory capacity is limited by low GFR and lower buffer capacity is associated with reduced excretion of ammonia and phosphate [15, 16].This poses a risk of acidosis in the infant unless phosphate and protein are incorporated into new cells during active growth, reducing the potential excretory load. Fractional excretion of sodium is inversely proportional to gestational age. (Fractional excretion of sodium is approximately 15–20 % at 28 weeks and slowly falls to 1–2 % by 35 weeks.)

Fluid and electrolyte status may be assessed clinically by consideration of history, physical examination, and laboratory profile. Changes in vital signs, chemistries, and acid–base monitoring of kidney are similar to those in older children and adults. The blood pressure response to reduced cardiac output may be attenuated in the neonate.

Maintenance fluid therapy needs special attention. Initial intravenous fluids consist of dextrose solution in sufficient concentration to maintain serum glucose level. Prophylactic parenteral nutrition is commenced immediately upon admission using a premixed solution of amino acids and trace elements in 5 % dextrose. (The exact rate and composition of these solutions vary with local nursery practice to provide glucose at 4–10 mg/kg/min.) [17, 18].

Metabolic Disorders in the Neonate

Acid–base disorders in neonates associated with electrolyte disorders [17, 18] raise specific questions different from later life. Metabolic acidosis with an increased anion gap occurs in a number of the inborn errors of metabolism, with a differential diagnosis that includes renal failure, and lactic acidosis from poor perfusion. Metabolic acidosis associated with a normal or increased anion gap usually follows bicarbonate loss from gastrointestinal or renal tract as in older patients [16]. Premature infants less than 32 weeks gestation frequently manifest a proximal renal tubular acidosis, as a result of bicarbonate losses from the immature proximal tubule [16, 17]. "Late metabolic acidosis of prematurity" results from metabolism of the sulfur-containing amino acids in high casein feedings; this condition usually occurs during the second and third week of life and resolves without the need for bicarbonate supplementation. Observation alone is justified if growth continues; however, bicarbonate supplementation is reasonable if weight gain is slow.

Metabolic alkalosis results from gain in base or loss of acid from the ECF space with subsequent generation of bicarbonate. As in older patients to maintain a metabolic alkalosis the distal nephron must have an increased capacity for bicarbonate reabsorption from the increased filtered bicarbonate load. Generation of bicarbonate or increase in bicarbonate reabsorptive capacity alone cannot generate a metabolic alkalosis, so searches are undertaken for potassium depletion or a decrease in effective arterial blood volume which is essential for perpetuation of metabolic alkalosis [17, 42]. (See also discussion of pyloric stenosis and congenital chloride diarrhea which follow.) In the rare situation where metabolic alkalosis is life-threatening, exogenous acid (arginine or lysine hydrochloride or rarely 0.1N HCl) can be used for correction, with the choice depending upon local experience.

As in adults urinary chloride is helpful clinically to distinguish between causes of metabolic alkalosis: Low urinary chloride (<10 mEq/l) usually results from volume and/or sodium depletion, such as chronic diuretic therapy, nasogastric suction, vomiting, pyloric stenosis, or secretory diarrhea or following acute correction of chronically compensated respiratory acidosis. In the early phases of diuretic therapy chloride excretion is elevated and may be a confounding issue. High urinary chloride concentration (>20 mEq/l) occurs with mineralocorticoid excess either primary or secondary, e.g., Bartter's syndrome or Gitelman syndrome or congenital chloride diarrhea. In primary mineralocorticoid excess circulating volume is increased while in secondary forms circulatory volume is decreased. Alkali administration particularly with low urine output or diminished renal function, or following large blood product transfusion with citrate buffer will lead to metabolic alkalosis particularly in the smaller infant.

Oligoanuria in the Nursery

Urine flow of less than 1 ml/kg/h in the nursery may occur as the result of prerenal causes, renal parenchymal disorders, or post renal causes. Although micturition in a healthy infant may be delayed until 24–48 h after birth, *low urine output in the critically ill infant* should be assessed at 8–12 h of life. Decreased cardiac output unresponsive to ECF expansion requires the institution of inotropic/chronotropic pressor agents such as dopamine 0.5–2 mcg/kg/min. If the cause of diminished urine output is uncertain from history and physical exam, place a urethral catheter. If urine output < 0.5 ml/kg/h or 50 ml/kg/day or the laboratory profile is otherwise suggestive of prerenal causes in the absence of cardiac failure or overt heart disease, a fluid challenge 10 ml/kg/h normal saline is given, with a repeat bolus if the urine output is not reestablished. Failure to promote a diuresis with fluid challenge and/or furosemide is an indication for urgent abdominal ultrasound to exclude renal, urethral, and bladder obstruction where further imaging modalities may be required.

Burns in Children

Continuous changes in the relative surface area of head and limbs during growth make it necessary to use age-related charts to allow accurate assessment of the burned surface area [9]. Calculation using the adult rule of nines, although reasonable in adolescents, can lead to significant errors in estimates in the younger child and infant [5, 9]. Mortality and morbidity depend on the extent and depth of the burn. The severity of the injury and potential problems during treatment depend on the burn agent—flame, electrical, hot liquid—associated injuries, and the potential for smoke inhalation and should be noted for inclusion in design of therapy. High fluid rate requires central access of at least one large bore line; two central lines are preferred in burns greater than 60 % body surface area. It is wise to discuss the extent of the burn and resuscitation planned with a specialized burn unit and plan for transfer to specialized treatment. The "Parkland formula" provides a good starting point for fluid therapy [9]. 4 ml Lactated Ringer solution/kg/%BSA are administered over the first 24 h; 50 % of the volume should be administered in the initial 8 h post burn (not the first 8 h of therapy, so it is important to start therapy as soon as possible) and the remaining 50 % over the next 16 h in children weighing greater than 10 kg. In infants weighing <10 kg, the requirement for maintenance dextrose leads to modification of the standard formula, using D5LR at 4 ml/kg/h to provide dextrose containing fluid together with LR at 3 ml/kg/% for resuscitation. The rate of infusion is varied to maintain pulse, BP within normal range for age, and a urine flow of 1 ml/kg/h. Vital signs, acid–base balance, and mental status are a reflection of adequate resuscitation. In the second 24 h, restoration of capillary integrity is followed by reabsorption of edema fluid leading to a diuresis. This allows maintenance of circulation and tissue perfusion using approximately half of the volume of D5RL that was used during the first day resuscitation. Oral supplementation as milk based formula, or artificial feedings may start as early as 48 h.

Colloid replacement can be used after 24–48 h as capillary integrity returns, using 5 % albumin to maintain serum albumin >2gm/dl [9]. Fresh frozen plasma is provided if coagulation problems are present and packed red blood cells to maintain the hematocrit at 24 % (8 g/dl Hgb).

Pyloric Stenosis

Treatment of pyloric stenosis exemplifies the correction of deficits associated with alkalosis in childhood. Therapy differs from most other causes of dehydration in the need for early potassium replacement (as soon as urine output is demonstrated). After volume expansion with 0.9 % saline if necessary, 0.45 or 0.9 % saline solution with added potassium chloride 30–40 mEq/l should be administered at a rate to provide correction of the deficit and maintenance over 24 h. Ongoing losses are minimized by using a nasogastric tube and withholding feedings to reduce vomiting. Both sodium and potassium should be repleted as the chloride salt because of the large chloride deficit. Although deficits may be repleted to normal electrolyte pattern by 12 h, it is preferable to delay surgery until electrolyte depletion has been complete for a period of some 12–24 h to allow optimal readjustment of cellular function.

Congenital Alkalosis of Gastrointestinal Origin

Metabolic alkalosis may result from prolonged chronic diarrhea with potassium deficit but is a feature of congenital chloride diarrhea [52], a condition in which the multiple stools with high chloride content lead to significant chloride and potassium depletion. Alkalosis results from ensuring volume depletion with significant concurrent potassium losses. Acute treatment of fluid and electrolyte abnormalities is similar to that for pyloric stenosis, with longer-term therapy with potassium chloride supplement in amount sufficient to maintain serum potassium and chloride levels while establishing adequate dietary intake and allowing transition to oral supplementation.

Perioperative Fluid Therapy

In patients without preexisting deficit or in whom the deficit has been repaired, supply adequate carbohydrate to spare protein breakdown (75–100 g glucose/m^2/24 h) together with administration of usual maintenance requirement of water and electrolytes. Intraoperative maintenance fluid is provided as isotonic fluid—normal saline or lactated Ringer's solution [53].

Young infants who are not vomiting should receive carbohydrate and sodium chloride mixture by mouth until 3–4 h prior to the operation. In the newborn deficits of water and electrolytes from vomiting or from intestinal obstruction should be replaced and stabilized as fully as possible before operation [53]. During surgery, blood, plasma, and saline are provided in sufficient volumes to maintain intravascular volume and to replace concurrent losses as determined by the surgeon and anesthesiologist intraoperatively. The most common error in administration of parenteral fluid during and after surgery is excessive administration dextrose in water [14, 53]. Little potassium is usually needed during this time, because of operative stress and tissue trauma which results in release of intracellular potassium with the potential for hyperkalemia. If shock was present preoperatively, acute renal dysfunction may further impair the ability to eliminate generated potassium loads produced or administered potassium.

Postoperative fluid intake should be limited to a maintenance requirement of 85 ml/100 kcal metabolized together with measured ongoing losses until the antidiuresis anticipated from response to surgery, and circulatory readjustment after anesthesia has occurred, unless the renal concentrating ability is impaired (sickle cell disease, chronic pyelonephritis, or obstructive uropathy) where replacement equal to measured urinary losses will require specific replacement.

Homeostasis in the Malnourished Child

Severe malnutrition caused by diarrheal dehydration is common in tropical countries. In temperate zones the cause is more commonly associated with chronic illness such as inflammatory bowel disease, malabsorption syndromes, chronic renal disease, cystic fibrosis and with after trauma or burns. Therapy should be adapted to meet the specific disturbances in body composition and the expected response to refeeding. Overexpansion of extracellular fluid space is accompanied by extracellular and presumably intracellular hypoosmolality, low serum protein levels, low serum sodium, potassium, calcium, and magnesium. Tetany may result from magnesium or calcium deficiency. Cardiac reserve is lowered and heart failure a common complication of aggressive fluid therapy [54].

Planning Replacement and Refeeding

It is particularly important to calculate replacement fluid and electrolyte on the basis of caloric requirements (indexed to calories provided rather than per kg/body weight) to avoid fluid overload and overt cardiac failure. Decrease in renal plasma flow and GFR occur with malnutrition, concentrating ability is impaired (limited production of urea impairs medullary gradient) and dilution the urine is limited by low sodium and potassium delivery to the distal tubule, diminishing water tolerance so that care for monitoring of weight and serum electrolytes is necessary. The ability to excrete an acid load is decreased by limitation to generation of titratable acidity (in the presence of a low phosphate), and low ammonia generation (low protein intake and anabolic state) together with potential increased bicarbonate loss with solute diuresis. It is important to frequently reassess and if necessary supplement with alkali (for the expected 4 mEq of acid generated by each 100 cal supplied) [41] during the time of refeeding. Care must be taken to concurrently supplement calcium and magnesium to prevent tetany. Refeeding results in intracellular shifts of phosphate, glucose, potassium, and magnesium which produce hypophosphatemia, hypoglycemia, hypokalemia, and hypomagnesemia resulting in neurologic, neuromuscular, pulmonary, cardiac, and hematologic complications which require close monitoring and supplementation [55].

Conditions Specific to the Premature Infant

A number of conditions specific to the immature infant occur during the adjustment of water and electrolyte homeostasis from a fetal status controlled by maternal and placental homeostatic mechanisms, through a phase of readjustment to extrauterine life, to homeostasis based on the growth coordinated with maturation of renal and hormonal function. Table 5.6 outlines potential problems, monitoring, and therapeutic considerations these conditions.

References

1. Friss-Hansen B. Body water compartments in children: changes during growth. Pediatrics. 1963;28:107–8.
2. Holliday MA, Segar WE. The maintenance need for water in parenteral fluid therapy. Pediatrics. 1957;19:823–32.
3. Friedman AL. Pediatric hydration therapy: historical review and a new approach. Nephrology forum. Kid Int. 2005;67:380–8.
4. Holliday M. The evolution of therapy for dehydration: should deficit therapy still be taught? Pediatrics. 1996;98:171–7.
5. Carvajal HF. Fluid resuscitation of pediatric burn victims: a critical appraisal. Pediatr Nephrol. 1994;8:357–66.
6. Carcello JA, Davis AL, Zaritsky A. Role of early resuscitation in pediatrics septic shock. JAMA. 1991;266:1242–5.
7. Pediatric advanced life support provider manual. In: Zartisky AL et al., editors. Dallas, TX: American Heart Association, Subcommittee on Pediatric Resuscitation; 2002.
8. Hammarlund K, Sedin G, Stromberg B. Trends epidermal water loss in newborn infants. VIII. Relation to gestational age and postnatal age inappropriate and small for gestational age infants. Acta Pediatr Scand. 1993;72:721–8.
9. Antoon A, Magoon K. Burn Injuries in childhood. In: Burg FD, Ingelfinger Jr, Wald ER, Pollin RA, editors, 17th ed. Philadelphia, PA: W.B. Saunders, Co. Publishers; 2002. p. 1064–9.
10. Wong C, Herrin JT. Fluid and Electrolytes. Chapter 7 in Manual of pediatric therapeutics, 7th ed. In: Graef JW, Wolfsdorf JI, Greenes DS, editors. Philadelphia, PA: Lippincott-Williams and Wilkins Publishers; 2008. p. 65–75.
11. Alderson P, Schierhout G, Roberts I, Bunn F. Colloids versus crystalloid for fluid resuscitation in critically ill patients. Cochrane Database Syst Rev 2000:CD000567.
12. Finfer S, Bellomo R, Boyce N, et al. A comparison of albumin and saline for fluid resuscitation in the intensive care unit. N Eng J Med. 2004;350:2247–53.
13. Joint Task Force on Advanced Pediatric Life-support. Shock. In: Gausche M, editor. APLS: the Pediatric Emergency Medicine Course; 1998. p. 61.
14. Holliday MA, Friedman AL, Segar WE, et al. Acute hospital induced hyponatremia in children: a physiologic approach. J Pediatr. 2004;145:584–7.
15. Lorenz JM. Fluid and electrolyte therapy in the newborn infant. In: Burg FD, Ingelfinger Jr, Wald ER, Pollin RA, editors. Pediatric therapeutics Gellis and Kagan 17th ed. W.B. Philadelphia, PA: Saunders, Co. Publishers; 2002. p. 29–36.
16. Guinard JP, Drucker A. Clinical neonatal nephrology. In: Barratt M, Avener E, Harmn WE, editors. Chap 64 in pediatric nephrology, 4th ed. Baltimore, MD: Lippincott Williams & Wilkins Publishers; 1999. p. 1051–66.
17. Lin PW, Simmons CF. Fluid and electrolyte management. In: Cloherty JP, Eichenwald EC, Stark AR, editos. Chap 9 in manual of neonatal care, 5th ed. Baltimore, MD: Lippincott Williams and Wilkins; 2003. p. 101–14.
18. Lorenez JM, Kleinman LI, Ahmed G, et al. Phases of fluid and electrolyte homeostasis in the extremely low birthweight infant. Pediatrics. 1995;96:484–9.
19. Zeigler EE, Forman SJ. Fluid intake, renal solute load, and border balance in infancy. J Pediatr. 1971;78:561–8.
20. Edelmann CM, Barnett HL, Troupkou V. Renal concentrating mechanisms in newborn infants. Effect of dietary protein and water content, role of urea and responsiveness to anti-diuretic hormone. J Clin Invest. 1960;39:1062.
21. Friedman JN, Goldman RD, Srivastava R, Parkin PC. Development of a clinical dehydration scale for use in children between 1 and 36 months of age. J Pediatr. 2004;145:201–7.
22. Edelman IS, Liebman J, O'Meara MP, Birkenfeld LW. Interrelations between serum sodium concentration, serum osmolarity and total exchangable sodium, total exchangeable potassium and total body water. J Clin Invest. 1958;37:1236–56.
23. Edelman IS, Litchman J. Anatomy of body water and electrolytes. Am J Med. 1959;27:256–77.
24. Holliday MA, Freidman AL, Wassner SJ. Extracellular fluid restoration in dehydration a critique of rapid versus slow. Pediatr Nephrol. 1999;13:292–7.
25. AAP Provisional Committee on Quality Improvement. Subcommittee On Acute Gastroenteritis: practice parameter: the management of acute gastroenteritis in children. Pediatrics. 1996;97:424–30.
26. Ellison DH, Berl T. The syndrome of inappropriate antidiuresis. N Eng J Med. 2007;356:2064–72.
27. Brion LP, Satlin LM. Clinical significance of developmental renal physiology. In: Polin RA, Fox WW, editors. Fetal and neonatal physiology. 2nd ed. Philadelphia, PA: WB Saunders; 1998.
28. Kaplan SL, Feigin RD. Syndrome of inappropriate antidiuretic hormone in children. Adv Pediatr. 1980;27:247–58.
29. Singh S, Bohn D, Carlotti AP, et al. Cerebral salt wasting: truce, fallacies, theories, and challenges. Crit Care Med. 2002;30:2575–9.
30. Androgue HJ, Madias NE. Hyponatremia. N Eng J Med. 2000;342:1581–9.
31. Ayus JC, Arieff AI. Hyponatremia and myelinolysis. Ann Intern Med. 1997;127:163.
32. Sterns RH. The treatment of hyponatremia: first, do no harm. Am J Med. 1990;88:557.
33. Karp BI, Laureno R. Pontine and extra pontine myelinolysis: the neurologic disorder following rapid correction of hyponatremia. Medicine (Baltimore). 1993;72:359.
34. Berl T. Hypernatremia. Clinical disorders of water metabolism. Kid Int. 1976;110:117.
35. Strange K. Regulation of solute and water balance and cell volume in the central nervous system. J Am Soc Nephrol. 1992;3:12.

36. Bruck E, Abal G, Aceto Jr T. Pathogenesis and pathophysiology of hypertonic dehydration with diarrhea. Am J Dis Child. 1968;115:122.
37. Roscelli JD, Yu CE, Southgate WM. Management of salt poisoning in an extremely low birthweight infant. Pediatr Nephrol. 1994;8:172–4.
38. Yang CW, Kim YS, Park IS, et al. Treatment of severe acute hypernatremia and renal failure by hemodialysis. Nephron. 1995;70:372–3.
39. Pazmino PA, Pazmino BP. Treatment of acute hypernatremia with hemodialysis. Am J Nephrol. 1993;13:260–5.
40. Saunders N, Balfe J, Laski B. Severe salt poisoning in an infant. J Pediatr. 1976;88:258–61.
41. Herrin JT. Renal tubular acidosis. pediatric nephrology. Chap 39. In: Avner ED, Harmon W, Niadeut PA editors. 5th ed. Philadelphia , PA: Lippincott Williams & Wilkins; 2004. p. 757–76.
42. Schwartz, G. Potassium. Chap in pediatric nephrology, 5th ed. In: Avner ED, Harmon WE, Niaduet P, editors. Philadelphia, PA: Lippincott Williams and Wilkins; 2004. p. 147–88.
43. Rodriguez-Soriano J. Potassium homeostasis and it's disturbances in children. Pediatr Nephrol. 1995;9: 364–74.
44. Tepper D, Aronson R. ECG interpretation for the noncardiologist: effects of potassium and calcium abnormalities. Hospital medicine; 1984. p. 111–23.
45. Pullen H, Doig A, Lambie AT. Intravenous potassium replacement therapy. Lancet. 1967;2:809–11.
46. Rose BD, Post TW. Hyperkalemia. In: Wonsiewicz M, McCullough K, Davis K, editors. Clinical physiology of acid-base and electrolyte disorders. New York: McGraw Hill; 2001. p. 888–930.
47. Simmons MA. Hypernatremia, intracranial hemorrhage, and bicarbonate administration in neonates. N Eng J Med. 1974;291:6.
48. Juppner H, Carpenter TO. Disorders of the parathyroid, hypocalcemia and hypercalcemia. In: Burg FD, Ingelfinger Jr, Wald ER, Pollin RA, editors. Pediatric therapeutics Gellis and Kagan 17th ed. Philadelphia, PA: W.B. Saunders, Co. Publishers; 2002. p. 687–92.
49. Rude RK. Magnesium homeostasis. In: Bilezikian JP, Raisz LG, Rodan GA, editors. Principles of bone biology. New York: Academic Press; 1996. p. 277–93.
50. Yoshioka T, Iitaka K, Ichikawa I. Body fluid compartments. In: Ichikawa I, editor. Pediatric textbook of fluids and electrolytes. Baltimore, MD: Williams and Wilkins; 1990. p. 14–20.
51. Baum M, Quigley R. Postnatal renal development. In: Seldin DW, Giebisch G, editors. Chapter 26 in the kidney physiology and pathophysiology. 3rd ed. Philadelphia, PA: Lippincott Williams and Wilkins; 2000. p. 703–25.
52. Kere J, Lohi H, Hoglund P. Genetic disorders of membrane transport. III congenital chloride diarrhea. Am J Physiol. 1999;276:G7–13.
53. McMahon Y, Ward JD, Boucek RJ, Hammon JW, Neblett WW, McDougal S, MacDonnell RC, Ichekawa I. Management of the patient immediately after surgery. In: Ichikawa I, editor. Pediatric textbook of fluids and electrolytes. Baltimore, MD: Williams and Wilkins; 1990. p. 459–69.
54. LaFrance JP, Leblanc M. Metabolic, electrolytes and nutritional concerns in critical illness. Crit Care Clin. 2005;21:305–27.
55. Kraft MD, Btaiche IF, Sacks GS. Review of the refeeding syndrome. Nutr Clin Pract. 2005;20:625–33.

Diuretic Therapy

6

Arohan R. Subramanya and David H. Ellison

Introduction

Excluding regional factors or lymphatic obstruction, edema is the clinical consequence of extracellular fluid (ECF) volume expansion. Edema occurs when dietary sodium intake exceeds renal Na excretion and is seen in a variety of disorders including heart failure, cirrhosis, and nephrotic syndrome. In each of these conditions, the total body sodium and water content is elevated; therefore, aside from treating the underlying disease, reducing sodium intake via modifications in diet is the first intervention in the approach to treating edema. Water restriction is usually not necessary when the underlying disease is mild and is usually only recommended when hyponatremia supervenes [1]. When these interventions are inadequate or not possible, diuretics are used to enhance renal sodium and water excretion.

Although diuretics are powerful drugs that are capable of rapidly improving life-threatening conditions such as acute pulmonary edema, they are obviously not perfect. Each class bears its own host of clinical side effects and chronic diuretic exposure often induces long-term adaptive changes in the kidney that ultimately lead to diuretic resistance. Fortunately, the current diverse armamentarium of pharmacologic agents permits the rational management of these conditions, allowing the clinician to tailor therapy to the specific needs of his or her patients.

The purpose of this chapter is to review the classes of diuretic agents and their mechanisms of action and to discuss their role in treating edema. Both generalized approaches and treatment of specific edematous states are discussed. Finally, we address the issue of diuretic resistance and treatment options for this complex problem.

Diuretic Classes

"Diuretic" is derived from the Greek word *diouretikos*, which means "to promote urine." Traditionally, the term has been reserved for agents that reduce ECF volume by enhancing urinary solute excretion [2]. The advent of new drugs that promote solute-free urinary water excretion, however, has necessitated a novel scheme of diuretic classification. Most of the diuretics that are used in clinical practice are *natriuretics*; i.e., they increase urine volume by inhibiting specific sodium transport pathways at defined anatomic sites along the nephron. *Osmotic diuretics*, in contrast, do not have a precise molecular target, and primarily force diuresis by

A.R. Subramanya, M.D.
Department of Medicine, Renal-Electrolyte Division, University of Pittsburgh School of Medicine, S832 Scaife Hall, 3550 Terrace St, Pittsburgh, PA 15261, USA

D.H. Ellison, M.D. (✉)
Division of Nephrology and Hypertension, Department of Medicine, Oregon Health and Science University, 3181 SW Sam Jackson Park Rd, Portland, OR 97239, USA
e-mail: ellisond@ohsu.edu

D.B. Mount et al. (eds.), *Core Concepts in the Disorders of Fluid, Electrolytes and Acid-Base Balance*,
DOI 10.1007/978-1-4614-3770-3_6,

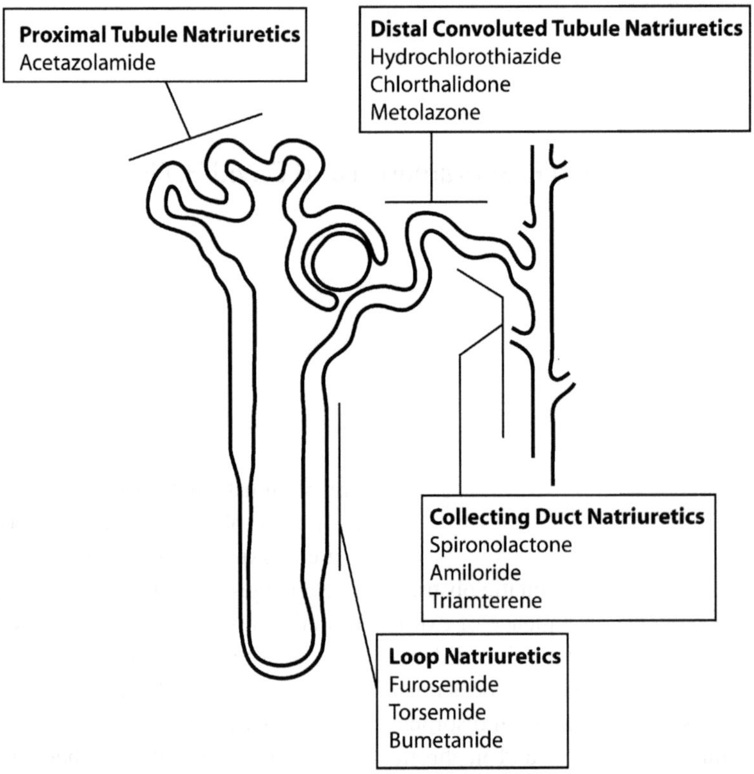

Fig. 6.1 Sites of natriuretic action along the nephron. Carbonic anhydrase inhibitors such as acetazolamide suppress sodium reabsorption in the proximal tubule. The loop diuretics (e.g., furosemide, torsemide, bumetanide) inhibit sodium chloride reabsorption in the thick ascending limb of the loop of Henle. Distal convoluted tubule natriuretics such as thiazides and thiazide-like diuretics inhibit NaCl reabsorption in the early and late distal convoluted tubule. Collecting duct natriuretics inhibit electrogenic sodium transport in the cortical collecting duct and the late distal tubule. Consequently the sites of action of DCT and collecting duct natriuretics overlap slightly

altering the osmotic pressure of the glomerular filtrate. *Aquaretics* constitute a new class of agents that increase the excretion of solute-free water by inhibiting vasopressin-mediated renal water reabsorption.

Natriuretics

Natriuretics are by far the most frequently used class of diuretics and are among the most commonly prescribed drugs (source: IMS Health). These agents promote a solute and water diuresis by inhibiting the movement of sodium from the tubular lumen to the blood. Four general subclasses of natriuretics primarily act on different sites of the nephron to facilitate sodium and water excretion. As noted in Fig. 6.1, these nephron segments are responsible for reabsorbing different fractions of the filtered sodium load, and each segment plays its own important role in controlling ECF volume homeostasis. In general, more proximal segments of the nephron reabsorb the bulk of sodium from the glomerular filtrate, while more distal segments "fine-tune" the urinary sodium content by reabsorbing smaller fractions of the total sodium load in a tightly regulated fashion. The molecular targets and anatomic sites of action of specific agents define many of their clinical properties, including their therapeutic uses, side effects, and chronic effects on nephron adaptation. Commonly used natriuretics and key pharmacologic aspects of their clinical use are summarized in Table 6.1.

Table 6.1 Commonly used natriuretics

Diuretic class	Maximum change in urinary fractional excretion of sodium[a] (%)	Oral dose range[b] (mg)	Onset of action	Oral bioavailability (%)	Duration of action	Elimination half-life ($t_{1/2}$) in normal adults (h)	Hepatic metabolism?	Route of excretion
Carbonic anhydrase inhibitors	5–6							
Acetazolamide		125–375	2 h	100	8–12 h	6–9	No	Renal (100 %)
Loop natriuretics	30							
Furosemide		20–320	0.5–2 h	50	6–8 h	0.5–1	Minimal	Renal, fecal
Torsemide		5–200	0.5–1 h	80–100	6 h	2–4	Yes (80 %)	Renal
Bumetanide		0.5–10	0.5–1 h	80–100	4–6 h	1–1.5	Yes	Renal
Ethacrynic acid		25–400	0.5 h	100	12 h	1	Yes (30 %)	Renal, fecal
Distal convoluted tubule natriuretics	5–12							
Hydrochlorothiazide		12.5–200	2 h	50–80	6–12 h	2.5–14	No	Renal (100 %)
Chlorthalidone		12.5–200	2 h	65	24–72 h	35–55	Yes	Renal, fecal
Metolazone		0.5–10	1 h	65	~ 24 h	20	Yes (~10 %)	Renal, fecal
Indapamide		1.25–5	1–2 h	~95	≤36 h	~14	Yes (~100 %)	Renal, fecal
Collecting duct natriuretics	3–5							
Spironolactone		50–400	Several days	65	2–3 days	1.6	Yes (~100 %)	Renal, fecal
Eplerenone		50–100	Several days	~65	2–3 days	5	Yes (~100 %)	Renal, fecal
Amiloride		5–20	2 h	15–25	24 h	6–9	No	Renal
Triamterene		50–250	2–4 h	30–70	7–9 h	~4.5	Yes	Renal, fecal

[a]Each value indicates the approximate maximal fractional excretion of sodium following acute administration of a maximally effective dose of natriuretic
[b]The maximum safe dose of diuretic is rarely indicated or advantageous, and may be associated with excessive side effects

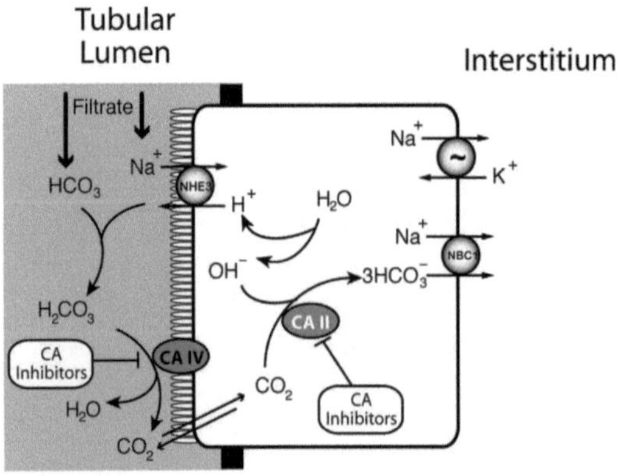

Fig. 6.2 Mechanism of action of carbonic anhydrase (CA) inhibitors. Diagram of a proximal tubule cell illustrating expression of CA IV in the luminal brush border and CA II in the cytoplasm. HCO_3 from the glomerular filtrate combines with protons extruded by the sodium hydrogen exchanger (NHE3) to form carbonic acid (H_2CO_3). CA IV breaks down H_2CO_3 to water and carbon dioxide, which freely diffuse across cell membranes. CA II then catalyzes the formation of intracellular bicarbonate (HCO_3) from cytoplasmic CO_2 and OH. HCO_3 is then transported into the interstitium by a basolateral sodium bicarbonate cotransporter (NBC1). CA inhibitors block the bicarbonate reabsorptive process by inhibiting luminal CO_2 formation and cytoplasmic HCO_3 generation by inhibiting CA IV and CA II. This ultimately suppresses vectorial sodium reabsorption across the proximal tubule apical and basolateral membranes (see text)

Proximal Tubule Diuretics (Carbonic Anhydrase Inhibitors)

Natriuretics that primarily act in the proximal tubule suppress renal sodium reabsorption through the inhibition of carbonic anhydrase (CA). Two isoforms of this enzyme are primarily responsible for reclaiming greater than 80 % of the filtered sodium bicarbonate load in the early proximal tubule (Fig. 6.2) [3]. During this process, protons secreted by proximal tubule cells into the tubular lumen combine with filtered bicarbonate to form carbon dioxide and water. This reaction is catalyzed by type IV CA expressed at the luminal surface of the proximal tubule [4]. CO_2 is lipid soluble and rapidly diffuses across the apical membrane of the proximal tubule. Once inside the proximal tubule cell, CO_2 combines with OH^- in the presence of type II CA to form HCO_3^-. Cytoplasmic bicarbonate ions are then moved across the basolateral membrane of the proximal tubule cell in a sodium-dependent manner via a Na^+-HCO_3^- cotransporter [5]. Thus, the net effect of this process is to reclaim bicarbonate and sodium from the glomerular filtrate while maintaining cellular isotonicity.

Although different carbonic anhydrase inhibitors exhibit different isoform specificities [6], these drugs have been shown to effectively suppress the activity of both type II and type IV CA. The inhibition of either or both of these enzymes results in reduced HCO_3^- reabsorption and a relative increase in luminal nonchloride anions [2]. This change in the anionic composition of the proximal tubule luminal fluid prevents the apical reabsorption of sodium cations, ultimately increasing distal Na^+ delivery [7].

In spite of the fact that CA inhibitors are capable of inhibiting proximal tubule Na^+ exit by 40–60 %, the natriuretic effect of these drugs is mild [8]. At most, proximal tubule natriuretics only enhance net sodium excretion by 3–5 % [9], except when combined with other agents (see below). This is largely due to enhanced sodium reabsorption by more distal nephron segments [10]. Since chloride is reabsorbed with sodium in both the thick ascending limb (TAL) of the loop of Henle, and the distal convoluted tubule, urinary chloride excretion is low in patients treated with CA inhibitors [11].

The principal effect of CA inhibition on the urinary electrolyte composition is to increase its bicarbonate and potassium content. As one might expect, CA inhibition increases urinary bicarbonate excretion by 25–30 %, elevating the urine pH, mimicking proximal renal tubular acidosis [7]. This is a direct consequence of the fact that downstream of the proximal tubule, bicarbonate is a poorly reabsorbable anion [7]. In concert with the increase in bicarbonaturia, acetazolamide increases potassium excretion [8]. Current evidence suggests that the kaliuretic effect is indirect, and largely derived from increased potassium secretion in the distal nephron due to a change in the lumen-negative voltage and flow induced by enhanced distal bicarbonate delivery [12].

Acetazolamide is the most commonly prescribed CA inhibitor in the United States. Used as monotherapy, it is a mild diuretic due to its aforementioned weak effect on natriuresis, and adaptive processes downstream of the proximal tubule quickly give rise to diuretic resistance. Acetazolamide, however, can be very useful in combination with natriuretics that block more distal NaCl transport pathways (see Sect. 12, below).

Aside from its use as a diuretic, acetazolmide has several other clinical uses. The bicarbonaturia associated with acetazolamide therapy is useful in the prevention of uric acid and cysteine nephrolithiasis [13]. Raising the pH of the tubular lumen via CA inhibition is a tactic commonly employed in the treatment of salicylate toxicity [14]. Due to the fact that aqueous humor formation in the eye is dependent on CA-mediated bicarbonate production, CA inhibitors [including dorzolamide and brinzolamide (topical) and acetazolamide and methazolamide (oral)] are commonly used to treat chronic open-angle glaucoma [6]. The increased respiratory drive associated with acetazolamide-induced bicarbonaturia makes it useful as a prophylactic for high-altitude mountain sickness and pulmonary edema [15].

Generally, acetazolamide and other CA inhibitors are well tolerated. All CA inhibitors are sulfonilamide derivatives, and should be avoided in patients with severe sulfa allergies. Serum potassium and bicarbonate levels need to be monitored due to the associated hypokalemia and metabolic acidosis that often accompany therapy. In contrast to its therapeutic utility in uric acid and cysteine stone formers, CA inhibition increases the risk of nephrolithiasis in patients with hypercalciuria due to the elevation in urine pH and increased calcium excretion [16]. CNS and other neurologic symptoms, such as drowsiness, fatigue, and paresthesias, are other known side effects.

Loop Diuretics

Commonly used loop diuretics in the United States include furosemide, bumetanide, torsemide, and ethacrynic acid (Table 6.1). The primary molecular target of these agents is the Na-K-2Cl cotransporter (NKCC2), which reabsorbs sodium, potassium, and chloride ions in the TAL of the loop of Henle [17]. Since this nephron segment is impermeable to water, NKCC2 plays a crucial role in generating the hypertonic medullary interstitium that is essential for efficient urinary concentration [18]. Twenty-five percent of the filtered NaCl load is reabsorbed by this cotransporter [17]; thus, inhibition of its transport activity leads to a marked increase in sodium chloride excretion. Indeed, the loop natriuretics constitute the most potent class of diuretics used in current clinical practice [2].

Loop diuretics bind to a site on NKCC2 exposed at the apical surface of the epithelium lining the lumen of the TAL [19]. Loop diuretic binding to the cotransporter interferes with the apical translocation of ions passing through the TAL; this increases the luminal NaCl and K content. The increase in luminal NaCl and K content correlates with a reduction in the medullary concentration gradient [18]. Consequently, the selective water-reabsorptive response to vasopressin during loop diuretic-mediated ECF volume contraction is diminished, ensuring that urine volume increases and urine osmolality approaches that of plasma.

In addition to increasing Na and Cl excretion via NKCC2 inhibition in the TAL, loop diuretics are powerful stimulators of renin release. This effect is a direct consequence of loop diuretic-induced changes in tubular fluid load sensing by the macula densa, a specialized group of epithelial cells anatomically positioned at the end of the TAL. Macula densa cells recognize alterations in fluid delivery by sensing changes in NaCl influx through NKCC2 cotransporters expressed at the tubular lumen [20]. A decrease in NKCC2-mediated NaCl entry activates local signaling cascades to trigger renin release from granular cells in the juxtaglomerular apparatus (JGA) [21]. Since the stimulus for renin release hinges on a decrease in NKCC2-mediated NaCl influx, direct inhibition of NKCC2 by loop diuretics dramatically augments the process [22]. The exaggeration in renin release seen with high-dose loop diuretic therapy may be harmful in some treatment scenarios. In two studies, 1–1.5 mg/kg intravenous boluses of furosemide given to patients with chronic heart failure (HF) caused a transient decline in hemodynamic parameters, resulting in a *worsening* of HF symptoms over the first hour of treatment [23, 24]. This finding was attributed to over-activation of the renin-angiotensin and/or sympathetic nervous systems [25]. Others have postulated that chronic loop diuretic-induced renin release may contribute to loop diuretic resistance [26]. Moreover, chronic deleterious over-activation of the intrarenal renin-angiotensin system by long-term diuretic use is a theoretical risk that could contribute to the development of chronic kidney disease [27]. Currently, efforts are being taken to develop agents that may block paracrine signaling from the macula densa to the renin-producing cells of the JGA. Such an inhibitor would in all likelihood attenuates the tendency of loop diuretics to overstimulate the renin-angiotensin system.

NKCC2-mediated NaCl cotransport in the macula densa is also an essential step in a critical renal homeostatic process, tubuloglomerular feedback (TGF). TGF is a negative feedback mechanism in which the glomerular filtration rate (GFR) is tightly controlled in response to changes in tubular fluid delivery to the macula densa. Luminal sodium chloride is sensed by the macula densa by way of its cotransport via NKCC2. The increase in intracellular NaCl then triggers a local signaling cascade involving adenosine [21]. This induces preglomerular vasoconstriction [28], decreasing the GFR and filtration fraction. Loop diuretics impede TGF by interfering with the NKCC2 sensing step; this makes the JGA much less effective at matching GFR with tubular fluid delivery to the TAL [29]. Thus, through the blockade of TGF, loop diuretics tend to maintain the GFR at a higher level than would occur if the TGF were not blocked.

In addition to their profound natriuretic and kaliuretic effects, loop diuretics enhance the urinary excretion of calcium and magnesium. Na-K-2Cl cotransport in the TAL generates a lumen-positive transepithelial voltage, largely owing to the recycling of intracellular potassium cations back into the tubular lumen via low- and high-conductance potassium channels [18]. This voltage gradient favors the paracellular reabsorption of calcium and magnesium. NKCC2 inhibition by loop diuretics dissipates the transepithelial voltage by disrupting the driving force for K^+ recycling; therefore, calcium and magnesium reabsorption decreases. Because of their hypercalciuric effects, loop diuretics are sometimes used to treat hypercalcemia in the volume-replete patient, although they are now generally reserved for prevention and treatment of hypervolemia in this setting [30].

Furosemide, bumetanide, and torsemide are absorbed from the gut within 30 min to 2 h following oral administration (Table 6.1). Delayed absorption may occur in the edematous patient due to bowel wall edema [31]; this problem is bypassed with intravenous therapy. Since the oral bioavailability of furosemide is as low as 50 %, when converting a patient from an intravenous to oral formulation, the dose is often doubled; the same does not hold for bumetanide and torsemide because the bioavailability is higher. Of these commonly used loop diuretics, furosemide is the only one which is cleared primarily by renal processes; in contrast, bumetanide and torsemide are largely metabolized in the liver. Consequently, the half-life of furosemide is increased in renal failure, whereas this is not the case for bumetanide or torsemide [32].

Owing to their efficacy, loop diuretics are among the most frequently prescribed drugs in the world. They are commonly used to treat most edematous conditions, including HF, renal failure, cirrhosis, and nephrotic syndrome. The treatment of these conditions is discussed in detail below (see Sect. 7, below).

Although the loop diuretics (particularly furosemide, bumetanide, and torsemide) are well tolerated, several adverse effects are associated with their clinical use. Due to their kaliuretic effects, hypokalemia is a common consequence of therapy, and serum potassium levels must be monitored regularly. Periodic replacement of magnesium and calcium may be required due to the enhanced urinary excretion of these divalent cations. As a consequence of increased sodium-dependent proton secretion and aldosterone activity, metabolic alkalosis is often observed in the setting of aggressive loop diuretic therapy [33].

Ototoxicity is the most common non-renal toxic effect observed with loop diuretic treatment, and is likely due to cross-reactivity against the secretory Na-K-2Cl isoform NKCC1, which is expressed in the lateral wall of the cochlear duct [34]. The hearing loss associated with loop diuretics is dependent on the peak level of drug in the bloodstream [35]. Consequently, this adverse effect is more commonly seen with intravenous therapy. Due to its renal clearance, intravenous furosemide must be administered with care to avoid ototoxicity in the patient with renal insufficiency. It has been recommended that furosemide infusion be no more rapid than 4 mg/min [36]. Ototoxicity may be more common with ethacrynic acid than the other loop diuretics. Although hearing loss is often reversible, permanent damage has been reported [36].

Like many other diuretics, furosemide, bumetanide, and torsemide are sulfonamide derivatives and should not be used in patients with severe sulfa allergies. Ethacrynic acid, on the other hand, is the only loop diuretic available in the United States that does not contain sulfa moieties, and is an effective alternative for the edematous sulfa allergic patient. The former manufacturer sold production rights for ethacrynic acid to another company; thus ethacrynic acid remains available as both an oral and intravenous preparation.

Distal Convoluted Tubule Diuretics

Thiazides, including chorothiazide and hydrochlorothiazide, and thiazide-like diuretics such as metolazone and chlorthalidone primarily act in the distal convoluted tubule (DCT). The major effect of these drugs is to suppress sodium chloride reabsorption in the DCT [37]. The molecular target of the DCT diuretics is the thiazide-sensitive Na-Cl cotransporter (NCC), which is responsible for reabsorbing approximately 5 % of the filtered NaCl load [37]. Given its anatomic position in the distal nephron, NCC plays an important role in "fine-tuning" the final concentration of NaCl in the urine. Consequently, in the setting of normal GFR, NCC-mediated NaCl reabsorption is one of the key renal mechanisms involved in the regulation of ECF volume [38].

Thiazides and thiazide-like diuretics are organic anions that bind to a luminally exposed site on NCC cotransporters expressed at the apical surface of DCT cells [39]. Thiazide binding interferes with the ability of NCC to translocate sodium and chloride ions from the DCT lumen. The increased natriuresis afforded by the DCT diuretics contracts ECF volume and reduces blood pressure, making them effective antihypertensive agents [40].

Structurally similar to CA inhibitors, thiazides also have modest inhibitory effects on proximal sodium transport. This proximal effect probably contributes little to the final urinary NaCl content [41]. It does, however, contribute to the changes in renal hemodynamics seen with thiazides. During *acute* administration, thiazides activate TGF, causing pre-glomerular vasoconstriction and a reduction in the glomerular filtration rate [42]. The ability of thiazides to inhibit CA likely plays some role in this process, since the decreased proximal Na reabsorption seen with CA inhibition increases sodium delivery to the loop of Henle and macula densa. The effect of thiazides to stimulate TGF is likely less of an issue during *chronic* administration, since the sustained reduction in ECF volume diminishes the delivery of solutes to the macula densa [43]. As one might expect, chronic thiazide treatment also enhances renin release due to decreased macula densa sodium chloride delivery [43].

When administered chronically, DCT diuretics decrease urinary calcium excretion, making them highly effective agents in the treatment of calcium nephrolithiasis [44]. Several mechanisms have been proposed to explain the hypocalciuric effect of thiazides. Recently, work in knockout mice lacking TRPV5, the major portal for calcium entry in the distal nephron, still exhibits thiazide-induced hypocalciuria due to enhanced calcium reabsorption [45]. This observation is likely a consequence of ECF volume contraction and enhanced proximal sodium-dependent calcium transport. Thus, the mechanism by which DCT diuretics exert their hypocalciuric effect is at least in part related to enhanced proximal calcium reabsorption. More recent studies, however, confirm an important effect of thiazide diuretics to reduce urinary calcium excretion, independent of changes in sodium balance [46]. In contrast to their pro-reabsorptive effects on calcium, chronic DCT diuretics increase urinary magnesium excretion

[47]. This may be due to the indirect effect of thiazides to suppress the expression of magnesium channels in the DCT, owing to structural effects [45]. Alternatively, thiazides might suppress magnesium reabsorption through the effects of the drug on the distal nephron transepithelial voltage [48].

DCT diuretics increase urinary potassium excretion [12]; this effect is largely due to the effects of thiazides and thiazide-like drugs on potassium secretion in the distal nephron. Chronic thiazide administration increases aldosterone concentrations, which facilitates distal potassium secretion via aldosterone-sensitive K channels in the late DCT and cortical collecting duct [12]. In addition, thiazides increase luminal sodium and chloride ionic content in the DCT; this tends to increase flow to downstream nephron segments and augment flow-dependent K secretion [49]. The hypomagnesemia seen with thiazide administration also likely contributes to the tendency for hypokalemia [50].

DCT diuretics are absorbed rather rapidly, reaching peak concentrations within 90 min to 4 h after ingestion [51]. The half-lives of DCT diuretics vary widely (Table 6.1). Of the agents commonly used in the United States, hydrochlorothiazide has a short half-life, while chlorthalidone and metolazone are longer-acting [51]. The extended half-life of chlorthalidone has been the subject of speculation that it may be a more potent diuretic and antihypertensive than hydrochlorothiazide [52]. A recent trial comparing the blood pressure lowering effects of these two drugs suggests that chlorthalidone might be a more effective antihypertensive agent, although the question of dose equivalency was difficult to resolve in this study [53].

The DCT diuretics have many clinical uses. In patients with normal GFR, thiazides are effective blood pressure-lowering agents commonly used to treat essential hypertension [54]. The guidelines of the Seventh Report of the Joint National Committee of Prevention, Detection, Evaluation, and Treatment of High Blood Pressure (JNC-7) recommend that thiazides should be first-line agents in the treatment of essential hypertension [55]. DCT diuretics are also commonly used as monotherapy to treat edematous disorders such as HF, but they are usually considered less potent than loop diuretics in achieving a substantial diuresis HF [26]. Thiazides and thiazide-like diuretics are, however, very effective in the treatment of edematous patients who have become resistant to loop diuretics (see Sect. 7, below). Owing to their hypocalciuric effects, the DCT diuretics are the treatment of choice for patients with idiopathic hypercalciuria and nephrolithiasis [44]. In nephrogenic diabetes insipidus, thiazides exert a paradoxical antidiuretic effect, and this has been used as an effective treatment of the disorder. Although the mechanism for the antidiuretic effect of thiazides remains unclear, these drugs appear to increase collecting duct water channel expression, increasing free water reabsorption [56, 57]. Other potential mechanisms include thiazide-induced TGF activation (as described above), which would reduce GFR and distal water delivery [42].

As with the other classes of diuretics, thiazides and thiazide-like diuretic agents are generally well tolerated, but several potential adverse effects deserve mention. Hyponatremia can be observed with all classes of diuretics, but is particularly common with DCT diuretic therapy [58]. In fact, hyponatremia can become severe enough in the setting of DCT diuretic therapy to become life threatening. There are at least three mechanisms which contribute to the hyponatremia that can accompany DCT diuretic therapy. First, the inhibition of solute reabsorption in the distal convoluted tubule impairs free water excretion (see above). Second, thiazides increase proximal Na reabsorption and inhibit TGF (see above); these effects impair solute and water delivery to the distal nephron, reducing free water clearance. Finally, thiazide treatment stimulates thirst centers in the brain, increasing water consumption [59]. Risk factors for thiazide-induced hyponatremia include female gender, low total body mass, and advanced age [58].

DCT diuretics induce disturbances related to glucose and lipid metabolism. DCT diuretics cause a dose-dependent increase in glucose intolerance [60, 61]. This observation was initially made in the 1950s, and was thought to be a complication only seen in patients treated with high doses of diuretics. More recent studies, however, have revealed that glucose intolerance may be seen even with lower doses of DCT diuretics. In ALLHAT, the largest blood pressure lowering randomized controlled trial conducted to date, the incidence of new-onset diabetes was significantly higher in the chlorthalidone-treated group compared to groups treated with amlodipine or lisinopril (11.9 % vs. 9.8 % or 8.1 %, respectively) [40]. The mechanism by which DCT diuretics cause glucose intolerance is not entirely clear, but may be related to the degree of diuretic-induced hypokalemia, which may alter insulin secretion by pancreatic beta cells and glucose uptake by muscle [62]. This was recently supported by a quantitative review of 59 clinical trials of thiazide diuretics in which blood glucose and potassium levels were reported; the results of this study suggested a dose-dependent inverse relationship between blood glucose and serum potassium levels in patients treated with thiazides [63]. Thus, the risk of new-onset diabetes associated with DCT diuretic therapy may be ameliorated if potassium levels are monitored closely and maintained within the normal range. The DCT diuretics also increase the levels of total cholesterol, low-density lipoprotein, and triglycerides, and reduce HDL. Although the mechanisms underlying the effects of these drugs on the lipid profile remain unclear, they are probably linked to those that lead to impaired glucose tolerance. Like the effects of DCT diuretics on blood glucose, their hyperlipidemic effects are dose dependent. In ALLHAT, the mean total cholesterol concentrations were higher in the group randomized to chlorthalidone, and averaged 2–3 mg/dl higher than the other treatment arms [40].

Cortical Collecting Tubule Natriuretics

Three pharmacologically distinct groups of drugs act to inhibit sodium reabsorption in the cortical collecting tubule: mineralocorticoid receptor antagonists (spirolactones), pteridines (triamterene), and pyrazine-carbonyl-guanidines (amiloride). These agents have a tendency to *minimize* potassium secretion rather than promote it, as is commonly seen with diuretics which act on other segments of the nephron. For this reason, the cortical collecting tubule natriuretics are collectively known as "potassium-sparing diuretics."

The site of action of potassium-sparing diuretics is the aldosterone-sensitive distal nephron (ASDN), which by current definitions includes the late distal convoluted tubule, connecting tubule, and cortical collecting duct [38]. This is the final site of sodium reabsorption in the kidney, and is responsible for reclaiming approximately 3 % of the filtered NaCl load. Ultimately, the effect of the potassium-sparing diuretics is to inhibit sodium transport by the aldosterone-sensitive epithelial sodium channel (ENaC). ENaC channels selectively reabsorb sodium ions, and their synthesis and expression at the apical surface of cells of the ASDN are tightly controlled by the mineralocorticoid hormone aldosterone [64]. The potassium-sparing effect of these diuretics is largely due to their ability to inhibit ENaC (Fig. 6.3); blocking the reabsorption of sodium cations in the collecting tubule decreases the lumen negativity of the segment, which diminishes the driving force for potassium and hydrogen ion secretion [65].

The *spirolactones* inhibit aldosterone action by binding to intracellular mineralocorticoid receptors in the ASDN. This causes the retention of mineralocorticoid receptors in the cytoplasm and prevents their nuclear translocation, rendering them unable to promote the transcription of aldosterone-induced gene products [66]. Because of their effects on gene transcription, the spirolactones have a delayed onset of action, and may not reach their peak natriuretic effects until several days after starting the drug [51]. Spironolactone has at least a tenfold higher binding affinity to the mineralocorticoid receptor than its newer cousin eplerenone, but has a greater tendency to activate the cytochrome P450 system [67]. Although the half-life of spironolactone is short, it has long-acting metabolites that greatly prolong its functional half-life. Although *amiloride* and *triamterene* are structurally different, both of these compounds bind directly to ENaC and inhibit its activity [68, 69]. At higher doses, amiloride inhibits multiple ion transport pathways, most notably the sodium hydrogen

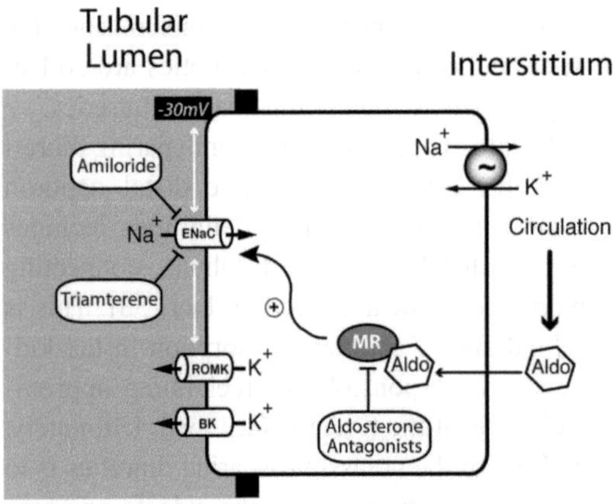

Fig. 6.3 Mechanisms of action of collecting duct natriuretics. Diagram of a connecting or cortical collecting duct cell illustrating major pathways for sodium entry and potassium secretion. In the collecting duct, sodium reabsorption via the epithelial sodium channel (ENaC) is electrogenic, and generates a lumen-negative voltage of −30 mV. This voltage provides the driving force for potassium secretion via the renal outer medullary potassium channel (ROMK). All collecting duct natriuretics ultimately suppress ENaC-mediated Na reabsorption. Their "potassium-sparing" effect derives from the reduced potassium secretion seen with the dissipation of the voltage gradient. Amiloride and triamterene block luminal Na^+ entry by binding to the channel, while the aldosterone antagonists such as spironolactone interfere with cell signaling processes that stimulate ENaC by blocking aldosterone binding to the mineralocorticoid receptor (MR)

exchangers; this effect however is not as relevant with respect to the low doses of the drug that are used in clinical practice. All of the potassium-sparing diuretics are weak natriuretics, increase sodium excretion in normal subjects by no more than 1–2 % [2]. In clinical practice, triamterene has weaker diuretic potency than either amiloride or spironolactone.

The mineralocorticoid receptor antagonists are effective natriuretics that reduce blood pressure in patients with hyperaldosteronism [70]. This is true for patients with primary aldosterone excess from either adrenal adenomas or bilateral adrenal hyperplasia, or secondary hyperaldosteronism from HF, cirrhosis, or nephritic syndrome. Conversely, spironolactone and eplerenone are ineffective in inducing a natriuresis in patients with a nonfunctional adrenal gland. With regard to the secondary hyperaldosteronemic disorders, spironolactone and eplerenone are particularly effective when used with loop diuretics and ACE inhibitors to treat HF [71, 72]. RALES and EPHESUS were two large randomized placebo-controlled trials in which patients with advanced HF were treated with spironolactone and eplerenone, respectively. In both trials, aldosterone antagonist therapy reduced the risk of all-cause mortality in patients with chronic HF and left ventricular dysfunction following acute myocardial infarction. Although a non-renal effect may confer the mortality-reducing benefits seen in these studies, a current debate exists in the literature as to whether the benefit of these agents is related to the prevention of hypokalemia, a known risk factor for sudden cardiac death hypokalemia [73].

In addition, owing to its inhibitory effect on aldosterone activity, spironolactone has been shown to be a more effective diuretic than furosemide in the treatment of cirrhotic ascites [74] (see Sect. 7, below).

Amiloride and triamterene are commonly used in combination with loop or thiazide diuretics to reduce potassium loss and the risk of hypokalemia. Amiloride has been used to treat primary hyperaldosteronism [75] or other potassium wasting states such as Liddle's, Bartter's, or Gitelman's syndrome [76, 77]; the weak potency of triamterene renders it incapable of treating these disorders. Amiloride has also been used to treat lithium-induced nephrogenic diabetes insipidus. The beneficial effect of amiloride in this disorder stems from its ability to block the intracellular entry of lithium ions through the ENaC pore [78].

The major adverse effect encountered with the use of spironolactone or eplerenone is hyperkalemia [79]. Patients that are particularly at risk for hyperkalemia include those with decreased GFR and those that are on active potassium supplementation. Consequently, prior to starting therapy with a mineralocorticoid receptor antagonist, all potassium supplements must be stopped and serum potassium levels should be monitored. Spironolactone exerts other endocrine effects due to its cross-reactivity with androgen and progesterone receptors [71, 80]. Gynecomastia is a common side effect in males; in RALES, the incidence was 10 % [71]. Other common symptoms in males include breast tenderness, decreased libido, and impotence. Females may experience breast tenderness, hirsutism, or irregular menses. Eplerenone, in contrast, appears to have greater specificity for the mineralocorticoid receptor. In EPHESUS, the incidence of impotence and gynecomastia in men taking eplerenone was not different from placebo [72].

Due to their potassium sparing effects, amiloride and triamterene can cause hyperkalemia, and should be avoided in patients with low GFR or those who are taking potassium supplements. Triamterene can promote the formation of renal stones by acting as a nidus for the precipitation of uric acid or calcium oxalate [81]. Consequently, this drug is contraindicated in stone formers. In addition, triamterene has been reported to be associated with acute kidney injury, particularly when used in combination with indomethacin [82, 83].

Osmotic Diuretics

Osmotic diuretics are substances that are freely filtered at the glomerulus but are poorly reabsorbed. The ability of these drugs to provoke a diuresis is dependent on their ability to generate an osmotic gradient within the tubular lumen. Thus, the osmotic diuretics do not exert their diuretic effects through a specific molecular target. Mannitol is the osmotic diuretic used most commonly in clinical practice. Mannitol infusion increases the urinary excretion of water, sodium, calcium, magnesium, and phosphorus [84, 85]. Once mannitol is freely filtered at the glomerulus, its presence in the proximal tubule lumen offsets the osmotic gradient that is usually generated by the net reabsorption of sodium through specific transport mechanisms. This minimizes proximal water reabsorption. As the glomerular filtrate travels down the nephron, non-reabsorbable mannitol ions replace sodium as the predominant element contributing to the urine osmolality. The relative displacement of sodium ions decreases the driving force for sodium reabsorption in multiple nephron segments including the thin loop of Henle and collecting duct; this results in a net increase in the fractional excretion of Na [84, 85]. In addition, cortical and medullary renal blood flow is increased [11, 86]. Cortical increases in renal blood flow contribute to an increase in the urine flow rate, resulting in a net diuresis. The increase in medullary renal blood flow "washes out" the papillary sodium and urea content; this impairs the urinary concentrating mechanism, perpetuating mannitol's diuretic effect [87].

Since mannitol cannot be absorbed from the GI tract [88], it is administered intravenously. It has a plasma half-life of approximately 2 h and is almost entirely cleared by the kidneys [89]. Its osmotic properties are beneficial as an acute treatment to lower increases in intraocular or intracranial pressure [90]. Mannitol is also used as prophylaxis against the dialysis disequilibrium syndrome, a disorder that typically occurs in patients with severe azotemia who are initiating hemodialysis [91, 92]. In this syndrome, patients develop postdialytic acute central nervous system symptoms, such as nausea, blurred vision, confusion, headaches, and seizures. The rapid removal of solutes such as urea results in the development of an osmotic gradient that favors the movement of water into brain cells [92]. This fluid shift leads to cerebral edema and neurological dysfunction. To reduce the magnitude of the osmotic gradient, mannitol is sometimes infused during the dialysis treatment to boost the plasma osmolality.

Many of the adverse effects of mannitol treatment are related to problems that can develop if it is poorly cleared from the circulation, or if too much of it is administered too quickly. Mannitol infusion increases the pulmonary capillary wedge pressure and can cause pulmonary edema in patients with impaired left ventricular function. Overzealous use acutely leads to dilution of the plasma bicarbonate and sodium concentrations, causing metabolic acidosis and hyponatremia [93]. In addition, acute high-dose mannitol infusion promotes the extracellular movement of potassium and causes hyperkalemia [94]. Prolonged mannitol treatment depletes total body potassium, leading to hypokalemia. Excessive losses of sodium and water cause volume depletion, and since electrolyte-free water is excreted

Table 6.2 V2 Receptor antagonists currently under development or in clinical use

Compound	Receptor	Route	Current status
Conivaptan (YM-087)	V1a+V2	Intravenous	FDA approved for treatment of euvolemic and hypervolemic hyponatremia
Tolvaptan (OPC 41–061)	V2	Oral	FDA approved for treatment of euvolemic and hypervolemic hyponatremia
Lixivaptan (VPA-985)	V2	Oral	Phase 3 clinical trials in hyponatremic patients with heart failure
Satavaptan (SR-121463)	V2	Oral	Phase 3 clinical trials in hyponatremic patients with ascites

in excess relative to sodium, hypernatremia develops [95]. In extreme cases of mannitol intoxication, the drug can be rapidly removed from the circulation with hemodialysis mannitol [96].

Aquaretics (Vasopressin Receptor Antagonists)

The vasopressin receptor antagonists promote the excretion of solute-free water, and thus are known as "aquaretics." One of these agents is currently available for intravenous administration. Oral analogues are currently the subject of clinical trials, designed to determine their efficacy and clinical use in various disease states. As discussed in detail below, they hold promise for serving as effective diuretics to treat edematous conditions accompanied by hyponatremia owing to the excessive release of arginine vasopressin (AVP, antidiuretic hormone).

The vasopressin receptor antagonists are competitive inhibitors of AVP action in water-reabsorptive segments of the nephron. The actions of AVP are carried out by two receptors, V1 and V2. V1 receptors are divided into two major subtypes. V1a receptors are expressed in multiple tissues, including vascular smooth muscle, platelets, and myocardium. V1b receptors are predominantly found in cells of the anterior pituitary gland. V2 receptors are predominantly localized to principal cells of the distal nephron, including the connecting tubule and cortical and medullary collecting duct [97]. During states of high osmolality or extreme ECF volume contraction, AVP is released from its storage centers in the posterior pituitary. Once the hormone binds to V2 receptors located at the basolateral membrane of distal nephron principal cells, it triggers a cyclic AMP-dependent signaling cascade that leads to an increase in the expression of aquaporin-2 water channels at the luminal surface. Ultimately, this enhances water reabsorption and normalizes the serum osmolality and extracellular fluid volume. Although some of the vasopressin receptor antagonists show cross-reactivity towards V1 receptors, all of the members of the class competitively inhibit AVP binding to V2 receptors; binding of the drug to these receptors thus decreases water reabsorption, enhancing free water excretion and urinary flow [97].

V2 receptor antagonists that are currently being clinically used or are under development for commercial use are listed in Table 6.2. To date, the Food and Drug Administration has only approved one member of the class, conivaptan, for clinical use in the United States. Conivaptan (YM-087) is a vasopressin receptor antagonist that exhibits activity towards both V1a and V2 receptors [98]. Clinical trials illustrate its diuretic potency. In one study performed in healthy volunteers, oral conivaptan increased urinary flow by sevenfold and reduced urinary osmolality from 600 mOsm/kg to less than 100 mOsm/kg within 2 h of administration [99]. In accordance with studies performed in laboratory animals, the peak effect of conivaptan was seen 2 h after giving the dose, and persisted for at least 6 h. Despite the oral efficacy seen in this study, there are concerns about its interactions with other drugs metabolized by the CYP3A4 pathway, so the agent has been developed for clinical use as an intravenous preparation only [97]. The primary FDA-approved indication for conivaptan use was for the treatment of euvolemic hyponatremia in hospitalized patients, but this has recently been hypervolemic hyponatremia, as well. The initial approval was based on a double-blinded placebo-controlled study of 56 patients with euvolemic hyponatremia. In this trial, a loading dose, followed by a 4-day continuous infusion at 20 or 40 mg/day increased the serum Na concentration at least 4 mEq/l from the baseline concentration at the start of the study [97]. Conivaptan was also shown to correct hyponatremia in decompensated CHF during 4 days of intravenous infusion [100].

Tolvaptan (OPC-41061) is an oral once-daily vasopressin receptor antagonist that exhibits higher selectivity for V2 receptors. This agent has received much attention due to several recent clinical studies evaluating its utility in hyponatremic and edematous disorders, particularly CHF. Although the drug is currently not FDA approved for the treatment of these conditions, it may become clinically available in the near future. In ACTIV in CHF [101], patients with New York Heart Association class III or IV HF were treated with between 30 and 90 mg of tolvaptan or placebo and were reassessed at 24 h or 7 weeks post treatment. In this study, the tolvaptan-treated patients exhibited decreased edema and body weight and a higher serum sodium compared to the placebo arm. No changes in serum potassium levels, heart rate, or blood pressure were noted. Although these findings illustrate the diuretic potency of tolvaptan, no significant difference in rate of rehospitalization was appreciated. These data were very recently echoed in two papers describing the short- and long-term results from the Efficacy of Vasopressin Antagonism in Heart Failure Outcome Study with Tolvaptan (EVEREST) [102, 103]. EVEREST was a large-scale randomized placebo-controlled trial that evaluated the effect of a 30 mg daily dose of tolvaptan on the outcomes of more than 4,000 patients with decompensated CHF. The aggregate results implicate tolvaptan as a safe and effective treatment that is capable of reducing some of the adverse symptoms of decompensated HF, when added to current pharmacologic standard of care. The observed improvement in CHF symptoms was related to the diuretic effect of tolvaptan, since the beneficial change in symptom score was driven by a reduction in body weight. It is important to note however that despite adequate power, there was no measurable beneficial effect of tolvaptan on the long-term composite primary end point of all-cause mortality or rehospitalization for HF.

The Studies of Ascending Levels of Tolvaptan (SALT-1 and SALT-2) were identical randomized double-blinded placebo-controlled trials conducted in parallel in Europe and the United States [104]. Both of these trials enrolled more than 200 hyponatremic patients with normal or expanded ECF volume, and randomized them to treatment with 15 mg tolvaptan per day or placebo. Based on the serum sodium levels, the dose could be increased to 30 or 60 mg/day. The results of these studies demonstrated that tolvaptan significantly increased the serum sodium concentration relative to patients receiving placebo. No significant changes in renal function, blood pressure, or heart rate were noted, and the serum Na concentration fell back to baseline within 7 days of stopping the drug. Consistent with other studies of vasopressin receptor antagonists, the observations from SALT-1 and SALT-2 suggest that tolvaptan may be an effective acute treatment for hyponatremia.

As mentioned above, tolvaptan is currently not FDA approved for the treatment of hyponatremia or CHF. It did, however, recently receive a "Fast-Track" designation from the FDA for the treatment of autosomal dominant polycystic kidney disease (ADPKD). The Fast-Track designation was granted on the basis of a current lack of effective treatments for ADPKD, and empiric evidence suggesting that vasopressin receptor antagonists may reduce cystic fluid accumulation, expansion, and rupture [105, 106]. Phase III clinical trials are currently being conducted to determine the role of tolvaptan in reducing ADPKD symptoms and disease progression.

The side effect profile of the vasopressin receptor antagonists continues to evolve. Major side effects that have been reported during treatment include dry mouth and thirst. As one might expect, hypernatremia has been observed; consequently, serum sodium levels should be closely monitored during treatment. Infusion site reactions are common during conivaptan therapy, occurring in greater than 63 % of subjects treated at a dose higher than 20 mg/day, according to the package insert. Conivaptan and tolvaptan are both primarily metabolized by the cytochrome P450 isoenzyme CYP3A4, and their concentrations may be increased by CYP3A4 inhibitors, including ketoconazole, indinavir, and clarithromycin [98]. Concomitant use of these agents is contraindicated. In addition, conivaptan and tolvaptan inhibit CYP3A4 activity, so their use with drugs that are metabolized by the isoenzyme (including some HMG CoA reductase inhibitors) should be avoided if possible. Conivaptan reduces the rate of digoxin clearance, and clinicians should be aware of the possibility that blood digoxin levels may rise. Tolvaptan, in contrast, does not significantly affect the serum digoxin concentration [97].

Clinical Use of Diuretics

General Concepts

Determinants of Maximal Diuresis

The change in urinary flow seen during the administration of a diuretic depends on many factors, including its mechanism of action, dose, kinetics of entry into the bloodstream, and delivery to its site of action.

In many cases, the site of action of a diuretic determines its potency. For example, loop diuretics are more potent than the DCT diuretics such as hydrochlorothiazide. This observation is largely related to the fact that loop diuretics inhibit a transport pathway responsible for reabsorbing up to 30 % of the filtered sodium load, while DCT diuretics inhibit a pathway responsible for reabsorbing only 5–10 %. Similarly, mineralocorticoid antagonists have a mild natriuretic effect due to the fact that they suppress a pathway responsible for reabsorbing only 3 % of the filtered Na load. There are, of course, exceptions to this rule. The carbonic anhydrase inhibitors, which reduce proximal tubule reabsorption, are only weakly natriuretic due to adaptive changes in the loop of Henle and DCT [10].

Diuretic efficacy is highly dependent on the kinetics of drug entry into the bloodstream. The dynamics of drug absorption may be perturbed in certain clinical situations, and this might result in a diminished effect. This is exemplified by the pharmacokinetics of furosemide. In normal individuals, the rate of furosemide absorption from the GI tract is not rapid, and a reservoir of drug can persist long after the diuretic is administered [51]. This reservoir provides a consistent source of diuretic that, when dosed appropriately, maintains the blood furosemide concentrations above the natriuretic threshold. In certain edematous states, however, impaired absorption from the gut may slow furosemide absorption to a point where it dips *below* the diuretic threshold, rendering it ineffective [31]. To compensate for this, switching to different loop diuretics with higher bioavailabilities, such as torsemide or bumetanide, might facilitate a brisker diuresis [107]. Another even more effective approach would be to switch to an intravenous loop diuretic preparation, which is of course 100 % bioavailable.

The effectiveness of a diuretic is also dependent on its rate of delivery to its site of action. In the case of furosemide, its rate of delivery to NKCC2 binding sites in the tubular lumen can be inferred by measuring the rate of urinary furosemide excretion. If the rate of urinary furosemide excretion is low, few binding sites are inhibited, leading to poor diuretic effectiveness. Conversely, a high rate of furosemide delivery will lead to diuretic inefficiency, since any furosemide molecules in excess of the total number of binding sites will be wasted as they move past their sites of action and into the collecting system. Brater established that diuretics such as furosemide have an *excretion rate of maximal efficiency*, i.e., a rate of diuretic delivery that is associated with a maximal natriuretic response [108]. This concept helps to explain why an orally administered dose of furosemide can be more effective than an equivalent single intravenous dose in individuals with normal GI absorption (Fig. 6.4). When a dose of furosemide is given as an intravenous bolus, the rate of diuretic excretion is very high early on in the time course, substantially greater than the rate of maximal

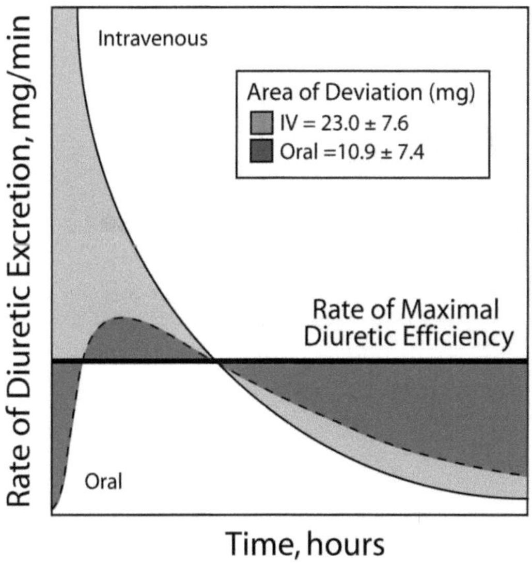

Fig. 6.4 Time course of urinary furosemide excretion following intravenous (*solid line*) and oral (*dashed line*) dosing. The curves are shown in relation to the furosemide excretion rate with maximal efficiency (*thick solid line*). Following a bolus intravenous dose, a large area of deviation from the max efficiency rate (*light gray shading*) is observed. This is greater than the area of deviation seen with the equivalent oral dose (*dark gray shading*), illustrating that the overall efficiency of oral dosing is greater than bolus intravenous dosing. Note: These findings are only relevant in individuals with normal gastrointestinal absorption kinetics. Adapted from ref. [108]

efficiency. This rate tapers down over time, but the curve quickly dips below the maximal efficiency rate. In contrast, oral administration of the same dose of diuretic reaches the bloodstream more gradually due to "absorption-limited" kinetics. Thus, a constant reservoir of furosemide is present in the GI tract, and when optimized, the rate of absorption into the bloodstream (and hence, the rate of furosemide delivery to its site of action in the urinary space) keeps the circulating level above the natriuretic threshold and close to the rate of maximal diuretic efficiency for a longer period. When the kidney becomes less responsive to a diuretic, however, the same situation may not hold true. For example, a patient with edema from heart failure may demonstrate an increased natriuretic threshold (above the horizontal line, in Fig. 6.4). In this case, an intravenous dose may be effective, when an oral dose is not, because the oral dose does not lead to serum levels above the natriuretic threshold.

With the exception of the mineralocorticoid receptor antagonists and aquaretics, all diuretics must access the tubule lumen to mediate their effects. Thus, they must be delivered to their site of action by either glomerular filtration or tubular secretion. Since most diuretics are tightly bound to albumin, they primarily access the urinary space via secretion, particularly in the proximal tubule. Loop and DCT diuretics and CA inhibitors are negatively charged, and they are transported into the tubular lumen via the proximal organic anion secretory pathway. Two basolateral organic anion transporters (OAT-1 and OAT-3) transport thiazides, loop diuretics, and CA inhibitors into the proximal tubule epithelial cell [109]. In order to facilitate this process, OAT-1 and OAT-3 exchange anions with intracellular α(alpha)-ketoglutarate. The pathways for the apical secretion of organic anions are less well defined, but likely involve voltage-driven mechanisms and/or urate countertransport [110]. Amiloride and triamterene are organic cations that are transported to the proximal tubule lumen via the organic cation transport pathway. Basolateral entry is mediated by OCTs, organic cation transporters that facilitate the diffusion of cations in either direction [111]. Apical efflux of organic cations is carried out by an organic cation/proton exchange mechanism.

These transport processes are relatively nonspecific, and a single transporter type can facilitate the movement of a variety of similarly charged molecules into the tubular lumen. Accordingly, any exogenous or endogenous substance that competes with a diuretic for one of these transport processes can potentially limit the efficient arrival of that diuretic to its site of action. For instance, cimetidine, an organic cation, has been shown to inhibit the tubular secretion of creatinine [112]. Several substances, including nonsteroidal anti-inflammatory drugs, probenecid, penicillins, and uremic anions, all compete with loop and thiazide diuretics for tubular secretion probenecid [113, 114]. In certain disease states, competition between different drugs or endogenous substances for transport to the tubular lumen

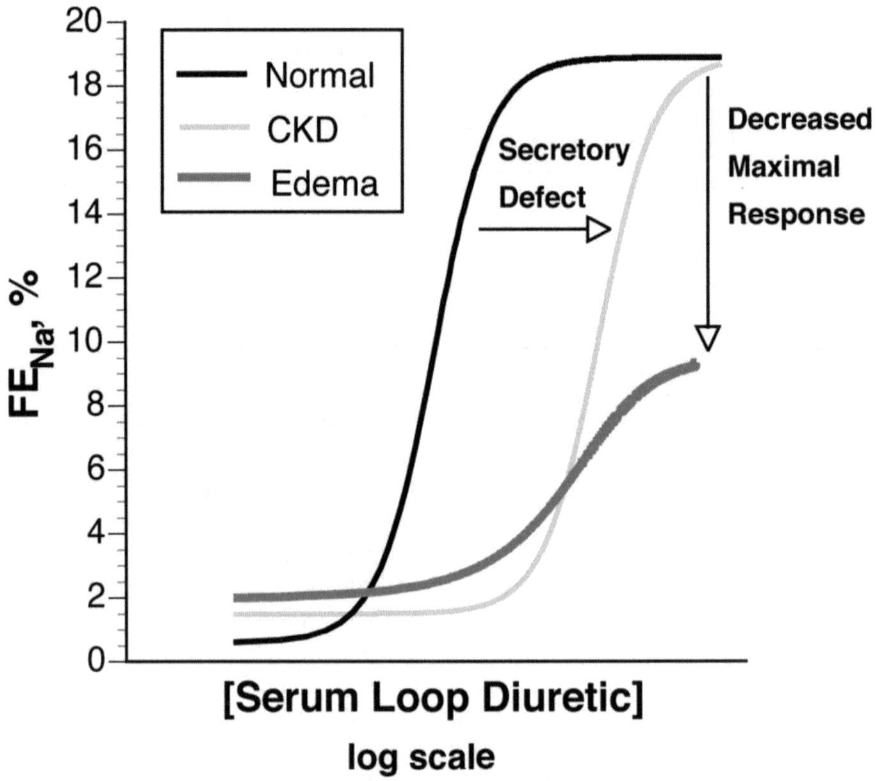

Fig. 6.5 Dose response for loop diuretics. The fractional sodium excretion (FENa) is plotted versus the logarithm of the serum diuretic concentration. In patients with chronic kidney disease (CKD) the curve is shifted to the right, but the maximal natriuresis is unchanged. In patients with edema, such as heart failure, the curve is shifted down and to the right

may lead to diuretic resistance. The prototypical example of such a condition is chronic kidney disease (CKD), in which diuretic delivery to the urine is impaired [32]. In CKD, impaired drug delivery shifts the diuretic dose response curve to the right, and a higher dose is required to achieve a diuretic effect (Fig. 6.5). This potentially could unmask the competitive effects of two different pharmacologic agents on an organic ion transport process, since a slight decrease in the rate of transport of the diuretic to the urinary space could make the tubular diuretic concentration fall beneath its threshold of effectiveness.

Diuretic Adaptation and Resistance

Typically, the brisk increase in urinary solute and water excretion following each dose of diuretic wanes during the first week of treatment. This phenomenon occurs because certain renal and systemic adaptations take place in response to diuretic therapy. Early on in treatment, diuretic adaptation helps to protect the body from ECF volume depletion and maintain volume homeostasis in the presence of daily diuretic dosing. Eventually, however, these adaptive changes can counteract the ability of the diuretic to reduce edema, and thus become a major cause of diuretic resistance.

Diuretic adaptations can be generally classified into immediate, short-term, and chronic changes [2]. *Immediate adaptations* refer to the instantaneous changes in sodium transport that the kidney undergoes *during* the period of diuretic-induced natriuresis. An example of an immediate diuretic adaptation would be the increased sodium reabsoprtion seen in the loop of Henle during active carbonic anhydrase inhibition by acetazolamide (see above). As discussed, this effect is a major factor that limits the natriuretic effectiveness of carbonic anhydrase inhibitors. Coadministration of a loop diuretic with a carbonic anhydrase inhibitor can limit sodium reabsorption in the TAL and counteract the immediate diuretic adaptations seen during CA inhibition.

Short-term adaptation refers to the tendency of sodium reabsorptive processes in the kidney to rebound once the drug concentration of a diuretic falls beneath the natriuretic threshold. This phenomenon is often referred to as "post-diuretic NaCl retention," and has been attributed to three factors. First, short-term changes occur in response to an acute decrease in ECF volume. These effects are both renal and systemic and involve the activation of the renin-angiotensin-aldosterone axis and sympathetic nervous system, changes in GFR, and suppression of atrial natriuretic peptide secretion (reviewed in ref. [115]). The net effect of these responses is to enhance renal NaCl retention in an effort to increase ECF volume. Second, the decline of a diuretic drug concentration to a level beneath the natriuretic threshold induces rebound effects at its direct site of action. For example, in the case of loop diuretics, the number of NKCC2 cotransporters expressed at the apical surface of the TAL increases in response to a reduction in intracellular chloride concentration [116]. While a loop diuretic is present in the lumen of the TAL at its appropriate therapeutic concentration, this cellular response is ineffective at increasing sodium reabsorption, since any NKCC2 cotransporter reaching the luminal surface of the TAL epithelium will be inhibited by the drug. Once the dose of loop diuretic drops beneath its therapeutic threshold, however, the inhibitory effect is unmasked and Na-K-2Cl cotransport will be increased to a higher rate than baseline. Third, post-diuretic NaCl retention occurs as a consequence of changes in sodium chloride reabsorption at nephron segments downstream of the diuretic's molecular site of action. In the case of loop diuretic therapy, the number of thiazide-sensitive cotransporters in the DCT increases as early as 60 min following the drug administration [117]. This effect is likely a consequence of changes in the luminal sodium chloride concentration, which activates molecular mechanisms that stimulate NCC synthesis and delivery to the DCT apical surface.

Chronic adaptations are those mechanisms that cause the "braking phenomenon," which refers to the tendency of daily dosed diuretics to lose their effectiveness over time as NaCl balance returns to neutral. The braking phenomenon is likely due to a combination of factors. These factors include those that contribute to post-diuretic NaCl retention, such as the chronic intermittent stimulation of the sympathetic nervous and renin-angiotensin-aldosterone systems from ECF volume contraction. But other, more long-term changes also take place. One of the most significant of these is the capacity of chronic diuretic therapy to induce structural changes in the epithelium lining the nephron. Specifically, chronic diuretic therapy can lead to both hypertrophy and hyperplasia of sodium chloride-reabsorbing cells [118, 119]. These effects act together to enhance the sodium chloride reabsorbing capacity of the nephron, which ultimately leads to the braking phenomenon. For instance, in the case of chronic loop diuretic infusion, as little as 7 days of continuous treatment with furosemide increases the number and size of distal convoluted cells in the kidney [118, 119]. Accordingly, this also increases the total number of active thiazide-sensitive NaCl cotransporters in the DCT [118, 120, 121]. These changes result in enhanced DCT sodium chloride reabsorption, which undermines the therapeutic effectiveness of loop diuretics and contributes to diuretic resistance. Since chronic loop diuretic therapy increases the fraction of thiazide-sensitive NaCl reabsorption, combining a low-dose thiazide with a loop diuretic can be a highly effective approach to counteracting resistance (see below).

Approach to the Treatment of Generalized Edema

Edema is a direct consequence of an increase in capillary hydrostatic pressure or permeability, an increase in interstitial oncotic pressure, or a

Table 6.3 Causes of generalized edema

Increased capillary hydrostatic pressure
Heart failure
Cirrhosis
Nephrotic syndrome
Drug-induced Minoxidil Diazoxide Calcium channel blockers (e.g., Nifedipine) Estrogens Corticosteroids
Premenstrual edema
Reduced capillary oncotic pressure
Cirrhosis
Malnutrition
Nephrotic syndrome
Protein-losing enteropathy
Increased interstitial oncotic pressure
Hypothyroidism
Increased microvascular permeability
Allergic reactions, anaphylaxis, angioedema
Sepsis
Bone marrow transplant [122]
Drug-induced Calcium channel blockers Interleukin-2 therapy

reduction in capillary oncotic pressure. Under any of these circumstances, a shift in vessel hemodynamics occurs, and fluid moves from the intravascular space to the interstitium. As with any clinical sign or symptom, the first step towards treatment is to identify the underlying clinical disorder. The differential diagnosis of generalized edema is broad and can be classified by the four major factors that dictate capillary hemodynamics (Table 6.3) [122].

Renal salt and water retention is crucial in the pathogenesis of generalized edema. In the case of acute kidney injury or CKD with reduced GFR, the retention of salt and water results primarily from renal parenchymal damage, which reduces the number of functional nephrons that are capable of excreting electrolytes and water. In all other disorders that result in generalized edema, the renal NaCl and water retention is a secondary, compensatory phenomenon. In these clinical situations, fluid movement from the intravascular space to the interstitium results in a reduction in capillary hydrostatic pressure and "effective" arterial blood volume (EABV). The reduction in EABV is sensed by the homeostatic mechanisms involved in the preservation of tissue perfusion and stimulates the reabsorption of sodium and water by the kidney. These mechanisms include neurohormonal responses to low intravascular blood volume that culminate in the release of catecholamines, renin, and vasopressin [123].

The treatment of generalized edema consists of four key interventions: optimizing treatment of the underlying disorder, dietary sodium and fluid restriction, measures to mobilize fluid from edematous tissues, and diuretic drug therapy.

Treating the Edema-Causing Disorder

Initial attempts at treating edema should be directed at identifying its underlying cause and optimizing disease management. In the case of HF, this might involve assessing cardiac function with diagnostic studies such as echocardiography, ruling out dietary indiscretion, medication noncompliance, or an ischemic insult to the myocardium which might have compromised cardiac output, or optimizing the medication regimen with inotropes or improved afterload reduction. The treatment of HF and other common edematous states is discussed in greater detail below.

Dietary Sodium and Fluid Restriction

As mentioned above, every patient with generalized edema suffers from excessive renal sodium and water retention, either from primary renal dysfunction or secondary compensatory homeostatic mechanisms directed towards preserving EABV. Consequently, patients with edema are sensitive to fluctuations in dietary sodium and water intake, and an acute ingestion of sodium above baseline can dramatically worsen an edematous state. Sodium restriction is an essential component in the management of ECF volume expansion. Typically, dietary sodium is restricted to 2 g (88 mEq) per day and should be sufficient for maintaining neutral sodium balance as long as measures are being taken to increase sodium excretion (i.e., diuretic therapy). Generally, in edematous states, negative fluid balance cannot be achieved solely by restricting dietary sodium, since the kidneys of patients with these disorders are unable to increase Na excretion above the level of Na intake. Thus, sodium restriction does not reverse the severity of edema, but rather only prevents the edema from worsening.

Common edematous disorders, such as HF, nephrotic syndrome, and cirrhosis, are in part caused by a defect in water excretion [124]. In each of these conditions, water can be retained in excess of sodium, leading to hypervolemic hyponatremia. Although fluid restriction is not indicated for edema in the absence of hyponatremia [1], fluid restriction should be recommended when hyponatremia supervenes. The typical inpatient recommendation of fluid restriction to 2 l/24 h is often not stringent enough, and restricting fluid intake to 1 or 1.5 l/24 h may be necessary to achieve the desired results. Realistically, fluid restriction is extremely difficult to accomplish in outpatients given multiple factors, the most important of which is the excess thirst caused by excess vasopressin release.

Mobilization of Edema

Once edema fluid transudes into the interstitium of peripheral tissues, it can be difficult to recruit back into the intravascular space. This is at least in part related to the pooling of fluid into gravity-dependent areas. By altering the effect of gravity, edema fluid can be moved from pooled compartments in the interstitium, thus leading to increased venous return. Bed rest can be highly effective in mobilizing edema fluid from peripheral tissues, although this may raise the risk for venous thrombosis . Alternatively, patients with leg edema can achieve a similar effect if they elevate their lower extremities above the level of the heart four times per day.

Compression stockings are also extremely helpful at minimizing dependent edema [125]. Knee or thigh-high compression stocking may be used to mobilize edema fluid; thigh-high stockings are generally less well tolerated due to patient discomfort, but are more effective at minimizing fluid accumulation in the legs than knee-high stockings. Patients should be measured by an expert to make sure that the appropriate level of compression is being attained. Often, moderate levels of compression (i.e., 30 mmHg) are needed to achieve satisfactory results. Depending on the clinical situation, higher levels of compression (50 mmHg) may be necessary.

Diuretic Therapy

As mentioned above, diuretics are associated with a host of side effects, potentially deleterious neurohormonal changes, and chronic renal adaptations that ultimately lead to resistance. Consequently, treatment of the underlying disease and dietary sodium restriction should be tried before initiating diuretic therapy.

In general, the goal of diuretic therapy in patients with ECF volume overload is to facilitate an efficient negative NaCl balance without compromising EABV. In order to accomplish this goal, volume removal needs to occur at a rate that allows for adequate vessel refilling from the interstitial space. This rate varies depending on the clinical situation. For instance, in the generalized edema seen in HF, fluid readily moves from the interstitium to the intravascular compartment. Therefore, 2 l of edema fluid can be removed per day without major concerns of intravascular volume depletion from inadequate refilling. In contrast, the rate of refilling in patients with cirrhosis and ascites can be slower, especially when peripheral edema is absent, and a negative fluid balance on the order of up to only 750 ml/day can be safely achieved without depleting intravascular volume [126]. Thus, in all outpatient and most inpatient situations where diuretic therapy is required, gentle but consistent fluid removal is the rule of thumb. *Life-threatening* pulmonary edema is the one major exception to this rule. In this situation, diuretics should be used more aggressively to facilitate the efficient and rapid removal of edema fluid.

Many patients will initially present to their physician with pedal edema or leg swelling. In the absence of severe cases or skin breakdown, peripheral edema should be viewed largely as a cosmetic issue and, by itself, is not an absolute indication for diuretic treatment. The key factor that should drive a clinician's decision to start therapy for peripheral edema is the underlying cause of the condition. If, for instance, the patient has developed pedal edema in the setting of known left ventricular dysfunction, it would be reasonable to consider starting diuretic therapy in order to avoid the development of pulmonary vascular congestion. Conversely, if the patient has peripheral edema related to the menstrual cycle, or drug-induced edema from agents such as calcium channel blockers, diuretic therapy is not an ideal early intervention.

In the outpatient setting, the goal of therapy should be to find the minimum dose of diuretic that consistently ensures a natriuretic response. Due to their effectiveness in ensuring a brisk diuresis, loop diuretics are often the initial treatment of choice for patients who present with significant generalized edema. Patients with normal GFR who are naïve to the effects of a loop diuretic can develop a natriuresis with as little as 10 mg of furosemide per day. In contrast, those with a reduced number of functioning nephrons, such as in CKD, may require a higher initial dose to experience an effective natriuresis [32]. In either case, one way a clinician can monitor for the effectiveness of a diuretic dose would be to simply ask the patient whether he/she experiences an increase in urine output within hours after taking an oral dose of loop diuretic [115]. In addition, any patient on diuretic therapy should be measuring his/her weight on a daily basis, preferably at the same time of the day. If the patient does *not* perceive a significant difference in urine output after each dose of diuretic, and if the patient's weight has not significantly changed within a few days of starting diuretic therapy, it is unlikely that the prescribed diuretic dose is generating a negative fluid balance. The initial management of edema in the outpatient setting should be conducted carefully, and both the volume status and blood chemistries (including the electrolytes, blood urea nitrogen, and creatinine) of the patient should be closely monitored to ensure that he/she is not developing intravascular volume depletion from overdiuresis or developing hypokalemia or other electrolyte abnormalities. Once the physical exam suggests euvolemia, the initial diuretic dose may need to be titrated to ensure neutral sodium and water balance, although this might not be necessary since the aforementioned short-term adaptive effects may allow the kidneys to adjust sodium excretion to match sodium intake over the initial 1–2 weeks of treatment [127, 128].

When a patient is hospitalized for edema, it is often useful to use loop diuretics intravenously to obviate problems associated with limited bioavailability. When switching from intravenous to oral doses however, it is generally recommended that twice the intravenous dose of furosemide be administered. In clinical settings where a maximum natriuretic response is necessary, continuous diuretic infusion appears to be more effective than bolus intermittent diuretic dosing. In a prospective randomized crossover trial that studied modes of diuretic administration in patients with HF, continuous furosemide infusion preceded by a loading dose produced a greater diuresis and natriuresis than a 24-h dose equivalent of furosemide given in boluses intermittently [129]. No significant differences in side effects were noted between the two groups. Similar findings were reported from a study of patients with CKD, in which bumetanide was administered either by bolus or infusion [130]. In this case, side effects were also reduced by the continuous infusion. The effectiveness of continuous loop diuretic infusion likely results from the fact that a constant supply of diuretic is being maintained in the bloodstream. This serves to clamp urinary furosemide levels at a concentration above the diuretic threshold, close to the concentration of maximal diuretic efficiency (Fig. 6.4). Moreover, continuous therapy has the benefit of minimizing the adaptive effect of post-diuretic NaCl retention, and therefore generally can facilitate negative fluid balance much more effectively than if an identical dose of intravenous diuretic was given intermittently over the same period of time [131].

A possible alternative to intravenous treatment is the use of diuretics that are better absorbed. Both torsemide and bumetanide are much more bioavailable than furosemide and their absorption is more consistent [132]. Bumetanide is very short acting, however, whereas torsemide's action is longer (Table 6.1). Unblinded data suggest that the use of torsemide to treat HF may be associated with a reduced rate of exacerbations [107]. In a blinded trial of patients with CKD, torsemide and furosemide were equally effective at reducing blood pressure [133]. Thus, despite pharmacokinetic differences, a clear demonstration of the superiority of specific loop diuretics awaits randomized trials.

Although loop diuretics are commonly prescribed as the initial therapy to treat generalized edema, other diuretic classes have specific uses in certain edema-causing disorders. These special clinical situations are discussed in the subsequent section (see below).

Diuretic Treatment of Specific Generalized Edematous States

Heart Failure

Heart failure with systolic dysfunction is characterized by impaired myocardial contractility, which leads to the sensing of low EABV by normally functioning homeostatic mechanisms. One of the most important contributors to the pathophysiology of HF is the kidney, which responds to elevations in catecholamines, vasopressin, and aldosterone by enhancing sodium and water retention. This increases blood volume, capillary hydrostatic pressure, and pulmonary vascular congestion in the face of poor left ventricular outflow. Initially, these effects increase venous return, helping to preserve cardiac output. Ultimately, however, the changes in intravascular pressure translate into the transudation of fluid into the interstitium, and edema.

Conventional management of systolic HF includes both measures shown to prolong life, such as angiotensin converting enzyme inhibitors (or alternatively angiotensin receptor blockers, or hydralazine + long-acting nitrates), beta adrenergic blocking drugs, and aldosterone blocking drugs (see below). Symptomatic interventions include digoxin and inotropes, such as dobutamine and milrinone. Diuretics are required whenever symptomatic HF is present and, although these drugs have not tested in controlled trials, observational studies and practical considerations suggest that they may reduce mortality and are clearly an essential aspect of treatment [134–136]. Mild HF may be treated with a single DCT diuretic such as hydrochlorothiazide or chlorthalidone. As HF symptoms progress, loop diuretics become the treatment of choice, owing to their effectiveness at increasing sodium and water excretion to remove edema fluid and maintain intravascular volume at acceptable levels.

Loop diuretics are an essential component of the treatment regimen for severe HF, owing to their effectiveness at controlling HF symptoms. However, they are not completely benign drugs. A recent study pointed out a dose-dependent association of loop diuretic use and all-cause mortality in patients with HF [137]. Although this effect might simply reflect a correlation between loop diuretic dose and more severe salt and water retention owing to worse disease state, other factors might play a role. This is supported by observations that the incidence of arrhythmic deaths is higher in patients using loop diuretics—an association which is likely related to the increased risk of diuretic-induced hypokalemia [138]. Moreover, as mentioned above, ample evidence suggests that loop diuretic therapy is associated with activation of the renin angiotensin aldosterone system, which aggravates salt and water retention and amplifies the fluid retentive state [26]. Finally, evidence suggests that loop diuretics exert their beneficial effect at the expense of reducing cardiac output [139], and care must be taken to dose diuretic appropriately and ensure that intravascular volume does not become so low as to compromise organ tissue perfusion. Indeed, it seems likely that, in the case of loop diuretic therapy, the very treatments that are employed to improve HF symptoms and quality of life accelerate disease progression as the HF becomes more severe.

For the reasons described above, chronic loop diuretic therapy in HF is commonly associated with diuretic resistance. Short-term adaptive effects can be minimized with twice-daily diuretic dosing, but over time chronic adaptations, including DCT cell hypertrophy and hyperplasia, overcome the ability of loop diuretics to facilitate adequate sodium and water excretion. Once a total furosemide dose of 240 mg orally per day is insufficient to maintain volume status, a DCT diuretic should usually be added to the regimen. Adding a DCT diuretic such as metolazone or chlorthalidone effectively counteracts the enhanced sodium chloride reabsorption caused by long-term DCT adaptation to chronic loop diuretic therapy [140–143]. In the setting of loop diuretic resistance, even adding a very low dose of metolazone (e.g., 2.5 mg orally every other morning) can have a surprisingly robust diuretic effect. Consequently, when initiating DCT diuretic therapy to counterbalance loop diuretic resistance, patients should monitor their weight carefully, potassium needs to be supplemented, and K^+ levels need to be followed to keep them from becoming volume depleted and hypokalemic. Typically, the DCT diuretic takes approximately 30 min to 1 h prior to the oral ingestion of loop diuretic to ensure that sodium transport pathways in the DCT are inhibited at the time the loop diuretic reaches the urinary space.

In addition to loop diuretic therapy, aldosterone receptor antagonists are commonly prescribed in severe (New York Heart Association Class IV) HF [144]. Low-dose diuretic treatment with either spironolactone or eplerenone has been shown to reduce mortality in patients with severe HF who are already on an ACE inhibitor and loop diuretic [71, 145]. The beneficial effects of the aldosterone antagonists are believed to be a consequence of their ability to suppress the neurohormonal activation of the renin-angiotensin-aldosterone system, but also may be related to their ability to attenuate renal potassium secretion and hypokalemia [71].

The utility of aquaretics in the treatment of HF is currently under investigation. From a pathophysiological point of view, V2 receptor antagonism makes good sense, since vasopressin levels are elevated early on in systolic HF, and their circulating concentrations correlate with the severity of disease [146]. The recent results from the EVEREST trial support the use of tolvaptan to increase free water excretion and improve symptoms in HF, although the results from this well-designed study did not detect a difference in all-cause mortality compared to placebo [103] (also, see above). Thus, the current evidence suggests that V2 receptor antagonists should not be incorporated into the pharmacologic standard of care for severe HF. Nevertheless, they may serve as a safe and effective therapy to facilitate relief from the symptoms of volume overload, in patients with hyponatremia and HF.

Acute Kidney Injury

Acute kidney injury (AKI) is defined as an abrupt decrease in renal function over 48 h, manifesting as an increase in the serum creatinine concentration of 0.3 mg/dl or 50 % above baseline, or the development of oliguria [147]. AKI can be classified in a number of different ways, but one of the most important distinctions is whether the renal failure associated with the insult is oliguric or nonoliguric. Oliguric renal failure, that is AKI associated with a total urine output of less than 400 ml/24 h, is associated with a markedly worse prognosis than the nonoliguric variety [148]. This is due to the fact that nonoliguric AKI is associated with fewer of the metabolic complications associated with renal failure and also is less likely to require dialysis.

Loop diuretic therapy has been proposed to serve as a potential treatment for AKI. The rationale for this idea was in part supported by studies suggesting that loop diuretics increase the degree of oxygenation of the renal medulla [149], possibly due to the inhibition of active transport in the TAL. In addition, since volume overload is commonly an indication for dialysis in patients with AKI, it was thought that loop diuretics might improve outcomes by minimizing the number of patients that require acute dialysis. Finally, it was also proposed that in many cases, loop diuretics could increase urinary flow and convert oliguric renal failure to nonoliguria, and thus could reduce the mortality associated with a low urine output state.

Multiple small randomized controlled trials used loop diuretic therapy as an intervention to treat acute renal failure [150, 151]. The results from these studies were negative; in each case, although loop diuretics were able to increase the urine output above the defined oliguric threshold, they did not improve patient mortality or reduce the need for dialysis. It is important to note, however, that these trials were small and statistically underpowered. More recently, Mehta et al. [152] conducted a large-scale multicenter retrospective analysis of the outcomes of all patients hospitalized in intensive care units with AKI who were seen in nephrology consultation over a 6-year period. In this study, diuretic treatment was associated with an increased risk of death and lack of recovery of renal function. Although these findings suggest that high-dose furosemide therapy *might* be harmful to patients with AKI, it is important to note that this was an observational study, and therefore the findings do not invoke causality. Indeed, a recent meta-analysis of nine acute renal failure trials encompassing 849 patients was unable to replicate the association between loop diuretic therapy and higher patient mortality [153]. Thus, the current state of the literature illustrates the need for large-scale, adequately powered randomized controlled trials to definitively establish the role of diuretics in AKI. Current evidence does suggest however that while loop diuretic therapy may not be harmful to critically ill patients with AKI, it does not lead to improved outcomes, and should not serve as a means to delay renal replacement therapy. Early nephrologist involvement—shortly after the onset of AKI—can be extremely helpful in determining the appropriate time course for initiating dialysis.

Cirrhosis

In cirrhosis, the initiating event that leads to volume expansion is the dilation of the splanchnic vasculature [154]. Coupled with the alterations in portal pressure and decreased plasma oncotic pressure from hypoproteinemia, these changes all contribute to ECF volume expansion. During this process, volume expansion in cirrhosis is associated with an up-regulation of the renin-angiotensin system, and circulating aldosterone concentrations increase. In addition, the perceived low EABV leads to an increase in vasopressin secretion from the posterior pituitary. Together, these neurohormonal changes lead to enhanced renal salt and water retention. Similar to the clinical situation seen in HF, as the disorder reaches its more advanced stages, excessive vasopressin release can lead to hyponatremia.

Owing to changes in the portal venous pressure, edema fluid tends to accumulate in the peritoneum. As volume overload progresses, peripheral edema is also observed. Ascites fluid tends to refill the intravascular space slowly, with a *maximum* rate of absorption of approximately 750 ml/day [126, 155]. For most patients with ascites however, the rate of reabsorption from the peritoneal space is significantly lower than this number. Thus, the clinician must devise an approach that will ultimately lead to net negative fluid balance while being mindful of the tendency of patients with this condition to refill their vasculature poorly. Moreover, the clinician must be especially careful not to diurese a patient with liver failure too aggressively due to the propensity to develop encephalopathy. Specifically, overzealous diuresis in cirrhosis can lead to azotemia, and the secondary hyperaldosteronism associated with this condition favors hypokalemia and increased renal ammoniagenesis during diuretic therapy hepatic encephalopathy [156]. Both the azotemia and increased ammonia levels can ultimately lead to mental status changes and overt encephalopathy. In light of these special considerations, patients with cirrhotic ascites need to be particularly mindful of their volume status. Close monitoring of the weight and regular clinic visits to track the GFR and electrolytes are essential. The importance of sodium restriction should be emphasized to the patient.

A reasonable initial daily negative fluid balance in a cirrhotic patient with ascites should total approximately 750 ml/24 h. Given the overactivity of the renin-angiotensin system in cirrhotic ascites, aldosterone receptor antagonists are the first-line diuretic of choice. Spironolactone is typically prescribed initially at a dose of up to 100 mg orally per day. If the patient does not appear responding to aldosterone receptor antagonist monotherapy, a loop diuretic such as furosemide may be added, usually starting at 20–40 mg orally per day. The American Society for the Study of Liver Disease recommends that the ratio of furosemide to spironolactone be

40 mg/100 mg [1]. In the setting of tense ascites requiring large-volume paracentesis, diuretic therapy may need to be adjusted to account for any fluid shifts that might occur following the bulk removal of peritoneal fluid. Aquaretic therapy may eventually be useful to facilitate a water diuresis in the cirrhotic patient with edema and hyponatremia, and studies are currently being conducted to confirm the safety and efficacy of this novel treatment modality.

Nephrotic Syndrome

Nephrotic edema poses unique problems to the clinician. Despite considerable effort, a unifying hypothesis that explains all of the pathophysiologic features of edema in the nephrotic syndrome has been elusive. Currently, a debate exists in the literature as to how edema is formed in the nephrotic syndrome. The traditional "underfill" hypothesis, which proposes that the underlying etiology is purely driven by hypoalbuminemia leading to secondary renal sodium retention, has been challenged by several pieces of evidence. An alternative "overflow" model suggests that a primary defect in renal sodium excretion drives ECF volume expansion and edema formation [157]. According to this hypothesis, the distal sodium reabsorptive machinery becomes less responsive to systemic mediators of sodium excretion, such as ANP, thus leading to an increase in the capillary hydrostatic pressure and transudation of fluid into the interstitium. More recently, the interstitial inflammation that often accompanies massive proteinuria has been proposed to be an additional factor that modulates sodium reabsorption in the nephrotic syndrome [158]. Given the heterogeneity of the various underlying glomerulopathies that give rise to the nephrotic syndrome, it seems likely that multiple factors may work together to generate the sodium-avid phenotype seen in patients with the disease.

Loop diuretics are the treatment of choice for edema in the nephrotic syndrome due to the fact that other diuretic classes are less capable of facilitating a clinically significant natriuretic effect. Massive proteinuria, the hallmark of the nephrotic syndrome, diminishes the effectiveness of loop diuretic therapy. When Brater and colleagues measured the diuretic efficiency of furosemide in nephrotic rats, sodium reabsorption was decreased relative to urinary furosemide excretion, compared to non-nephrotic controls [159]. This finding illustrates that, compared to their efficacy in some edematous disorders, loop diuretics are less capable of provoking a natriuresis in the nephrotic syndrome. The authors suggested that this observation may be due to the fact that a large fraction of the furosemide that enters the loop of Henle during diuretic therapy remains bound to albumin and is therefore unable to inhibit Na-K-2Cl cotransport. Yet work by the same group later showed that albumin binding to loop diuretics in the tubule lumen is *not* a major contributor to diuretic resistance; agents that reduce diuretic binding to albumin had no substantial effect on diuretic efficacy in nephrotic patients [160]. Hypoalbuminemia also may act to diminish the effectiveness of loop diuretics. Once loop diuretics are absorbed into the bloodstream, they become largely bound to albumin. A low serum albumin level diminishes the total blood concentration of loop diuretic and increases its volume of distribution. Therefore, less diuretic will be conveyed by the renal circulation to the nephron, and less will be extruded by basolateral-to-apical proximal tubule organic anion transport into the tubule lumen for delivery to the TAL. This scenario provides the rationale for infusing albumin together with loop diuretics to patients with substantial hypoalbuminemia, a suggestion that has received some support in the literature [161–165]. Yet there is little evidence that such an approach is useful, if the serum albumin concentration exceeds 2 g/dl [165].

Three important clinical practice points come to mind when one considers the various pathophysiologic factors that make nephrotic edema more resistant to diuretic treatment. First, since both loop diuretic drug delivery and efficiency are diminished in the nephrotic syndrome, clinicians may need to use a higher dose to achieve the desired natriuretic effect. Second, since the "overfill" mechanism suggests that the distal nephron is less able to adjust its sodium

Table 6.4 Ceiling doses of loop diuretics

	Furosemide		Bumetanide		Torsemide	
	i.v.	p.o.	i.v.	p.o.	i.v.	p.o.
Renal insufficiency						
GFR 20–50 ml/min	80–160	160	4–8	4–8	50	50
GFR < 20 ml/min	200	240	8–10	8–10	8–10	100
Severe acute renal failure[a]	500	NA	12	NA	200	NA
Nephrotic syndrome	120	240	3	3	20–50	20–50
Cirrhosis	40–80	80–160	1	1–2	10–20	20
Congestive heart failure	40–80	80–160	1–2	1–2	10–20	20

Ceiling dose indicates the dose that produces the maximal increase in FE_{Na}. Larger doses may increase net daily natriuresis by increasing the duration of natriuresis without increasing the maximal rate. All doses in milligrams. (Based on Brater DC: Diuretic therapy. N Engl J Med. 1998;339:387–95)

[a]This dose is not usually recommended; instead, a continuous infusion may be utilized. NA, not available

reabsorptive capacity to changes in volume, incorporating combination loop and DCT diuretic therapy early in treatment may protect the patient from volume overload. Finally, when hypoalbuminemia is severe, combining loop diuretic treatment with intravenous albumin infusion may help to improve glomerular hemodynamics [162] and facilitate loop diuretic delivery to its site of action. When considering any or all of these approaches, one should always keep the underlying clinical disorder in mind. Like many heterogeneous syndromes, measures that did not work well in one case of nephrotic syndrome may be exceedingly effective under a different set of circumstances and glomerular pathologies.

Chronic Kidney Disease

CKD typically increases extracellular fluid volume, even in the absence of overt edema [166]. Although CKD alone typically does not cause edema, its presence greatly complicates the treatment of edema owing to heart failure, cirrhosis, or nephrotic syndrome. In addition, the dependence of hypertension on salt intake is enhanced as CKD progresses [167]. Therefore, salt restriction and diuretics are central features of the treatment of hypertension in patients with CKD. Diuretics also stimulate K^+ and H^+ excretion by increasing distal NaCl and fluid delivery through the distal nephron. Thus, loop diuretics are useful in patients with CKD to prevent or treat the hyperkalemia and acidosis that can often occur, especially during concomitant use of drugs that block the renin-angiotensin-aldosterone axis.

Ceiling doses of loop diuretics have been evaluated (Table 6.4). Ceiling doses are those that produce a maximal increase in fractional Na^+ excretion. A further increase in dose may produce a further modest increase in Na^+ loss by prolonging the duration of the natriuresis, but repeating the ceiling dose is preferable to avoid diuretic toxicity. In CKD, ceiling doses are higher than normal, for a number of reasons. Increasing the dose of furosemide above the ceiling increases the plasma level sharply with the possibility of precipitating ototoxicity [35].

Although many factors in patients with CKD conspire to limit the response of the kidney to loop diuretics [168], only a few can be addressed therapeutically. The first is drug effects that limit diuretic effectiveness. Several drugs, most commonly the nonsteroidal anti-inflammatory drugs, compete with loop diuretics for proximal secretion and thereby diminish diuretic efficacy [114, 169]. The second is the effect of CKD on the loop diuretic dose response curve (Fig. 6.5). As discussed above, CKD is associated with a shift in the loop diuretic dose response to the right. This means that a higher dose of diuretic is necessary to elicit the same increase in fractional sodium excretion [170]. The practitioner should exercise caution in such patients, however, because furosemide is metabolized by the kidneys and can accumulate in renal failure. Therefore, when needed for prolonged, high-dosage therapy in CKD, bumetanide or torsemide may be preferred because they are metabolized by the liver and do not accumulate.

A strategy in diuretic resistant patients with CKD is to combine a loop with a distal acting diuretic, such as a thiazide. Wollam et al. [171] compared increasing the dose of furosemide or adding a thiazide to a group of mildly azotemic hypertensive subjects. Doubling the furosemide dosage had little effect, whereas hydrochlorothiazide normalized the BP. This beneficial effect on BP and body fluid accumulation was associated, however, with a sharp increase in the serum creatinine. In more severe CKD, adding a DCT diuretic remains effective. In a group of patients with stage 4–5 CKD (mean GFR = 13 ml/min), a thiazide significantly increased urinary sodium excretion above the rates obtained by a loop diuretic alone [172].

References

1. Runyon BA. Practice guidelines Committee AAftSoLD. Management of adult patients with ascites due to cirrhosis. Hepatology. 2004;39(3):841–56.
2. Okusa MD, Ellison DH. Physiology and pathophysiology of diuretic action. In: Alpern RJ, Hebert SC, editors. The kidney: physiology and pathophysiology. 4th ed. Amsterdam: Elsevier; 2008. p. 1051–984.
3. Schwartz GJ. Physiology and molecular biology of renal carbonic anhydrase. J Nephrol. 2002;15 Suppl 5:S61–74.
4. Schwartz GJ, Kittelberger AM, Barnhart DA, Vijayakumar S. Carbonic anhydrase IV is expressed in H(+)-secreting cells of rabbit kidney. Am J Physiol Renal Physiol. 2000;278(6):F894–904.
5. Soleimani M, Aronson PS. Ionic mechanism of Na+-HCO-3 cotransport in rabbit renal basolateral membrane vesicles. J Biol Chem. 1989;264:18302–8.
6. Pastorekova S, Parkkila S, Pastorek J, Supuran CT. Carbonic anhydrases: current state of the art, therapeutic applications and future prospects. J Enzyme Inhib Med Chem. 2004;19(3):199–229.
7. DuBose TD, Lucci MS. Effect of carbonic anhydrase inhibition on superficial and deep nephron bicarbonate reabsorption inthe rat. J Clin Invest. 1983;71:55–65.
8. Ellison DH, Okusa MD, Schrier RW. Mechanisms of diuretic action. In: Schrier RW, editor. Diseases of the kidney and urinary tract. Philadelphia: Wolters Kluwer/Lippincott Williams & Wilkins; 2007. p. 2122–50.
9. Cogan MG, Maddox DA, Warnock DG, Lin ET, Rector Jr FC. Effect of acetazolamide on bicarbonate reabsorption in the proximal tubule of the rat. Am J Physiol. 1979;237:F447–54.
10. Lorenz JN, Schultheis PJ, Traynor T, Shull GE, Schnermann J. Micropuncture analysis of single-nephron function in NHE3-deficient mice. Am J Physiol. 1999;277(3 Pt 2):F447–53.
11. Buckalew Jr VM, Walker BR, Puschett JB, Goldberg M. Effects of increased sodium delivery on distal tubular sodium reabsorption with and without volume expansion in man. J Clin Invest. 1970;49:2336–44.
12. Velázquez H, Wright FS. Control by drugs of renal potassium handling. Ann Rev Pharmacol Toxicol. 1986;26:293–309.
13. Neto M, Pilloff B, Simon J. Dissolution of renal uric acid calculus with allopurinal and alkalization of urine: a case report. J Urol. 1976;115(6):740–1.
14. Prescott LF, Balali-Mood M, Critchley JA, Johnstone AF, Proudfoot AT. Diuresis or urinary alkalinization for salicylate poisoning? British Med J. 1982;285:1383–6.
15. Grissom CK, Roach RC, Sarnquist FH, Hackett PH. Acetazolamide in the treatment of acute mountain sickenss: clinical efficacy and effect on gas. Ann Intern Med. 1992;116:461–5.
16. Parfitt AM. Acetazolamide and sodium bicarbonate induced nehrocalcinosis and nephrolithiasis; relationship to citrate and calcium excretion. Arch Intern Med. 1969;124:736–40.
17. Shankar SS, Brater DC. Loop diuretics: from the Na-K-2Cl transporter to clinical use. Am J Physiol Renal Physiol. 2003;284(1):F11–21.
18. Reeves WB, Andreoli TE. Sodium chloride transport in the loop of Henle, distal convoluted tubule, and collecting duct. In: Alpern RJ, Hebert SC, editors. The kidney: physiology and pathophysiology. Amsterdam: Elsevier; 2008. p. 849–88.
19. Isenring P, Forbush III B. Ion and bumetanide binding by the Na-K-Cl cotransporter. Importance of transmembrane domains. J Biol Chem. 1997;272:24556–62.
20. Obermüller N, Kunchaparty S, Ellison DH, Bachmann S. Expression of the Na-K-2Cl cotransporter by macula densa and thick ascending limb cells of rat and rabbit nephron. J Clin Invest. 1996;98:635–40.
21. Schnermann J, Homer W. Smith Award lecture. The juxtaglomerular apparatus: from anatomical peculiarity to physiological relevance. J Am Soc Nephrol. 2003;14(6):1681–94.
22. Skott O, Briggs JP. Direct demonstration of macula densa-mediated renin secretion. Science. 1987;237(4822):1618–20.
23. Francis GS, Siegel RM, Goldsmith SR, Olivari MT, Levine B, Cohn JN. Acute vasoconstrictor response to intravenous furosemide in patients with chronic congestive heart failure. Ann Intern Med. 1985;103:1–6.
24. Larsen FF. Haemodynamic effects of high or low doses of furosemide in acute myocardial infarction. Eur Heart J. 1988;9(2):125–31.

25. Goldsmith SR, Francis G, Cohn JN. Attenuation of the pressor response to intravenous furosemide by angiotensin converting enzyme inhibition in congestive heart failure. Am J Cardiol. 1989;64:1382–5.
26. Ellison DH. Diuretic therapy and resistance in congestive heart failure. Cardiology. 2001;96(3–4):132–43.
27. Hawkins RG, Houston MC. Is population-wide diuretic use directly associated with the incidence of end-stage renal disease in the United States? A hypothesis. Am J Hypertens. 2005;18(6):744–9.
28. Sun D, Samuelson LC, Yang T, et al. Mediation of tubuloglomerular feedback by adenosine: evidence from mice lacking adenosine 1 receptors. Proc Natl Acad Sci USA. 2001;98(17):9983–8.
29. Wright FS, Schnermann J. Interference with feedback control of glomerular filtration rate by furosemide, triflocin, and cyanide. J Clin Invest. 1974;53:1695–708.
30. Body JJ. Hypercalcemia of malignancy. Semin Nephrol. 2004;24(1):48–54.
31. Vasko MR, Brown-Cartwright D, Knochel JP, Nixon JV, Brater DC. Furosemide absorption altered in decompensated congestive heart failure. Ann Intern Med. 1985;102:314–8.
32. Brater DC. Diuretic therapy. N Engl J Med. 1998;339:387–95.
33. Cannon PJ, Heinemann HO, Albert MS, Laragh JH, Winters RW. "Contraction" alkalosis after diuresis of edematous patients with ethacrynic acid. Ann Intern Med. 1965;62:979–90.
34. Mizuta K, Adachi M, Iwasa KH. Ultrastructural localization of the Na-K-Cl cotransporter in the lateral wall of the rabbit cochlear duct. Hear Res. 1997;106(1–2):154–62.
35. Ryback LP. Ototoxicity of loop diuretics. Otolaryngol Clin North Am. 1993;26:829–44.
36. Star RA. Ototoxicity. Academic Press: San Diego; 1997. p. 637–42.
37. Reilly RF, Ellison DH. Mammalian distal tubule: physiology, pathophysiology, and molecular anatomy. Physiol Rev. 2000;80(1):277–313.
38. Meneton P, Loffing J, Warnock DG. Sodium and potassium handling by the aldosterone-sensitive distal nephron: the pivotal role of the distal and connecting tubule. Am J Physiol Renal Physiol. 2004;287(4):F593–601.
39. Beaumont K, Vaughn DA, Fanestil DD. Thiazide diuretic drug receptors in rat kidney: identification with [3H]metolazone. Proc Natl Acad Sci. 1988;85:2311–4.
40. ALLHAT Officers and Coordinators for the ALLHAT Collaborative Research Group. Major outcomes in high-risk hypertensive patients randomized to angiotensin-converting enzyme inhibitor or calcium channel blocker vs diuretic: the antihypertensive and lipid-lowering treatment to prevent heart attack trial (ALLHAT). JAMA. 2002;288(23):2981–97.
41. Kunau Jr RT, Weller DR, Webb HL. Clarification of the site of action of chlorothiazide in the rat nephron. J Clin Invest. 1975;56(2):401–7.
42. Okusa MD, Erik A, Persson G, Wright FS. Chlorothiazide effect on feedback-mediated control of glomerular filtration rate. Am J Physiol. 1989;257:F137–44.
43. Walter SJ, Shirley DG. The effect of chronic hydrochlorothiazide administration on renal function in the rat. Clin Sci (Lond). 1986;70(4):379–87.
44. Prevention and treatment of kidney stones. A consensus conference. JAMA. 1988;260:977–81.
45. Nijenhuis T, Vallon V, van der Kemp AW, Loffing J, Hoenderop JG, Bindels RJ. Enhanced passive Ca2+ reabsorption and reduced Mg2+ channel abundance explains thiazide-induced hypocalciuria and hypomagnesemia. J Clin Invest. 2005;115(6):1651–8.
46. Belge H, Gailly P, Schwaller B, et al. Renal expression of parvalbumin is critical for NaCl handling and response to diuretics. Proc Natl Acad Sci USA. 2007;104(37):14849–54.
47. Ljunghall S, Backman U, Danielson BG, Fellstrom B, Johansson G, Wikstrom B. Calcium and magnesium metabolism during long-term treatment with thiazides. Scand J Urol Nephrol. 1981;15(3): 257–62.
48. Ellison DH. Divalent cation transport by the distal nephron: insights from Bartter's and Gitelman's syndromes. Am J Physiol Renal Physiol. 2000;279(4):F616–25.
49. Pluznick JL, Wei P, Carmines PK, Sansom SC. Renal fluid and electrolyte handling in BKCa-beta1−/− mice. Am J Physiol Renal Physiol. 2003;284(6): F1274–9.
50. Huang CL, Kuo E. Mechanism of hypokalemia in magnesium deficiency. J Am Soc Nephrol. 2007;18(10):2649–52.
51. Brater DC. Diuretic pharmacokinetics and pharmacodynamics. In: Seldin DW, Giebisch G, editors. Diuretic agents: clinical physiology and pharmacology. San Diego: Academic Press; 1997. p. 189–208.
52. Carter BL, Ernst ME, Cohen JD. Hydrochlorothiazide versus chlorthalidone: evidence supporting their interchangeability. Hypertension. 2004;43(1):4–9.
53. Ernst ME, Carter BL, Goerdt CJ, et al. Comparative antihypertensive effects of hydrochlorothiazide and chlorthalidone on ambulatory and office blood pressure. Hypertension. 2006;47(3):352–8.
54. Austin PC, Mamdani MM, Tu K, Zwarenstein M. Changes in prescribing patterns following publication of the ALLHAT trial. JAMA. 2004;291(1): 44–5.
55. Chobanian AV, Bakris GL, Black HR, et al. The seventh report of the joint national committee on prevention, detection, evaluation, and treatment of high blood pressure: the JNC 7 report. JAMA. 2003;289(19):2560–72.
56. Kim GH, Lee JW, Oh YK, et al. Antidiuretic effect of hydrochlorothiazide in lithium-induced nephrogenic diabetes insipidus is associated with upregulation of aquaporin-2, Na–Cl co-transporter, and epithelial sodium channel. J Am Soc Nephrol. 2004;15(11):2836–43.

57. Cesar KR, Magaldi AJ. Thiazide induces water absorption in the inner medullary collecting duct of normal and Brattleboro rats. Am J Physiol. 1999;277(5 Pt 2):F756–60.
58. Chow KM, Szeto CC, Wong TY, Leung CB, Li PK. Risk factors for thiazide-induced hyponatraemia. QJM. 2003;96(12):911–7.
59. Friedman E, Shadel M, Halkin H, Farfel Z. Thiazide-induced hyponatremia: reproducibility by single dose rechallenge and an analysis of pathogenesis. Ann Intern Med. 1989;110:24–30.
60. Harper R, Ennis CN, Sheridan B, Atkinson AB, Johnston GD, Bell PM. Effects of low dose versus conventional dose thiazide diuretic on insulin action in essential hypertension. BMJ. 1994;309:226–30.
61. Carlsen JE, Kober L, Torp-Pedersen C, Johansen P. Relation between dose of bendrofluazide, antihypertensive effect, and adverse biochemical effects. BMJ. 1990;300:975–8.
62. Helderman JH, Elahi D, Andersen DK, et al. Prevention of the glucose intolerance of thiazide diuretics by maintenance of body potassium. Diabetes 1983;32:106–11.
63. Zillich AJ, Garg J, Basu S, Bakris GL, Carter BL. Thiazide diuretics, potassium, and the development of diabetes: a quantitative review. Hypertension. 2006;48(2):219–24.
64. Schild L. The epithelial sodium channel: from molecule to disease. Rev Physiol Biochem Pharmacol. 2004;151:93–107.
65. McCormick JA, Bhalla V, Pao AC, Pearce D. SGK1: a rapid aldosterone-induced regulator of renal sodium reabsorption. Physiology (Bethesda). 2005;20:134–9.
66. Couette B, Lombes M, Baulieu E-E, Rafestin-Oblin M-E. Aldosterone antagonists destablilize the mineralocorticoid receptor. Biochem J. 1992;282:697–702.
67. Delyani JA. Mineralocorticoid receptor antagonists: the evolution of utility and pharmacology. Kidney Int. 2000;57(4):1408–11.
68. Busch AE, Suessbrich H, Kunzelmann K, et al. Blockade of epithelial Na+ channels by triamterene-underlying mechanisms and molecular basis. Pflugers Arch. 1996;432:760–6.
69. Kashlan OB, Sheng S, Kleyman TR. On the interaction between amiloride and its putative alpha-subunit epithelial Na+ channel binding site. J Biol Chem. 2005;280(28):26206–15.
70. Liew D, Krum H. Aldosterone receptor antagonists for hypertension: what do they offer? Drugs. 2003;63(19):1963–72.
71. Pitt B, Zannad F, Remme WJ, et al. The effect of spironolactone on morbidity and mortality in patients with severe heart failure. Randomized Aldactone Evaluation Study Investigators. N Engl J Med. 1999;341(10):709–17.
72. Pitt B, Williams G, Remme W, et al. The EPHESUS trial: eplerenone in patients with heart failure due to systolic dysfunction complicating acute myocardial infarction. Eplerenone Post-AMI Heart Failure Efficacy and Survival Study. Cardiovasc Drugs Ther. 2001;15(1):79–87.
73. Ahmed A, Zannad F, Love TE, et al. A propensity-matched study of the association of low serum potassium levels and mortality in chronic heart failure. Eur Heart J. 2007;28(11):1334–43.
74. Perez-Ayuso RM, Arroyo V, Planas R, et al. Randomized comparative study of efficacy of furosemide versus spironolactone in nonazotemic cirrhosis with ascites. Relationship between the diuretic response an the activity of the renin-aldosterone system. Gastroenterology. 1983;84:961–8.
75. Griffing GT, Cole AG, Aurecchia SA, Sindler BH, Komanicky P, Melby JC. Amiloride for primary hyperaldosteronism. Clin Pharmacol Ther. 1982; 31:56–61.
76. Colussi G, Rombola G, De Ferrari ME, Macaluso M, Minetti L. Correction of hypokalemia with antialdosterone therapy in Gitelman's syndrome. Am J Nephrol. 1994;14(2):127–35.
77. Botero-Velez M, Curtis JJ, Warnock DG. Brief Report: Liddle's syndrome revisited-a disorder of sodium reabsorption in the distal tubule. N Engl J Med. 1994;174:178–8078.
78. Batlle DC, von Riotte AB, Gaviria M, Grupp M. Amelioration of polyuria by amiloride in patients receiving long-term lithium therapy. N Engl J Med. 1985;312(7):408–14.
79. Juurlink DN, Mamdani MM, Lee DS, et al. Rates of hyperkalemia after publication of the randomized aldactone evaluation study. N Engl J Med. 2004; 351(6):543–51.
80. Rose LI, Underwood RH, Newmark SR, Kisch ES, Williams GH. Pathophysiology of spironolactone-induced gynecomastia. Ann Intern Med. 1977;87: 398–403.
81. Ettinger B, Oldroyd NO, Sorgel F. Triamterene nephrolithiasis. JAMA. 1980;244(21):2443–5.
82. Weinberg MS, Quigg RJ, Salant DJ, Bernard DB. Anuric renal failure precipitated by indomethacin and triamterene. Nephron. 1985;40:216–8.
83. Favre L, Glasson P, Vallotton MB. Reversible acute renal failure from combined triamterene and indomethacin: a study in healthy subjects. Ann Intern Med. 1982;96:317–20.
84. Wong NLM, Quamme GA, Sutton RAL, Dirks JH. Effects of mannitol on water and electrolyte transport in dog kidney. J Lab Clin Med. 1979;94: 683–92.
85. Stinebaugh BJ, Bartow SA, Eknoyan G, Martinez-Maldonado M, Suki WN. Renal handling of bicarbonate:effectof mannitol diuresis. Am J Physiol. 1971;220:1271–4.
86. Morris CR, Alexander EA, Bruns FJ, Levinsky NG. Restoration and maintenance of glomerular filtration by mannitol during hypoperfusion of the kidney. J Clin Invest. 1972;51:1555–64.
87. Atherton JC, Hai MA, Thomas S. Depletion of medullary urea concentration gradient in rat kidney during osmotic diuresis. J Physiol. 1968;194(1):21P–2.
88. Better OS, Rubinstein I, Winaver JM, Knochel JP. Mannitol therapy revisited (1940–1997). Kidney Int. 1997;51:886–94.

89. Weiner IM. Diuretics and other agents employed in the mobilization of edema fluid. In: Gilman AG, Rall TW, Nies AS, Taylor AS, editors. The pharmacological basis of therapeutics. 8th ed. New York: Pergamon Press; 1990. p. 713–42.
90. Quon DK, Worthen DM. Dose response of intravenous mannitol on the human eye. Ann Opthalmol. 1981;13:1392–3.
91. Gong G, Lindberg J, Abrams J, Whitaker WR, Wade CE, Gouge S. Comparison of hypertonic saline solutions and dextran in dialysis-induced hypotension. J Am Soc Nephrol. 1993;3:1808–12.
92. Arieff AI. Dialysis disequilibrium syndrome: current concepts on pathogenesis and prevention. Kidney Int. 1994;45:629.
93. Oster JR, Singer I. Hyponatremia, hyposmolality, and hypotonicity: tables and fables. Arch Intern Med. 1999;159(4):333–6.
94. Moreno M, Murphy C, Goldsmith C. Increase in serum potassium resulting from the administration of hypertonic mannitol and other solutions. J Lab Clin Med. 1969;73:291.
95. Gipstein RM, Boyle JD. Hypernatremia complicating prolonged mannitol diuresis. N Engl J Med. 1965;272:1116.
96. Doi K, Ogawa N, Suzuki E, Noiri E, Fujita T. Mannitol-induced acute renal failure. Am J Med. 2003;115(7):593–4.
97. Greenberg A, Verbalis JG. Vasopressin receptor antagonists. Kidney Int. 2006;69(12):2124–30.
98. Verbalis JG, Ghali JK, Gross P. Efficacy and safety of vasoptressin antagonist conivaptan in patients with euvolemic hyponatremia evaluated in a phase III clinical trial. J Clin Oncol. 2006;24:8550.
99. Palm C, Pistrosch F, Herbrig K, Gross P. Vasopressin antagonists as aquaretic agents for the treatment of hyponatremia. Am J Med. 2006;119(7 Suppl 1): S87–92.
100. Zeltser D, Rosansky S, van Rensburg H, Verbalis JG, Smith N. Assessment of the efficacy and safety of intravenous conivaptan in euvolemic and hypervolemic hyponatremia. Am J Nephrol. 2007;27(5): 447–57.
101. Gheorghiade M, Gattis WA, O'Connor CM, et al. Effects of tolvaptan, a vasopressin antagonist, in patients hospitalized with worsening heart failure: a randomized controlled trial. JAMA. 2004;291(16): 1963–71.
102. Gheorghiade M, Konstam MA, Burnett Jr JC, et al. Short-term clinical effects of tolvaptan, an oral vasopressin antagonist, in patients hospitalized for heart failure: the EVEREST clinical status trials. JAMA. 2007;297(12):1332–43.
103. Konstam MA, Gheorghiade M, Burnett Jr JC, et al. Effects of oral tolvaptan in patients hospitalized for worsening heart failure: the EVEREST outcome trial. JAMA. 2007;297(12):1319–31.
104. Schrier RW, Gross P, Gheorghiade M, et al. Tolvaptan, a selective oral vasopressin V2-receptor antagonist, for hyponatremia. N Engl J Med. 2006;355(20):2099–112.
105. Wang X, Gattone II V, Harris PC, Torres VE. Effectiveness of vasopressin V2 receptor antagonists OPC-31260 and OPC-41061 on polycystic kidney disease development in the PCK rat. J Am Soc Nephrol. 2005;16(4):846–51.
106. Bennett WM. V2 receptor antagonists in cystic kidney diseases: an exciting step towards a practical treatment. J Am Soc Nephrol. 2005;16(4):838–9.
107. Murray MD, Deer MM, Ferguson JA, et al. Open-label randomized trial of torsemide compared with furosemide therapy for patients with heart failure. Am J Med. 2001;111(7):513–20.
108. Kaojarern S, Day B, Brater DC. The time course of delivery of furosemide into urine: an independent determinant of overall response. Kidney Int. 1982;22:69–74.
109. Sweet DH, Bush KT, Nigam SK. The organic anion transporter family: from physiology to ontogeny and the clinic. Am J Physiol Renal Physiol. 2001; 281(2):F197–205.
110. Sekine T, Miyazaki H, Endou H. Molecular physiology of renal organic anion transporters. Am J Physiol Renal Physiol. 2006;290(2):F251–61.
111. Wright SH. Role of organic cation transporters in the renal handling of therapeutic agents and xenobiotics. Toxicol Appl Pharmacol. 2005;204(3):309–19.
112. Somogyi AA, Hovens CM, Muirhead MR, Bochner F. Renal tubular secretion of amiloride and its inhibition by cimetidine in humans and in an animal model. Drug Metab Dispos. 1989;17(2):190–6.
113. Rose HJ, Pruitt AW, McNay JL. Effect of experimental azotemia on renal clearance of furosemide in the dog. J Pharmacol Exp Ther. 1976;196:238–47.
114. Brater DC. Effects of probenecid on furosemide response. Clin Pharmacol Ther. 1978;24:548–54.
115. Ellison DH, Wilcox CS. Diuretics. In: Taal MW, Chertow GM, Marsden PA, Skorecki K, Yu ASL and Brenner BM, editors. Brenner and Rector's The Kidney. Philadelphia, Elsevier; 2008. p. 1646–78.
116. Gagnon E, Bergeron MJ, Brunet GM, Daigle ND, Simard CF, Isenring P. Molecular mechanisms of Cl− transport by the renal Na(+)-K(+)-Cl− cotransporter. Identification of an intracellular locus that may form part of a high affinity Cl(−)-binding site. J Biol Chem. 2004;279(7):5648–54.
117. Chen ZF, Vaughn DA, Beaumont K, Fanestil DD. Effects of diuretic treatment and of dietary sodium on renal binding of 3H-metolazone. J Am Soc Nephrol. 1990;1:91–8.
118. Ellison DH, Velázquez H, Wright FS. Adaptation of the distal convoluted tubule of the rat: structural and functional effects of dietary salt intake and chronic diuretic infusion. J Clin Invest. 1989;83:113–26.
119. Kaissling B, Bachmann S, Kriz W. Structural adaptation of the distal convoluted tubule to prolonged furosemide treatment. Am J Physiol. 1985;248: F374–81.
120. Kaissling B, Stanton BA. Adaptation of distal tubule and collecting duct to increased sodium delivery. I. Ultrastructure. Am J Physiol. 1988;255:F1256–68.

121. Stanton BA, Kaissling B. Adaptation of distal tubule and collecting duct to increased sodium delivery. II. Na+ and K+ transport. Am J Physiol. 1988;255:F1269–75.
122. Cahill RA, Spitzer TR, Mazumder A. Marrow engraftment and clinical manifestations of capillary leak syndrome. Bone Marrow Transplant. 1996; 18(1):177–84.
123. Schrier RW. Body fluid volume regulation in health and disease: a unifying hypothesis. Ann Intern Med. 1990;113:155–9.
124. Schrier RW, Gurevich AK, Cadnapaphornchai MA. Pathogenesis and management of sodium and water retention in cardiac failure and cirrhosis. Semin Nephrol. 2001;21(2):157–72.
125. Clement DL. Management of venous edema: insights from an international task force. Angiology. 2000;51(1):13–7.
126. Pockros PJ, Reynolds TB. Rapid diuresis in patients with ascites from chronic liver disease: the importance of peripheral edema. Gastroenterology. 1986;90(6):1827–33.
127. Rose BD. Diuretics. Kidney Int. 1991;39:336–52.
128. Bock HA, Stein JH. Diuretics and the control of extracellular fluid volume: role of counterregulation. Semin Nephrol. 1988;8(3):264–72.
129. Lahav M, Regev A, Ra'anani P, Thodor E. Intermittent administration of furosemide vs continuous infusion preceded by a loading dose for congestive heart failure. Chest. 1992;102:725–31.
130. Rudy DW, Voelker JR, Greene PK, Esparza FA, Brater DC. Loop diuretics for chronic renal insufficiency: a continuous infusion is more efficacious than bolus therapy. Ann Intern Med. 1991;115:360–6.
131. Ellison DH. Adaptation to diuretic drugs. In: Seldin DW, Giebisch G, editors Diuretic agents: clinical physiology and pharmacology. San Diego: Academic Press; 1997. p. 209–32.
132. Vargo DL, Kramer WG, Black PK, Smith WB, Serpas T, Brater DC. Bioavailability, pharmacokinetics, and pharmacodynamics of torsemide and furosemide in patients with congestive heart failure. Clin Pharmacol Ther. 1995;57:601–9.
133. Vasavada N, Saha C, Agarwal R. A double-blind randomized crossover trial of two loop diuretics in chronic kidney disease. Kidney Int. 2003;64(2): 632–40.
134. Shah MR, Stevenson LW. Searching for evidence: refractory questions in advanced heart failure. J Card Fail. 2004;10(3):210–8.
135. Stevenson LW, Nohria A, Mielniczuk L. Torrent or torment from the tubules? Challenge of the cardiorenal connections. J Am Coll Cardiol. 2005;45(12):2004–7.
136. Shah MR, Flavell CM, Weintraub JR, et al. Intensity and focus of heart failure disease management after hospital discharge. Am Heart J. 2005;149(4):715–21.
137. Eshaghian S, Horwich TB, Fonarow GC. Relation of loop diuretic dose to mortality in advanced heart failure. Am J Cardiol. 2006;97(12):1759–64.
138. Cooper HA, Dries DL, Davis CE, Shen YL, Domanski MJ. Diuretics and risk of arrhythmic death in patients with left ventricular dysfunction. Circulation. 1999;100(12):1311–5.
139. Stampfer M, Epstein SE, Beiser GD, Braunwald E. Hemodynamic effects of diuresis at rest and during intense upright exercise in patients with impaired cardiac function. Circulation. 1968;37(6):900–11.
140. Channer KS, McLean KA, Lawson-Matthew P, Richardson M. Combination diuretic treatment in severe heart failure: a randomised controlled trial. Br Heart J. 1994;71:146–50.
141. Knauf H, Mutschler E. Diuretic effectiveness of hydrochlorothiazide and furosemide alone and in combination in chronic renal failure. J Cardiovasc Pharmacol. 1995;26:394–400.
142. Fliser D. Loop diuretics and thiazides—the case for their combination in chronic renal failure [editorial]. Nephrol Dial Transplant. 1996;11(3):408–10.
143. Ellison DH. Intensive diuretic therapy: high doses, combinations, and constant infusions. In: Seldin DW, Giebisch G, editors. Diuretic agents: clinical physiology and pharmacology. San Diego: Academic Press; 1997. p. 281–300.
144. Hunt SA. ACC/AHA 2005 guideline update for the diagnosis and management of chronic heart failure in the adult: a report of the American College of Cardiology/American Heart Association Task Force on Practice Guidelines (writing committee to update the 2001 guidelines for the evaluation and management of heart failure). J Am Coll Cardiol. 2005;46(6):e1–82.
145. Pitt B, Remme W, Zannad F, et al. Eplerenone, a selective aldosterone blocker, in patients with left ventricular dysfunction after myocardial infarction. N Engl J Med. 2003;348(14):1309–21.
146. Schrier RW, Cadnapaphornchai MA, Ohara M. Water retention and aquaporins in heart failure, liver disease and pregnancy. J R Soc Med. 2001;94(6): 265–9.
147. Mehta RL, Kellum JA, Shah SV, et al. Acute Kidney Injury Network: report of an initiative to improve outcomes in acute kidney injury. Crit Care. 2007;11(2):R31.
148. Anderson RJ, Linas S, Berns AS, et al. Nonoliguric acute renal failure. N Engl J Med. 1977;296: 1134–8.
149. Heyman SN, Rosen S, Epstein FH, Spokes K, Brezis ML. Loop diuretics reduce hypoxic damage to proximal tubules of the isolated perfused rat kidney. Kidney Int. 1994;45(4):981–5.
150. Allison MEM, Shilliday I. Loop diuretic therapy in acute and chronic renal failure. J Cardiovasc Pharmacol. 1993;22 Suppl 3:S59–70.
151. Brown CB, Ogg CS, Cameron JS. High dose frusemide in acute renal failure: a controlled trial. Clin Nephrol. 1981;15:90–6.
152. Mehta RL, Pascual MT, Soroko S, Chertow GM. Diuretics, mortality, and nonrecovery of renal

function in acute renal failure. JAMA. 2002;288(20):2547–53.
153. Ho KM, Sheridan DJ. Meta-analysis of frusemide to prevent or treat acute renal failure. BMJ. 2006;333(7565):420.
154. Schrier RW, Ecder T. Gibbs memorial lecture. Unifying hypothesis of body fluid volume regulation: implications for cardiac failure and cirrhosis. Mt Sinai J Med. 2001;68(6):350–61.
155. Shear L, Ching S, Gabuzda GJ. Compartmentalization of ascites and edema in patients with hepatic cirrhosis. N Engl J Med. 1970;282(25):1391–6.
156. Wright G, Jalan R. Management of hepatic encephalopathy in patients with cirrhosis. Best Pract Res Clin Gastroenterol. 2007;21(1):95–110.
157. Schrier RW, Fassett RG. A critique of the overfill hypothesis of sodium and water retention in the nephrotic syndrome. Kidney Int. 1998;53(5):1111–7.
158. Rodriguez-Iturbe B, Herrera-Acosta J, Johnson RJ. Interstitial inflammation, sodium retention, and the pathogenesis of nephrotic edema: a unifying hypothesis. Kidney Int. 2002;62(4):1379–84.
159. Voelker JR, Jameson DM, Brater DC. In vitro evidence that urine composition affects the fraction of active furosemide in the nephrotic syndrome. J Pharmacol Exp Ther. 1989;250:772–8.
160. Agarwal R, Gorski JC, Sundblad K, Brater DC. Urinary protein binding does not affect response to furosemide in patients with nephrotic syndrome. J Am Soc Nephrol. 2000;11(6):1100–5.
161. Mattana J, Patel A, Ilunga C, Singhal PC. Furosemide-albumin complexes in refractory nephrotic syndrome and chronic renal failure [letter] [see comments]. Nephron. 1996;73(1):122–3.
162. Fliser D, Zurbruggen I, Mutschler E, et al. Coadministration of albumin and furosemide in patients with the nephrotic syndrome [in process citation]. Kidney Int. 1999;55(2):629–34.
163. Blendis L, Wong F. Intravenous albumin with diuretics: protean lessons to be learnt? [editorial; comment]. J Hepatol. 1999;30(4):727–30.
164. Gentilini P, Casini-Raggi V, Di Fiore G, et al. Albumin improves the response to diuretics in patients with cirrhosis and ascites: results of a randomized, controlled trial. J Hepatol. 1999;30(4):639–45.
165. Brater DC, Chalasani N, Gorski JC, et al. Effect of albumin-furosemide mixtures on response to furosemide in cirrhotic patients with ascites. Trans Am Clin Climatol Assoc 2001;112:108–15; discussion 16.
166. Mitch WE, Wilcox CS. Disorders of body fluids, sodium and potassium in chronic renal failure. AmJMed. 1982;72:536–50.
167. Koomans HA, Roos JC, Boer P, Geyskes GG, Mees EJ. Salt handling in patients with chronic renal insufficiency. Miner Electrolyte Metab. 1982;7(3):134–45.
168. Wilcox CS. New insights into diuretic use in patients with chronic renal disease. J Am Soc Nephrol. 2002;13(3):798–805.
169. Chennavasin P, Seiwell R, Brater DC. Pharmacokinetic-dynamic analysis of the indomethacin-furosemide interaction in man. J Pharmacol Exp Ther. 1980;215:77–81.
170. De Nicola L, Minutolo R, Bellizzi V, et al. Achievement of target blood pressure levels in chronic kidney disease: a salty question? Am J Kidney Dis. 2004;43(5):782–95.
171. Wollam GL, Tarazi RC, Bravo EL, Dustan HP. Diuretic potency of combined hydrochlorothiazide and furosemide therapy in patients with azotemia. Am J Med. 1982;72:929–38.
172. Fliser D, Schröter M, Neubeck M, Ritz E. Coadministration of thiazides increases the efficacy of loop diuretics even in patients with advanced renal failure. Kidney Int. 1994;46:482–8.

Renal Acidification Mechanisms

7

I. David Weiner, Jill W. Verlander, and Charles S. Wingo

Introduction

Maintaining acid–base homeostasis is critical for normal health. Acid–base disorders lead to such clinical problems as growth retardation in neonates and children, nausea and vomiting, electrolyte disturbances, increased susceptibility to cardiac arrhythmias, decreased cardiovascular catecholamine sensitivity, bone disorders including osteoporosis and osteomalacia, recurrent nephrolithiasis, skeletal muscle atrophy, paresthesias, and coma in adults.

The kidneys have two major functions in acid–base homeostasis: (1) reabsorbing filtered bicarbonate and (2) generating new bicarbonate. In the typical adult, the kidneys filter ~4,200 mmol/day of bicarbonate. Renal epithelial cells reabsorb almost all of this in a process termed bicarbonate reabsorption. Kidneys also produce new bicarbonate in a process termed "bicarbonate generation." Kidneys can also excrete alkalis, including bicarbonate and organic anions, a process that is necessary for recovery from chronic respiratory acidosis and metabolic alkalosis. Organic anion excretion is also important for prevention of renal stone formation.

I.D. Weiner, M.D. (✉)
Department of Medicine, University of Florida College of Medicine and North Florida/South Georgia Veterans Health System, 1600 SW Archer Rd, Gainesville, FL 32610, USA
e-mail: david.weiner@medicine.ufl.edu

J.W. Verlander, D.V.M.
Division of Nephrology, Hypertension and Transplantation, Department of Medicine, University of Florida College of Medicine, Gainesville, FL, USA
e-mail: jill.verlander@medicine.ufl.edu

C.S. Wingo, M.D.
Division of Nephrology, Department of Medicine, University of Florida, Gainesville, FL, USA

North Florida/South Georgia Vetrans Health System, Gainesville, FL, USA
e-mail: charles.wingo@medicine.ufl.edu

Bicarbonate Reabsorption

Bicarbonate reabsorption involves coordinated processes in multiple nephron segments (Fig. 7.1). The majority of bicarbonate reabsorption occurs in the proximal tubule. The thin descending limb of Henle's loop reabsorbs little and the thick ascending limb reabsorbs moderate amounts of bicarbonate. The remainder of filtered bicarbonate is reabsorbed in the distal convoluted tubule (DCT), connecting segment (CNT), and the collecting duct.

Proximal Tubule

General Transport Mechanisms

Proximal tubule bicarbonate reabsorption involves four distinct processes (Fig. 7.2) [1]. Protons (H^+) are secreted into the luminal fluid by the apical Na^+/H^+ exchanger, NHE-3, and by an apical H^+-ATPase. NHE-3 is responsible for

D.B. Mount et al. (eds.), *Core Concepts in the Disorders of Fluid, Electrolytes and Acid-Base Balance*, DOI 10.1007/978-1-4614-3770-3_7, © Springer Science+Business Media New York 2013

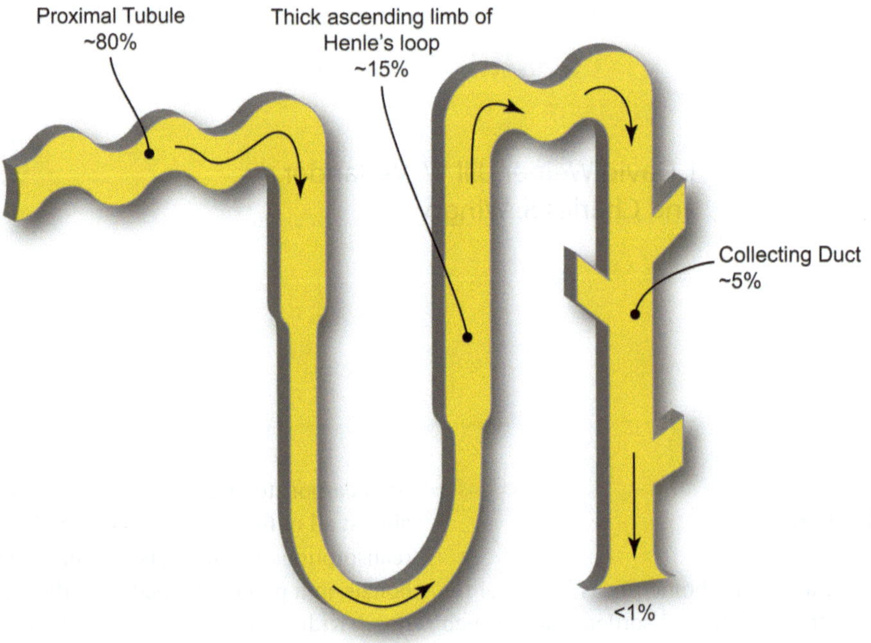

Fig. 7.1 Distribution of bicarbonate reabsorption in the kidney. Bicarbonate is freely filtered at the glomerulus, resulting in filtered bicarbonate load equal to GFR multiplied by serum bicarbonate concentration. The proximal tubule reabsorbs the majority of filtered bicarbonate, the TAL reabsorbs 10–15% of filtered bicarbonate, and the distal tubule and collecting duct reabsorb essentially all remaining bicarbonate. Under normal conditions in humans, urinary bicarbonate is less than 1% of filtered bicarbonate

60–70% of apical H^+ secretion and H^+-ATPase accounts for most of the remainder. Secreted H^+ and luminal HCO_3^- combine to form carbonic acid (H_2CO_3), which dissociates to water (H_2O) and carbon dioxide (CO_2). The dehydration reaction is catalyzed by carbonic anhydrase IV (CA IV), which is present in the proximal tubule brush border membrane. Luminal CO_2 moves across the apical plasma membrane, at least partly through AQP1-mediated transport. Cytosolic CO_2 is hydrated, forming carbonic acid, in a process catalyzed by cytosolic carbonic anhydrase II (CA II). Cytosolic carbonic acid spontaneously dissociates to H^+ and HCO_3^-, which regenerates the secreted H^+. Cytosolic HCO_3^- is transported across the basolateral plasma membrane, primarily by the sodium-coupled, electrogenic bicarbonate cotransporter, NBCe1, in the S1 and S2 segments of the proximal tubule and by a basolateral Na^+-dependent, Cl^-/HCO_3^- exchanger in the S3 segment, although NBCe1 may also contribute in the S3.

In addition, there is a small component of bicarbonate secretion in the proximal tubule, which is termed bicarbonate "backleak." Quantitatively, bicarbonate backleak is less important in the early proximal tubule than in late proximal tubule segments, and involves both paracellular and transcellular components. The transcellular component is developmentally regulated, with less in newborn than in adult animals, and hormonally regulated, with AngII decreasing bicarbonate backleak [2, 3].

Regulation of Proximal Tubule Bicarbonate Reabsorption

Extracellular Acid–Base

Several conditions alter proximal tubule bicarbonate transport. Both metabolic and respiratory acidosis increase and alkalosis decreases bicarbonate

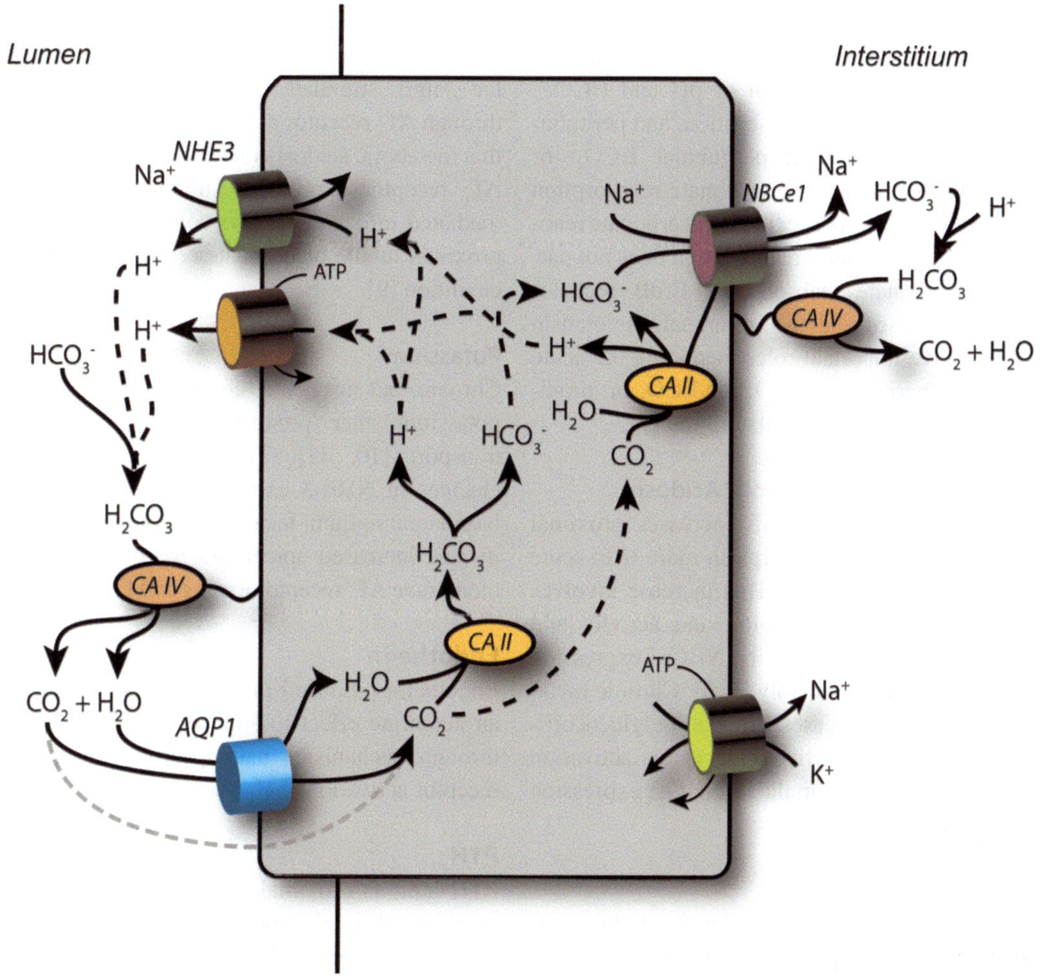

Fig. 7.2 Proximal tubule HCO_3^- reabsorption involves integrated function of multiple proteins. H^+ are secreted by both the Na^+/H^+ exchanger, NHE-3, and by H^+-ATPase, and titrate luminal HCO_3^- to H_2CO_3. Luminal H_2CO_3 dehydration to H_2O and CO_2 is accelerated by luminal carbonic anhydrase activity mediated by CA IV. CO_2 enters the cell via AQP1 and, most likely, via diffusive movement, where its hydration to H_2CO_3 is accelerated by cytoplasmic CA II. H_2CO_3 rapidly dissociates to H^+ and HCO_3^-, thereby "replenishing" the secreted cytosolic H^+. Cytosolic HCO_3^- exits across the basolateral plasma membrane primarily by the $Na^+(HCO_3^-)_3$ cotransporter, NBCe1. Basolateral CA II and CA IV facilitate HCO_3^- transport

reabsorption and the effects of chronic acid–base disturbances are greater than observed with acute disturbances. Luminal bicarbonate concentration regulates proximal tubule bicarbonate reabsorption. Increased luminal bicarbonate concentration increases bicarbonate reabsorption and decreased luminal bicarbonate decreases it. These parallel changes are a part of glomerular–tubular balance in which filtered load regulates tubular reabsorption.

Mechanism by Which Extracellular pH Regulates Proximal Tubule Bicarbonate Reabsorption

Recent studies show that extracellular HCO_3^- and pCO_2 directly regulate proximal tubule bicarbonate transport, but that pH, independent of its association with extracellular HCO_3^- and pCO_2, does not. In particular, studies using out-of-equilibrium solutions, in which pH, HCO_3^- and pCO_2 can be separately and independently altered, show that peritubular HCO_3^-, independent of pH and pCO_2, decreases bicarbonate reabsorption, whereas peritubular pCO_2, independent of pH and HCO_3^-, increases bicarbonate reabsorption, and peritubular pH, independent of peritubular HCO_3^- or pCO_2, has no effect on bicarbonate reabsorption [4]. These effects are specific to bicarbonate reabsorption, because fluid reabsorption does not parallel bicarbonate reabsorption. ErbB receptor tyrosine kinases and the intrarenal angiotensin system have important roles mediating the acute effects of peritubular HCO_3^- and CO_2 on proximal tubule bicarbonate reabsorption [1].

Chronic Effects of Metabolic Acidosis

Chronic metabolic acidosis increases proximal tubule bicarbonate reabsorption more than acute metabolic acidosis does. This increase involves increased NHE-3 expression and activity and increased H^+-ATPase activity; NBCe1 expression does not change detectably [5, 6]. Chronic metabolic acidosis increases circulating glucocorticoids, and glucocorticoid receptor activation increases acidosis-stimulated NHE-3 expression and apical trafficking.

Luminal Flow Rate

Altered rates of glomerular filtration induce parallel changes in proximal tubule bicarbonate reabsorption, a form of glomerulotubular feedback. This is mediated at least partly by flow-dependent changes in proximal tubule transport [7]. Several factors enable flow-dependent regulation. Increased flow minimizes changes in luminal bicarbonate concentration; the resultant higher luminal bicarbonate concentrations thereby enables increased rates of luminal bicarbonate reabsorption. Increasing luminal flow also directly increases apical plasma membrane NHE-3 insertion; this may partially involve proximal tubule brush border microvilli functioning as flow sensors, with drag force transmitted through the actin filament altering cytoskeletal elements and regulating transport.

Angiotensin II

Low concentrations of AngII increase and high concentrations inhibit bicarbonate reabsorption [8]. The effects on bicarbonate transport are greatest in the S1 segment, but are also present in S2 and S3 segments. Both luminal and peritubular AngII stimulate bicarbonate reabsorption through AT_1 receptor activation. The observation that metabolic acidosis increases proximal tubule AT_1 receptor expression suggests that AngII-mediated effects may also contribute to altered proximal tubule bicarbonate reabsorption in this condition [9].

Potassium

Chronic, but not acute, changes in extracellular potassium alter proximal tubule bicarbonate transport [10, 11]. These responses involve changes in NHE-3 expression and activity and basolateral sodium–bicarbonate cotransport activity and increased apical and basolateral plasma membrane AT_1 receptor expression [12, 13].

Endothelin

Endothelin produced in the proximal tubule has an autocrine effect to stimulate NHE-3 activity through mechanisms that appear to require ET-B receptor activation [14].

PTH

PTH inhibits proximal tubule bicarbonate reabsorption through mechanisms that involve decreased apical Na^+/H^+ exchange activity, decreased NHE-3 apical expression, total protein and mRNA expression, and decreased basolateral Na-HCO3 transport activity [15].

Transporters Involved in Proximal Tubule Bicarbonate Reabsorption

Na^+/H^+ Exchangers

Na^+/H^+ exchangers (NHE) are expressed widely in the kidney, where they function in intracellular pH regulation and transepithelial bicarbonate reabsorption. NHE use the extracellular-to-intracellular Na^+ gradient generated by ubiquitous Na^+-K^+-ATPase to drive electroneutral H^+ secretion and Na^+ uptake with a stoichiometry of 1:1. Although Na^+ and H^+ are the preferred ions, NHE can also transport either Li^+ or NH_4^+ [16]; involvement of NH_4^+ enables Na^+/NH_4^+ exchange, which is important in proximal tubule NH_4^+ secretion.

NHE-3 is the primary NHE in the proximal tubule apical membrane, although NHE-2 and

NHE-8 may contribute to a minor extent [1]. NHE-3 mediates the majority of the apical H^+ secretion necessary for luminal bicarbonate reabsorption. In addition, coupling of NHE-3 to Cl^-/base and Cl^-/anion exchangers enables NaCl reabsorption, and thereby facilitates H_2O reabsorption.

NHE-3 expression and activity are regulated by hormones through a variety of mechanisms, including transcription, protein synthesis, phosphorylation, trafficking, and protein–protein interactions. The most widely studied hormones regulating NHE-3 are parathyroid hormone, dopamine and AngII. Both PTH and dopamine inhibit NHE-3 activity, whereas AngII has a biphasic effect, stimulating at low concentrations and inhibiting at high concentrations. These effects involve multiple intracellular signaling pathways, including protein kinase A, protein kinase C, and phosphatidylinositol-3-kinase.

Changes in the NHE-3's subcellular location are another important regulatory mechanism. NHE-3 exists in a variety of subcellular domains in proximal tubule cells, including microvilli, intermicrovillar clefts, endosomes, and cytoplasmic vesicles; only NHE-3 in microvilli is functionally active in transepithelial transport. Redistribution among these sites is regulated by renal sympathetic nerve activity, glucocorticoids, insulin, AngII, dopamine, and PTH [17]. NHE-3 subcellular distribution involves protein kinase A, dynamin, NHERF-1, clathrin-coated vesicles, calcineurin homologous protein-1, ezrin phosphorylation, G-protein alpha subunits, and G-protein beta-gamma dimers.

H^+-ATPase

The second major transporter in proximal tubule apical H^+ secretion is the vacuolar H^+-ATPase. In the proximal tubule, H^+-ATPase is expressed in the brush border microvilli, the base of the brush border, and apical invaginations between clathrin-coated domains as well as in endosomes, lysosomes, and cytoplasmic vesicles. It mediates a substantial component, but not all, of proximal tubule H^+ secretion not mediated by NHE-3 [18]. In addition, H^+-ATPase acidifies proximal tubule endosomes and lysosomes, senses endosomal pH, and is involved in recruiting trafficking proteins to acidified vesicles. Proximal tubule H^+-ATPase activity is increased a variety of conditions, including AngII, increased luminal flow and chronic metabolic acidosis [19].

NBCe1 (SLC4A4)

The electrogenic sodium–bicarbonate cotransporter, NBCe1, is present in the basolateral plasma membrane in the proximal tubule and is the primary means of basolateral HCO_3^- exit [20]. The critical role of NBCe1 is demonstrated by the development of proximal RTA in individuals with mutations in the NBCe1 gene [20, 21]. The mechanism through which NBCe1 mediates increased basolateral bicarbonate exit in conditions of increased transepithelial transport is only partially understood. In metabolic acidosis, transport activity increases, but total protein expression does not [6]. Phosphorylation can regulate NBCe1 activity, raising the possibility that posttranslational modifications are a primary regulatory mechanism [22].

Carbonic Anhydrase II

Carbonic anhydrases are zinc metalloenzymes that catalyze the reversible hydration of CO_2, forming carbonic acid (H_2CO_3), reaction 1 in the equation:

$$CO_2 + H_2O \overset{1}{\Leftrightarrow} H_2CO_3 \overset{2}{\Leftrightarrow} H^+ + HCO_3^-$$

Dissociation of carbonic acid to H^+ and HCO_3^- (reaction 2) is rapid. Consequently, carbonic anhydrases facilitate the rate-limiting step in conversion of CO_2 and H_2O to H^+ and HCO_3^-.

CA II is the predominant carbonic anhydrase in the kidney, accounting for ~95% of total renal carbonic anhydrase activity, and is the predominant carbonic anhydrase in the proximal tubule. CA II is expressed in the kidney predominantly in the cytoplasm of proximal tubule cells and in intercalated cells in the collecting duct. In the mouse kidney, CA II is also expressed in collecting duct principal cells.

CA IV

CA IV is a membrane-associated carbonic anhydrase isoform expressed in the proximal tubule and in intercalated cells in the collecting duct. In the proximal tubule, CA IV is expressed in both apical and basolateral plasma membranes where it facilitates HCO_3^- interconversion with CO_2 and thereby contributes to bicarbonate reabsorption. CA IV interacts with proximal tubule NBCe1, which may facilitate proximal tubule bicarbonate reabsorption [23].

Loop of Henle

The thick ascending limb of the loop of Henle (TAL) reabsorbs ~15–20% of the filtered bicarbonate load. Overall, TAL bicarbonate reabsorption is similar to that in the proximal tubule [24]. Cytosolic H^+ is secreted predominantly by an apical Na^+/H^+ exchange activity. The TAL expresses two NHE isoforms, NHE-2 and NHE-3; NHE-3 is the predominant isoform involved in bicarbonate reabsorption. Vacuolar H^+-ATPase is also present, but has at most a minor role in TAL bicarbonate reabsorption. Secreted H^+ reacts with luminal HCO_3^- to form H_2CO_3, which dissociates to CO_2 and H_2O, possibly catalyzed by luminal CA IV. CO_2 likely enters the cell across the apical plasma membrane through mechanisms which may involve both AQP1-mediated CO_2 transport and a component of diffusive CO_2 movement. Cytoplasmic CA II then catalyzes intracellular CO_2 hydration to form H_2CO_3, which dissociates to H^+ and HCO_3^-, thereby replenishing the H^+ secreted across the apical plasma membrane. Multiple proteins likely mediate basolateral bicarbonate exit, including AE2 and Cl^- channels [24, 25]. Although NBCn1 is highly expressed in the TAL basolateral plasma membrane, it is unlikely to contribute directly to bicarbonate reabsorption as the electrochemical gradient for NBCn1-mediated transport favors sodium-coupled bicarbonate uptake.

Regulation of TAL Bicarbonate Reabsorption

Various physiologic conditions regulate TAL bicarbonate reabsorption. Acute and chronic metabolic acidosis increase and acute metabolic alkalosis inhibits TAL bicarbonate reabsorption [24]. The effect of metabolic alkalosis on TAL bicarbonate reabsorption appears to depend on the experimental model. When induced by intravenous $NaHCO_3$ administration, TAL bicarbonate reabsorption decreases; when induced by chronic hypokalemia, luminal bicarbonate reabsorption does not change [24], and chloride-depletion metabolic alkalosis decreases bicarbonate reabsorption.

Several hormones regulate TAL bicarbonate reabsorption [24]. AngII stimulates TAL bicarbonate reabsorption through activation of AT_1 receptors. Glucocorticoid receptors are present in the TAL and their activation is necessary for bicarbonate reabsorption [24]. High concentrations of mineralocorticoids stimulate bicarbonate reabsorption, but their absence does not alter basal transport. AVP inhibits bicarbonate reabsorption by decreasing apical Na^+/H^+ exchange activity [26].

Recent studies show that cytokines regulate TAL bicarbonate transport [27]. Lipopolysaccharide (LPS) inhibits transport; this effect involves the cytokine receptor, TLR4. Luminal LPS activates the mTOR pathway and peritubular LPS functions through the MEK/ERK pathway to inhibit bicarbonate reabsorption.

Renal medullary tonicity is another important regulatory mechanism; increased tonicity inhibits and decreased tonicity stimulates bicarbonate reabsorption through mechanisms involving altered apical NHE-3-mediated Na^+/H^+ exchange activity [28]. Medullary tonicity's effect is separate from AVP's effect on TAL bicarbonate transport.

Several ion transporters regulate TAL bicarbonate reabsorption. Inhibiting the apical Na^+-K^+-$2Cl^-$ cotransporter, NKCC2, increases bicarbonate reabsorption [24]. This likely involves decreased apical Na^+ entry, which decreases intracellular Na^+, thereby increasing the Na^+ uptake gradient for apical Na^+/H^+ exchange-mediated bicarbonate reabsorption. Blocking basolateral Na^+/H^+ exchange activity inhibits apical NHE-3, which inhibits bicarbonate reabsorption [29]. This may result from changes in the actin cytoskeleton that decreases apical plasma membrane NHE-3 insertion.

Paracellular HCO_3^- Transport

Although the TAL has a significant paracellular Cl^- permeability which can also transport bicarbonate, the paracellular permeability of HCO_3^- relative to Cl^- is 10% or less [24]; consequently, transepithelial voltage does not regulate bicarbonate reabsorption significantly and paracellular bicarbonate backleak is relatively minimal.

Distal Convoluted Tubule

The DCT is an important site for bicarbonate reabsorption. The DCT contains both DCT cells and intercalated cells. DCT cells express apical NHE-2 and inhibiting NHE-2 decreases bicarbonate reabsorption [30]. Basolateral bicarbonate exit is thought to occur by Cl^-/HCO_3^- exchange, possibly AE2, and may also involve a basolateral Cl^- channel with partial HCO_3^- permeability [31]. Cytosolic CA II is present and likely facilitates bicarbonate reabsorption, but apical CA IV is not present. Intercalated cells comprise only a very small proportion of cells in the DCT, and the majority are type A and type C (non-A, non-B) intercalated cells. The role of intercalated cells is discussed below.

Collecting Duct

The collecting duct is the site of the final regulation of urinary acid excretion. It contributes to acid–base homeostasis by both reabsorbing and secreting bicarbonate, by protonating titratable acids and by secreting ammonia. These functions are regulated and are mediated by specific transporters in specific epithelial cell types, which vary in type and frequency along the collecting duct.

Collecting Duct Segments

The collecting duct begins with the initial collecting tubule (ICT), distal to the connecting segment (CNT). Although the CNT has a different embryonic origin than the ICT and the remainder of the collecting duct, we discuss it here because its intercalated cell types and acid–base transport mechanisms are similar to those in the collecting duct. Medullary collecting duct segments are defined by the kidney region where they reside: outer medullary collecting duct in the outer stripe (OMCDo), outer medullary collecting duct in the inner stripe (OMCDi), and inner medullary collecting duct (IMCD). In the IMCD, the most proximal portion, located in the base of the inner medulla, is called either IMCD1 or initial IMCD (IMCDi). The IMCD in the papilla is either called the terminal IMCD (IMCDt) or divided into IMCD2 and IMCD3, with IMCD3 being the most distal part.

Cell Composition

Collecting ducts contain several distinct epithelial cell subtypes. Two main cell types are present, intercalated and principal cells, with ~60–65% of cells from ICT into the OMCD being principal cells and ~35–40% intercalated cells. At least three distinct intercalated cell subtypes exist; the type A intercalated cell, the type B intercalated cell and a third, distinct intercalated cell type, the non-A, non-B intercalated cell (Fig. 7.3). The proportion of collecting duct cells that are intercalated cells decreases in the initial IMCD and intercalated cells are almost completely absent from the terminal IMCD. The IMCD3 epithelium is composed of IMCD cells, a cell type distinct from both intercalated cells and principal cells. The CNT contains intercalated cells and a cell type specific to the CNT, the connecting segment cell, as well as principal cells in some species.

Type A Intercalated Cell

The type A intercalated cell secretes H^+ and reabsorbs luminal bicarbonate, and is found in the CNT, ICT, CCD, OMCD and the initial IMCD. Bicarbonate reabsorption involves integrated activity of multiple proteins (Fig. 7.4). Apical H^+ secretion involves both H^+-ATPase and H^+-K^+-ATPase. H^+-ATPase is abundant in the apical plasma membrane and in apical cytoplasmic tubulovesicles in type A intercalated cells, and apical redistribution of H^+-ATPase between cytoplasmic vesicles and the apical plasma

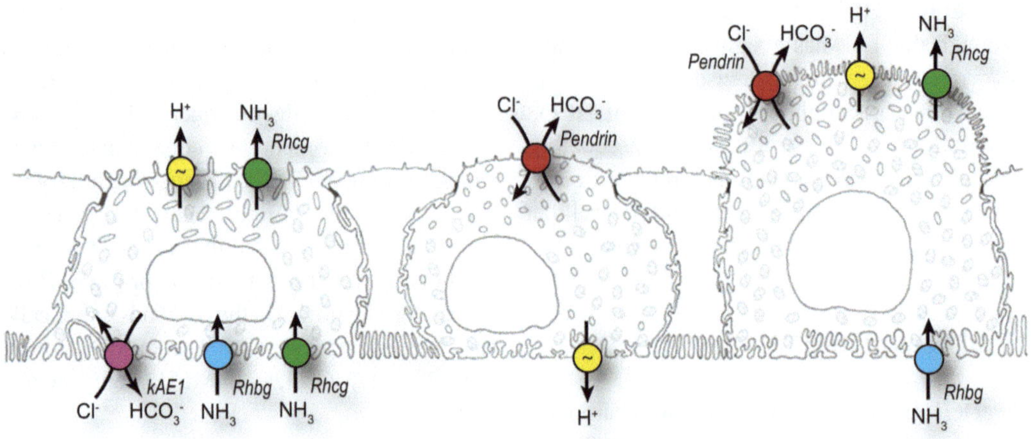

Fig. 7.3 Intercalated cell subtypes. The distal nephron, i.e., the connecting segment, initial collecting tubule, CCD, OMCD, and IMCD, has multiple distinct cell types. Three intercalated cell types can be distinguished based on differential expression in different plasma membrane domains of several proteins involved in renal acid–base transport, including H^+-ATPase, AE1, pendrin, Rhbg, and Rhcg. Figure modified from an original provided by Ki-Hwan Han, M.D., Ph.D., Ewha Womans University, Seoul, South Korea

membrane enables regulated apical proton secretion in response to physiologic perturbations [32]. Another mechanism of H^+ secretion involves electroneutral H^+/K^+ exchange mediated by H^+-K^+-ATPase proteins [33]. At least two isoforms of the catalytic, α-subunit are present. One, $HK\alpha_1$, is similar to the α-isoform responsible for gastric acid secretion, whereas the other, $HK\alpha_2$, is similar to the α-isoform in the colon. K^+ reabsorbed via apical H^+-K^+-ATPase can either recycle across the apical plasma membrane or exit the cell across the basolateral plasma membrane.

Bicarbonate exit is mediated by a truncated isoform of the erythrocyte anion exchanger, kAE1 (Slc4a1), present in the basolateral plasma membrane. Cl^- that enters the cell via basolateral Cl^-/HCO_3^- exchange exits via a basolateral Cl^- channel, presumably ClC-Kb in humans and ClC-K2 in rodents [34, 35]. Cytoplasmic carbonic anhydrase II (CA II) is abundant in type A intercalated cells [36] and catalyzes intracellular by conversion of CO_2 and H_2O to H^+ and HCO_3^-. Membrane-associated carbonic anhydrase is present in the apical region (CA IV) and, at least in mouse and rabbit, in the basolateral region (CA XII) of intercalated cells.

Type B Intercalated Cell

The type B intercalated cell is almost exclusively located in the CNT through CCD and is capable of bicarbonate secretion and Cl^- reabsorption. It contains basolateral H^+-ATPase and apical pendrin (SLC26A4), an electroneutral Cl^-/HCO_3^- exchanger [37]. H^+-ATPase is also present in vesicles throughout the cell, but ultrastructural studies using immunogold localization show it is absent from the apical plasma membrane. Type B intercalated cells express both $HK\alpha_1$ and $HK\alpha_2$ [33] and functional studies suggest there is apical Sch28080-sensitive, H^+-K^+-ATPase activity in both rabbit and mouse B intercalated cells [38, 39]. The type B cell also has cytoplasmic CA II, but its abundance is less than in type A intercalated cells [36]. Basolateral Cl^-/HCO_3^- exchange activity is present in all type B intercalated cells [40], but the molecular identity of this activity and its physiologic role have not been determined.

Non-A, Non-B or Type C Intercalated Cell

A third intercalated cell subtype is present, and is found primarily in the DCT, CNT, and ICT. In particular, it expresses apical H^+-ATPase and apical pendrin, but not basolateral AE1, and thus

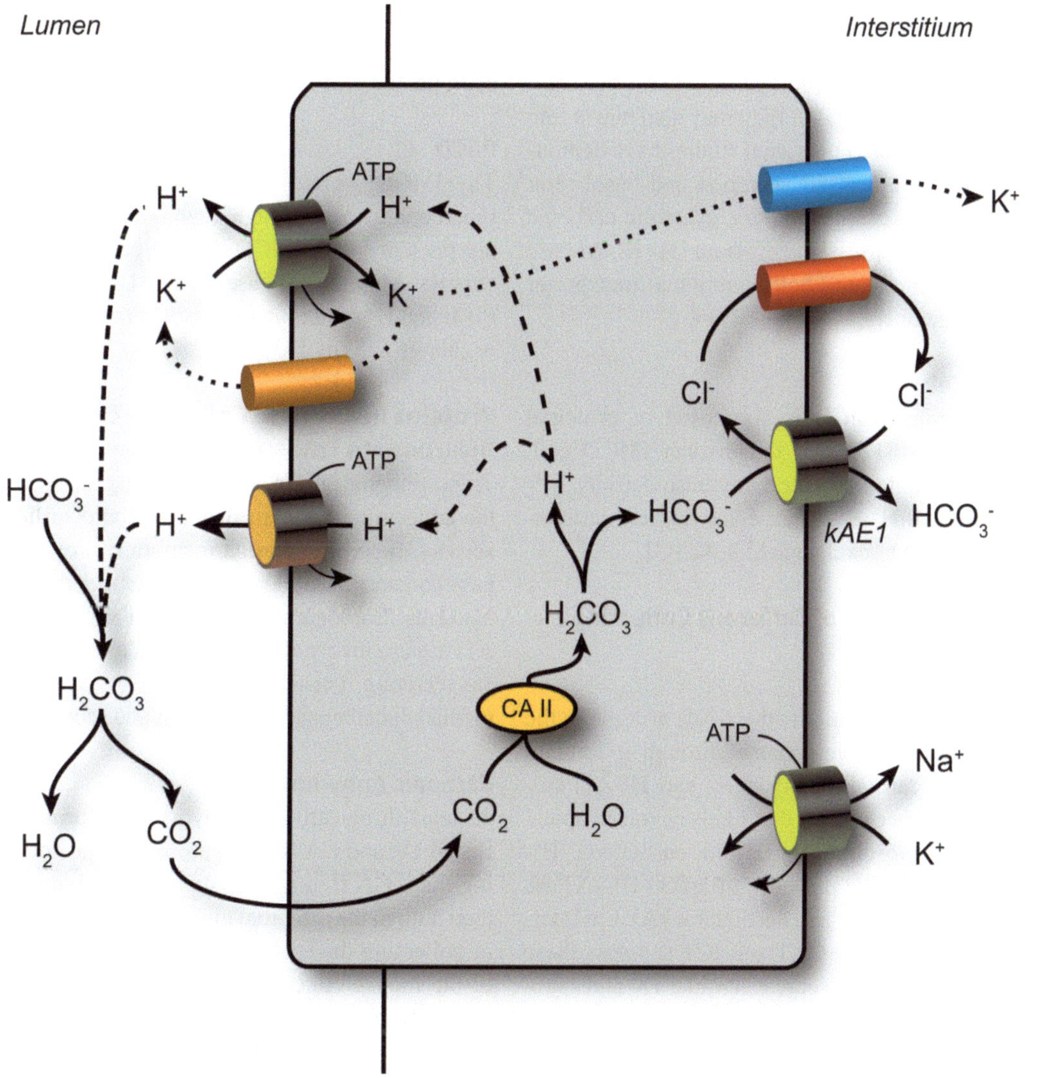

Fig. 7.4 Bicarbonate reabsorption by the type A intercalated cell. The type A intercalated cell is present from the connecting segment through the initial IMCD. Two families of H^+ transporters, H^+-ATPase and H^+-K^+-ATPase, are present in the apical plasma membrane. Secreted H^+ titrate luminal HCO_3^- to form H_2CO_3, which dehydrates to water (H_2O) and CO_2. Luminal carbonic anhydrase activity, most likely mediated by CA IV, is variably present in the collecting duct (see text for details). Cytosolic H^+ and HCO_3^- are formed from CA II-accelerated hydration of CO_2 and rapid dissociation of H_2CO_3. Cytosolic HCO_3^- exits across the basolateral plasma membrane via the anion exchanger, AE1. Cl^- that enters via kAE1 recycles via a basolateral Cl^- channel. K^+ that enters via apical H^+-K^+-ATPase can either recycle via an apical, Ba^+-sensitive K^+ channel or be reabsorbed via a basolateral Ba^+-sensitive K^+ channel. A basolateral Na^+/H^+ exchanger is present, but does not contribute to bicarbonate reabsorption and is not shown

differs fundamentally from both A-type and B-type intercalated cells (Fig. 7.3). This cell type was initially termed a "non-A, non-B cell" because it did not have features consistent with either recognized intercalated cell subtype; alternative names include "non-A, non-B intercalated cell" or "Type C intercalated cell." Studies of the developing mouse kidney indicate that the non-A, non-B intercalated cells in the CNT arise from separate foci than type B intercalated cells [41].

Principal Cells

Principal cells are widely recognized for their major role in transepithelial sodium, potassium and water transport, but they may also play a role in acid secretion. Functional studies have demonstrated both apical H^+ secretion and basolateral Cl^-/HCO_3^- exchange activity, cytosolic carbonic anhydrase, expression of both H^+-K^+-ATPase alpha-subunits and both ammonia transporter family members, Rhcg and Rhbg.

IMCD Cell

The terminal IMCD is composed of principal cells (in IMCD2) and the distinct IMCD cell, which exhibits carbonic anhydrase activity, H^+-ATPase and H^+-K^+-ATPase activity and basolateral Cl^-/HCO_3^- exchange [33, 42, 43].

Functional Role of Different Collecting Duct Segments

CNT-ICT

Under basal conditions, the CNT, at least in the rabbit, secretes bicarbonate through a luminal chloride-, carbonic anhydrase- and H^+-ATPase-dependent mechanism that likely involves apical pendrin, cytosolic CA II and basolateral H^+-ATPase [44]. The presence of apical H^+-ATPase and H^+-K^+-ATPase and basolateral kAE1 in intercalated cells in the CNT and ICT suggests these segments can also secrete luminal H^+ and reabsorb luminal HCO_3^-.

CCD

The CCD has an important role in acid–base homeostasis because of the ability to both reabsorb and secrete bicarbonate [45]. The basal direction of bicarbonate transport varies among species, but both net bicarbonate absorption and secretion can be induced in response to systemic acid or alkali loading. The ability to secrete bicarbonate, which is not found in the OMCD or IMCD, correlates with the presence of type B intercalated cells in the CCD and its absence in more distal collecting duct segments.

OMCD

The OMCD is responsible for approximately 40–50% of the net acid secretion in the collecting duct. Acid secretion is largely mediated by intercalated cells, which are essentially of a single subtype, the type A intercalated cell.

IMCD

The IMCD secretes H^+ and reabsorbs luminal bicarbonate even though few intercalated cells are present in the IMCD. IMCD cells appear to express both H^+-ATPase- and H^+-K^+-ATPase-mediated H^+ secretion and basolateral Cl^-/HCO_3^- exchange activity [43, 46].

Proteins Involved in Collecting Duct H^+/Bicarbonate Transport

Transepithelial proton and bicarbonate transport in the collecting duct is mediated by the coordinate activity of specific plasma membrane proton and bicarbonate transporters and carbonic anhydrase isoforms. Carbonic anhydrases and vacuolar H^+-ATPase are involved in both proton and bicarbonate secretion, but distinct Cl^-/HCO_3^- exchangers mediate bicarbonate reabsorption and secretion.

Carbonic Anhydrase

At least three carbonic anhydrase isoforms, CA II, CA IV, and CA XII, are present in the collecting duct. CA II is a cytosolic form and is abundant both in the proximal tubule, discussed above, in collecting duct intercalated cells and, at least in the mouse collecting duct, in principal cells. Although not as abundant as in A cells, CA II is present in type B and C (non-A, non-B) intercalated cells as well.

CA IV is an extracellular, membrane-associated carbonic anhydrase tethered to the membrane through a glycosylphosphatidylinositol lipid (GPI) anchoring protein, and is expressed apically in the majority of cells in rabbit OMCD and IMCD and in type A intercalated cells in the CCD [23]. By catalyzing dehydration of carbonic acid, luminal CA IV accelerates bicarbonate reabsorption [47]. Metabolic acidosis increases CA IV mRNA expression in response to metabolic acidosis, suggesting increased CA IV protein and activity facilitate increased rates of bicarbonate reabsorption [23].

Carbonic anhydrase XII (CA XII) is another extracellular, membrane-associated carbonic anhydrase [23]. CA XII has a single transmembrane spanning region, which differs from CA IV. CA XII is expressed in the collecting duct, although there may be significant species differences in cellular distribution. Basolateral CA XII immunoreactivity has been reported in principal cells in human kidney, but in the mouse basolateral CA XII immunoreactivity is present in type A intercalated cells in the CCD and OMCD [48].

H^+-ATPase

Electrogenic apical H^+ secretion in acid-secreting intercalated cells and basolateral H^+ transport by bicarbonate-secreting intercalated cells is mediated by the vacuolar H^+-ATPase. Vacuolar H^+-ATPase is a complex, multi-subunit protein, with distinct isoforms and splice variants identified for many of the H^+-ATPase subunits [32]. In the collecting duct, H^+-ATPase is most abundant in intercalated cells. Intercalated cells in the medullary collecting ducts and type A intercalated cells in the CCD contain H^+-ATPase in the apical plasma membrane and in an apical cytoplasmic vesicle pool [49]. Acid secretion is regulated in large part by redistribution of H^+-ATPase between the cytoplasmic vesicle pool and the plasma membrane; changes in total H^+-ATPase expression are not a major mechanism regulating H^+ secretion [32]. H^+-ATPase is also present in the apical region of principal cells and connecting segment cells, but it is less abundant than in intercalated cells. The role of apical H^+-ATPase in nonintercalated cells has not been clearly defined; it may be involved in endosomal trafficking and fusion, and in the OMCDi it can also mediate luminal proton secretion [50].

H^+-K^+-ATPase

H^+-K^+-ATPases (Type IIC P-ATPases) also mediate apical H^+ secretion in the collecting duct [33]. The active pump is a heterodimer composed of α- and β- subunits. The α-subunit is an integral membrane protein with multiple transmembrane domains and is the catalytic portion of the enzyme. The β-subunit has only a single membrane spanning region and is necessary for targeting to the plasma membrane and for transport function. Two isoforms of the α-subunit have been identified. $HK\alpha_1$, the gastric isoform, forms heterodimers with its specific β-subunit, HKβ. Three splice variants of $HK\alpha_2$, the colonic isoform, have been identified in the kidney. $HK\alpha_2$ forms heterodimers with the β_1-subunit of Na^+-K^+-ATPase.

Both $HK\alpha_1$ and $HK\alpha_2$ and HKβ are expressed throughout the collecting duct. In general, these subunits are more abundant in intercalated cells than in principal cells. Both $HK\alpha_1$ and $HK\alpha_2$ isoforms are present in type A and type B intercalated cell subtypes. Immunohistochemistry results vary with respect to the precise cellular distribution of the $HK\alpha_1$ and $HK\alpha_2$ isoforms. Apical $HK\alpha_1$ immunoreactivity has been found in AE1-positive (type A) and AE1-negative intercalated cells in both rat and rabbit kidney [51], whereas in the human kidney, diffuse $HK\alpha_1$ immunoreactivity has been observed in both intercalated and principal cells [52]. $HK\alpha_2$ immunoreactivity was found exclusively in the connecting segment cell in rabbit in one study, exclusively in the OMCD principal cell in rat in another [53, 54], and another study found the splice variant, $HK\alpha_{2c}$, in both intercalated cells, principal cells, and connecting segment cells from the CNT through the initial IMCD in rabbit kidney [55].

Multiple physiologic conditions alter H^+-K^+-ATPase expression and activity. Metabolic acidosis increases $HK\alpha_1$ and $HK\alpha_2$ mRNA and H^+-K^+-ATPase activity in the CCD, suggesting that apical H^+-K^+-ATPase contributes to H^+ secretion [33]. In the rat, metabolic alkalosis, which increases CCD bicarbonate secretion, also increases H^+-K^+-ATPase activity, suggesting that a basolateral H^+-K^+-ATPase activity may contribute to bicarbonate secretion [56]. However, studies have identified apical, but not basolateral, H^+-K^+-ATPase activity in the type B intercalated cells in mouse and rabbit kidney [38, 57]. In addition, chronic mineralocorticoid administration, possibly through potassium-dependent mechanisms, increases $HK\alpha_2$ mRNA and H^+-K^+-ATPase activity [33].

kAE1 (Slc4a1)

The basolateral anion exchanger in intercalated cells in the medullary collecting duct and in type A intercalated cells in the cortex is a truncated splice variant of AE1, also known as band 3 protein, the anion exchanger found in erythrocytes. In the human, rat, and mouse kidney AE1 is expressed almost entirely in the basolateral plasma membrane. In the rabbit kidney under basal conditions, AE1 is present in intracellular multivesicular bodies, as well as in the basolateral plasma membrane; metabolic acidosis decreases intracellular AE1 and increases basolateral AE1, suggesting AE1 trafficking contributes to regulated bicarbonate reabsorption [49].

Pendrin (Slc26a4)

Pendrin is an electroneutral Cl^-/HCO_3^- exchanger expressed in the CNT, ICT, and CCD exclusively in type B and non-A, non-B intercalated cells. Under basal conditions, pendrin is predominantly expressed in the apical plasma membrane in non-A, non-B intercalated cells and in subapical cytoplasmic vesicles in type B intercalated cells [58]. Although mineralocorticoid treatment increases apical plasma membrane pendrin in both B and non-A, non-B intercalated cells, other conditions associated with increased pendrin expression, such as dietary Cl^- deficiency, increase apical plasma membrane pendrin expression only in the type B intercalated cell largely by subcellular redistribution from intracellular vesicles [59]. Pendrin also mediates an important role in extracellular fluid volume and blood pressure regulation. This involves both transcellular Cl^- reabsorption and, through luminal alkalinization due to HCO_3^- secretion, activation of the principal cell epithelial Na^+ transporter, ENaC [60].

Other Anion Transporters

Cl^- entering via basolateral kAE1 recycles across the basolateral plasma membrane. The potassium–chloride cotransporter, KCC4, is basolateral in acid-secreting intercalated cells, and appears to facilitate chloride exit [61]. In addition, the Cl^- channel, ClC-K2, is present in the basolateral plasma membrane of intercalated cells and likely also contributes to basolateral Cl^- exit [62].

Several other anion transporters, including anion exchangers and sodium bicarbonate cotransporters, are present in the collecting duct. AE2 (Slc4a2) is expressed in collecting ducts, particularly in the basolateral plasma membrane of inner medullary collecting duct cells in the terminal IMCD [63]. Slc26a7 can mediate basolateral Cl^-/HCO_3^- exchange in OMCD intercalated cells, and its expression increases with acid-loading [64]. NBCn1 (Slc4a7) is an electroneutral sodium–bicarbonate cotransporter in the basolateral plasma membrane in IMCD cells, where it appears to contribute to intracellular pH regulation [65]. Another product of the SLC4A7 gene, termed NBC3 in some studies, is found in the apical region of OMCD intercalated cells and type A intercalated cells in the CCD and in the basolateral region of type B intercalated cells; in OMCDi intercalated cells it regulates intracellular pH regulation and does not appear to contribute to bicarbonate transport [66, 67]. NBCe2 (Slc4a5), an electrogenic sodium–bicarbonate cotransporter, is apical in intercalated cells in the medullary collecting duct [68].

Regulation of Collecting Duct Acid–Base Transport

The collecting duct is the final site controlling renal acid–base regulation. It responds quickly to physiologic conditions to increase acid or bicarbonate excretion as needed to maintain systemic acid–base homeostasis.

Acidosis

The collecting duct response to the challenge of excreting an increased acid load includes acute and chronic adaptations and involves all segments of the collecting duct and the connecting segment. The known mechanisms include alterations in the abundance, subcellular location, and activity of the major proteins involved in proton and bicarbonate transport.

Increased acid secretion in the collecting duct during metabolic acidosis is primarily mediated by H^+-ATPase [32]. Both metabolic and respiratory acidosis increase apical H^+-ATPase activity and apical plasma membrane H^+-ATPase in acid-secreting collecting duct intercalated cells.

Redistribution of H^+-ATPase from a subapical vesicle pool to the apical plasma membrane is the primary means of activation of proton secretion, and involves vesicular trafficking via SNARE proteins and Rab GTPases. In most experimental models of metabolic acidosis, renal H^+-ATPase mRNA and protein expression do not change.

During metabolic acidosis, AE1 mRNA and protein expression increases. In rats and mice, AE1 is present in the basolateral membrane under basal conditions and the subcellular distribution does not change with metabolic acidosis. In rabbits fed a normal diet, AE1 is located in intracellular multivesicular bodies and the basolateral plasma membrane in type A intercalated cells; metabolic acidosis increases AE1 immunoreactivity in the basolateral plasma membrane and reduces intracellular AE1, suggesting that altered subcellular distribution contributes to increased bicarbonate reabsorption [49].

During ammonium chloride loading, pendrin expression in type B and non-A, non-B intercalated cells decreases in parallel with decreased apical Cl^-/HCO_3^- exchange activity in type B intercalated cells in the CCD [69]. Reduced bicarbonate secretion by B cells during acid-loading thus contributes to increased net bicarbonate reabsorption by the CCD.

Carbonic anhydrase activity and the expression of CA II and CA IV in the collecting duct are increased by metabolic acidosis [23]. CA IV expression is upregulated in the OMCD, whereas CA II expression is upregulated in the CNT, CCD, and OMCD.

The collecting duct response to respiratory acidosis is similar to metabolic acidosis. Respiratory acidosis stimulates structural changes in OMCD and CCD type A intercalated cells consistent with translocation of H^+-ATPase from the apical vesicle pool to the apical plasma membrane [70]. Respiratory acidosis also stimulates NEM-sensitive ATPase activity and bicarbonate reabsorption in isolated CCDs, consistent with activation of H^+-ATPase mediated proton secretion. At least in part, the increase in bicarbonate reabsorption with respiratory acidosis is due to increased H^+-K^+-ATPase-mediated H^+ secretion. In addition, chronic respiratory acidosis increases kAE1 mRNA. Pendrin expression is downregulated during respiratory acidosis, which likely decreases bicarbonate secretion.

How the collecting duct "senses" changes in extracellular pH is under continued investigation and likely involves regulatory mechanisms other than simple direct effects of extracellular pH on the collecting duct. Importantly, in vivo acid–base changes cause greater adaptations than equivalent in vitro changes, suggesting that mechanisms other than extracellular pH have direct effects on collecting duct acid–base transport [71]. One regulatory mechanism may involve the family of proton-activated G protein-coupled receptors. One of these, GPR4 is abundantly expressed in the kidney, particularly in the collecting duct, and GPR4 gene deletion increases urine pH, decreases titratable acid and net acid excretion, causes development of spontaneous non-gap metabolic acidosis and impairs the normal increase in net acid excretion in response to metabolic acidosis [72]. Thus, GPR4 may mediate an important role in renal acid–base homeostasis.

Alkalosis

Metabolic alkalosis also induces coordinated changes in collecting duct acid–base transport. In the OMCD of bicarbonate-loaded animals, bicarbonate reabsorption is less than in control animals, and in the IMCD, bicarbonate loading abolishes acid secretion. In the CCD, bicarbonate loading in animals induces net bicarbonate secretion. Importantly, the renal response to metabolic alkalosis involves luminal Cl^--dependent HCO_3^- secretion, a process that likely involves pendrin-mediated Cl^- reabsorption and HCO_3^- secretion.

The cellular response to alkalosis in OMCD and CCD type A cells entails essentially the reverse of the processes that stimulate acid secretion. H^+-ATPase is redistributed from the apical plasma membrane into the apical vesicle pool, and basolateral AE1 immunoreactivity decreases. Alkalosis increases apical plasma membrane pendrin expression in type B and non-A, non-B intercalated cells [73]. However, pendrin expression, subcellular location and functional activity are also regulated by factors other than acid–base status, including mineralocorticoids and chloride balance [74]. The role of pendrin as the primary bicarbonate transporter involved in CCD bicarbonate secretion and its dependence on luminal chloride availability provides a mechanistic explanation for the importance of chloride in correction of metabolic alkalosis [75].

Hormonal Regulation of Collecting Duct Acid–Base Transport

In addition to extracellular pH, multiple other factors regulate collecting duct acid–base transport. Several hormones and receptors regulate bicarbonate transport in the collecting duct, including mineralocorticoids, angiotensin II, and endothelin.

Aldosterone is an important regulator of collecting duct bicarbonate transport. Both in vivo and in vitro mineralocorticoids increase OMCD bicarbonate reabsorption [76]. This involves, at least in vitro, increased H^+-ATPase activity and apical translocation in OMCD intercalated cells [77]. Mineralocorticoids also increase CCD pendrin-mediated bicarbonate secretion through mechanisms involving increased mRNA and protein expression, pendrin redistribution from cytoplasmic vesicles to the apical plasma membrane of B-type intercalated cells, and increased plasma membrane pendrin in non-A, non-B intercalated cells without subcellular redistribution [78], indicating that mineralocorticoids exhibit cell-specific effects.

Angiotensin II (AngII) is an important regulator of ion transport in the proximal tubule and thick ascending limb. Its effects on collecting duct acid–base transport, however, are unclear. AngII has been reported to increase H^+-ATPase activity in CCD and OMCD acid-secreting intercalated cells and pendrin-mediated chloride reabsorption in some studies and to decrease bicarbonate reabsorption and H^+-ATPase activity in other studies.

Endothelin has important effects on collecting duct acid–base transport which are mediated partly by nitric oxide. Dietary protein intake stimulates urinary acidification through a process involving H^+-ATPase activation, which is mediated by endothelin and nitric oxide [79]. Endothelin-1 (ET-1) is synthesized in native collecting duct and cultured collecting duct cells. Endothelin receptors A and B (ET-A and ET-B) are present in the collecting duct, but ET-B predominates. In vitro metabolic acidosis normally increases acid secretion by type A cells and decreases bicarbonate secretion by type B cells. ET-B, in conjunction with nitric oxide synthase, regulates the type B intercalated cell response to metabolic acidosis, whereas the ET-B receptor, but not nitric oxide synthase, regulates the type A cell response.

The calcium-sensing receptor is another important regulator of collecting duct H^+ secretion. It is present in the apical membrane in IMCD and in type A intercalated cells and mediates luminal Ca^{2+}-stimulation of H^+-ATPase [80]. Luminal acidification stimulated by this pathway may increase urinary calcium-salt solubility and thereby minimize development of nephrolithiasis.

Bicarbonate Generation

Renal acid–base homeostasis requires new bicarbonate generation in order to replace bicarbonate consumed in buffering endogenous and exogenous acid loads. There are two major components of bicarbonate generation, titratable acid excretion and ammonia excretion. Renal regulation of acid–base homeostasis also involves organic anion excretion, which is physiologically equivalent to bicarbonate excretion because organic acids can be metabolized into alkali equivalents.

Titratable Acid Excretion

Titratable acids are solutes in the urine that buffer secreted protons, enabling H^+ excretion without substantial changes in urine pH. Titratable acid excretion comprises ~30–40% of net acid excretion under basal conditions. Metabolic acidosis increases titratable acid excretion by as much as 50% above baseline, thereby contributing to recovery from this acid–base disorder (Fig. 7.5). However, the role of increased titratable acid excretion is quantitatively less than that of ammonia in response to metabolic acidosis [81].

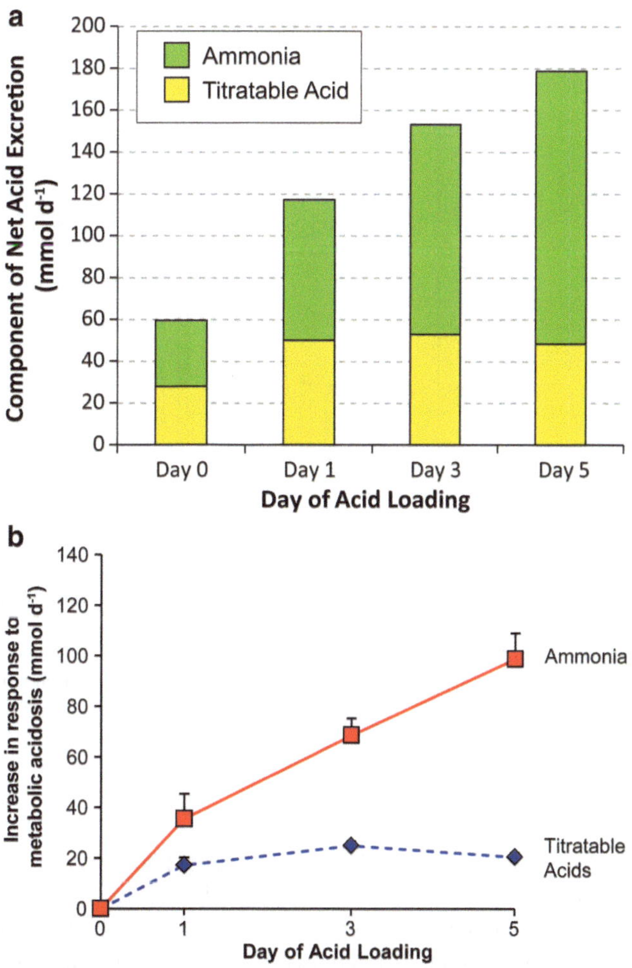

Fig. 7.5 Relative roles of titratable acid and ammonia excretion in basal net acid excretion and in the response to metabolic acidosis. Normal human volunteers were acid-loaded with ~2 mmol/kg/day of ammonium chloride and changes in urinary ammonia and titratable acid excretion were quantified. Data recalculated from [81]

Multiple solutes contribute to titratable acid excretion [82]. Figure 7.6 shows the relative contributions of major urinary buffers, taking into account the amount excreted under basal conditions and the p*K*a. Ammonia is frequently considered a urinary buffer, but because of its high p*K*a it does not contribute substantially to titratable acid excretion. Phosphate is the predominant titratable acid, typically accounting for more than 50% of total titratable acid. Citrate and creatinine also contribute to titratable acid excretion, but to a lesser extent. Although sulfate is excreted in relatively large amounts, because of its low p*K*a′ it does not effectively buffer secreted H^+ and therefore does not contribute significantly to titratable acid excretion.

Phosphate as a Titratable Acid

The amount of phosphate excreted that functions as a titratable acid is determined by filtered load, renal tubular reabsorption and urine pH. Plasma phosphate is almost completely filtered at the glomerulus; renal tubular phosphate reabsorption and urine pH are the major factors regulating titratable acid excretion in the form of phosphate.

Phosphate exists in serum in equilibrium between two molecular forms, $H_2PO_4^-$ and HPO_4^{2-}. The relative amount of these two forms is determined by the formula:

$$10^{\mathrm{pH}-6.8} = \left[\mathrm{HPO_4}^{2-}\right]/\left[\mathrm{H_2PO_4}^{-}\right]$$

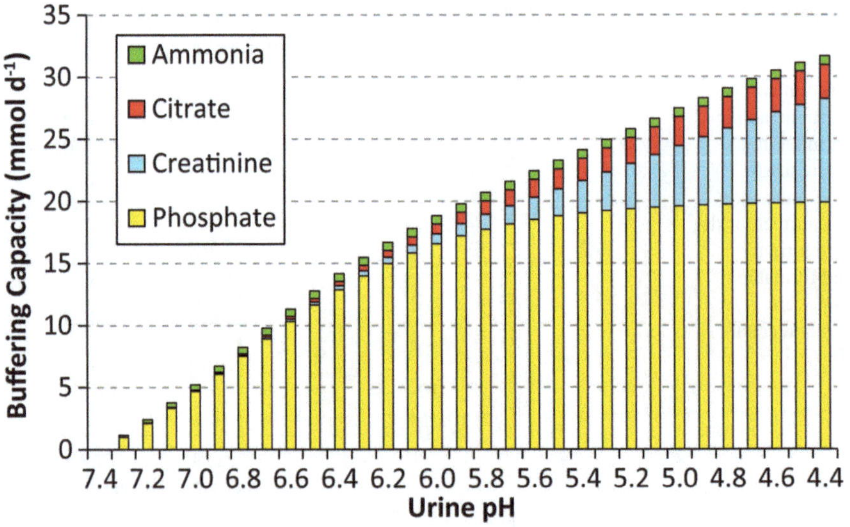

Fig. 7.6 Relative contribution of various urinary buffers to titratable acid excretion. Ability of various urinary buffers to contribute to titratable acid excretion depends on their urinary excretion rate, p*K*a and final urine pH. Figure shows buffering capacity of each of four major urinary buffers, phosphate, creatinine, citrate and ammonia at differing urine pH. Rates were calculated with daily excretion rate and p*K*a, respectively, for phosphate, 25 mmol/day and 6.8; creatinine, 11 mmol/day and 4.9; citrate, 3 mmol/day and 5.6; and ammonia, 40 mmol/day and 9.15

Accordingly, at pH 7.4, ~80% of filtered phosphate is HPO_4^{2-} and 20% is $H_2PO_4^-$. Titratable acid excretion in the form of phosphate thus reflects the amount of filtered HPO_4^{2-} that is not reabsorbed and that buffers H^+ secreted in the proximal tubule, loop of Henle, distal tubule, and the collecting duct.

Regulation of renal tubular phosphate transport is a complex process, and is discussed in more detail elsewhere. Here, we review only the factors that regulate this process in response to acid–base disorders.

The proximal tubule is the primary site of phosphate reabsorption and where metabolic acidosis and other acid–base disorders regulate renal phosphate transport. Minimal phosphate reabsorption occurs distal to the proximal tubule, and distal sites do not regulate phosphate excretion. Acute and chronic metabolic acidosis decrease proximal tubule phosphate reabsorption through a variety of mechanisms [83]. There is decreased apical Na^+-dependent phosphate transport which appears due in part to decreased NaPi-IIa protein and mRNA expression. In acute metabolic acidosis, changes in NaPi-IIa subcellular distribution decrease phosphate reabsorption. PTH likely contributes to decreased phosphate reabsorption in metabolic acidosis; metabolic acidosis increases PTH release, which inhibits proximal tubule phosphate reabsorption. Finally, metabolic acidosis decreases proximal tubule luminal pH, and luminal acidification independently inhibits proximal tubule phosphate uptake.

Multiple phosphate transporters, including NaPi-IIa, NaPi-IIc, and Pit-2 are present in the proximal tubule apical plasma membrane. The central role of NaPi-IIa in the response to metabolic acidosis was shown in studies in which NaPi-IIa deletion prevents changes in phosphate excretion with metabolic acidosis [83]. Whether NaPi-IIc changes with metabolic acidosis is unclear as some studies find decreased expression and others do not [83, 84]. Pit-2 expression, although regulated by dietary phosphate availability, is not altered in metabolic acidosis in phosphate replete conditions, but does increase in response to metabolic acidosis in conditions of phosphate depletion [84].

Acidosis-induced changes in phosphate excretion depend on systemic phosphate availability. When dietary phosphate is restricted, basal phosphate excretion is greatly reduced, metabolic acidosis-induced changes in urinary phosphate excretion are blunted [84] and there is a lack of change in NaPi-IIa protein and mRNA abundance.

Finally, metabolic acidosis alters extrarenal phosphate transport. Metabolic acidosis increases small intestinal Na^+-dependent phosphate uptake through increased expression of the apical phosphate transporter, NaPi-IIb [85] and it increases bone-derived phosphate release [86]. These extrarenal effects may enable increased urinary phosphate excretion without developing changes in systemic phosphate concentration.

Other Urinary Buffers

Creatinine, although typically used to assess glomerular filtration, has a p*K*a of ~4.9 and is excreted in sufficient quantities, ~11 mmol/day, that it can contribute to titratable acid excretion [82]. This is particularly true in conditions when urinary pH is 5.5 or less, when creatinine can account for as much as 20% of titratable acid excretion. Uric acid is excreted in most individuals in such small amounts, ~4 mmol/day, as to limit is role as a titratable acid. In ketoacidosis, β-hydroxybutyric acid and acetoacetic acid excretion increases, which increases titratable acid excretion. However, because ketoacids can be metabolized to bicarbonate, their loss in the urine has no net effect on acid–base homeostasis.

Organic Anion Excretion

Many organic anions are present in urine and can contribute to acid–base homeostasis. In general, their role in acid–base homeostasis is not as titratable acids, but as alkali equivalents, because their metabolism produces bicarbonate. Some, however, such as citrate and uric acid, can function both as titratable acids and as metabolizable organic anions.

Citrate Excretion

Citrate is important both for acid–base homeostasis and to prevent nephrolithiasis. The latter function relates to citrate's ability to complex calcium, thereby decreasing urinary ionized calcium and minimizing calcium-containing stone formation. In this chapter we discuss citrate's role in acid–base homeostasis.

Citrate exists in four molecular forms, citrate^{3-}, citrate^{2-}, citrate^{1-}, and citric acid. The p*K*as for the interconversion of these molecular forms are 5.6, 4.3, and 2.9, respectively. In plasma almost all citrate is in the form of citrate^{3-}. In urine, the two major molecular forms are citrate^{3-} and citrate^{2-}, with the relative amounts of each determined by pH. Unless specified explicitly, we use the term citrate to refer to all molecular forms.

Citrate has two roles in acid–base homeostasis, as a urinary buffer contributing to titratable acid excretion and as a substrate for the tricarboxylic acid cycle. Because the interconversion of citrate^{3-} and citrate^{2-} has a p*K*a′ of 5.6, at a urine pH of 6 ~30% of urinary citrate is in the form of citrate^{2-} and is able to function as a titratable acid (see Fig. 7.6). In the tricarboxylic acid cycle, citrate metabolism results in HCO_3^- generation. Thus, citrate excretion is functionally equivalent to HCO_3^- excretion. Because the majority of urinary citrate is citrate^{3-}, not citrate^{2-}, the predominant effect of variations in citrate excretion are in its role in the tricarboxylic acid cycle and thereby as an alkali equivalent. Multiple factors regulate renal citrate excretion [87]. Metabolic acidosis decreases and alkalosis increases citrate excretion. Hypokalemia reduces citrate excretion through mechanisms independent of systemic pH. Both the carbonic anhydrase inhibitor, acetazolamide, and high dietary protein or NaCl intake decrease excretion.

Renal tubular citrate transport determines citrate excretion. In humans, plasma citrate levels average ~0.1 mM, and changes in plasma levels are not an important regulatory mechanism.

Plasma citrate is essentially completely filtered at the glomerulus and the proximal tubule reabsorbs 65–90% of filtered citrate, with reabsorption paralleling changes in the filtered load. There also is basolateral proximal tubule citrate uptake, but no evidence for citrate secretion [87]. Instead, citrate transported into proximal tubule epithelial cells, whether across apical or basolateral plasma membranes, is metabolized as a component of renal oxidative metabolism. There does not appear to be a significant component of citrate transport in other renal sites.

Proximal tubule apical citrate uptake is a secondarily active process, involving electrogenic cotransport of three Na^+ with $citrate^{2-}$, and is dependent on basolateral Na^+-K^+-ATPase activity. Apical citrate transport is believed to be mediated by the sodium–dicarboxylate cotransporter, NaDC-1, an integral membrane protein expressed in apical plasma membrane in the proximal tubule and in the small intestine.

Multiple mechanisms regulate proximal tubule citrate transport [87]. First, because the transported citrate form is $citrate^{2-}$, the increased luminal acidification present in metabolic acidosis shifts the buffer reaction, $citrate^{3-} + H^+ \leftrightarrow citrate^{2-}$, towards $citrate^{2-}$, thereby facilitating an increased citrate uptake. Metabolic acidosis also increases NaDC-1 expression [88]. Both hypokalemia and starvation, which decrease citrate excretion, increase citrate transport activity measured in brush border membrane vesicles [87].

Basolateral citrate transport in the proximal tubule is responsible for ~20% of total uptake and has different characteristics than apical transport. Uptake is pH-independent, Na^+-dependent and electroneutral, appears to involve cotransport of three Na^+ per one $citrate^{3-}$ and appears to be mediated by NaDC-3 [89].

Other Organic Anions

Humans excrete 26–52 mEq/day of organic anions other than citrate under normal conditions. Because organic anions can be metabolized to bicarbonate, organic anion excretion is functionally equivalent to alkali excretion and contributes to acid–base regulation. The extent of change in organic anion excretion with acid–base disturbances is not clear. Some studies show that acid or alkali loading do not alter urinary organic anion excretion, whereas other, more recent, studies show that alkali loading increases and a ketogenic, acid-producing diet decreases organic anion excretion [90, 91]. Studies in experimental animal models indicate an important role for organic anions in acid–base homeostasis. In the rat, changes in organic anion excretion in response to acid–base loading can be as much as 40% of the change in net acid excretion [92].

Ammonia Metabolism

Renal ammonia metabolism and transport is the predominant component of basal net acid excretion and is the predominant component of the renal response to most acid–base disorders, with changes in renal ammonia excretion that typically greatly exceed changes in titratable acid excretion (Fig. 7.5). Ammonia metabolism involves integrated function of multiple portions of the kidney. Only a minimal amount of urinary ammonia derives from glomerular filtration. Instead, ammonia is produced by the kidney and is then selectively transported into either the urine or into the renal vein.

Ammonia's selective transport into either the urine, where it can be excreted, or into the renal interstitium and then into the renal veins, resulting in return to the systemic circulation, determines its effect on acid–base homeostasis. Ammonia excreted into the urine as NH_4^+ results in equimolar new bicarbonate formation. Ammonia returned to the systemic circulation is metabolized by the liver; this process utilizes equimolar amounts of bicarbonate, thereby consuming the bicarbonate produced during ammoniagenesis. Selective transport of ammonia into either the urine or the renal vein involves integrated transport in the proximal tubule, thick ascending limb of the loop of Henle, and the collecting duct (Fig. 7.7).

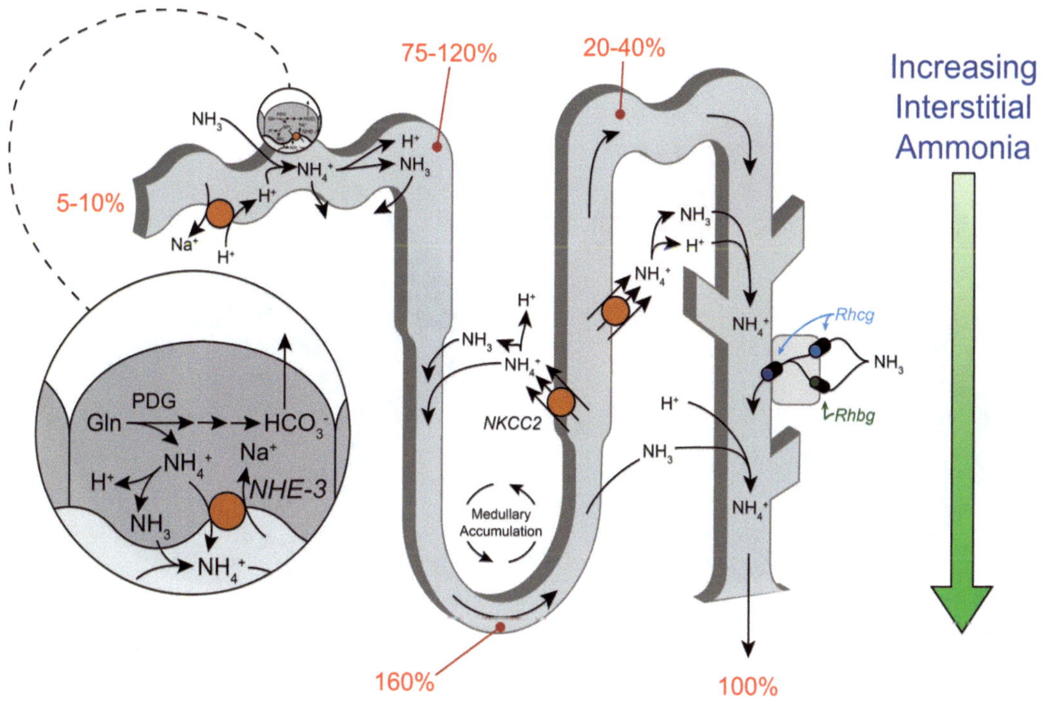

Fig. 7.7 Summary of renal ammonia metabolism. The proximal tubule produces ammonia, as NH_4^+, from glutamine. NH_4^+ is then secreted preferentially into the luminal fluid, primarily by NHE-3. It is then reabsorbed by the TAL, primarily by NKCC2. This results in ammonia delivery to the distal nephron accounting for ~20% of final urinary ammonia; the remaining ~80% is secreted in the collecting duct through parallel NH_3 and H^+ transport. Numbers in *red* indicate proportion of total urinary ammonia present at the indicated sites under baseline conditions

Ammonia Chemistry

Ammonia exists in two molecular forms, NH_3 and NH_4^+. The relative amounts of each are governed by the buffer reaction: $NH_3 + H^+ \leftrightarrow NH_4^+$. This reaction occurs essentially instantaneously and has a p*Ka*′ under biologically relevant conditions of ~9.15. Accordingly, the majority of ammonia is present as NH_4^+; at pH 7.4 only ~1.7% of total ammonia is present as NH_3. Because most biological fluids exist at a pH substantially below the p*Ka*′ of this buffer reaction, small changes in pH cause exponential changes in NH_3 concentration, but almost no change in NH_4^+ concentration.

NH_3, although uncharged, has an asymmetric arrangement of positively charged hydrogen nuclei surrounding a central nitrogen; as a result NH_3 is a polar, albeit uncharged, molecule (Fig.7.8). This molecular polarity causes NH_3 to have limited lipid solubility and consequently a finite permeability across plasma membranes.

NH_4^+ also has limited permeability across lipid bilayers. However, in aqueous solutions NH_4^+ and K^+ have nearly identical biophysical characteristics [93], which enables NH_4^+ to be transported at the K^+-transport site of many proteins [94].

Ammonia Production

Ammonia is produced by almost all renal epithelial cells, but the proximal tubule is the primary site [93]. In particular, the glomeruli, S1, S2, S3, descending thin limb of the loop of Henle, medullary and cortical thick ascending limb of the loop of Henle, DCT, CCD, OMCD, and IMCD all have the capability to synthesize ammonia, with glutamine being the primary metabolic substrate. Rates of ammoniagenesis increase in

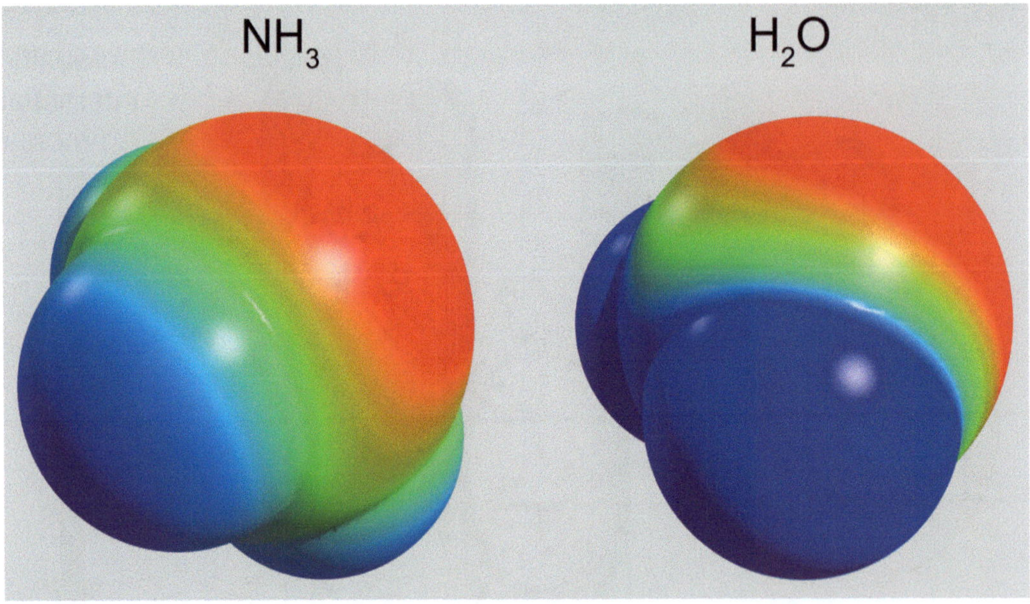

Fig. 7.8 Molecular polarity of NH_3 and H_2O. Space-filling model of NH_3 and H_2O with surface pseudocolored according to predicted electrostatic charge (red indicates negative charge and blue indicates positive charge). Models generated using Avogadro, version 1.0.1

response to metabolic acidosis in the S1 and S2 proximal tubule segments, and under specific conditions in the S3 segment [93]. Taking into consideration the production rates per unit length and the relative lengths of the different nephron segments, the proximal tubule accounts for 60–70% of total renal ammonia production under basal conditions and almost all of the increase with metabolic acidosis.

Multiple pathways for ammoniagenesis are present in the proximal tubule (Fig. 7.9). The predominant ammoniagenic pathway involves phosphate-dependent glutaminase (PDG). PDG is a mitochondrial enzyme which metabolizes glutamine to glutamate, producing NH_4^+. Glutamine can also be metabolized by γ-glutamyl transpeptidase (γ-GT), also known as phosphate-independent glutaminase, although this is unlikely to be a major mechanism of renal ammoniagenesis. Glutamate then undergoes further metabolism through multiple pathways. The major pathways involve either glutamate dehydrogenase (GDH), mediating conversion to α-ketoglutarate (α-KG) with release of NH_4^+, or transamination via glutamate-oxaloacetate transaminase (GOT) to aspartate. GDH-mediated metabolism of glutamate to form α-KG is the predominant mechanism, and is regulated in parallel with changes in total renal ammoniagenesis.

Glutamate can also be converted back to glutamine via the enzyme glutamine synthetase [93]. Because this reaction utilizes NH_4^+ as a co-substrate, it results in decreased net NH_4^+ formation. Glutamine synthetase is expressed in the proximal tubule of the rat and mouse, primarily in late proximal tubule segments. Metabolic acidosis decreases glutamine synthetase activity, but not protein expression, in the rat kidney and decreases both activity and expression in the mouse kidney.

α-KG can be metabolized through α-KG dehydrogenase and succinate dehydrogenase, forming oxaloacetic acid (OAA). OAA can serve as a substrate for phosphoenolpyruvate carboxykinase (PEPCK) to form phosphoenolpyruvate (PEP), when can then be utilized for gluconeogenesis. Conditions which increase ammonia, such as metabolic acidosis, increase flux through this pathway and stimulate renal gluconeogenesis. Pyruvate can also be metabolized by pyruvate dehydrogenase (PDH), forming HCO_3^- and acetyl-CoA (AcCoA).

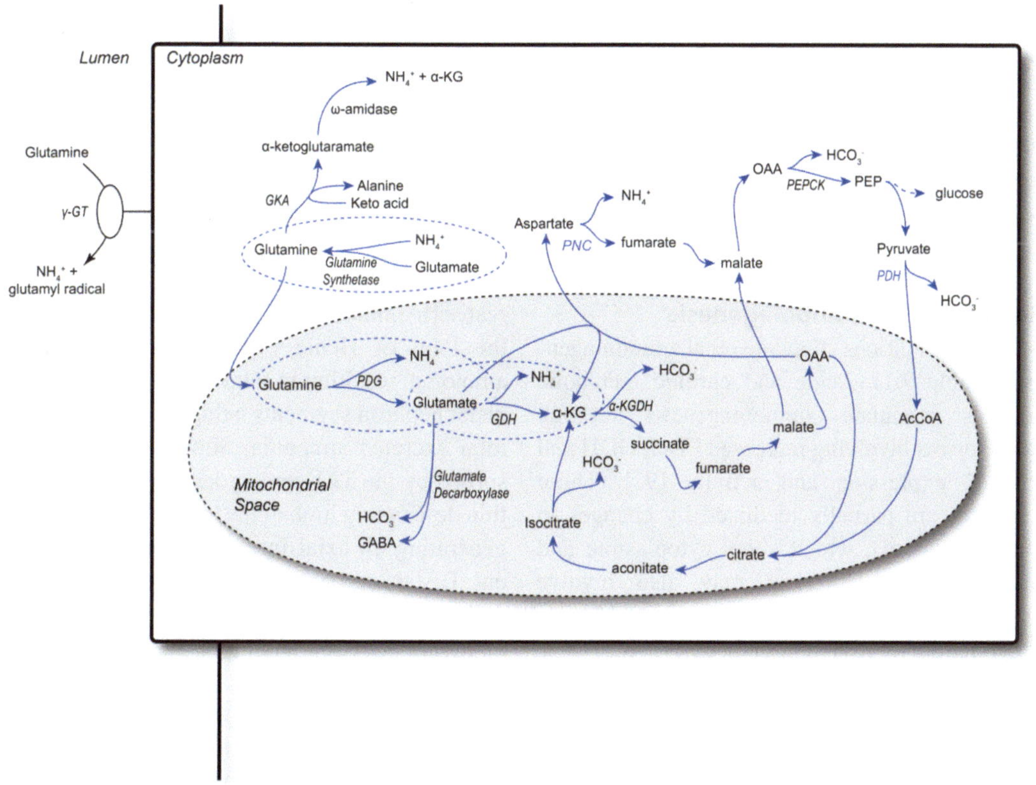

Fig. 7.9 Mechanisms of ammoniagenesis. Multiple pathways for enzymatic ammonia production originating from glutamine metabolism are present in the proximal tubule. Glutamine metabolism through PDG and GDH and involving PEPCK is the quantitatively most significant component of renal ammoniagenesis and the primary pathway stimulated in response to metabolic acidosis

Glutamine Transport in Ammoniagenesis

Glutamine is the primary metabolic source for renal ammoniagenesis [95]. Under conditions of normal acid–base balance, the kidneys extract very little glutamine, less than 3% of delivered glutamine. However, acute metabolic acidosis rapidly increases plasma glutamine levels. This results primarily from increased skeletal muscle glutamine release. In parallel renal glutamine uptake increases. With chronic metabolic acidosis, renal extraction increases to as much as 50% of delivered glutamine, even though plasma glutamine levels actually decrease. Increased renal glutamine utilization is balanced by increased skeletal muscle and liver glutamine release.

Filtered glutamine is almost completely reabsorbed in the PCT. Apical glutamine transport is Na^+-dependent and is likely to be mediated by the Na^+-dependent neutral amino acid transporters B^0AT1 (SLC6A19) and B^0AT3 (SLC6A18) [96]. Under basal conditions, relatively little of the glutamine reabsorbed in the proximal tubule is metabolized, and instead is transported across the basolateral membrane resulting in net glutamine reabsorption. Chronic metabolic acidosis increases renal glutamine extraction, increases basolateral glutamine transport and increases basolateral SNAT3 (also known as SN1 or SLC38A3) protein expression [96]. Although multiple other amino acid transporters are present in the kidney, the only transporter other than SNAT3 whose expression is altered is y^+-LAT1, whose expression decreases, suggesting that it does not contribute to increased glutamine uptake in this condition [96].

Mitochondrial glutamine uptake involves a specific transporter-mediated mechanism. This uptake is *trans*-stimulated and *cis*-inhibited by alanine and is stimulated by metabolic acidosis [93]. The transporter appears to have an apparent molecular weight of 41.5 kDa and may also transport asparagine. This protein's molecular identity has not been identified.

Table 7.1 Known stimuli of renal ammonia metabolism

Acidosis
Hypokalemia
Glucocorticoids
Mineralocorticoids
Cyclic AMP (cAMP)
Circulating nondialyzable factor

Regulation of Ammoniagenesis

Multiple conditions stimulate renal ammoniagenesis (Table 7.1). Acute and chronic metabolic acidosis stimulate ammoniagenesis through mechanisms involving increased PDG, GDH and PEPCK expression and activity [97]. These increases are partially mediated by changes in extracellular pH, which alters cytoplasmic and mitochondrial pH. They may also involve increased presence of a small, nondialyzable factor which increases ammoniagenesis [98].

Chronic hypokalemia increases ammoniagenesis through mechanisms involving increased enzyme expression and activity similar to those identified for chronic metabolic acidosis. Acute changes in extracellular K^+ also regulate proximal tubule ammoniagenesis; these effects are directly mediated by extracellular K^+ and, because they can be observed within 45 min of change in extracellular K^+, likely do not require changes in protein expression. Ammoniagenesis can be modulated independently of acid–base status by a variety of factors, including TCA cycle intermediates, hormones that increase cAMP, prostaglandin F2 alpha, insulin, growth hormone, angiotensin II (AngII), corticosteroids, aldosterone, and tubular flow rate [97]. Increasing evidence suggests an important role for AngII, acting through both the AT_1 and AT_2 receptors, to regulate ammoniagenesis [9].

Ammonia Transport

Renal ammonia transport requires integrated transport mechanisms involving most renal epithelial cells [93]. In the proximal tubule, ammonia is secreted preferentially into the luminal fluid, although there is some transport across the basolateral membrane. Late proximal tubule segments, such as the S3 segment, can also reabsorb ammonia. The thick ascending limb of the loop of Henle (TAL) reabsorbs luminal ammonia, resulting in total ammonia delivery to distal nephron segments being only ~20–40% of total excreted ammonia. Some ammonia reabsorbed by the TAL undergoes recycling into the thin descending limb of the loop of Henle (DTL), generating an axial interstitial ammonia gradient. Distal segments then secrete ammonia; the collecting duct is the site of the majority of ammonia secretion and involves parallel H^+ and NH_3 secretion.

Ammonia produced in the proximal tubule is secreted preferentially into the tubule lumen, although there is some transport across the basolateral membrane [93]. Preferential apical secretion is due to multiple factors, including luminal acidification, which facilitates "trapping" of secreted NH_3 as NH_4^+, and NHE-3 mediated Na^+/NH_4^+ exchange. An apical Ba^{2+}-sensitive K^+ channel and a NH_3 transport component also appear to be involved in ammonia secretion.

The proximal tubule also can reabsorb luminal ammonia; this appears to occur primarily in the late proximal tubule. These portions of the proximal tubule express glutamine synthetase, which catalyzes the reaction of NH_4^+ with glutamate to form glutamine. Metabolic acidosis converts late proximal tubule ammonia transport from net reabsorption to net secretion; the molecular mechanisms that underlie this conversion involve decreased glutamine synthetase-mediated NH_4^+ metabolism.

The TAL reabsorbs luminal ammonia through integrated apical and basolateral plasma membrane transporters. Apical NH_4^+ transport primarily involves the apical Na^+-K^+-$2Cl^-$ cotransporter, NKCC2; an apical K^+/NH_4^+ antiporter and an amiloride-sensitive NH_4^+-conductance are also present, but quantitatively contribute very little to transepithelial ammonia movement [93]. Cytosolic ammonia exit involves basolateral Na^+/NH_4^+ exchange mediated by NHE-4 and a "bicarbonate shuttle" pathway involving NBCn1 [93].

Some of the ammonia absorbed by the medullary thick ascending limb (TAL) of the loop of Henle undergoes recycling into the thin descending limb (TDL), resulting in countercurrent amplification of medullary interstitial ammonia concentration. Ammonia recycling predominantly involves NH_3 transport, but a small component of NH_4^+ transport is also present.

The net effect of ammonia transport in the TAL and the TDL is twofold: development of an axial ammonia concentration in the medullary interstitium and net ammonia reabsorption such that ammonia delivery to the distal tubule is only ~20–40% of final urinary ammonia content.

Collecting duct ammonia secretion mediates the majority of distal nephron ammonia secretion. Although transport could theoretically involve either NH_3 or NH_4^+ transport, multiple studies show that collecting duct ammonia secretion involves parallel NH_3 and H^+ transport, with little-to-no pH-independent NH_4^+ permeability [94]. H^+ secretion involves both H^+-ATPase and H^+-K^+-ATPase; these proteins have been discussed in detail in prior portions of this chapter. Cytosolic carbonic anhydrase activity is necessary for ammonia secretion, probably through a role in supplying cytosolic H^+ for secretion [93].

The presence or absence of luminal carbonic anhydrase activity has an important role in collecting duct ammonia secretion. In the absence of luminal carbonic anhydrase activity, the luminal H^+ concentration increases above equilibrium due to delayed dissociation of H_2CO_3. This is termed a luminal "disequilibrium pH." Because the $H^+ + NH_3 \leftrightarrow NH_4^+$ reaction occurs rapidly, the increased luminal H^+ concentration in the absence of luminal carbonic anhydrase activity shifts the ammonia buffer reaction towards NH_4^+, decreasing the luminal NH_3 concentration and thereby increasing the transepithelial gradient for NH_3 secretion. Detailed studies show a luminal disequilibrium pH in the inner stripe of the OMCD and the terminal IMCD of the rat kidney, in the rabbit CCD and outer stripe of OMCD, but not in the inner stripe of OMCD in the rabbit [93]. Thus, a luminal disequilibrium pH facilitates ammonia secretion, although it may inhibit bicarbonate reabsorption.

The Rh glycoproteins, Rh B Glycoprotein (Rhbg) and Rh C Glycoprotein (Rhcg), are critical for collecting duct NH_3 transport [93]. Rhcg is an NH_3-specific transporter expressed from the DCT through the IMCD of the human, rat and mouse kidney in intercalated cells, principal cells, DCT cells and CNT cells, but not in nonintercalated cells in the IMCD or the B-type intercalated cell. Multiple gene deletion studies, utilizing both global and renal epithelial cell-specific deletion, demonstrate Rhcg's essential role in both basal and acidosis-stimulated ammonia excretion [93]. Because Rhcg deletion results in impaired ammonia and thus net acid excretion, but an intact, or even exaggerated, ability to decrease urine pH in response to an acid load, we suggest that the clinical condition associated with Rhcg deletion should be termed "incomplete distal RTA, type 2," to differentiate it from "classic" incomplete distal RTA in which the ability to decrease urine pH in response to an acid load is impaired.

Rhbg is another member of the Rh glycoprotein family with an important role in distal ammonia secretion [93]. Similar to Rhcg, Rhbg is an ammonia-specific transporter. Rhbg is expressed in the same cells that express Rhcg, with the significant difference that that Rhbg has only basolateral expression, in contrast to the apical and basolateral expression of Rhcg. Although initial studies did not identify an effect of Rhbg gene deletion on the response to NH_4Cl-induced metabolic acidosis, more recent studies found that intercalated cell-specific Rhbg deletion impairs renal ammonia excretion.

Another mechanism for basolateral ammonia uptake involves basolateral Na^+-K^+-ATPase [99]. In particular, in the IMCD the basolateral Na^+-K^+-ATPase contributes to basolateral NH_4^+ uptake. Intracellular NH_4^+ dissociates to H^+ and NH_3, which are then secreted across the apical membrane. However, in the CCD basolateral Na^+-K^+-ATPase does not contribute to ammonia secretion, and its role in the OMCD has not been

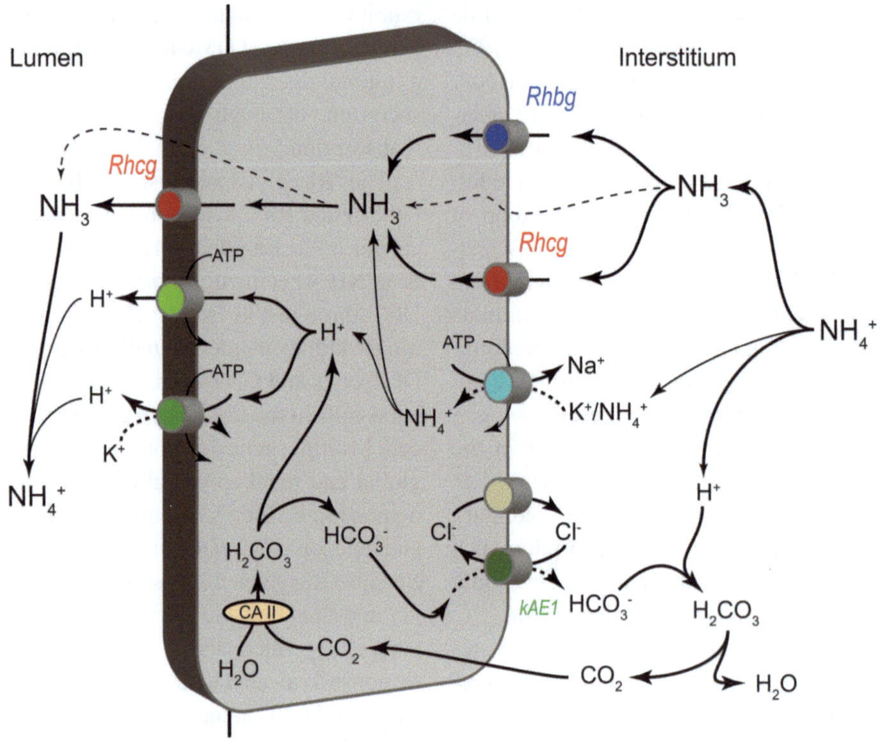

Fig. 7.10 Detailed model of collecting duct ammonia transport. Interstitial NH_4^+ is in equilibrium with NH_3 and H^+. NH_3 is transported across the basolateral membrane, predominantly by Rhcg, but also possibly partly by Rhbg. In the IMCD, basolateral Na^+-K^+-ATPase transports NH_4^+. Intracellular NH_3 is secreted across the apical membrane by apical Rhcg. H^+-ATPase and H^+-K^+-ATPase secrete H^+, which combines with luminal NH_3 to form NH_4^+, which is "trapped" in the lumen. Intracellular H^+ is generated by CA II-accelerated CO_2 hydration that forms carbonic acid, which dissociates to H^+ and HCO_3^-. Basolateral Cl^-/HCO_3^- exchange transports HCO_3^- across the basolateral membrane; HCO_3^- combines with H^+ released from NH_4^+, to form carbonic acid, which dissociates to CO_2 and water. This CO_2 can recycle into the cell, supplying the CO_2 used for cytosolic H^+ production. The net result is NH_4^+ transport from the peritubular space into the luminal fluid

reported [93]. Overall, collecting duct ammonia secretion involves the integrated function of a number of proteins (Fig. 7.10).

Specific Proteins Involved in Renal Ammonia Metabolism

Phosphate-Dependent Glutaminase

The initial enzymatic step in the majority of renal ammoniagenesis involves PDG, which catalyzes the reaction, L-glutamine + $H_2O \rightarrow$ L-glutamate$^-$ + NH_4^+. Metabolic acidosis increases proximal tubule PDG activity; these increases derive from increased protein synthesis and correlate with increased mRNA expression [93]. Increased mRNA expression results from gene stabilization involving an 8-nt AU-repeat sequence which functions as a pH-response element [95].

Glutamate Dehydrogenase

GDH is a mitochondrial enzyme that catalyzes the reaction, L-glutamate$^-$ + H_2O + NAD^+ (or $NADP^+$) $\rightarrow$ α-KG^{2-} + NH_4^+ + NADH (or NADPH) + H^+. Two GDH isoforms are products of two different genes; GLUD1 is widely expressed, whereas GLUD2 appears to be a neural and testicular specific isoform. In the kidney GDH is a product of the GLUD1 mRNA. Metabolic acidosis stimulates renal GDH activity, protein and mRNA (GLUD1) expression by increasing GLUD1 gene stability [100].

PEPCK

Renal PEPCK is a cytosolic enzyme that is the product of the PCK1 gene. In the kidney, as in extrarenal sites, including liver, adipose tissue and small intestine, PEPCK is a key enzyme in gluconeogenesis through its role in conversion of oxaloacetate into phosphoenolpyruvate and CO_2. It also mediates an important role in the renal response to metabolic acidosis which is coincident with increased renal gluconeogenesis. The adaptive increase in PEPCK activity and protein expression result from increased protein synthesis and mRNA expression. In contrast to PDG and GDH, the increased PEPCK mRNA expression involves increased gene transcription [100].

NHE-3

The proximal tubule apical NHE, NHE-3, secretes NH_4^+ through binding of NH_4^+ at the H^+ binding site. Evidence supporting this includes the observation that proximal tubule brush border membrane vesicles exhibit NH_4^+/Na^+ exchange activity, that combining a low luminal Na^+ concentration with a Na^+/H^+ exchange inhibitor decreases ammonia secretion and the observation that the Na^+/H^+ exchange inhibitor, EIPA, blunts ammonia secretion when alternative secretory pathways are blocked [93]. Because the TAL reabsorbs NH_4^+, whereas NHE-3 is involved in NH_4^+ secretion, NHE-3 probably does not mediate an important role in TAL ammonia transport.

K^+ Channels

At a molecular level, K^+ and NH_4^+ have nearly identical biophysical characteristics, enabling essentially all K^+ channels to transport NH_4^+ [94]. In the renal proximal tubule, the nonspecific K^+ channel inhibitor, barium, inhibits ammonia transport. Multiple K^+ channels are present in the apical membrane of the proximal tubule; which of these are involved in proximal tubule ammonia transport is not known currently. In the TAL, K^+ channels can contribute to luminal NH_4^+ uptake when apical Na^+-K^+-$2Cl^-$ cotransport is inhibited [93]. However, NKCC2 inhibitors completely inhibit TAL ammonia transport, suggesting that apical K^+ channels are unlikely to mediate a quantitatively important role in TAL ammonia transport [93].

Na^+-K^+-$2Cl^-$ Cotransport

NKCC1 is a widely expressed member of the Na^+-K^+-$2Cl^-$ cotransporter family, and in the kidney it is present in the basolateral membrane of A-type intercalated cells in the outer and inner medullary collecting duct cells [93, 94]. Because peritubular bumetanide, an inhibitor of NKCC1, does not alter OMCD ammonia secretion, NKCC1 appears unlikely to mediate a quantitatively important role in OMCD ammonia secretion. In the IMCD, although NH_4^+ and K^+ compete for a common binding site on NKCC1, inhibiting NKCC1 does not appear to significantly alter peritubular NH_4^+ uptake. Thus, NKCC1 appears unlikely to mediate a substantial role in renal ammonia secretion.

NKCC2 is a kidney-specific isoform expressed in the apical plasma membrane of the TAL and is the major mechanism for ammonia reabsorption in the thick ascending limb of the loop of Henle [93, 94]. Luminal NH_4^+ competes for binding with K^+ to the K^+-transport site, enabling alterations in luminal K^+ in hypokalemia and hyperkalemia to alter net NH_4^+ transport and lead to alterations in medullary interstitial ammonia concentration. TAL ammonia reabsorption increases with metabolic acidosis and involves transcriptionally mediated increases in NKCC2 expression. The ability of NH_4^+ to be transported at the K^+ binding site of NKCC2 may also contribute to TAL NaCl transport [93].

Na^+-K^+-ATPase

Na^+-K^+-ATPase is present in the basolateral plasma membrane of renal epithelial cells, and its expression is greatest in the medullary thick ascending limb of the loop of Henle, with lesser expression in the cortical thick ascending limb, DCT, CCD, MCD, and the proximal tubule [93, 94]. NH_4^+ competes with K^+ at the K^+-binding site of Na^+-K^+-ATPase, enabling Na^+-K^+-ATPase-mediated basolateral NH_4^+ uptake. In the inner medulla, Na^+-K^+-ATPase is critical for IMCD ammonia and acid secretion, and in hypokalemia, decreased interstitial K^+ concentrations, by facilitating increased NH_4^+ uptake by Na^+-K^+-ATPase, enable increased rates of NH_4^+ secretion independent of changes in Na^+-K^+-ATPase expression [93]. In the cortex, in contrast, interstitial ammonia concentrations are substantially less than the transporter's K_m, and even in the presence of high ammonia concentrations, pharmacologically inhibiting Na^+-K^+-ATPase does not alter CCD ammonia secretion, indicating that Na^+-K^+-ATPase's role in ammonia secretion may be limited to the IMCD [93, 94].

H^+-K^+-ATPase

H^+-K^+-ATPase proteins transport NH_4^+. The majority of evidence suggests NH_4^+ binds to and is transported at the K^+ binding site. However, potassium deficiency increases expression of the colonic H^+-K^+-ATPase and this has been postulated to mediate increased NH_4^+ secretion via binding of NH_4^+ to and transport at the H^+ binding site [93, 94].

Aquaporins

The aquaporin family is an extended family of proteins that transport H_2O. Because both H_2O and NH_3 have similar molecular sizes and charge distribution, several studies have examined the role of aquaporins in NH_3 transport. Importantly, many, but not all aquaporins can transport ammonia [101], but their specific role in renal ammonia transport has not been studied in detail.

Carbonic Anhydrase

Carbonic anhydrase, in addition to its role in bicarbonate reabsorption, also contributes to ammonia secretion. Direct studies have shown that inhibiting carbonic anhydrase, presumably CA II, almost completely inhibits OMCD ammonia secretion [93]. In contrast, CA IV, although functioning to increase bicarbonate reabsorption, likely decreases collecting duct ammonia secretion through its effects to prevent a luminal disequilibrium pH. Apical CA IV expression has been demonstrated in the rabbit CCD type A intercalated cell, in the rabbit OMCD and IMCD, in the human CCD and OMCD, but not in the rat collecting duct. This pattern is inconsistent with evidence of luminal disequilibrium pH in the rat CCD and OMCD, but is consistent with the evidence of luminal disequilibrium pH in the rabbit CCD and OMCD outer stripe segments [93].

Rh Glycoproteins

Rh glycoproteins are mammalian orthologues of Mep/AMT proteins, ammonia transporter family proteins present in yeast, plants, bacteria, and many other organisms. Three mammalian Rh glycoproteins have been identified to date, Rh A glycoprotein (RhAG/Rhag), Rh B Glycoprotein (RhBG/Rhbg), and Rh C Glycoprotein (RhCG/Rhcg). By convention, Rh A Glycoprotein is termed RhAG in human tissues and is termed Rhag in nonhumans; a similar terminology is used for RhBG/Rhbg and RhCG/Rhcg.

RhAG/Rhag

Rh A glycoprotein (RhAG/Rhag) is a component of the Rh complex, which consists of the nonglycosylated Rh proteins, RhD and RhCE in humans and Rh30 in nonhuman mammals, in association with RhAG/Rhag. RhAG mediates electroneutral, NH_3 transport. However, RhAG/Rhag is an erythrocyte and erythroid-precursor specific protein, and studies in the human kidney found no evidence of renal RhAG expression [94].

RhBG/Rhbg

The kidneys express basolateral Rhbg immunoreactivity in the DCT, CNT, ICT, CCD, OMCD, and IMCD. In general, both intercalated and principal cells express Rhbg, with greater expression in intercalated cells than in principal cells [93, 102]. The exceptions to this rule are the IMCD, where only intercalated cells express Rhbg, and the CCD B-type intercalated cell, which does not express Rhbg detectable with immunohistochemistry.

RhBG/Rhbg transports ammonia and the ammonia analogue, methylammonia, but does not appear to have other known substrates. Different studies have reached different conclusions regarding the exact ammonia species, NH_3 or NH_4^+, transported. Most studies show that Rhbg mediates electroneutral, Na^+- and K^+-independent, NH_3 transport, while another has identified both electroneutral NH_3 and electrogenic NH_4^+

transport. In all of these studies, the affinity for ammonia, when examined, was ~2–4 mM.

A variety of evidence indicates that Rhbg is critical to normal renal ammonia excretion [93, 102]. In the mouse, metabolic acidosis increases both mRNA and protein expression, and intercalated cell-specific Rhbg gene deletion impairs the normal increase in renal ammonia excretion in response to metabolic acidosis. Under basal conditions, Rhbg deletion does not alter urinary ammonia excretion, but maintenance of normal ammonia excretion appears to require adaptive changes in glutamine synthetase expression, suggesting that Rhbg contributes to basal ammonia excretion. Another study examining mice with global Rhbg deletion found normal responses to acid-loading, but used a different method of acid-loading, NH_4Cl, and observed a substantially smaller increase in urinary ammonia excretion. Thus, Rhbg appears to contribute to ammonia excretion, but compensatory adaptations can mask this role under both basal conditions and in response to mild stimulation of urinary ammonia excretion.

RhCG/Rhcg

RhCG/Rhcg is widely expressed in multiple ammonia transporting/metabolizing organs. In the kidney, Rhcg expression parallels Rhbg's expression, i.e., in the DCT, CNT, ICT, CCD, OMCD, and IMCD [93, 102]. Intercalated cell expression exceeds principal cell expression in the DCT, CNT, ICT, CCD, and OMCD, and in the IMCD Rhcg is expressed only in intercalated cells.

In all species reported, including human, rat, and mice, Rhcg exhibits both apical and basolateral immunoreactivity. Apical Rhcg immunoreactivity, at least in the rat and mouse kidney, involves expression in both the apical plasma membrane and in subapical sites. Metabolic acidosis increases apical plasma membrane and decreases subapical Rhcg expression, suggesting that trafficking between these two sites is an important regulatory mechanism. Basolateral Rhcg expression is ~20% of total cellular expression, at least in the rat OMCD in the inner stripe. In the mouse there are significant strain-specific variations in the extent of basolateral Rhcg expression and these differences correlate with the ability to excrete ammonia in response to acid-loading.

Multiple studies have addressed the molecular ammonia species transported by RhCG/Rhcg [93, 102]. Some studies suggest that RhCG/Rhcg mediates electroneutral NH_3 transport while others have reported both NH_3 and NH_4^+ transport. The explanation for these differing observations is unclear at present.

Rhcg's expression parallels ammonia excretion in multiple models [102]. Chronic metabolic acidosis significantly increases Rhcg protein expression in both the OMCD and the IMCD, but not in the cortex. In models of reduced renal mass, where there is increased single nephron ammonia secretion, there are widespread changes in Rhcg apical and basolateral expression. Cyclosporine A nephropathy is associated with decreased Rhcg expression, which likely contributes to impaired ammonia excretion and development of metabolic acidosis.

At least two distinct mechanisms contribute to increased Rhcg expression in these models [93, 102]. First, there is increased Rhcg protein expression, which, because Rhcg mRNA expression does not change, suggests regulation through posttranscriptional mechanisms. Second, there are changes in Rhcg's subcellular location. Under basal conditions, Rhcg is located in both the apical and basolateral plasma membrane and in subapical sites in both principal cells and intercalated cells. In response to chronic metabolic acidosis, particularly in the intercalated cell, apical plasma membrane expression increases and cytoplasmic expression decreases. However, in different cell types the predominant mechanism of Rhcg response differs, with subcellular distribution changes being the predominant adaptive response in the OMCD intercalated cell and increased protein expression being the predominant mechanism in the OMCD principal cell.

Chronic metabolic acidosis also increases basolateral plasma membrane Rhcg expression. This increase does not appear to involve redistribution from cytoplasmic sites to the basolateral plasma membrane.

Most recently, genetic deletion studies have confirmed the key role of Rhcg in renal ammonia excretion. Global Rhcg deletion decreases basal ammonia excretion and impairs urinary ammonia excretion in response to metabolic acidosis. Collecting duct-specific Rhcg deletion demonstrated identical findings, indicating that Rhcg deletion impaired collecting duct ammonia secretion, rather than an indirect effect of extrarenal Rhcg deletion. Moreover, Rhcg deletion decreases transepithelial ammonia permeability in perfused collecting duct segments and decreases apical membrane NH_3 permeability.

Nonglycosylated Rh Proteins

The nonglycosylated Rh proteins, RhD and RhCE in humans and Rh30 in nonhumans, are present in erythrocytes in a multimeric complex with RhAG. RhCE appears to neither transport ammonia or its analogue, methylammonia, nor alter transport by RhAG. Structural models suggest that the arrangement of key amino acids is sufficiently different in RhCE and RhD that they either do not transport ammonia or that they do so by mechanisms different from those used by the glycosylated Rh glycoproteins and their bacterial orthologues.

Acknowledgments The authors dedicate this chapter to the many talented investigators with whom we have been fortunate to work, the superb mentors who have supported, encouraged and, in many cases, enabled our scientific endeavors, and to our wonderful spouses and families who have supported all aspects of our lives. The preparation of this chapter was supported in part by funds from NIH R01-DK-45788, RO1-DK-49750, RO1-DK-82680 and Department of Veterans Affairs 1I01BX000818.

References

1. Boron WF. Acid-base transport by the renal proximal tubule. J Am Soc Nephrol. 2006;17:2368–82.
2. Quigley R, Baum M. Developmental changes in rabbit proximal straight tubule paracellular permeability. Am J Physiol Renal Physiol. 2002;283: F525–31.
3. Liu FY, Cogan MG. Angiotensin II stimulation of hydrogen ion secretion in the rat early proximal tubule. Modes of action, mechanism, and kinetics. J Clin Invest. 1988;82:601–7.
4. Zhou Y, Zhao J, Bouyer P, Boron WF. Evidence from renal proximal tubules that HCO3- and solute reabsorption are acutely regulated not by pH but by basolateral HCO3- and CO2. Proc Natl Acad Sci U S A. 2005;102:3875–80.
5. Ambuhl PM, Amemiya M, Danczkay M, et al. Chronic metabolic acidosis increases NHE3 protein abundance in rat kidney. Am J Physiol. 1996; 271:F917–25.
6. Kwon TH, Fulton C, Wang W, et al. Chronic metabolic acidosis upregulates rat kidney Na-HCO cotransporters NBCn1 and NBC3 but not NBC1. Am J Physiol Renal Physiol. 2002;282:F341–51.
7. Wang T. Flow-activated transport events along the nephron. Curr Opin Nephrol Hypertens. 2006;15: 530–6.
8. Schuster VL, Kokko JP, Jacobson HR. Angiotensin II directly stimulates sodium transport in rabbit proximal convoluted tubules. J Clin Invest. 1984; 73:507–15.
9. Nagami GT, Kraut JA. Acid-base regulation of angiotensin receptors in the kidney. Curr Opin Nephrol Hypertens. 2010;19:91–7.
10. Rector Jr FC, Bloomer HA, Seldin DW. Effect of potassium deficiency on the reabsorption of bicarbonate in the proximal tubule of the rat kidney. J Clin Invest. 1964;43:1976.
11. Chan YL, Biagi B, Giebisch G. Control mechanisms of bicarbonate transport across the rat proximal convoluted tubule. Am J Physiol Renal Physiol. 1982;242:F532–43.
12. Elkjar ML, Kwon TH, Wang W, et al. Altered expression of renal NHE3, TSC, BSC-1, and ENaC subunits in potassium-depleted rats. Am J Physiol Renal Physiol. 2002;283:F1376–88.
13. Fryer JN, Burns KD, Ghorbani M, Levine DZ. Effect of potassium depletion on proximal tubule AT1 receptor localization in normal and remnant rat kidney. Kidney Int. 2001;60:1792–9.
14. Laghmani K, Preisig PA, Moe OW, Yanagisawa M, Alpern RJ. Endothelin-1/endothelin-B receptor-mediated increases in NHE3 activity in chronic metabolic acidosis. J Clin Invest. 2001;107:1563–9.
15. Sasaki S, Marumo F. Mechanisms of inhibition of proximal acidification by PTH. Am J Physiol Renal Physiol. 1991;260:F833–8.
16. Kinsella JL, Aronson PS. Interaction of NH4+ and Li+with the renal microvillus membrane Na+-H+ exchanger. Am J Physiol. 1981;241:C220–6.
17. McDonough AA, Biemesderfer D. Does membrane trafficking play a role in regulating the sodium/hydrogen exchanger isoform 3 in the proximal tubule? Curr Opin Nephrol Hypertens. 2003;12: 533–41.
18. Wang T, Yang CL, Abbiati T, et al. Mechanism of proximal tubule bicarbonate absorption in NHE3 null mice. Am J Physiol. 1999;277:F298–302.
19. Brown D, Paunescu TG, Breton S, Marshansky V. Regulation of the V-ATPase in kidney epithelial

cells: dual role in acid-base homeostasis and vesicle trafficking. J Exp Biol. 2009;212:1762–72.
20. Romero MF. Molecular pathophysiology of SLC4 bicarbonate transporters. Curr Opin Nephrol Hypertens. 2005;14:495–501.
21. Pushkin A, Kurtz I. SLC4 Base (HCO3-, CO32-) transporters: classification, function, structure, genetic diseases, and knockout models. Am J Physiol Renal Physiol. 2006;290:F580–99.
22. Espiritu DJD, Yang VL, Bernardo AA, Arruda JAL. Regulation of renal Na+/HCO3- cotransporter stimulation by CO2: role of phosphorylation, exocytosis and protein synthesis. J Membr Biol. 2004;199: 39–49.
23. Purkerson JM, Schwartz GJ. The role of carbonic anhydrases in renal physiology. Kidney Int. 2007;71:103–15.
24. Capasso G, Unwin R, Rizzo M, Pica A, Giebisch G. Bicarbonate transport along the loop of Henle: molecular mechanisms and regulation. J Nephrol. 2002;15 Suppl 5:S88–96.
25. Weinstein AM, Krahn TA. A mathematical model of rat ascending Henle limb. II. Epithelial function. Am J Physiol Renal Physiol. 2009;298:F525–42.
26. Good DW. Inhibition of bicarbonate absorption by peptide hormones and cyclic adenosine monophosphate in rat medullary thick ascending limb. J Clin Invest. 1990;85:1006–13.
27. GoodDW,GeorgeT,WattsIIIBA.Lipopolysaccharide directly alters renal tubule transport through distinct TLR4-dependent pathways in basolateral and apical membranes. Am J Physiol Renal Physiol. 2009;297:F866–74.
28. Good DW, Di Mari JF, Watts III BA. Hyposmolality stimulates Na(+)/H(+) exchange and HCO(3)(-) absorption in thick ascending limb via PI 3-kinase. Am J Physiol Cell Physiol. 2000;279:C1443–54.
29. Good DW, George T, Watts III BA. Basolateral membrane Na+/H+exchange enhances HCO3- absorption in rat medullary thick ascending limb: evidence for functional coupling between basolateral and apical membrane Na+/H+exchangers. Proc Natl Acad Sci U S A. 1995;92:12525–9.
30. Wang T, Hropot M, Aronson PS, Giebisch G. Role of NHE isoforms in mediating bicarbonate reabsorption along the nephron. Am J Physiol Renal Physiol. 2001;281:F1117–22.
31. Weinstein AM. A mathematical model of rat distal convoluted tubule. I. Cotransporter function in early DCT. Am J Physiol Renal Physiol. 2005;289: F699–720.
32. Blake-Palmer KG, Karet FE. Cellular physiology of the renal H+ATPase. Curr Opin Nephrol Hypertens. 2009;18:433–8.
33. Gumz ML, Lynch IJ, Greenlee MM, Cain BD, Wingo CS. The renal H+-K+-ATPases: physiology, regulation, and structure. Am J Physiol Renal Physiol. 2010;298:F12–21.
34. Kobayashi KATS, Uchida SHIN, Mizutani SHUK, Sasaki SEI, Marumo FUMI. Intrarenal and cellular localization of CLC-K2 protein in the mouse kidney. J Am Soc Nephrol. 2001;12:1327–34.
35. Kobayashi K, Uchida S, Okamura HO, Marumo F, Sasaki S. Human CLC-KB gene promoter drives the EGFP expression in the specific distal nephron segments and inner ear. J Am Soc Nephrol. 2002; 13:1992–8.
36. Kim J, Tisher CC, Linser PJ, Madsen KM. Ultrastructural localization of carbonic anhydrase II in subpopulations of intercalated cells of the rat kidney. J Am Soc Nephrol. 1990;1:245–56.
37. Wall SM. Recent advances in our understanding of intercalated cells. Curr Opin Nephrol Hypertens. 2005;14:480–4.
38. Weiner ID, Milton AE. H+-K+-ATPase in rabbit cortical collecting duct B-type intercalated cell. Am J Physiol. 1996;270:F518–30.
39. Lynch IJ, Rudin A, Xia SL, et al. Impaired acid secretion in cortical collecting duct intercalated cells from H, K-ATPase-deficient mice: role of HK isoforms. Am J Physiol Renal Physiol. 2008;294:F621–7.
40. Weiner ID, Weill AE, New AR. Distribution of Cl-/HCO3- exchange and intercalated cells in the rabbit cortical collecting duct. Am J Physiol. 1994;267: F952–64.
41. Song HK, Kim WY, Lee HW, et al. Origin and fate of pendrin-positive intercalated cells in developing mouse kidney. J Am Soc Nephrol. 2007;18: 2672–82.
42. Kleinman JG, Bain JL, Fritsche C, Riley DA. Histochemical carbonic anhydrase in rat inner medullary collecting duct. J Histochem Cytochem. 1992; 40:1535–45.
43. Weill AE, Tisher CC, Conde MF, Weiner ID. Mechanisms of bicarbonate transport by cultured rabbit inner medullary collecting duct cells. Am J Physiol. 1994;266:F466–76.
44. Tsuruoka S, Schwartz GJ. Mechanisms of HCO(-)(3) secretion in the rabbit connecting segment. Am J Physiol. 1999;277:F567–74.
45. McKinney TD, Burg MB. Bicarbonate transport by rabbit cortical collecting tubules. Effect of acid and alkali loads in vivo on transport in vitro. J Clin Invest. 1977;60:766–8.
46. Wall SM, Knepper MA. Acid-base transport in the inner medullary collecting duct. Semin Nephrol. 1990;10:148–58.
47. Tsuruoka S, Schwartz GJ. HCO3- Absorption in rabbit outer medullary collecting duct: role of luminal carbonic anhydrase. Am J Physiol. 1998;274: F139–47.
48. Purkerson JM, Schwartz GJ. Expression of membrane-associated carbonic anhydrase isoforms IV, IX, XII, and XIV in the rabbit: induction of CA IV and IX during maturation. Am J Physiol Regul Integr Comp Physiol. 2005;288:R1256–63.
49. Verlander JW, Madsen KM, Cannon JK, Tisher CC. Activation of acid-secreting intercalated cells in rabbit collecting duct with ammonium chloride loading. Am J Physiol. 1994;266:F633–45.

50. Weiner ID, Frank AE, Wingo CS. Apical proton secretion by the inner stripe of the outer medullary collecting duct. Am J Physiol Renal Physiol. 1999;276:F606–13.
51. Wingo CS, Madsen KM, Smolka A, Tisher CC. H-K-ATPase immunoreactivity in cortical and outer medullary collecting duct. Kidney Int. 1990;38: 985–90.
52. Kraut JA, Helander KG, Helander HF, Iroezi ND, Marcus EA, Sachs G. Detection and localization of H+-K+-ATPase isoforms in human kidney. Am J Physiol Renal Physiol. 2001;281:F763–8.
53. Fejes-Toth G, Naray-Fejes-Toth A. Immunohistochemical localization of colonic H-K-ATPase to the apical membrane of connecting tubule cells. Am J Physiol Renal Physiol. 2001;281:F318–25.
54. Sangan P, Kolla SS, Rajendran VM, Kashgarian M, Binder HJ. Colonic H-K-ATPase beta-subunit: identification in apical membranes and regulation by dietary K depletion. Am J Physiol. 1999;276: C350–60.
55. Verlander JW, Moudy RM, Campbell WG, Cain BD, Wingo CS. Immunohistochemical localization of H-K-ATPase alpha2C subunit in rabbit kidney. Am J Physiol Renal Physiol. 2001;281:F357–65.
56. Gifford JD, Rome L, Galla JH. H+-K+-ATPase activity in rat collecting duct segments. Am J Physiol. 1992;262:F692–5.
57. Lynch IJ, Greenlee MM, Gumz ML, Rudin A, Xia SL, Wingo CS. Heterogeneity of H-K-ATPase-mediated acid secretion along the mouse collecting duct. Am J Physiol Renal Physiol. 2010;298:F408–15.
58. Wall SM, Hassell KA, Royaux IE, et al. Localization of pendrin in mouse kidney. Am J Physiol Renal Physiol. 2003;284:F229–41.
59. Verlander JW, Kim YH, Shin W, et al. Dietary Cl(-) restriction upregulates pendrin expression within the apical plasma membrane of type B intercalated cells. Am J Physiol Renal Physiol. 2006;291:F833–9.
60. Wall SM, Pech V. The interaction of pendrin and the epithelial sodium channel in blood pressure regulation. Curr Opin Nephrol Hypertens. 2008;17:18–24.
61. Boettger T, Hubner CA, Maier H, Rust MB, Beck FX, Jentsch TJ. Deafness and renal tubular acidosis in mice lacking the K-Cl co-transporter Kcc4. Nature. 2002;416:874–8.
62. Palmer LG, Frindt G. Cl- channels of the distal nephron. Am J Physiol Renal Physiol. 2006;291: F1157–68.
63. Frische S, Zolotarev AS, Kim YH, et al. AE2 Isoforms in rat kidney: immunohistochemical localization and regulation in response to chronic NH4Cl loading. Am J Physiol Renal Physiol. 2004;286: F1163–70.
64. Sun X, Petrovic S. Increased acid load and deletion of AE1 increase Slc26a7 expression. Nephron Physiol. 2008;109:29–35.
65. Praetorius J, Kim YH, Bouzinova EV, et al. NBCn1 Is a basolateral Na+-HCO3- cotransporter in rat kidney inner medullary collecting ducts. Am J Physiol Renal Physiol. 2004;286:F903–12.
66. Kwon TH, Pushkin A, Abuladze N, Nielsen S, Kurtz I. Immunoelectron microscopic localization of NBC3 sodium-bicarbonate cotransporter in rat kidney. Am J Physiol Renal Physiol. 2000;278: F327–36.
67. Yip KP, Tsuruoka S, Schwartz GJ, Kurtz I. Apical H(+)/base transporters mediating bicarbonate absorption and pH(i) regulation in the OMCD. Am J Physiol Renal Physiol. 2002;283:F1098–104.
68. Damkier HH, Nielsen S, Praetorius J. Molecular expression of SLC4-derived Na+-dependent anion transporters in selected human tissues. Am J Physiol Regul Integr Comp Physiol. 2007;293:R2136–46.
69. Wagner CA, Finberg KE, Stehberger PA, et al. Regulation of the expression of the Cl-/anion exchanger pendrin in mouse kidney by acid-base status. Kidney Int. 2002;62:2109–17.
70. Verlander JW, Madsen KM, Tisher CC. Effect of acute respiratory acidosis on two populations of intercalated cells in rat cortical collecting duct. Am J Physiol. 1987;253:F1142–56.
71. Gifford JD, Ware MW, Luke RG, Galla JH. HCO3-transport in rat CCD: rapid adaptation by in vivo but not in vitro alkalosis. Am J Physiol. 1993;264: F435–40.
72. Sun X, Yang LV, Tiegs BC, et al. Deletion of the pH sensor GPR4 decreases renal acid excretion. J Am Soc Nephrol. 2010;21:1745–55.
73. Frische S, Kwon TH, Frokiaer J, Madsen KM, Nielsen S. Regulated expression of pendrin in rat kidney in response to chronic NH4Cl or NaHCO3 loading. Am J Physiol Renal Physiol. 2003;284: F584–93.
74. Quentin F, Chambrey R, Trinh-Trang-Tan MM, et al. The Cl-/HCO3- exchanger pendrin in the rat kidney is regulated in response to chronic alterations in chloride balance. Am J Physiol Renal Physiol. 2004;287:F1179–88.
75. Galla JH, Gifford JD, Luke RG, Rome L. Adaptations to chloride-depletion alkalosis. Am J Physiol. 1991;261:R771–81.
76. Stone DK, Seldin DW, Kokko JP, Jacobson HR. Mineralocorticoid modulation of rabbit medullary collecting duct acidification. A sodium-independent effect. J Clin Invest. 1983;72:77–83.
77. Winter C, Schulz N, Giebisch G, Geibel JP, Wagner CA. Nongenomic stimulation of vacuolar H+-ATPases in intercalated renal tubule cells by aldosterone. Proc Natl Acad Sci U S A. 2004;101: 2636–41.
78. Verlander JW, Hassell KA, Royaux IE, et al. Deoxycorticosterone upregulates PDS (Slc26a4) in mouse kidney: role of pendrin in mineralocorticoid-induced hypertension. Hypertension. 2003;42: 356–62.
79. Wesson DE. Regulation of kidney acid excretion by endothelins. Kidney Int. 2006;70:2066–73.
80. Renkema KY, Velic A, Dijkman HB, et al. The calcium-sensing receptor promotes urinary acidification to prevent nephrolithiasis. J Am Soc Nephrol. 2009;20:1705–13.

81. Elkinton JR, Huth EJ, Webster Jr GD, McCance RA. The renal excretion of hydrogen ion in renal tubular acidosis. Am J Med. 1960;36:554–75.
82. Hamm LL, Simon EE. Roles and mechanisms of urinary buffer excretion. Am J Physiol. 1987;253: F595–605.
83. Nowik M, Picard N, Stange G, et al. Renal phosphaturia during metabolic acidosis revisited: molecular mechanisms for decreased renal phosphate reabsorption. Pflugers Arch. 2008;457:539–49.
84. Villa-Bellosta R, Sorribas V. Compensatory regulation of the sodium/phosphate cotransporters NaPi-IIc (SCL34A3) and Pit-2 (SLC20A2) during Pi deprivation and acidosis. Pflugers Arch. 2009;459: 499–508.
85. Stauber A, Radanovic T, Stange G, Murer H, Wagner CA, Biber J. Regulation of intestinal phosphate transport II. Metabolic acidosis stimulates Na+-dependent phosphate absorption and expression of the Na+-Pi cotransporter NaPi-IIb in small intestine. Am J Physiol Gastrointest Liver Physiol. 2005;288:G501–6.
86. Lemann Jr J, Bushinsky DA, Hamm LL. Bone buffering of acid and base in humans. Am J Physiol Renal Physiol. 2003;285:F811–32.
87. Unwin RJ, Capasso G, Shirley DG. An overview of divalent cation and citrate handling by the kidney. Nephron Physiol. 2004;98:15–20.
88. Aruga S, Wehrli S, Kaissling B, et al. Chronic metabolic acidosis increases NaDC-1 mRNA and protein abundance in rat kidney. Kidney Int. 2000;58: 206–15.
89. Burckhardt BC, Burckhardt G. Transport of organic anions across the basolateral membrane of proximal tubule cells. Rev Physiol Biochem Pharmacol. 2003;146:95–158.
90. Lemann Jr J, Lennon EJ, Goodman AD, Litzow JR, Relman AS. The net balance of acid in subjects given large loads of acid or alkali. J Clin Invest. 1965; 44:507–17.
91. Hood VL. pH regulation of endogenous acid production in subjects with chronic ketoacidosis. Am J Physiol Renal Physiol. 1985;249:F220–6.
92. Cheema-Dhadli S, Lin SH, Halperin ML. Mechanisms used to dispose of progressively increasing alkali load in rats. Am J Physiol Renal Physiol. 2002;282:F1049–55.
93. Weiner ID, Verlander JW. Role of NH3 and NH4+ transporters in renal acid-base transport. Am J Physiol Renal Physiol. 2011;300:F11–23.
94. Weiner ID, Hamm LL. Molecular mechanisms of renal ammonia transport. Annu Rev Physiol. 2007;69:317–40.
95. Taylor L, Curthoys NP. Glutamine metabolism: role in acid-base balance. Biochem Mol Biol Educ. 2004;32:291–304.
96. Verrey F, Singer D, Ramadan T, Vuille-dit-Bille R, Mariotta L, Camargo S. Kidney amino acid transport. Pflugers Arch. 2009;458:53–60.
97. Tannen RL, Sahai A. Biochemical pathways and modulators of renal ammoniagenesis. Miner Electrolyte Metab. 1990;16:249–58.
98. Alleyne GA, Barnswell J, McFarlane-Anderson N, Alexander JE. Renal ammoniagenic factor in the plasma of rats with acute metabolic acidosis. Am J Physiol. 1981;241:F112–6.
99. Wall SM. Ammonium transport and the role of the Na, K-ATPase. Miner Electrolyte Metab. 1996; 22:311–7.
100. Curthoys NP, Gstraunthaler G. Mechanism of increased renal gene expression during metabolic acidosis. Am J Physiol Renal Physiol. 2001; 281:F381–90.
101. Musa-Aziz R, Chen LM, Pelletier MF, Boron WF. Relative CO2/NH3 selectivities of AQP1, AQP4, AQP5, AmtB, and RhAG. Proc Natl Acad Sci U S A. 2009;106:5406–11.
102. Weiner ID, Verlander JW. Molecular physiology of the Rh ammonia transport proteins. Curr Opin Nephrol Hypertens. 2010;19:471–7.

Core Concepts and Treatment of Metabolic Acidosis

8

Michael R. Wiederkehr and Orson W. Moe

Physiology of Acid Handling

Regulation of H^+ concentration within discreet limits is vital to all living organisms. Acid–base disturbances imply that the imposed stresses have exceeded the capacity of the normal homeostatic mechanisms, that the primary regulatory responses is impaired, or both. In metabolic acidosis, both acid overproduction and acid underexcretion stem from a wide variety of causes. The clinician's duty is to understand this failure of physiology and institute the appropriate intervention to rectify the imbalance. This section will highlight basic concepts of acid–base physiology to provide the foundation for discussion of treatment of metabolic acidosis.

Acid–Base Chemistry

Acidemia signifies low blood pH, whereas acidosis refers to excess acid in the body, which is not an easy entity to measure (Fig. 8.1). Acidosis does not invariably induce acidemia. There are numerous clinical scenarios of discordance between acidosis and acidemia such as mixed acid–base disorders (metabolic acidosis and respiratory alkalosis) [1], high protein induced positive acid balance (normal plasma pH and bone buffering) [2], and potassium deficiency (total body acidosis with extracellular alkalemia) [3].

M.R. Wiederkehr, M.D.
Department of Nephrology, Baylor University Medical Center, 3500 Gaston Avenue, Dallas, TX 75246, USA

O.W. Moe, M.D. (✉)
Center for Mineral Metabolism and Clinical Research, UT Southwestern Medical Center, 5323 Harry Hines Blvd., Dallas, TX 75390-8885, USA
e-mail: orson.moe@utsouthwestern.edu

Normal H^+ concentration in body fluid is 40 nmol/L, usually expressed as the negative base-10 logarithm (*p*): 40×10^{-9} M or 4×10^{-8} M translates to $-\log(4)-\log\ 10^{-8}$ which is $-0.6+8=7.4$. The normal range of pH is extremely narrow and represents five orders of magnitude lower than concentration of HCO_3^- and many other electrolytes in the body fluid (10^{-3} M). Figure 8.2 highlights the magnitude of the size of the pool of physiologic fluid being regulated and the size of the flux that traverses this pool. For H^+, there is about 1.6×10^{-6} mol of H^+ in total body water (TBW) compared to 5×10^{-2} mol of nonvolatile H^+ added to this pool. One can envision that exquisite regulation is critical. It is imperative for clinicians to have a solid understanding of CO_2 chemistry because the HCO_3^- anion is a major H^+ acceptor in the extracellular fluid (ECF). The high capacity and open nature of CO_2 removal by ventilation renders HCO_3^- a unique buffer, and HCO_3^- and CO_2 are the two variables that clinicians manipulate.

A typical arterial blood gas has a pH of 7.40 ± 2, pCO_2 of 40 ± 2 mmHg (5.3 ± 2 kPa), and HCO_3^- of 24 ± 2 mEq/L. A typical venous blood gas carries a much lower oxygen tension, a lower pH (7.35), a higher pCO_2 (45 mmHg), and a

D.B. Mount et al. (eds.), *Core Concepts in the Disorders of Fluid, Electrolytes and Acid-Base Balance*, DOI 10.1007/978-1-4614-3770-3_8, © Springer Science+Business Media New York 2013

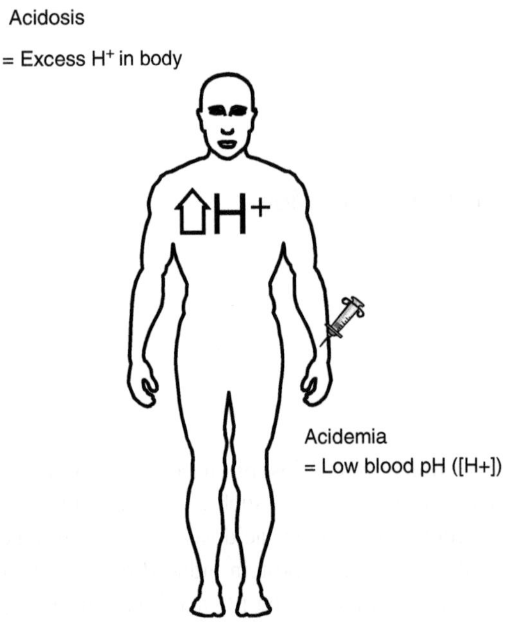

Fig. 8.1 Concept of acidosis. Acidosis refers to excess amount of H^+ in the body and is not a readily measurable parameter. Acidemia on the other hand is a clinical biochemical measurement of plasma H^+ concentration. The two are frequently associated but not synonymous

slightly higher HCO_3^- (26 mmHg). The arterial blood gas electrode measures H^+ and pCO_2, HCO_3^- is *calculated* using Karl Hasselbalch's transformation of the well-known Henderson equation (Fig. 8.3) [4]. The chemical (calorimetric) method measures CO_2 generated from HCO_3^- plus dissolved CO_2, but the latter component is minimal, typically only 1 mEq/L [5].

Acid–Base Biology

In understanding any homeostatic system, one has to consider the relative magnitude of the flux and the pool. The metabolism of a normal daily diet and the products of endogenous metabolic processes yield a net acid production of approximately 0.7–1 mEq H^+ per kg body weight. Thus, in an average person on a standard western diet, every day roughly 50–70 mEq H^+ is added to a pool of H^+ in TBW containing no more than 1.6×10^{-3} mmol. With this differential magnitude between flux and pool, H^+ regulation (pH homeostasis) necessitates buffers, which sequester H^+ from imparting harm to cells before removal from the body is achieved. Figure 8.4 illustrates the importance of both bicarbonate and nonbicarbonate buffers in the immediate defense against volatile (mainly CO_2) and nonvolatile (organic and inorganic) acids, prior to excretion by lungs and kidneys. Buffers are present in the intra- and extracellular milieu. An acid load is handled slightly more by intracellular buffers (IC to EC ~60:40), whereas an alkali load slightly more by extracellular buffers (IC to EC ~30:70). The most important contributor for both compartments is the HCO_3^- buffer system, which removes H^+ when HCO_3^- is metabolized to CO_2 and H_2O. Other extracellular buffers (e.g., phosphate, albumin, and hemoglobin) and intracellular buffers (proteins, phosphate, and bone carbonate/apatite) become more relevant with progression of acidosis and depletion of HCO_3^-. This open system is highly effective, allowing for rapid adjustment of pCO_2 by alveolar ventilation (Fig. 8.5).

Open buffer systems differ from closed ones in two major aspects. Instead of having a constant sum of acid and base, one component is held constant—either acid or base. As a result, the maximum buffer capacity of an open system is not at the p*K* of the acid–base pair, but at either end of the pH, depending on whether the acid or base is the open species (Fig. 8.5). This means that the HCO_3^-/CO_2 system is more effective against alkalemia than acidemia. The open buffer in the urine is ammonia (NH_3), which is titrated to ammonium NH_4^+. The advantage of an open buffer system can be illustrated by an example of an assault to the tune of 10 mmol H^+ delivered to 1 L of fluid with the following composition: pH = 7.40, HCO_3^- = 24 mM, and pCO_2 = 40 mmHg (representing a normal ECF). If the CO_2/HCO_3^- system were operating as a *closed* buffer system, the resultant chemistry is: pH = 6.20, HCO_3^- = 14 mM, pCO_2 = 372 mmHg. This is obviously highly undesirable. An alternative scenario is when the CO_2 species is kept "*open*" by ventilation and thus prevented from accumulating. In fact, it is clamped at a lower level at 30 mmHg.

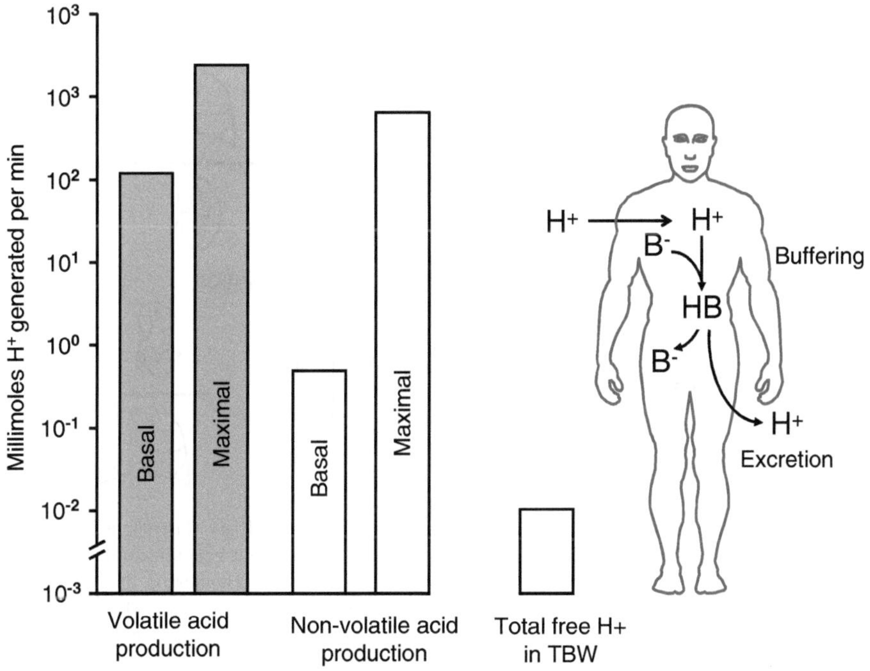

Fig. 8.2 Relative size of H^+ flux and H^+ pool in a 70 kg human. The total pool of H^+ in total body water (TBW) is no more than 1.6×10^{-3} mmol. This is infinitesimally small compared to the flux of H^+ added to and excreted from TBW from both nonvolatile (organic and inorganic) and volatile (CO_2) acid. The colossal difference between the flux and the pool implies that a mismatch between addition and excretion of H^+ from the body for a short period of time will yield disastrous consequences. This obligates a dual system of defense. The *right panel* shows the first step being buffering which has to be near instantaneous to sequester the H^+ followed by the slower excretion of the H^+ which by itself does not have fast enough response rate and accuracy to regulate body pH on a minute-to-minute time scale

The end result of the very same assault by protons (acid) is: pH = 7.30, HCO_3^- = 14 mM, and pCO_2 = 30 mmHg. The enormous power of the open buffer system cannot be overemphasized.

Likewise, urinary buffers can be classified as open and closed; their characteristics are summarized in Table 8.1. Since final urine contains very little HCO_3^-, the only open buffer of importance in the urine is NH_3. Closed buffers include any species that can accept H^+ at physiologic urinary pH. Table 8.2 is an incomplete list of urinary anions intended to illustrate their ability to serve as urinary H^+ buffers. Phosphate, creatinine, and urate are three examples of H^+ acceptors that have p*K*s able to accept H^+ at the urinary pH and in sufficient quantities to permit significant H^+ excretion. These urinary buffers have two limitations. First, their low p*K*s require the renal uroepithelium to generate and maintain a very low urinary pH. Second, their excretion rates cannot be upregulated to any significant degree to accommodate increased H^+ excretion. Thus, by far the most important urinary buffer is ammonia (NH_3) which has a p*K* of 9, allowing it to be fully titrated with H^+ except under conditions of massive bicarbonaturia (Table 8.1). It reflects an open system with enormous capacity to increase ammoniagenesis, as high as 200–300 mmol/day [6]. The generation of the major regulated urinary buffer requires delivery of nitrogen-containing substrate to the kidney from the liver, thereby involving adequate hepatic function for acid–base homeostasis, in collaboration with kidneys and lungs (Fig. 8.6). The liver provides the nitrogen-containing substrate glutamine for the proximal tubule to synthesize ammonia [7]. The deamination/deamidation of glutamine yield

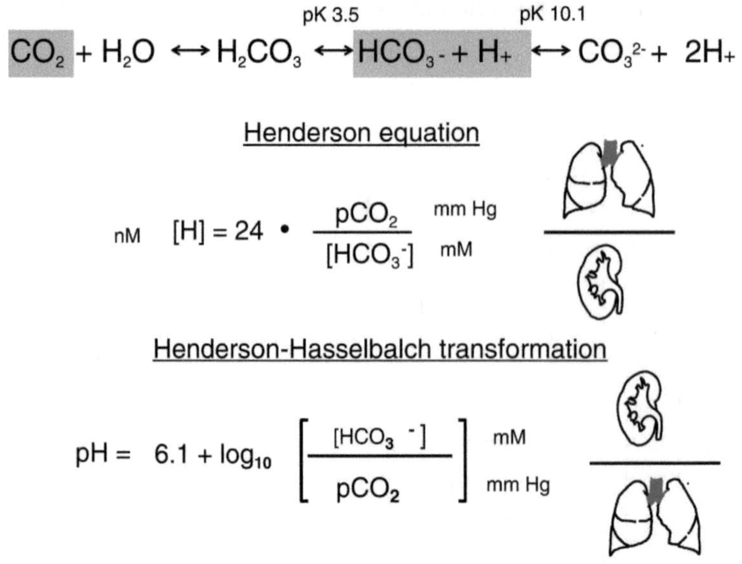

Fig. 8.3 Fundamental acid–base equations. CO_2 chemistry is of central importance because the HCO_3^- ion is quantitatively most significant in the ECFV and the open nature of this buffer system due to ventilatory CO_2 removal renders it unique. The hydration of carbon dioxide yields a strong acid (pK=3.50) that dissociates into HCO_3^- and H^+. Note that HCO_3^- will not be an effective H^+ acceptor if CO_2 is not removed by ventilation. The further dissociation into CO_3^{2-} is limited in body fluids as the pK is high (10.1). Therapeutic provision of CO_3^{2-} buffers two H^+s but generates only one CO_2. The equation by Lawrence Henderson describes the relationship between the concentrations of H^+, HCO_3^-, and CO_2 in the units stated. The transformation of the same equation by Karl Hasselbalch converts the unit of $[H^+]$ to the clinically friendly pH. Both equations can be used to conceptualize the relative roles of the kidney and the lung in setting plasma pH

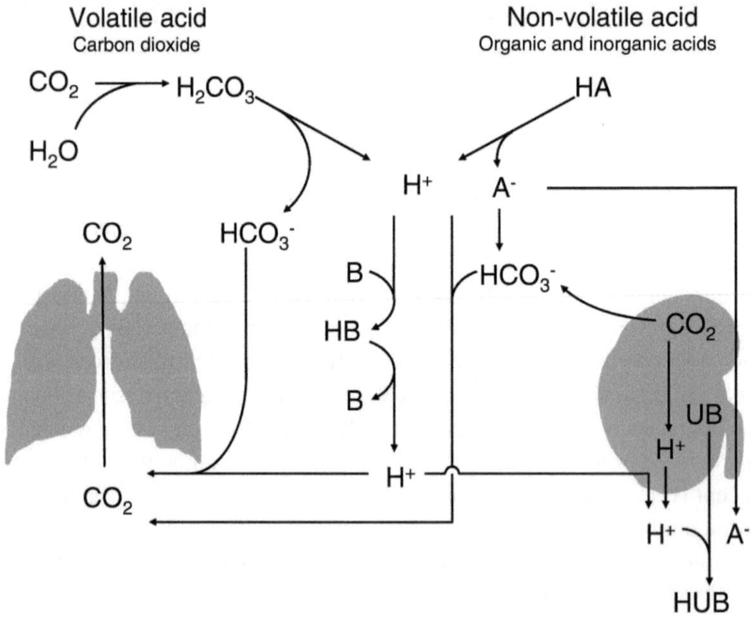

Fig. 8.4 Integrated excretion of volatile and nonvolatile acid load. Part of the metabolic CO_2 is carried in the blood as HCO_3^-. The H^+ produced by either volatile or nonvolatile acid is buffered in the blood by non-HCO_3^- buffers (B) and eventually excreted in either the lung or the kidney. Nonvolatile acids can provide an anion that is may or may not be metabolizable. Metabolizable anions (e.g., lactate, ketoanions) can potentially replenish the consumed HCO_3^- while non-metabolizable anions (e.g., phosphate, sulfate) are excreted unchanged in the kidney. External balance of addition of nonvolatile acid mandates renal excretion of the H^+ mostly carried by a urinary buffer (UB)

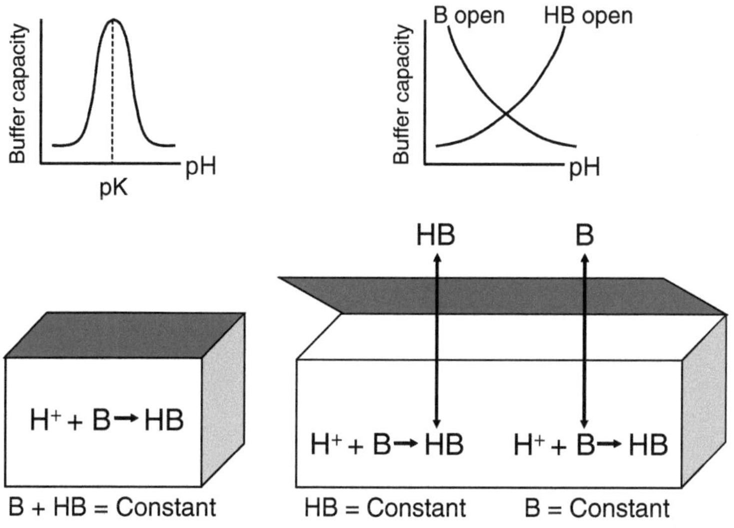

Fig. 8.5 Closed vs. open buffer systems. In a closed buffer system (*left*), the total concentration of the acid (H^+ donor HB) and the base (H^+ acceptor B) is constant. B is generically depicted without a charge because B can be a cation, neutral, or anion. In an open buffer system (*right*), one component (HB or B) is in constant exchange with another compartment, so its concentration is kept relatively constant. The bicarbonate buffer system in blood and urine is an example of constant HB (carbonic acid/carbon dioxide). The ammonia buffering system in the urine is an example of constant B (NH_3). In a closed system, the highest buffer capacity is around the p*K* of the buffer (e.g., phosphate at pH 6.8), whereas in an open buffer system, the highest buffer capacity is at either end of the pH depending on whether the acid (HB) or the base (B) is the open species

Table 8.1 Classification of urinary buffers

Ammonia	Others
Open	Closed
High p*K*	Low p*K*s
High capacity	Low capacity
Dedicated to acid–base	Multiple functions

two NH_3 molecules, which are then protonated to NH_4^+ and excreted as buffered acid in the urine. The metabolism of the remaining carbon skeleton (α(alpha)-ketoglutarate^{2-}) to neutral end products (CO_2, glucose, water) yields two HCO_3^- equivalents which are then added back to the blood. It has been suggested that acid–base homeostasis depends primarily on hepatic urea production vs. renal NH_4^+ secretion [8]. This model predicts that in states of acidosis, the liver shifts from urea to glutamine synthesis, with subsequent delivery to the kidney. However, some experimental data support the dissociation of acid–base from hepatic urea metabolism or even *augmented* urea production in the setting of low plasma HCO_3^- [9–12]. In fact, it appears more likely that ammonia per se is the primary driving force for urea synthesis, rather than pH. Another role of the liver is the metabolism of anions from organic anions (lactate and ketoanions) to neutral end products, thereby consuming H^+ and producing HCO_3^- equivalents. A non-metabolizable anion such as phosphate, sulfate, formate, oxalate, or hippurate is excreted unchanged. It does not consume H^+ during its handling by the body.

In addition to secreting H^+ into the urinary space to be carried by buffers, a major task of the kidneys is to reabsorb the enormous amount of HCO_3^- filtered (Fig. 8.7). Regardless of whether the kidney is in a mode of base conservation (acid load to the organism) or base excretion (base load to the organism), the renal tubule is charged with the task of reabsorption of the filtered HCO_3^-—a much larger quantity than the daily fluctuations in acid or base load. Figure 8.8 summarizes the normal urinary acid–base constituents.

Table 8.2 Urinary potential H^+ acceptors other than NH_3

Anion	p*K*	Estimated excretion rate (mmol/day)
Phosphate[a]	12.3/6.8/2.1	20–30
Creatinine	4.9	12
Urate	5.6	4–6
Citrate[a]	5.6/4.3/2.9	5–15
Chloride	−8.0	100–200
Sulfate	−3.0	15–30
Acetate	4.75	0.1–3.7
Acetoacetate	3.8	<0.1
β(beta)-OH-butyrate	4.7	<0.1
Formate	3.8	0.04–0.73
Fumarate	3.0	0.05–0.3
Glycolate	3.8	1–2.2
Lactate	3.1	0.3–0.4
Oxalate	4.2/1.2	0.1–0.5
Proprionate	4.9	<0.1
Succinate	5.6/4.2	0.3–1.2

The first category is anions with p*K*s that allow titration by H^+ in physiologic urine pH and also have excretion rates that support adequate amount of H^+ excretion. The second category is highly abundant anions but with p*K*s so low that they do not allow significant H^+ buffering under physiologic or pathophysiologic urine pH. The third category represents anions with such low excretion rates that they are not effective buffers irrespective of their p*K*

Modified from Moe OW, Preisig PA. Dual role of citrate in mammalian urine. Curr Opin Nephrol Hypertens. 2006;15:419–24. Used with permission.

[a]Multiple p*K*s

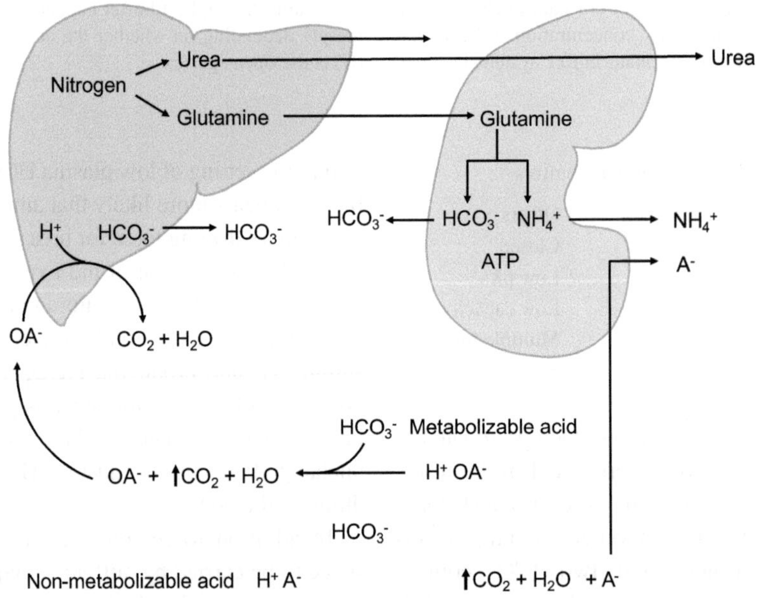

Fig. 8.6 Liver and kidney in acid–base homeostasis. The bottom equations show the acid addition to the body. HOA represents metabolizable organic acids such as lactic or ketoacids. HA represents non-metabolizable acids such as phosphoric or sulfuric acid. HA is largely inorganic but can also be organic such as hippuric acid. In both equations, the H^+ released instantly decomposes HCO_3^- which releases CO_2 to be excreted by the lungs. Metabolizable organic anions can be converted into neutral end products such as CO_2+H_2O in the liver thereby replenishing the decomposed HCO_3^-. The liver converts nitrogenous waste into nontoxic end products. The incorporation of nitrogen into urea earmarks it for excretion in the urine as a neutral acid–base substance. The liver cannot send toxic NH_4^+/NH_3 directly to the kidney via the blood stream. However, it can send glutamine to the kidney and the metabolism of glutamine generates ATP, acid, and base. The polarized renal epithelium partitions the excretion of acid into the urine and the base into the plasma which regenerates the decomposed HCO_3^-. Non-metabolizable anions (A^-) are excreted unchanged in the urine

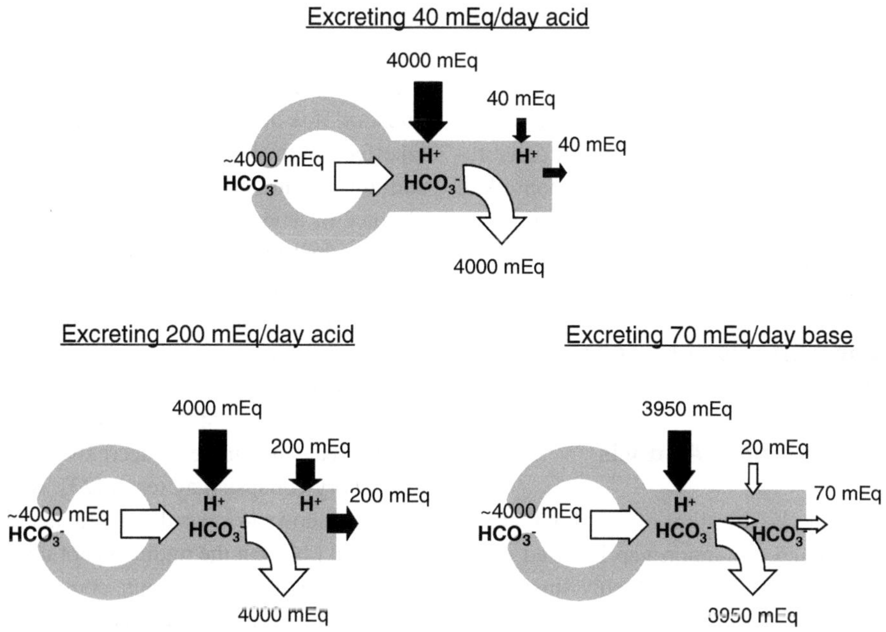

Fig. 8.7 The kidney is a H^+-secreting organ. The kidney has to reclaim a filtered load of HCO_3^- that far exceeds the usual day-to-day fluctuations of acid or base excretion under physiologic conditions. Because of this role, the kidney is always in a H^+-secreting mode. The figure depicts three physiologic conditions: a small acid (*top*), a large acid (*bottom left*), or a base load (*bottom right*) is being excreted

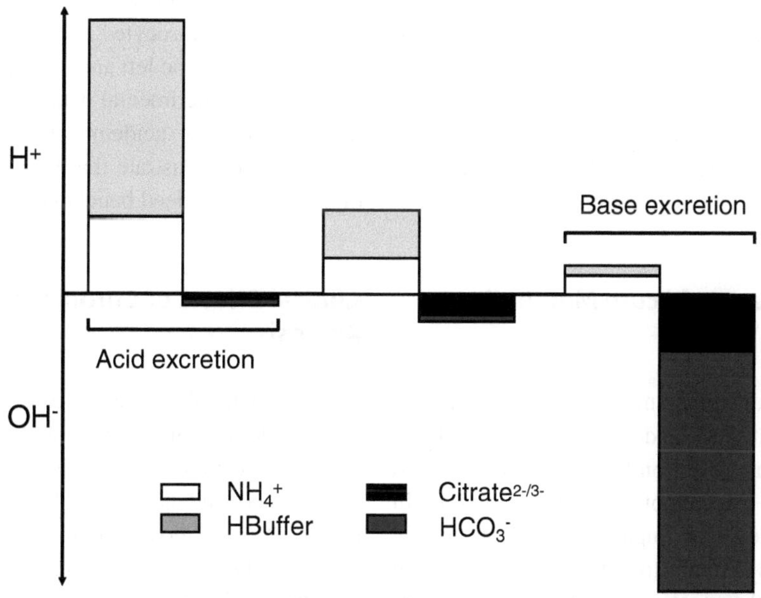

Fig. 8.8 Acid–base components in urine. Free H^+ in urine is extremely low. Most H^+ are carried by urinary buffers which can be divided into NH_3 (high p*K*, open, high capacity, and highly regulated) and all others (low p*K*, closed, lower capacity, and less regulated). Free OH– in urine is also extremely low. Urinary base composed of HCO_3^- and organic anions of which citrate2–/3– is the most abundant. Citrate2–/3– is more important than HCO_3^- in the day-to-day regulation of base excretion because there is very little bicarbonaturia. However, HCO_3^- has a much higher capacity than citrate2–/3– and assumes a pivotal role in situations where high urinary base excretion is required

Urinary acid consists of NH_4^+ and titratable acids, which embraces all other species that carry H^+. Free H^+ is negligible from the standpoint of external acid–base balance. Under increased acid loading, NH_4^+ is the main upregulated constituent. Urinary base is mostly citrate. Upon alkali loading, urinary citrate increases, yet never reaches the magnitude of bicarbonaturia.

Causes and Effects of Metabolic Acidosis

Causes of Metabolic Acidosis

The traditional classification of metabolic acidosis into anion and non-anion gap is based on an empirical calculation. It undoubtedly streamlines the diagnostic process, but the binary division can potentially be very misleading. An alternative categorization into overproduction and under-excretion acidosis has been proposed. While clinicians routinely measure neither acid production nor excretion, this classification is conceptually harder to grasp but it encourages more pathophysiologic reasoning. In general, bearing in mind the many exceptions, overproduction acidoses tend to elevate the anion gap while under-excretion acidoses tend to maintain a normal anion gap, but many exceptions abound. Table 8.3 provides a list of causes of metabolic acidoses.

Clinical Effects of Acute Metabolic Acidosis

All protein functions and biologic reactions are pH-dependent to some degree. From a teleologic viewpoint, any deviation from normal intra- and extracellular pH cannot be inconsequential. In reality, the negative impact of an acute fall in plasma pH is difficult to determine. The arterial pH remains the most common clinical convention of measuring acid–base status, but it does not tell the entire story. Changes in venous pH at the tissue level lead to variable and smaller disturbances in arterial pH. Also, for a given abnormality in arterial pH, it is difficult to discern the corresponding disturbance in intracellular pH. When acute metabolic acidosis is encountered in the setting of some catastrophic illness with extensive circulatory and metabolic consequences, it is impossible to isolate any detrimental effects of the low pH in isolation. For example, sodium lactate buffered to pH of 7.4 in the absence of acidosis can cause a decrease in cardiac contractility in animal models [13].

The cardiovascular system is a major target of acute metabolic acidosis [14]. Acute lowering of arterial pH decreases cardiac contractility in whole animals and in isolated heart preparations [15–18]. The responsiveness of adrenergic receptors to circulating catecholamines is decreased [19–22], and circulatory collapse may result [23]. Acidosis has also been shown to lower the ventricular fibrillation threshold [24], but the finding is not uniform [25–27]. The peripheral venous congestions shifts plasma volume to the pulmonary circulation and may enhance susceptibility to pulmonary edema [28]. Acute acidemia has profound effects on oxygen transport. Acidemia shifts the oxygen–hemoglobin dissociation curve (P50) to the right (decreases affinity for oxygen) [29] which should enhance O_2 delivery in tissue. However, an associated fall in erythrocyte 2,3-bisphosphoglycerate shifts the P50 to the left and negates the pH effect [30]. While experimental data showing the deleterious effects of acidemia is solid, it remains difficult to demonstrate that therapeutic reversal of a low pH is indeed beneficial.

Clinical Effects of Chronic Metabolic Acidosis

Chronic metabolic acidosis leads to bone resorption and demineralization through osteoclast activation and osteoblast inhibition. Bone resorption is activated and new bone formation impaired [31, 32]. Acidosis inhibits synthesis of $1,25(OH)_2D_3$ [33] and decreases sensitivity of parathyroid hormone (PTH) to ionized calcium [34]. The homeostatic relationships between blood ionized calcium, PTH, and $1,25(OH)_2D_3$ is deranged with a net effect of exaggerated bone dissolution [2]. In 14 young adults with long-standing metabolic acidosis due to distal renal tubular acidosis (RTA), bone histomorphometry

Table 8.3 Causes of metabolic acidosis

Overproduction	Anion gap	Comments
Lactic acid Type A lactic acidosis (hypoxia) Shock: septic, cardiogenic, hemorrhagic, anaphylactic Hypoxemia: respiratory failure intoxications: carbon monoxide, cyanide Severe anemia, methemoglobinemia Type B lactic acidosis Drugs Metformin Nucleoside-analogue reverse transcriptase inhibitors Acute thiamine deficiency Seizure, severe exertion Toxin related Ethanol, ethylene glycol, methanol, salicylate Liver failure Large solid tumor, lymphoma, and leukemia Hereditary enzyme deficiencies	Usually elevated	In catastrophic situations of massive overproduction acidosis and circulatory impairment, renal acid excretion is also compromised. However, this is of little relevance as the acid generation rate far exceeds the normal maximal renal acid excretion capacity $NaHCO_3$ therapy has no proven benefit
Ketoacids Insulin-dependent diabetes mellitus Starvation Ethanol induced	Usually elevated	In chronic mild ketoacidosis with normal GFR, ketoanions are excreted hence plasma levels are low and anion gap is normal $NaHCO_3$ therapy possibly benefits
Other acids Ethylene glycol–glycolic, glyoxalic, and oxalic acid Methanol–formic acid Toluene-derived hippuric acid Propylene glycol Pyroglutamate D-Lactic acidosis Fleet Phospho-soda	Usually elevated except hippuric acidosis	Hippurate is filtered and secreted so plasma levels rarely accumulate $NaHCO_3$ therapy likely benefits
Intestinal alkali loss Ileal conduits and ureterosigmoidostomies Chronic diarrhea: Malabsorption, ileostomy, colostomy, enteric fistulae, jejunal loop	Usually normal	Intestinal alkali loss per se with completely normal renal acid excretion is unlikely to cause sustained metabolic acidosis $NaHCO_3$ therapy will benefit
Under-excretion	**Anion gap**	**Comments**
Renal tubular acidosis (RTA) Proximal Distal hypokalemic Distal hyperkalemic RTA of renal failure (low nephron mass)	Usually normal	In near end stage CKD when GFR is extremely low, anions of inorganic acids accumulate and elevated the anion gap

and densitometry revealed lower bone mass and a significantly decreased bone formation rate [35]. Children with distal RTA have stunted growth and short stature [36]. Interestingly, even in the absence of overt metabolic acidosis, the acid generated by a standard western high protein, low potassium diet (with accompanying low alkali) may in fact promote demineralization of bone, even in the absence of overt clinical metabolic acidosis [37]. This “eubicarbonatemic” metabolic acidosis may be responsible for negative calcium and phosphorus balance and negative bone mineral density, especially in postmenopausal women [38–40].

Chronic metabolic acidosis induces protein catabolism through the ubiquitin–proteasome pathway and the growth hormone/IGF-1 axis [41, 42]. In healthy adults, chronic metabolic acidosis suppresses albumin synthesis, increases glucocorticoid levels and urinary nitrogen excretion, and induces growth hormone insensitivity [43, 44]. It also reduces thyroid hormones with elevated TSH [45]. In patients with azotemia, the direct effects of metabolic acidosis are harder to discern in the background of multiple abnormalities that may not all be controlled. Negative calcium balance has been described in chronic renal failure [46]. Growth hormone resistance was first documented in uremic children with stunted growth and low body mass [47]. Adults on dialysis or pre-dialysis exhibit growth hormone insensitivity [48], and the metabolic response to IGF-1 is impaired [49]. The thyroid hormone axis is also affected, with low plasma T3 and T4, a normal TSH, and a blunted response to TRH [50]. Finally, metabolic acidosis induces lower insulin secretion and insulin resistance [51].

Hypoalbuminemia is a major predictor of mortality in dialysis patients [52, 53]. Whether chronic metabolic acidosis per se produces hypoalbuminemia in this population remains a matter of controversy, as results have been inconsistent [34, 54–57].

Clinical Assessment of Acid–Base Disorders

Relationships between H^+, CO_2, and HCO_3^-

Figure 8.9 is a plot of the Henderson relationship between H^+, CO_2, and HCO_3^-, using pCO_2 isobars. The arrows describe metabolic acidosis with

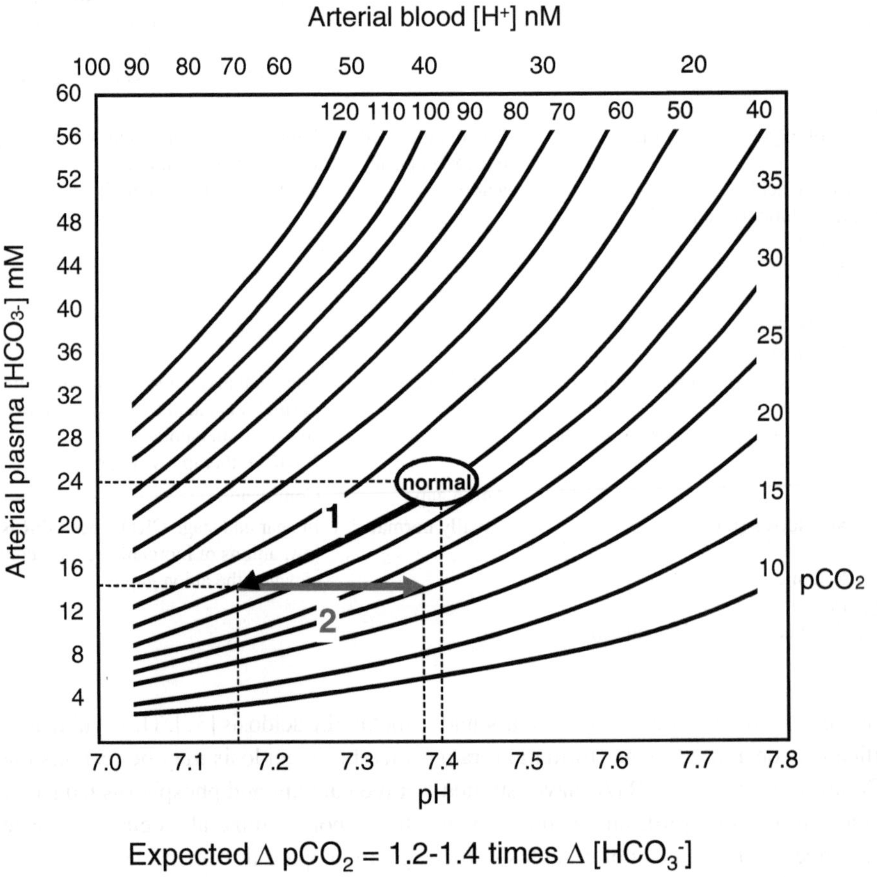

Fig. 8.9 Metabolic acidosis and respiratory compensation. Relationship of pH (H^+), plasma [HCO_3^-], and pCO_2 as described by the Henderson equation is shown pictorially. Each pCO_2 is depicted as an isobar. Metabolic acidosis is a primary fall in [HCO_3^-] that produces a drop in pH (*1*). Respiratory compensation lowers pCO_2 and returns pH towards normal (*2*)

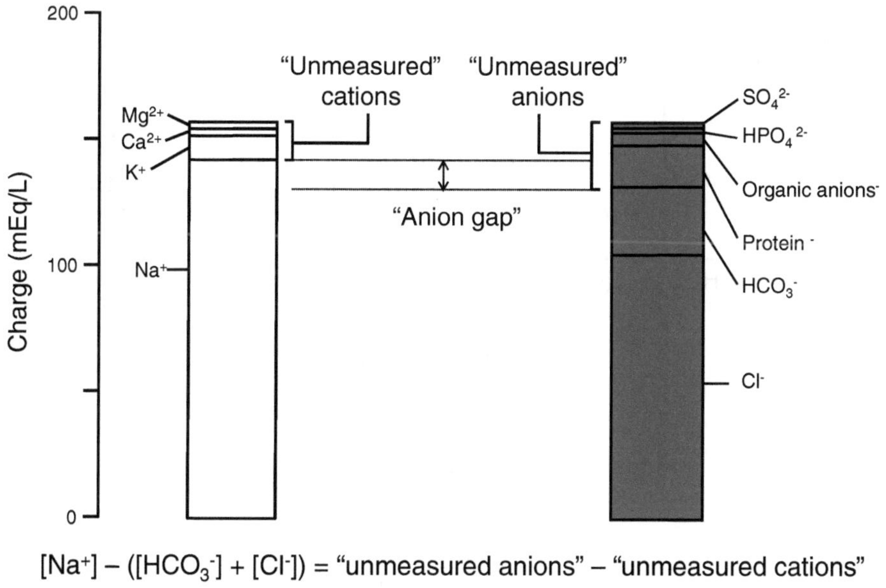

Fig. 8.10 Plasma cations and anions. The clinically accepted misnomer "anion gap" is actually the difference between unmeasured anions (anions that are not represented by HCO_3^- and Cl^-) and unmeasured cations (cations not represented by Na^+). The clinical anion gap can be elevated by increased unmeasured anions or decreased unmeasured cations. An increase in anions dissociated from acid added to the body fluid manifests itself as an increase in *unmeasured* anions. All else being equal, the "anion gap" will rise by the exact amount. This is a highly idealized situation

respiratory compensation. Several clinical parameters particularly relevant to metabolic acidosis are given due consideration. The respiratory compensation in metabolic acidosis lowers the $PaCO_2$ by about 1.2–1.5 mmHg for every mEq/L decrease in serum bicarbonate concentrations. Of the many formulas that help assess whether compensation has occurred or whether a mixed acid–base disorder is present, two are particularly popular: (1) Expected $pCO_2 = 1.5 \times HCO_3^- + 8 \pm 2$ (Winter's formula) and (2) pCO_2 = last two digits of pH × 100. In addition to the terms in the Henderson equation, we will discuss plasma anion gap, plasma osmolar gap, urinary anion gap (UAG), and urinary osmolar gap.

The Plasma Anion Gap

The term "plasma anion gap" is an unfortunate misnomer of an empirical numerical entity that is in fact the sum of concentrations of all cations other than Na^+ minus the sum of concentrations of all anions other than Cl^- and HCO_3^- (in mEq/L) [58, 59]. For the clinician, however, the term anion gap remains a practical substitute. Electroneutrality dictates equality of cations and anions so any addition of anions from invading acids elevates the anion gap (Fig. 8.10). The normal range varies widely and depends on the methodology, but is typically 6–12, as Na^+ exceeds the sum of Cl^- and HCO_3^-. An increased anion gap is due to either an elevated level of unmeasured anions or decreased level of unmeasured cations. A decreased anion gap is the effect of increased cations (such as positively charged paraproteins) or reduced anions (such as negatively charged albumin). Empirically, each 1 g/dL drop in albumin reduces the anion gap by about 3. Figure 8.11 demonstrates how the addition of acid (HA) or removal of base ($NaHCO_3$) from the body may, or may not, lead to a rise in anion gap.

A critical step is the translation of the biochemical diagnosis of metabolic acidosis to the clinical diagnosis of the underlying cause. The anion gap is useful in the context of metabolic acidosis. The degree of change (Δ(delta)) of bicarbonate vs. the anion gap is useful in classifying

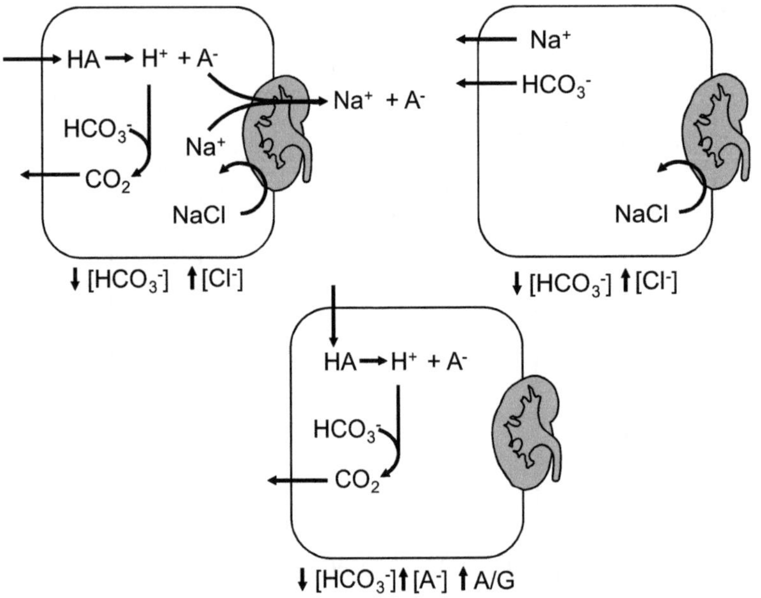

Fig. 8.11 Genesis of "non-anion gap" vs. "anion gap" metabolic acidosis. *Top left panel* shows addition of HA to the body leading to decomposition of HCO_3^-. The anion of the acid A^- is excreted as a Na^+ salt leading to obligatory Na^+ depletion triggering NaCl retention by the kidney. *Top right panel* depicts loss of $NaHCO_3$, which are valuable ECF ions, compensatory NaCl retention ensues. Both scenarios will lower plasma [HCO_3^-] and raise plasma [Cl^-] without changing the anion gap. The *bottom panel* shows HCO_3^- decomposition by HA with accumulation of A^- in the body leading to an anion gap

complex AB disorders. When Δ(delta) HCO_3^- = Δ(delta) AG, it is referred to as pure AG metabolic acidosis. When Δ(delta) HCO_3^- is greater than Δ(delta) AG, it is referred to as mixed AG/non-AG metabolic acidosis. When the Δ(delta) HCO_3^- is less than Δ(delta) AG, the metabolic acidosis may be mixed with metabolic alkalosis. While this concept streamlines and standardizes, one should not lose sight of the underlying pathophysiologic process. This is imperative as a number of pitfalls exist. The anion gap is certainly not as straightforward as conventionally presented.

The anion gap depends on three parameters, and inaccuracies of measurement in any of the three lead to errors. One hurdle is that the normal anion gap spans a range. Thus, a patient with a formally "normal" anion gap may have a modest elevation that goes undetected. Differences in volume of distribution (Vd) may render the relationship of Δ(delta)HCO_3^- and Δ(delta)AG not reciprocal [58, 60]. If HA is added to the ECF space, but H^+ is taken up into cells (larger Vd for H^+ than HA or A^-), then Δ(delta)HCO_3^- will be less than Δ(delta)AG. There is also continuous urinary excretion of A^-. Excretion of NH_4A will rid the plasma of A^-, regenerate the decomposed HCO_3^-, and restore normality. In contrast, excretion of NaA will not correct the acidosis but removes A^- from plasma, such that the fall in plasma HCO_3^- is accompanied by little or no rise in AG [59].

Ketoacidosis is a classical example of combination of AG and NAG metabolic acidosis depending on the speed, severity, volume status, and GFR. In conditions of low-grade ketoacid generation, normal circulating volume, and preserved GFR, the increased ketoacid production is accompanied by increased renal acid excretion so that ketoanions are excreted in the urine with Na^+, K^+, and largely NH_4^+. Hence, plasma ketoanions are either normal or slightly increased. The metabolic acidosis is of the NAG type. When ketoacid generation is overwhelming, plasma ketoanions accumulate and the acidosis becomes more of an AG type. With volume expansion and improved GFR, these accumulated ketoanions are excreted resulting in loss of potential HCO_3^-, which is tantamount to urinary loss of $NaHCO_3$; the acidosis once again reverts to the NAG type.

Chronic kidney disease (CKD) is typically a combination of AG/NAG acidosis [61]. The limited renal H^+ excretion leads to H^+ retention and consumption of HCO_3^- that cannot be fully regenerated by the kidneys. However, GFR is of sufficient magnitude to excrete A^- (Fig. 8.11, top left) and a NAG acidosis ensues. In later stages of CKD, A^- excretion is also reduced and a mixed NAG/AG acidosis occurs. Full quantitative equivalence of Δ(delta)HCO_3^- and Δ(delta)AG is difficult to ascertain because of A^- excretion and, because of the chronic nature of the acidosis, ECF HCO_3^- no longer be the sole buffer. Bone carbonate buffer can never be accounted for using plasma chemistry.

Toluene poisoning typically follows inhalation of the organic solvent and represents an overproduction of organic acidosis [62]. The metabolite of toluene is the strong hippuric acid whose anion is not metabolized but rapidly cleared by the kidney by glomerular filtration–tubular secretion as Na^+, K^+, and NH_4^+ salt. The classic biochemical picture is a NAG acidosis. In contrast, metabolic acidosis from overproduction of pyroglutamic acid results in AG acidosis because the fraction excretion of pyroglutamate is extremely low due to tubular reabsorption [59]. Hippuric and pyroglutamic acid overproduction are examples of organic acidoses with nonmetabolizable anions.

Plasma Osmolar Gap

Like the anion gap, there is really no osmolar gap in the plasma. The utility of the osmolar gap is in estimating whether there are any significant amount of osmoles in the extracellular space unaccounted for by Na^+ (plus accompanying anion), urea, and glucose. Table 8.4 summarizes some of the clinical conditions where an osmolar gap heralds the abundant presence of a low molecular weight substance such an alcohol or acetone in plasma. Several points are noteworthy. First, the small alcohol per se may not be toxic other than the inebriating effect at higher doses. However, two such alcohols with hydroxyl groups on the α(alpha)-carbons can be oxidized to carboxyl groups with low pK (H^+ donor). The anion represents the end product of metabolism, as it cannot regenerate decomposed HCO_3^-. Ethylene glycol and methanol are such examples (Table 8.4). Second, the chemical concentration of an alcohol can be predicted from the osmolar gap. Allowing about 7–10 mOsm/L for an osmolar gap that normally exists, every additional 10 mOsm of "excess osmoles" represent "*X*" mg/dL of the alcohol ("*X*" = molecular weight of the alcohol in grams). A caveat is that this deduction assumes that only a single species of alcohol was ingested. This may not be the case! Alcohols with hydroxyl groups on β(beta)-carbon such as isopropanol will not be metabolized to an acid but rather to a ketone. Thus, acidosis will not ensue (Table 8.4). Alcohols such as ethanol are metabolized to an acid (acetic acid) but the further metabolism of acetate consumes an H^+ yielding a base equivalent. Acetic acid does therefore not produce a net acid load.

Urinary Anion Gap

In analogy to the plasma anion gap, the urinary anion gap (UAG = urine $[Na^+] + [K^+] - [Cl^-]$) refers to the "sum of concentrations of all cations other than Na^+ and K^+ minus the sum of concentration of all anion other than Cl^-" (Fig. 8.12). Halperin and coworkers first used it to estimate urinary NH_4^+ concentrations [63, 64], later confirmed by Batlle and coworkers using urinary excretion rates [65]. Figure 8.12 illustrates the utility of this simple laboratory test that can be quickly obtained from a spot urine. Na^+, K^+, and NH_4^+ constitute the bulk of the cations while Cl^- is the major anion in normal urine. When the kidney escalates acid excretion by increasing urinary NH_4Cl, the rise in urine $[Cl^-]$ or $U_{Cl-}V$ will render the UAG more negative. Efforts have been made to empower this test to be more quantitative, but several limitations precluded its success. The

Table 8.4 Substances that elevate the plasma osmolar gap

Substance	MW (g)	Formula	mOsm for each 100 mg/dL	mg/dL for each 10 mOsm	Remarks
Ethylene glycol	62	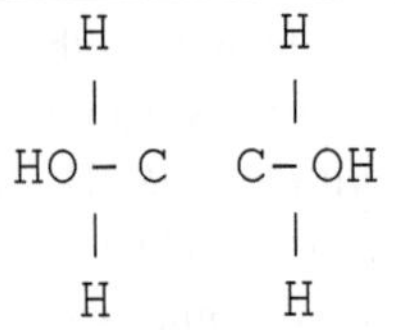	16	62	Metabolized to a series of strong acids whose anions are end products. Causes metabolic acidosis. As anion gap increases, osmolar gap decreases
Methanol	32	CH_3-OH	31	32	Metabolized to formic acid. Causes metabolic acidosis as formate is not metabolized. As anion gap increases, osmolar gap decreases
Isopropanol	60	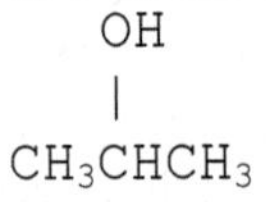	17	60	Metabolized to acetone and not to a carboxylic acid because of the –OH is on a β(beta)-carbon
Propylene glycol	76	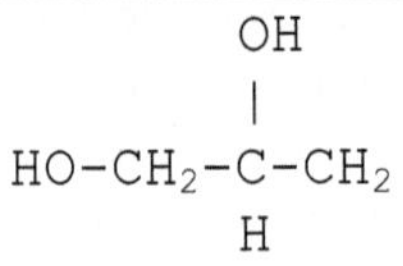	13	76	Oxidation of the –OH on the α(alpha)-carbon yields lactic acid. Lactate is metabolized to a base equivalent
Acetone	58	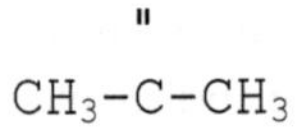	17	58	Similar to isopropanol
Ethanol	46	CH_3-CH_2-OH	22	46	Metabolized to acetic acid. Acetate is metabolized to a base equivalent. No net acid is generated
Mannitol	182	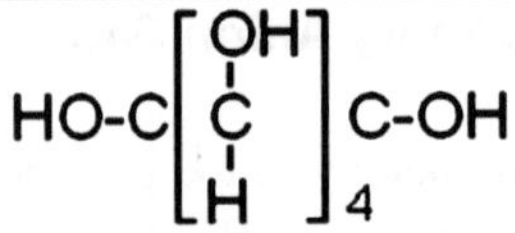	5.5	182	Not metabolized Excreted in kidneys

The gray column indicates that if the unaccounted osmolar gap is from a single alcohol, the chemical concentration of that alcohol in mg/dL is approximately the same (numerically) as the molecular weight of the alcohol

normal UAG depends on the excretion of a large number of solutes that varies from individual to individual and from day to day. There is really no normal reference range. However, the biggest drawback of the UAG is the excretion of anions from the invading acid (Figs. 8.11 and 8.12), which adds a significant quantity of "unmeasured" anions to the urine (e.g., β(beta)-OH-butyrate, acetoacetate, hippurate), thus yielding a positive UAG (Fig. 8.12) and the erroneous assumption of inadequate urinary ammonium excretion. One method to detect the excretion of $NH_4^+ + A^-$ is via the urinary osmolar gap.

Urinary Osmolar Gap

The urinary osmolar stems from the same principle as the plasma osmolar gap—the difference between predicted and measured osmolality. Normally, most of the osmoles in the urine are accounted for by electrolytes and urea [66, 67]. When other osmoles are present in significant amounts, a "gap" appears. Examples include glycosuria or mannitol in the urine. The same deduction can be applied to the detection of NH_4A as in the typical case of overproduction acidosis of toluene overdose where the kidney increases

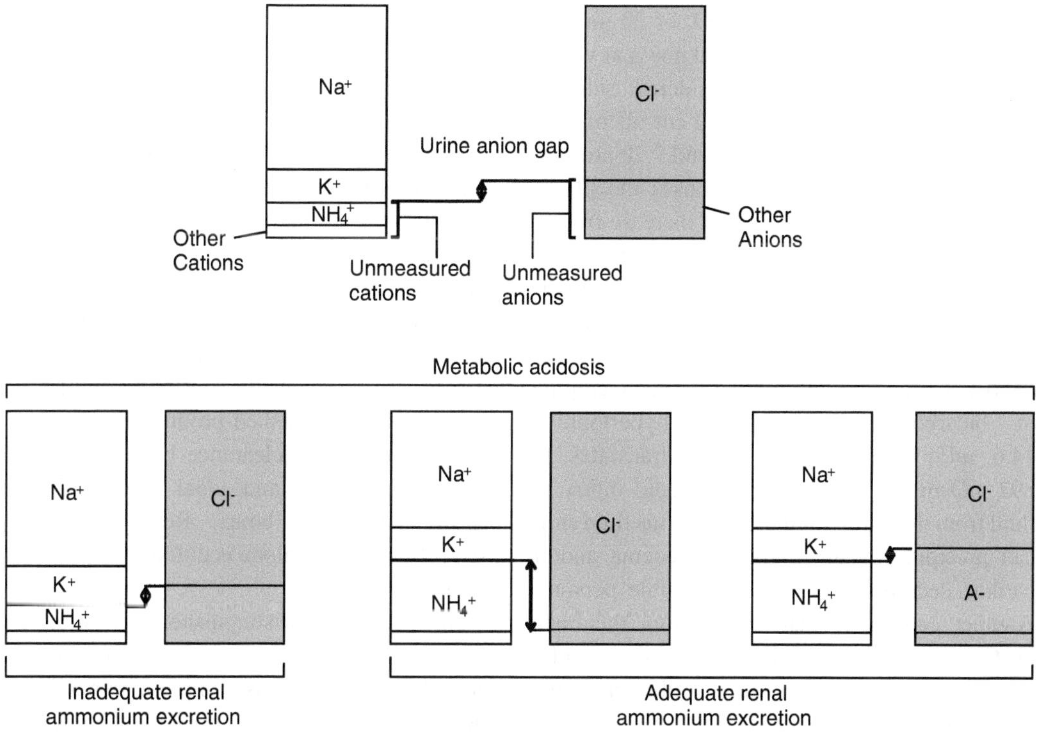

Fig. 8.12 Urinary anion gap (UAG) in estimating urinary ammonium. The clinical term "urinary anion gap" is in fact the sum of all cations not represented by Na^+ and K^+ minus the sum of all anions not represented by Cl^-. *Top panel* represents a typical normal individual where the UAG is a small positive number. The *bottom panels* represent three scenarios with metabolic acidosis where the expected renal response is elevated NH_4^+ excretion. The *left panel* represents inadequate NH_4^+ excretion with a positive UAG. The *middle* and *right panels* represent adequate NH_4^+ excretion. The negative UAG in the *middle panel* reflects the high NH_4^+ in the urine while the *right panel* shows a positive UAG despite high urinary NH_4^+ because of the additional urinary anion A^- from the invading acid

NH_4^+ excretion and the hippurate is removed very efficiently (Fig. 8.11). NH_4^+ hippurate will contribute to osmoles in the urine. A similar situation can be seen in chronic low-grade ketonuria where the ketoanions are excreted as NH_4^+ salts. When the osmolar gap is due to NH_4^+ salts, the NH_4^+ concentration can be approximated as half of the gap.

Treatment of Metabolic Acidosis

Acute Buffer Replacement: General Consideration

In the treatment of patients with metabolic acidosis, we distinguish between acute "catastrophic" metabolic acidosis typically seen in the emergency department or intensive care unit and conditions of chronic and indolent metabolic acidosis usually encountered in the outpatient setting. The principal biochemical defect of low plasma $[HCO_3^-]$ indicates consumption of the major plasma buffer HCO_3^- by the invading acid that cannot be rectified by the kidney's ability to regenerate the decomposed HCO_3^-. The central tenets of therapy are threefold: replacement of HCO_3^-, arrest of the increased acid generation, and reversal of the kidney's impairment in excreting the excess acid, if such exists. The first and most important principle is that simply replacing HCO_3^- (or equivalent buffer) without attempting to arrest the underlying disturbance is unacceptable. All efforts must be directed to reversing the condition that led to the overproduction of acid.

An example of an acute catastrophic acidosis is an unresponsive patient with a combined metabolic and respiratory acidosis. An arterial blood gas reveals a pH of 6.90, a pCO_2 of 20 mmHg, and a HCO_3 of 4 mEq/L. It is unknown at which target pH the patient can be considered "safe." A consensus rather than data-based cut-off of 7.10 is often suggested, but pH 7.15 and 7.20 are also used. If HCO_3 administration raises the pH to 7.20, then the serum HCO_3 must increase from 4 to 7.6 mEq/L—assuming ventilation maintains the pCO_2 at 20 mmHg. Using a volume of distribution (Vd) for HCO_3 of 50 % body weight, a 70 kg person will require 127 mEq HCO_3, or almost 3 ampoules of $NaHCO_3$. Each ampule of bicarbonate is markedly hypertonic—44.6 mEq $NaHCO_3$ in 50 mL translates to 892 mOsm/L—which triggers a rapid influx of fluid from the extravascular space. This fluid shift can precipitate acute pulmonary edema and/or cardiac decompensation in susceptible persons. Another caution is that replenishing the open HCO_3/CO_2 system implicitly necessitates adequate alveolar perfusion and ventilation. If the rise in extracellular HCO_3^- is offset by a simultaneous rise in pCO_2, then the benefit on extracellular pH is diminished or even negated. Since CO_2 enters cells much more rapidly than transporter-mediated HCO_3, extracellular hypercapnea can acidify cells despite a rise in extracellular HCO_3. Thus, intracellular acidosis due to rapid infusion of $NaHCO_3$ (often in large amounts) during resuscitation efforts in cardiopulmonary arrest may be the pathophysiologic basis why it is not only ineffective but also potentially harmful.

One needs to understand the dynamics of the combined clearance of acid by metabolism and respiration. In a patient without ventilatory support and impending ventilatory failure, there is security from having higher plasma HCO_3. Picture a patient with a severe but compensated metabolic acidosis (pCO_2 = 16 mmHg, HCO_3 = 6 mM, pH 7.19) who develops ventilatory failure. An acute rise of pCO_2 to 40 will cause the pH to fall to 6.79 while the same pCO_2 at HCO_3 = 12 mM will have a pH of 7.1.

Observations in animals and humans with the two commonest states of endogenous organic acidoses have observed an alkali pH-driven rise in lactic acid and keto acid production [68]. Other potential concerns are worsening hemodynamics and paradoxical cerebral spinal fluid (CSF) and intracellular acidosis [69–71]. Simply treating the acidosis with base is not only of little benefit, as ongoing production of the organic anion is overwhelming, but also potentially deleterious.

These considerations highlight the limitations of sodium bicarbonate therapy, especially for an organic metabolic acidosis, as it is a manifestation of an underlying pathologic process and not a disease in itself. The focus of therapy should therefore be on reversing the pathophysiologic process, not on alkali therapy. Successful treatment leads to diminished production of organic acids and enhanced clearance by liver and kidneys, with hepatic and renal regeneration of bicarbonate within hours. Replenishment of extracellular buffer alone is unlikely to provide a benefit.

This needs to be distinguished from situations where a non-metabolizable anion cannot be converted to bicarbonate, as in mineral hyperchloremic acidoses, or when non-metabolizable organic acids are overwhelmingly generated, as with certain alcohol poisonings (oxalate and formate anions from ethylene glycol and methanol, respectively). These patients could benefit from exogenous alkali therapy, since endogenous (renal) regeneration of bicarbonate occurs only slowly over several days.

Acute Bicarbonate Administration in Lactic Acidosis

During anaerobic glycolysis, pyruvate is converted to lactic acid instead of entering the Krebs cycle. Tissues producing lactic acid have high rates of glycolysis, which include skeletal muscle, gut, brain, skin, and red blood cells. The liver, and to a lesser extent, the kidneys (roughly 20–30 %) metabolize lactate and ultimately regenerate bicarbonate through gluconeogenesis or oxidation in the Krebs cycle. Thus, despite a daily production of lactic acid in the range of about 1,000 mmol/day (15–20 mmol/kg BW), blood lactate levels are maintained less than 1 mM. Two types of lactic acidoses are commonly distinguished (Table 8.3). Type A can be broadly defined as the result of tissue hypoxia while Type B lactic acidosis is not a problem of oxygen deficit, but rather conditions of either high lactic acid production or low lactic acid uptake and metabolism.

Two randomized controlled trials of $NaHCO_3$ therapy in critically ill patients with severe (type A) lactic acidosis have shown increase in blood pH and HCO_3^- with sodium bicarbonate, but without change in hemodynamic parameters [72, 73]. Neither study looked at differences in outcome. Intubated dogs with induced hypoxic lactic acidosis (FiO_2 of 8 %; PaO_2 25–30 mmHg) given $NaHCO_3$ had a greater increase in gut lactic acid production and serum lactate levels and further decrease in arterial pH and plasma HCO_3 levels. Intracellular pH in the liver was lower in the $NaHCO_3$-treated animals, and hemodynamic parameters worse [74]. Conversely, in another study of dogs with lactic acidosis from hemorrhagic shock treatment with $NaHCO_3$ increased lactate levels and pCO_2, but cardiac output and blood pressure improved [75]. In ventilated pigs receiving lactic acid infusion, $NaHCO_3$ reduced mean arterial pressure but did not affect cardiac output [76]. In pigs with hemorrhagic shock receiving hemastarch alone or in combination with $NaHCO_3$, both blood pressure and cardiac output remained unchanged, but blood lactic acid levels were increased [77]. Thus, most human and animal studies suggest either no benefit or worse hemodynamics with $NaHCO_3$.

Several arguments have been put forth against the administration of $NaHCO_3$ in lactic acidosis. There is evidence that acidemia impedes lactic acid production, and alkalemia enhances it [78–80]. In one study, bicarbonate produced intracellular acidosis by diffusion of CO_2 through cell membranes in vitro [70], but in another study, this effect was only observed with non-bicarbonate buffers [81]. As HCO_3^- binds H^+, more H^+ is released from non-bicarbonate buffers to increase CO_2 production. The measured CO_2 release after HCO_3^- infusion interestingly correlates with the hemoglobin and albumin concentration [82] and with the degree of intracellular acidosis [83]. Bicarbonate therapy may also lead to a drop in ionized calcium with a resultant negative inotropic effect on the heart [84]. Hypocalcemia in the setting of hyperkalemia may precipitate cardiac arrhythmia. Hypertonic $NaHCO_3$ can lead to fluid overload, potentially impairing alveolar ventilation or precipitating acute cardiac decompensation. Finally, the relentless production of large amounts of lactic acid, especially in the setting of reduced hepatic (and renal) clearance, is often overwhelmingly larger than the amount of alkali that can be infused. A uniformly dire prognosis ensues unless the underlying process is recognized and reversed. The current data do not support a beneficial role of $NaHCO_3$ therapy for lactic acidosis.

Treatment of Lactic Acidosis Not Associated with Circulatory Collapse

Type B lactic acidosis is a much more heterogeneous group than type A (Table 8.3). The acidosis tends to be less fulminant, and it carries a better overall prognosis. It may respond to specific therapy, for example, IV thiamine for lactic acidosis in patients with alcoholism or malignancy. Thiamine pyrophosphate is a cofactor for pyruvate dehydrogenase necessary for conversion of pyruvate to acetyl CoA. In thiamine deficiency, pyruvate accumulates and is metabolized to lactic acid. In HIV infected patients receiving therapy with nucleoside-analogue reverse transcriptase inhibitors (zidovudine and stavudine), lactic acidosis develops due to direct mitochondrial toxicity. Affected individuals present with chronic and asymptomatic hyperlactatemic states [85]. The biguanides metformin and phenformin act partly by activating the pyruvate dehydrogenase enzyme complex and inhibiting the transport of mitochondrial reducing agents. It enhances anaerobic metabolism and conversion of pyruvate to lactic acid. Lactic acidosis develops in susceptible patients and is contraindicated in patients with congestive heart failure, acute kidney injury or CKD (creatinine greater than 1.5 mg/dL in men or greater than 1.4 mg/dL in women), chronic lung disease with hypoxia, and with preexisting metabolic acidosis. It should be withheld for 48 h after administration of an intravenous contrast agent. In phenformin-induced lactic acidosis in dogs, mortality was no different in $NaHCO_3$ versus NaCl-treated animals [86]. A retrospective analysis of 300 patients with biguanide-induced lactic acidosis (phenformin, buformin, and metformin) showed no difference in outcomes for patients receiving $NaHCO_3$ therapy [87]. However, renal replacement therapy (RRT) is highly effective, as discussed below. In patients with seizures, lactic acidosis usually dissolves within a few hours following the episode and base therapy is not necessary.

Patients with fulminant liver failure invariably develop renal failure (hepatorenal syndrome type I) with profound metabolic acidosis and electrolyte disturbances, including hyperkalemia. The patient will expire within hours or days unless emergent liver transplantation is arranged. A patient with less severe liver failure can often be saved with RRT in anticipation of a liver transplant. The scenario is quite different for chronic liver disease where patients often exhibit some degree of renal impairment; however, progression is slow and may even extend over months to years (hepatorenal syndrome type II). The acid–base derangement is usually a combination of respiratory alkalosis (central stimulation) and metabolic acidosis due to a combination of reduced hepatic metabolism of lactic acid (anion gap) and renal failure (mainly non-anion gap). Depending on the predominating disorder, the patient presents with either acidemia or alkalemia, though the latter is more common. Regardless, alkali therapy is not advocated in these patients.

Bicarbonate Therapy in the Setting of Cardiopulmonary Resuscitation

The American Heart Association's (AHA) guidelines on the use of sodium bicarbonate during Advanced Cardiac Life Support (ACLS) have undergone an evolution. It was previously erroneously assumed that cardiac arrest victims would benefit from $NaHCO_3$ to improve cardiac function and outcome. Thus, guidelines published in 1974 mandated automatic IV bicarbonate in victims of cardiac arrest. These recommendations changed in 1986 based on published data on the ineffectiveness of such treatment and on potential adverse side effects, stating that "$NaHCO_3$ should be used, if at all, only after application of more definitive and better substantiated interventions," and furthermore: "$NaHCO_3$ therapy, although not recommended, can be considered in specific clinical circumstances such as documented preexisting metabolic acidosis with or without hyperkalemia" [88].

These recommendations were left essentially unchanged until the year 2000, when following addendum was added: "Adequate ventilation and CPR, not bicarbonate, are the major 'buffer agents' in cardiac arrest. $NaHCO_3$ is not recommended for routine use in cardiac arrest patients" [89]. Nevertheless, it does list several indications for appropriate use of $NaHCO_3$, including "... known, preexisting hyperkalemia, HCO_3-responsive acidosis; tricyclic antidepressant overdose; or urine alkalinization in aspirin or other drug overdose situation; and intubated and ventilated patients with long arrest interval, or return of circulation after a long arrest interval" [89]. Finally, the 2006 guidelines further caution against the use by citing the lack of evidence from animal data to support the use of bicarbonate in cardiac arrest and list the potential adverse effects: reduced coronary perfusion pressure, hypertonicity, hypernatremia, metabolic alkalosis, reduced oxygen release by hemoglobin, paradoxical intracellular acidosis in myocardial and cerebral cells, and inactivation of administered catecholamines [74, 90–92]. The guidelines do list exceptions where the use may be justified: "... preexisting metabolic acidosis, hyperkalemia, or tricyclic antidepressant overdose..." but admits that "...clinical experience is greatly limited and outcome studies are lacking" [93]. An evaluation of nine studies on $NaHCO_3$ in cardiac arrest in humans found inconsistent benefit [94]. A beneficial effect may be hidden by the heterogeneity of the human subjects. Under controlled cardiac arrest situations in animals, several studies documented a higher resuscitation rate with various base therapies (including $NaHCO_3$) compared to normal saline [95, 96], but others failed to find a benefit [97–99]. Thus, current data do not support the use of $NaHCO_3$ in cardiopulmonary resuscitation.

Bicarbonate Therapy in Ketoacidosis

The keto acids, β(beta)-hydroxybutyric acid and acetoacetic acid, are produced through incomplete oxidation of fat. This condition is commonly encountered in subjects with insulin-dependent diabetes mellitus. Other causes include starvation, especially in pregnant women and children (Table 8.3). In alcoholism, ketoacidosis may develop due to a combination of starvation, stimulated lipolysis due to a high catecholamine state, and reduced gluconeogenesis due to depleted NAD^+.

During ketogenesis, acetoacetic acid is produced and converted enzymatically to β(beta)-hydroxybutyrate and non-enzymatically to acetone. The enzymatic conversion requires NAD^+. The normal ratio of β(beta)-hydroxybutyrate to acetoacetate is 2:1, but the ratio increases with worsening ketoacidosis due to an increase in the $NADH^{2+}/NAD^+$ ratio. As the nitroprusside test *only* detects acetoacetate, with progressive ketoacidosis, the test becomes weaker and may become negative. Conversely, with appropriate therapy, the test becomes more positive, indicating an improvement in ketoacidosis (lower $NADH^{2+}/NAD^+$ ratio). At physiologic pH, both ketoacids completely dissociate, consume HCO_3^-, and produce an anion gap. With successful treatment, pH and serum HCO_3^- increase and the anion gap closes. Elevated serum acetone levels may persist as they are primarily excreted by ventilation yielding the characteristic odor. Acetone is not an acid and does not produce an anion gap, though it will contribute to the osmolar gap. It is important to realize that ketoacidosis does not elevate the anion gap if the glomerular filtration rate is sufficiently preserved. Renal excretion of the organic anion with sodium (Na^+A^-) results in hyperchloremic metabolic acidosis. Diabetic ketoacidosis is typically a combination of anion gap *and* hyperchloremic metabolic acidosis. In patients who initially present with a high anion gap, HCO_3^- may be rapidly generated with insulin therapy as the ketone bodies undergo hepatic metabolism. In fact, in patients with lower levels of ketone bodies, recovery from acidosis was slower compared to patients with higher levels [100]. Thus, in patients with a markedly elevated anion gap, aggressive alkali therapy may potentially precipitate "overshoot" metabolic alkalosis.

On the other hand, in patients with a substantial component of hyperchloremia due to a high renal excretion of ketoacid anions with sodium, potassium, and ammonium, therapy with $NaHCO_3$ is more justified [101]. The vast majority of severe cases of ketoacidosis occur in diabetic patients. Treatment is primarily volume expansion and intravenous insulin. Bicarbonate therapy will aid in the normalization of blood chemistry. Whether alkali therapy will improve morbidity or mortality in these patients is not proven. In diabetic rats with ketoacidosis, administration of $NaHCO_3$ lead to worsening hemodynamics and blood lactate levels [102]. In 18 patients with starvation ketogenesis and a 1-week intake each of $NaHCO_3$, NaCl, and NH_4Cl, urinary excretion and blood levels of ketone bodies were significantly *less* during the NH_4Cl phase compared to the $NaHCO_3$ phase, suggesting (but not proving) that systemic pH regulates and modifies ketone acid production [103]. In a prospective study of 16 patients with severe diabetic ketoacidosis and lactic acidosis (mean pH 7.1, plasma HCO_3^- 7 mEq/L), treatment with intravenous $NaHCO_3$ led to quicker recovery of metabolic acidosis, with no difference in complication rate, but a delayed decrease in serum lactate levels [104]. Another prospective trial of ten patients with diabetic ketoacidosis (mean pH 7.3, serum HCO_3^- 7.5 mEq/L) found no difference in recovery of systemic and cerebrospinal metabolic acidosis, and similar rate of decline of serum ketones [105]. A double-blind, randomized placebo-controlled study of 20 patients with profound diabetic ketoacidosis (mean pH 7.0 and 7.1, serum HCO_3^- 3 mEq/L) had a quicker recovery rate of metabolic acidosis in the $NaHCO_3$-treated group, but no difference in complications or hemodynamics [106]. A counterproductive effect of $NaHCO_3$ treatment was seen in a study of seven

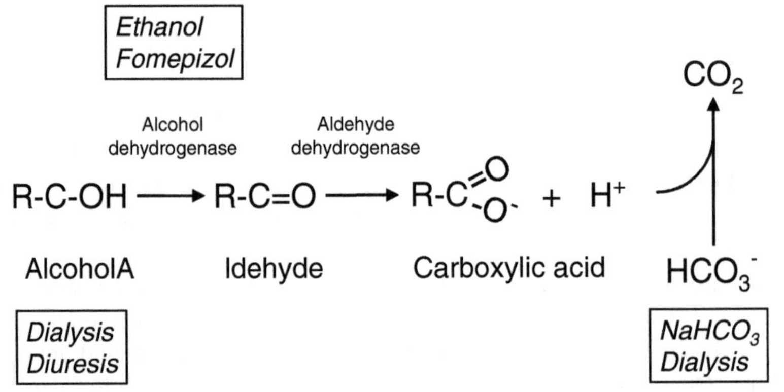

Fig. 8.13 Intoxication of a generic alcohol (RCOH), its metabolism, and treatment strategies. The hydroxyl group at the α(alpha)-carbon is metabolized sequentially into aldehyde and a strong carboxylic acid. The ill effects can stem from the alcohol itself but the enormous acid generation is the main culprit for morbidity. Treatment modalities (*boxed text*) include: (1) Removal of alcohol most effectively by dialysis. (2) Arrest of alcohol dehydrogenase by direct inhibition by fomepizol or competitive reaction by ethanol to the harmless metabolizable end product of acetic acid. (3) Replacement of decomposed HCO_3^- by infusion and/or dialysis

patients (three treated: mean pH 7.0, serum HCO_3^- 2 mEq/L; four untreated: mean pH 7.3, serum HCO_3^- 14 mEq/L) where quicker recovery from metabolic acidosis was seen with alkali therapy, but alkali administration augmented ketone production and resolution of ketosis took longer [107].

Retrospective analyses with a total of 247 patients with diabetic ketoacidosis found no difference in acidosis recovery or complication rate [108–111], with one study reporting a lower pH of the cerebrospinal fluid in the bicarbonate group [108]. In all cited studies, there was no difference in the glucose recovery rate. In summary, there may be quicker recovery from metabolic acidosis [104, 106], but no clinical benefit was derived. Some studies found CSF acidosis with HCO_3^- therapy, while others did not. However, CSF pH did not correlate with the level of consciousness, recovery or complication rate, and is therefore of no clinical importance. Finally, there remains the concern that base therapy impedes recovery from metabolic acidosis, be it lactic acidosis [78, 86, 104] for reasons discussed above, or ketoacidosis [107].

In conclusion, despite better biochemical resolution, there is insufficient data supporting superior outcome in using $NaHCO_3$ in diabetic ketoacidosis. However, unlike lactic acidosis of hypoperfusion, where adverse effects of $NaHCO_3$ therapy have been described, judicious use may be justified in situations of substantial ketonuria (predominantly hyperchloremic acidosis). $NaHCO_3$ is not indicated for ketoacidosis associated with starvation or alcoholism.

Treatment of Poisons

Intoxications due to ethylene glycol, methanol, ethanol, salicylate, and toluene are frequently accompanied by variable degrees of acidosis due to endogenously produced lactic and ketoacids, or toxin-derived metabolites such as glycolic acid, glyoxalic acid, and oxalic acid with ethylene glycol, formic acid with methanol, and hippuric acid with toluene poisoning (Tables 8.3 and 8.4).

Ethanol intoxication is best treated with thiamine and dextrose, provision of nutrients, cessation of ethanol intake, and general medical support. Methanol (wood alcohol) and ethylene glycol (antifreeze) intoxications often represent an acute life-threatening emergency because of the large amounts of strong acid produced and their treatment is urgent. Figure 8.13 summarizes the strategies for treating poisoning by alcohols that lead to non-metabolizable acid production.

As there is no chance of regeneration of the decomposed buffer, $NaHCO_3$ therapy is probably beneficial. Other treatment includes charcoal and forced dieresis, but the principal therapy is inhibition of alcohol dehydrogenase by ethanol or fomepizole, thus inhibiting formation of toxic metabolites (and metabolic acidosis) and enabling renal or dialytic clearance. Acute hemodialysis is highly effective in removing either alcohol or their toxic metabolites and should be used with a relatively low threshold, as the complication rate from a single hemodialysis treatment is minimal. Note that the osmolar gap is only present initially with the parent alcohol and subsequently disappears with the formation of carboxylic acids. Thus, *as the anion gap increases, the osmolar gap decreases*. Another alcohol frequently encountered is isopropanol (wood alcohol). It is converted to acetone, but since there is no α(alpha)-carbon, it cannot form a carboxyl group and release H^+. While it causes a persistent osmolar gap and a positive test for ketones, no elevation in the anion gap or metabolic acidosis is observed.

Salicylate poisoning induces metabolic acidosis predominantly due to the accumulation of lactic and keto acids and, to a much lesser extent, due to salicylic acid or other organic acids. Respiratory alkalosis frequently coexists, especially in adults. The more severe the acidosis, the more non-ionized (undissociated) salicylate is present. It becomes a neurotoxin as it diffuses into brain cells. Other complications include hypokalemia, hypoglycemia, non-cardiogenic pulmonary edema, renal failure, and bleeding. The nitroprusside test may be falsely positive, and salicylate may interfere with the measurement of chloride with certain machines, producing factitious hyperchloremia (and a nonexisting or even negative anion gap). A nasogastric tube provides access for gastric lavage and activated charcoal. To minimize neurotoxicity by minimizing undissociated (non-ionized) salicylic acid, treatment of metabolic acidosis is paramount. For example, by raising the systemic pH from 7.1 to 7.4, the amount of undissociated salicylic acid is cut in half. If renal function is preserved, forced alkaline diuresis is achieved with intravenous sodium bicarbonate. A goal of maintaining the urine pH between 7.0 and 7.5 produces a highly effective renal excretion of the acid. Excessive alkalemia must be avoided, however, as it may precipitate seizures. Adult patients in particular may already present with alkalemia due to hyperventilation.

Toluene is a component of certain glues and paint thinners. Inhalation of toluene leads to a classic hyperproduction of metabolic acidosis because of the metabolism of toluene to hippuric acid, which is readily excreted by the kidney with Na^+, K^+, and NH_4^+. The result is non-anion gap metabolic acidosis and K^+ depletion. Treatment consists of K^+ and HCO_3^- replacement.

Propylene glycol (PG) is a colorless and odorless solvent of some commonly administered drugs and may be the cause of an unexplained anion gap metabolic acidosis with an osmolar gap. It is typically seen in ICU patients receiving a particular drug at a high-dose intravenously, especially in the setting of reduced kidney function. PG was initially felt to be innocuous and has been approved by the Food and Drug Administration as a vehicle for various intravenous and topical compounds. It is metabolized to lactic acid by alcohol dehydrogenase in the liver. The acceptable serum level of propylene glycol remains unknown. A single-center, prospective study of patients admitted to intensive care over a 3-month period identified 44 patients receiving high-dose intravenous benzodiazepines. Twenty-one received the PG-containing benzodiazepines lorazepam or diazepam, and 23 received midazolam (non-PG solvent). Of the 21 patients, 4 had metabolic evidence of PG toxicity (19 %). The authors found metabolic abnormalities (anion gap and/or decreased bicarbonate, elevated osmolarity, elevated lactic acid) at levels ranging from 58 to 127 mg/dL, and toxicity (renal failure, hypotension) at levels ranging from 104 to 144 mg/dL [112].

About half of PG is excreted unchanged by the kidney, the remainder undergoes hepatic metabolism to glycolic acid and lactic acid. The normal half-life in adults is between 1.4 and 3.3 h [113]. Formal studies in patients with liver or renal failure are not available, but it is likely that the drug

Table 8.5 Intravenous medications containing propylene glycol (PG)

Drug	Concentration of therapeutic drug (mg/mL)	Percentage, PG (v/v)	mmoles (mg) PG/mL drug
Lorazepam[a]	2	80	11 (830)
Phenobarbital	65	70	9.2 (702)
Diazepam[a]	5	40	5.4 (413)
Phenytoin	50	40	5.4 (414)
TMP/SMX[a,b]	16:80	40	5.3 (400)
Etomidate[a]	2	35	4.8 (363)
Nitroglycerin[a]	5	30	6.8 (518)
Esmolol	250	25	3.4 (258)

[a]Case reports published
[b]Trimethoprim-sulfamethoxazole

accumulates under these conditions and may produce significant toxicity. It is typically seen in ICU patients receiving a particular drug at a high-dose intravenously. Also at risk are patients with reduced hepatic alcohol dehydrogenase, including children under the age of 4, pregnant women, and those receiving treatment with disulfiram or metronidazole [114]. Due to its small molecular weight, extracorporeal removal of PG by hemodialysis is highly effective and has been used successfully. In less severe cases, simply withdrawal of the drug and administration of IV fluids is helpful [115].

Published case reports include benzodiazepines, in particular, lorazepam and diazepam [115, 116], etomidate [117], nitroglycerin [118], and possibly trimethoprim-sulfamethoxazole [119]. Table 8.5 shows various compounds containing PG, their concentrations, and millimoles of PG delivered with each milliliter of the therapeutic drug. This could provide a helpful guide for the clinician suspecting PG poisoning in a patient with an unexplained osmolar and anion gap metabolic acidosis. The osmolar gap is a surrogate marker for circulating PG as few hospitals have the capability of measuring PG serum concentrations. In fact, a linear correlation between osmolar gap (OG, in mOsm/L) and the serum concentration of PG (in mg/dL) exists. In nine critically ill patients receiving high-dose intravenous lorazepam, the relationship was empirically defined as: $[PG] = (6.5 \times OG) - 82$ [120]. Treatment is supportive.

Strictly speaking, pyroglutamic acidosis is not a poisoning but a heightened state of endogenous acid production usually secondary to the ingestion of a toxin [59, 121]. The diagnosis is often subtle. The best clinical clue is an anion gap metabolic acidosis without an obvious cause. The clinical setting is sepsis, renal, and/or hepatic dysfunction, though they must not be present. Acetaminophen ingestion is by far the most frequent culprit, but reports with flucloxacillin and vigabatrin have been published [122–124]. The pathophysiology is largely due to glutathione depletion (which activates the glutamyl cycle) and a decreased metabolism of pyroglutamic acid [59, 121]. Treatment consists of *N*-acetylcysteine to replenish glutathione stores, although there is no clinical evidence that this regimen works better than simple withdrawal of the causative drug (acetaminophen).

Contrast-induced nephropathy (CIN) is a well-established entity, rare in patients with normal kidney function, but much more common in individuals with underlying CKD, in particular, when associated with significant comorbidities, such as congestive heart failure, diabetes mellitus, or paraproteinemia. The pathogenesis of contrast-induced renal tubular injury is complex and incompletely understood, though felt to be at least partly due to intrarenal vasoconstriction and/or generation of antioxidants and free radicals. However, prophylactic use of vasodilating agents (dopamine, theophylline, and fenoldopame), or antioxidants (*N*-acetylcysteine), has failed to demonstrate a benefit. Volume expansion with saline dilutes the contrast load and increases renal perfusion. It is a well-established and proven strategy to prevent CIN and has become the standard of care. However, since the originally published study by Merten et al. in 2004, much excitement was generated on the infusion of sodium bicarbonate as a more effective approach [125]. While the mechanism is not understood, it is hypothesized that it protects against free radicals. Since then, many small, but only a few larger and well-controlled, randomized trials on the benefit of sodium bicarbonate in CIN have been published. Two recent meta-analyses thoroughly reviewed all available evidence. Both concluded that the sum of data do *not* suggest an advantage of sodium bicarbonate over saline for this entity [126, 127].

Use of Non-bicarbonate Buffers

THAM

Tromethamine (*tris*-hydroxymethyl-aminomethane, or trometamol, or THAM) is a sodium-free amino alcohol able to buffer both nonvolatile acid ($THAM + H^+ \rightarrow THAM^+$; p*Ka* 7.8) and volatile acid ($THAM + H_2CO_3 \rightarrow THAM^+ + HCO_3^-$). Tromethamine distributes in both the extra- and intracellular space. It is rapidly excreted in the kidney, and capable of generating HCO_3^- and lowering pCO_2, which theoretically improves intracellular acidosis. Rats resuscitated from ventricular fibrillation, THAM improved cardiac parameters and prolonged survival compared to HCO_3^- [128]. Despite the theoretical advantages, human data is limited. In an uncontrolled trial of ten ventilated ICU patients with acute lung injury and persistent acidemia (mean pH 7.14), infusion of THAM (0.55 mmol/kg/h) improved pH and reduced pCO_2 [129]. Twelve patients with ARDS receiving permissive hypercapnia (target pCO_2 80 mmHg) were randomized to THAM or no intervention. The group receiving THAM had less depression of myocardial contractility than the control group [130]. Side effects of THAM include dose-dependent respiratory depression due to reduced pCO_2 in the cerebrospinal fluid and hypoglycemia [131]. THAM is commercially available, indicated in adults for use in metabolic acidosis during cardiac bypass surgery or cardiac arrest. It is also used to correct excess acidity of stored blood preserved with citric acid.

Tribonat is a buffer mixture of THAM, sodium bicarbonate disodium phosphate, and acetate. It is not available in the United States. A randomized, double-blind controlled trial of 502 patients with asystole or ventricular receiving either Tribonat or normal saline found no difference in patient outcome [132].

Dichloroacetate

Dichloroacetate was investigated in clinical trials but remains unavailable in the United States. This compound exerts multiple effects on pathways of glucose and lipid metabolism. It is a stimulator of pyruvate dehydrogenase and thus accelerates oxidation of lactate. In diabetic patients receiving oral dichloroacetate, fasting glucose, cholesterol and triglycerides, and plasma lactate levels were all lowered [133]. In children with congenital lactic acidosis, 6 months therapy with oral dichloroacetate blunted the postprandial increase in lactic acid, though no benefits on neurologic or other clinical parameters were seen [134]. In dogs with lactic acidosis due to either phenformin or hepatectomy ("type B" lactic acidosis), arterial pH and bicarbonate, cardiac index, and blood lactate levels all improved with dichloroacetate, and mortality was reduced. The same laboratory showed that intravenous dichloroacetate given to hypoxic lactic acidosis in dogs ("type A" lactic acidosis) improved arterial pH and HCO_3^- while serum lactic acid remained stable. However, there was no difference in hemodynamic parameters [135]. A more recent study using a similar experimental setting confirmed these findings [136]. Unfortunately, human studies have been disappointing. In several trials, Stacpoole and colleagues administered dichloroacetate to hypotensive patients. Blood lactic acid and pH improved, but hemodynamic parameters, and ultimately survival, were not affected [137–139].

Carbicarb

Carbicarb is a compound containing equimolar quantities of sodium bicarbonate and sodium carbonate. Carbonate is the stronger base and buffers H^+ to generate HCO_3^- ($H^+ + CO_3^{2-} \rightarrow HCO_3^-$). Thus, CO_3^{2-} produces one CO_2 for every $2H^+$ buffer. From a quantitative point of view, it is difficult to fathom how this is advantageous since buffer-generated CO_2 is orders of magnitude smaller than endogenous CO_2 production. Also, both carbonate and bicarbonate have similar risks for hypervolemia and hypertonicity. Carbicarb has been extensively tested in animals, but in only one human trial. It is not commercially available in the United States. Dogs with hypoxia-induced lactic acidosis were given either bicarbonate or Carbicarb. Arterial and intracellular (liver) pH, lactic acid, oxygen consumption, and cardiac stroke volume all improved with carbicarb but deteriorated with bicarbonate [140, 141]. In dogs with hemorrhagic shock, both bicarbonate and carbicarb improved blood chemistries but there was no cardiovascular benefit [142]. Similar results were found in rats with hemorrhagic shock [143] or ammonium-chloride induced metabolic acidosis [144]. Rates of successful resuscitation and hemodynamics were no different in animals with cardiac arrest compared to either bicarbonate or normal saline [26, 95, 145]. Only one human trial has ever been performed. Acidotic surgical patients derived no benefit of Carbicarb treatment over standard sodium bicarbonate infusion [146]. In summary, while there may be theoretical benefits of Carbicarb, clinical trials failed to demonstrate an advantage.

Renal Replacement Therapy

RRT is performed in critically ill patients with refractory or progressive lactic acidosis and multiorgan failure regardless of the degree of renal failure. The two common types of RRT, hemodialysis (HD), and veno-venous hemodiafiltration (CVVHDF) differ dramatically in their technical application. Both methods are highly effective in improving biochemical profiles. To date, neither has proven superior or more efficacious in determining the course of illness or outcome in several well-conducted clinical trials. When evaluating "efficacy," one has to differentiate end points as improvement in intermediate parameters, such as metabolic and hemodynamic profiles, from actual survival. Critically ill patients are a diverse population with an exceedingly high mortality. While it remains difficult to show a survival benefit of continuous renal replacement therapy (CRRT) vs. intermittent hemodialysis, it should not deter the clinician from using CRRT in the intensive care unit.

RRT allows for direct infusion of large amounts of $NaHCO_3$ while controlling volume status and electrolyte. Rats receiving large amounts of $NaHCO_3$ to maintain a serum HCO_3^- level >20 mEq/L [147], survival was prolonged compared to an equimolar infusion of NaCl. Ultimately, however, no difference in mortality was achieved. A report of two patients with sepsis receiving massive isotonic HCO_3^- infusion with simultaneous ultrafiltration had marked improvement of lactic acidosis, but eventually could not be saved [148].

A common belief is that RRT, in particular CVVHDF, facilitates removal of lactate anion, which derives a clinical benefit. The normal daily production of lactic acid is in the order of 10^3 mmol. To maintain a constant blood concentration below 1 mmol, the same amount (10^3 mmol) requires clearance. In addition, lactic acid production is up to tenfold increased during critical illness (10^4 mmol/day). In ten patients with stable blood lactic acid levels while undergoing CVVHDF, calculated dialysate clearance was less than 5 % of metabolic clearance [149]. This demonstrates that even during CVVHDF, serum lactate levels are ultimately determined by production and endogenous elimination. It underlines the prerogative that treatment of the underlying condition is imperative in determining outcome. Furthermore, it demonstrates that lactic acidosis per se should never be an indication to initiate RRT, though this remains widespread practice. CVVHDF influences multiple clinical parameters—electrolytes, acid–base, fluid status, and hemodynamics, to name a few—and to attribute a successful outcome to any single parameter is inherently flawed. A 7-year review of 200 patients with acute renal failure and lactic acidosis receiving HCO_3^--based CVVHDF, blood pH, and serum [HCO_3^-] improved rapidly with therapy, and in 45 % of patients lactic acidosis resolved. However, mortality was 71.5 %, and neither the severity of the acidosis nor arterial lactic acid levels predicted survival, but rather patient age, mean arterial pressure, and APACHE II scores [150].

In diabetic ketoacidosis, RRT is typically not necessary unless the patient is in acute renal failure with cardiac or respiratory decompensation due to volume overload or has refractory metabolic acidosis despite optimal medical management. The same criteria apply as for other indications to initiate RRT. There are no published trials or observations.

For lactic acidosis associated with some intoxications, RRT can be very beneficial in removing the toxin. An example is the biguanide metformin. It is readily dialyzable by either hemodialysis or CVVHDF, and several reports have been published [151–153].

Peritoneal dialysis in critical illness has been shown to be less efficacious and cannot be recommended. In an open randomized comparison of 70 patients with severe infection and sepsis assigned to either peritoneal dialysis or CVVHDF, the mortality rate was 47 % for the peritoneal group vs. 15 % for the CVVHDF group. Furthermore, acidosis resolved quicker and dialysis could be discontinued earlier in the group receiving CVVHDF. The cost of dialysis per survivor was less than half that of peritoneal dialysis [154].

D-Lactic Acidosis

This is an unusual form of lactic acidosis occurring in patients with small bowel malabsorption and bacterial overgrowth, often in the setting of short-bowel syndrome after resection or after bypass surgery. A large carbohydrate load is delivered to the colon providing substrate for bacterial fermentation to both L- and D-lactic acid (humans are only able to synthesize the L-form). Following systemic absorption, L-lactate is rapidly metabolized by its dehydrogenase providing the base to neutralize the H^+ absorbed. However, D-lactate accumulates due to its much slower metabolism [155]. Serum lactic acid levels are normal by standard testing as D-lactate is not detected. This requires a specific D-lactic dehydrogenase assay. Patients present with crampy abdominal pain and diarrhea and an osmolar and anion gap. They may exhibit acute encephalopathy, probably a direct neurotoxic effect of D-lactate. Some patients present without associated acid–base abnormalities or a near-normal anion gap with hyperchloremia (the drop in serum bicarbonate is larger than the anion gap). The likely explanation is the renal excretion of Na^+—or K^+—D-lactate. Another scenario is gastrointestinal absorption of H^+ without D-lactate in exchange for Na^+ or K^+. Management includes restriction of carbohydrates and oral antibiotics such as vancomycin [156, 157].

Fleet Phospho-Soda

The potential dangers of Fleet Phospho-soda laxatives for bowel preps were initially described more than 30 years ago but have, until recently, been largely ignored or forgotten [158, 159]. In most cases, an individual presents with nonspecific symptoms of malaise, nausea, and weakness several days or weeks after a bowel prep, and renal failure is detected incidentally after electrolyte abnormalities have resolved. Rarely, patients present dramatically with profound hyperphosphatemia, severe hypocalcemia, a high anion gap metabolic acidosis, hypernatremia, hypokalemia, tetany and seizures, cardiac arrhythmias, and acute renal failure, it may even by fatal [160, 161]. The pathophysiologic process is the rapid intestinal absorption of phosphate with complexation to serum calcium.

The acid load from an enema is appreciated by the following analysis (Fig. 8.14): One adult-size Fleet Phospho-soda enema contains 164 mmol of phosphate with a molar ratio of $H_2PO_4^-$ to HPO_4^{2-} of 5:1, or about 137 mmol $H_2PO_4^-$ and 27 mmol HPO_4^{2-} [162]. Because the average urine pH on a typical Western diet is about 5.5, about 95 % of the phosphorus is excreted as $H_2PO_4^-$ (ratio monovalent to divalent 20:1) so complete renal excretion will render this an alkali load (Fig. 8.14). However, because of the swift and high capacity absorption of phosphorus through the colonic epithelium, at a physiologic pH of 7.4, only 20 % is monovalent (ratio 1:4). This translates to about

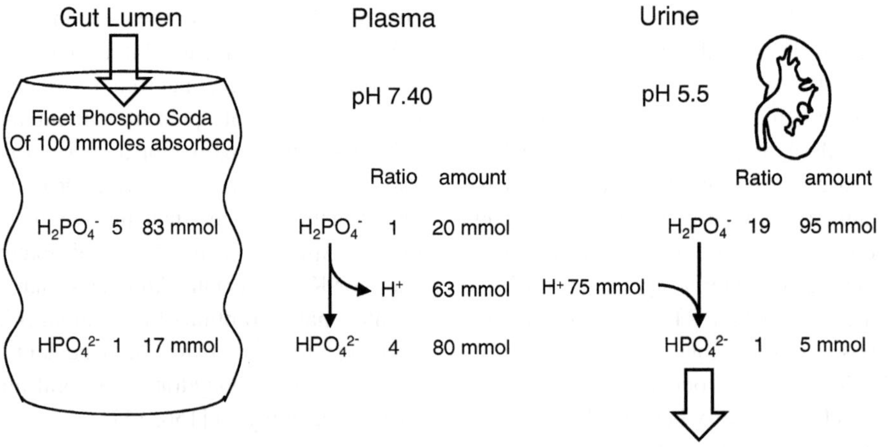

Fig. 8.14 Acid–base effects of a Fleet Phospho-soda. For every 100 mmol of phosphate absorbed with a monovalent to divalent ratio of 5:1, full absorption into the plasma at pH 7.4 will result in a H^+ gain of 63 mmol. If these same 100 mmol are excreted in the urine with a pH of 5.5, there will be 75 mmol of H^+ loss, which results in a net 12 mmol (75–63 mmol) of H^+ loss. With complete urinary excretion, the Fleet Phospho-soda is an alkali load. However, during disequilibrium—after absorption and before excretion—or in the face of impaired excretion, it imparts a large acid load to the organism

33 mmol HPO_4^{2-} and 131 mmol $H_2PO_4^-$, resulting in an *acid*, rather than alkali load for the organism. Fleet Phospho-soda bowel prep for endoscopy constitutes 75 mL Na_3PO_4, providing 9.7 g or 310 mmol of elemental phosphorus, or 195 mmol of H^+ prior to renal excretion. This explains why some individuals develop severe metabolic acidosis and a substantial anion gap. While this more commonly occurs in persons with some degree of renal impairment, smaller body size, or advanced age, it has been described in persons with normal serum creatinine. Nevertheless, in the absence of risk factors, and in particular in persons with an adequate GFR, clinical symptoms are much less likely, despite marked (transient) hyperphosphatemia. In one investigation, blood was drawn immediately after receiving oral sodium phosphate colon preparation in 32 patients with a serum creatinine below 1.5 mg/dL, Hyperphosphatemia greater than 8.0 mg/dL was seen in 28 %, and hypocalcemia less than 8.0 mg/dL in 6 % of patients. None of these patients were clinically symptomatic [163]. A review of 21 cases of acute renal failure following colonoscopy preceded by oral sodium phosphate bowel cleansing found a female predominance (81 %) and previous use of an angiotensin-converting enzyme inhibitor or angiotensin-2 receptor blocker (67 %). Mean baseline serum creatinine was 1.0 mg/dL; patients presented with acute kidney injury with a mean creatinine of 3.9 mg/dl, typically one month after colonoscopy. At follow-up after 16.7 months, 4 patients were dialysis-dependent while the remaining 17 patients had CKD with a mean creatinine of 2.4 mg/dL [164].

Treatment is supportive. In the absence of neurological or cardiac symptoms, hypocalcemia should not be treated because of concomitant hyperphosphatemia. Bicarbonate should be avoided even with severe acidosis, as administration of an alkalinizing agent would lower ionized calcium even more, and the risk of calcium phosphate precipitation increases with a higher pH. Acute hemodialysis should only be necessary if the patient becomes oliguric or anuric and is thus unable to excrete the phosphorus load, correct the acidosis, or becomes hemodynamically unstable. Renal failure is typically transient, but larger case reports and our own experience indicate that permanent renal impairment, even dialysis dependence, is not uncommon. The pathophysiologic mechanism appears to be obstructive calcium phosphate crystalluria and subsequent intratubular nephrocalcinosis [165]. The term *acute phosphate nephropathy* has been proposed for this entity.

Chronic Kidney Disease

With progressive loss of nephron mass in renal failure, the combination of insufficient production and excretion of ammonium but adequate excretion of inorganic acids lead to a modest degree of hyperchloremic (non-anion gap) acidosis. Some degree of hyperkalemia often coexists, further impeding ammonia production [166]. As renal failure progresses, typically at a GFR below 30 mL/min, retention of organic anions such as sulfuric acid, phosphoric acid, and uric acid produces a mixed hyperchloremic and anion gap acidosis. The increase in AG is rarely more than 4–6 mEq/L, and HCO_3^- usually stabilizes between 12 and 20 mEq/L, likely due to some degree of buffering by bones. At the other extreme are functionally anephric patients with a pure anion gap acidosis. However, the drop in bicarbonate (Δ(delta)HCO_3^-) is often less than the increment in anion gap (Δ(delta)AG), again probably due to non-bicarbonate buffers such as bones.

The first recommendations pertaining metabolic acidosis published by the National Kidney Foundation (NKF) addressed specifically hemodialysis patients, stating that a "pre-dialysis or stabilized serum bicarbonate levels should be maintained at or above 22 mmol/L" [167]. More recent recommendations include CKD stages 3–5. "A goal of equal or greater than 22 mmol/L should be attained, if necessary, with supplemental alkali salts … serum level of total CO_2 should be measured every 12 months in CKD stage 3, and every 3 months in stage 4 or 5 (pre-dialysis)" [168]. In essence, the NKF recommends a target serum HCO_3 level of 22 mEq/L or greater for all CKD patients, including dialysis patients. Robust evidence for these recommendations is lacking. Rather, the NKF guidelines rely on extrapolations from (mostly non-randomized) data in dialysis patients and expert opinion. The United Kingdom Renal Association specifies different targets for pre-ESRD patients ("within normal range"), hemodialysis patients (20–26 mEq/L), and peritoneal dialysis patients (25–29 mEq/L).

In earlier stages of CKD, maintaining potassium aids in managing acidosis, since hyperkalemia inhibits renal ammoniagenesis. This is accomplished by avoiding hyperkalemia-provoking medications, such as nonsteroidal anti-inflammatory drugs, beta-blockers if appropriate, and distal sodium channel blockers such as trimethoprim and the potassium-sparing diuretics amiloride and triamterene. Diuretics induce delivery of sodium to the collecting duct and promote both renal hydrogen ion and potassium excretion. In some patients, the combination of the mineralocorticoid fludrocortisone with a diuretic corrects hyperkalemia and acidosis with minimal effect on blood pressure and fluid status.

The choice of phosphate binder is relevant. Both calcium acetate and calcium carbonate provide base supplementation, whereas sevelamer binds HCO_3^- from alkaline secretions by bile and pancreas, as well as organic anions, leading to a loss of "potential" HCO_3^- [169]. The chloride released in the process of anion exchange also drives Cl^-/HCO_3^- exchange in the colon to lose even more HCO_3^-. Indeed, dialysis patients ingesting sevelamer have lower pre-dialysis bicarbonate levels than patients on the calcium containing binders [170]. In reviewing determinants of metabolic acidosis in 190 hemodialysis patients, the three key factors were a high nitrogen appearance (high-protein intake), a low dialysis dose (*Kt*/*V*), and choosing sevelamer over calcium carbonate as the choice of phosphate binder [171].

For oral base replacement therapy, citrate has to be avoided as it carries the risk of aluminum toxicity due to enhanced gastrointestinal absorption of dietary aluminum [172, 173]. Also, in the vast majority of patients with CKD, potassium salts should be avoided to minimize the risk of hyperkalemia. This leaves $NaHCO_3$ as the only safe option. As outlined in Table 8.2, $NaHCO_3$ tablets provide only 3.8 or 7.6 mEq of base per pill, resulting in significant cost and pill burden for patients, and may challenge compliance. An alternative is baking soda, which is cheap, readily available, and able to provide a large amount of base. A typical alkali dose for patients with CKD (dialysis or non-dialysis) is 0.5–1.0 mEq/kg body weight. For an average 70 kg person, twice daily ½ flat teaspoons will provide this amount (Table 8.6).

Table 8.6 Forms of alkali replacement

Brand	Composition	HCO_3 equivalents
ARM and HAMMER®	Baking soda ($NaHCO_3$)	70 mEq per flat teaspoon
Brioschi®, Neut®	$NaHCO_3$	7.6 or 3.8 mEq/tablet
Shohl's®, Bicitra®	Na^+ citrate/citric acid	1 mEq/mL
Polycitra®	Na^+ citrate/K^+ citrate/citric acid	2 mEq/mL
Polycitra-K®	K^+ citrate/citric acid	2 mEq/mL
K-Lyte®, Klor-Con®	K^+HCO_3/K^+ citrate	50 or 25 mEq/tablet
Urocit-K®	K^+ citrate	10 or 5 mEq/tablet

In dialysis patients, adjustment of dialysate HCO_3^- is an effective way of improving acidosis. Bicarbonate has completely replaced acetate as the dialysis buffer of choice as it offers better hemodynamic stability [174]. Standard dialysate HCO_3^- concentrations are typically around 35 mEq/L—often insufficient to provide lasting correction of acidosis. Higher dialysate HCO_3^- has been used successfully. In 38 patients treated with a 42 mEq/L dialysate HCO_3^- concentration over 3 months, pre-dialysis serum HCO_3^- was greater than 23 mEq/L in 75 % of patients. There were no adverse effects, in particular, no alkalemia (bicarbonate > 30 mEq/L), hypoxia, or hypercarbia [175]. Similarly, increasing dialysate from 30 to 40 mmol/L in 46 hemodialysis patients resulted in a higher pre-dialytic arterial pH and was well tolerated [57].

What are the benefits of improving serum HCO_3^- in various stages of CKD? In non-dialysis patients, a recent retrospective cohort study of more than 5,000 patients in various stages of CKD investigated the association of serum bicarbonate level and progression of kidney disease. The authors found that a serum bicarbonate level ≤22 mEq/L was associated with 54 % increased hazard of progression of CKD compared to the reference group (HCO_3 25–26 mEq/L). The results were similar when using other outcome measures such as a 30 % decrease in estimated GFR or doubling of serum creatinine [176]. To date, only one rigorously conducted, randomized controlled trial of the effect on oral sodium bicarbonate supplementation in metabolic acidosis on progression of CKD has been released. Over a 2-year period, 134 patients with a *measured* creatinine clearance (24 h urine collection) between 15 and 30 mL/min (CKD stage IV) and serum bicarbonate 16–20 mL/min received oral sodium bicarbonate to a goal serum bicarbonate ≥23 mEq/L. The proportion of patients with rapid decline of kidney function was significantly less, and fewer patients reached ESRD in the bicarbonate group. In addition, nutritional parameters improved. No adverse effects were observed, in particular, no worsening of blood pressure control or development of edema or heart failure [177]. The results were highly significant: To calculate the benefit in clinically relevant terms, only four patients required bicarbonate supplementation to prevent one patient from reaching dialysis over the observed period of 2 years.

In dialysis patients, three randomized controlled trials provide information. Sixty peritoneal dialysis patients were randomized to receive oral $NaHCO_3$ (2.7 g/day) over 12 months. Serum HCO_3 improved from 25 to 28 mEq/L, as did measures of nutrition and protein metabolism [178]. Twenty-one hemodialysis patients were randomized to receive either a dialysate HCO_3 of 33 mEq/L resulting in an average pre-dialysis serum HCO_3 of 16 mEq/L or a dialysate HCO_3 of 40–48 mEq/L with the goal to achieve a pre-dialysis serum HCO_3 of 24 mEq/L. After 18 months, the treatment group had lower PTH levels and improved markers of bone turnover on bone biopsy [179]. In the third trial, both oral $NaHCO_3$ (1 mEq/kg body weight) and increased dialysate HCO_3 (40 mEq/L vs. 35 mEq/L) were used for 4 months. The treatment group achieved a pre-dialysis serum HCO_3 of 20 mEq/L vs. 17 mEq/L in the control arm, but no difference was identified in nutritional indicators (albumin and nPCR) or intact PTH [180]. In all three trials, the interventions did not result in adverse effects on weight or blood pressure. A smaller non-randomized trial of 14 hemodialysis patients receiving oral Na citrate for 4 weeks (pre-dialysis HCO_3 26.7 mmol/L), followed by 4 weeks of equimolar NaCl (pre-dialysis HCO_3 20.2 mmol/L), improved growth hormone insensitivity, increased and normalized plasma-free T3 concentration, and improved serum albumin levels. It had no effect on measured cytokines [56].

For hemodialysis patients, larger and more long-term studies are required to better study the effects of sustained normalization of pH by alkali supplementation, or the effects of *intra*dialytic alkalemia plus progressive *inter*dialytic acidosis using high dialysis bicarbonate, on clinical outcomes. For instance, there is at least theoretical concern, based on animal studies, that a higher pH potentiates vascular and soft tissue calcification in the setting of a high calcium phosphorus product [181]. Indeed, an analysis of 12,000 US hemodialysis patients found the lowest mortality associated with a serum HCO_3 level between 20 and 22.5 mEq/L, a mildly acidotic range [182]. In a multinational analysis of 7,000 patients, an *inverse* correlation was found between pre-dialytic midweek HCO_3 and normalized protein catabolic rate (nPCR), serum albumin, and phosphorus levels. Mild metabolic acidosis was associated with less hospitalizations (best at HCO_3 21.1–22.0 mEq/L) and lower mortality (best at HCO_3 20.1–21.0 mEq/L). Outcomes were worse at both the high (>27 mEq/L) and very low (<17 mEq/L) range, demonstrating that the *association* between serum bicarbonate and survival follows a U-shaped curve [183].

Spuriously low HCO_3 in dialysis patients has been reported if bloods samples were transported to a centralized reference laboratory, as compared to processing locally the same day (total CO_2 17 mEq/L vs. 22 mEq/L, respectively) [184]. It is speculated that delayed processing results in CO_2 loss, estimated at about 2.5 mEq/L/h [185].

Following renal transplantation, persistent hyperchloremic metabolic acidosis is frequently observed in patients with chronic allograft nephropathy, though it is typically mild. The mechanism includes a tubular defect for distal acidification and a state of hypoaldosteronism [186]. The calcineurin inhibitors cyclosporine and tacrolimus carry the risk of long-term irreversible nephrotoxicity, which contribute to allograft nephropathy, decreased GFR, hyporeninemic hypoaldosteronism, hypertension, and tubular dysfunction with associated hyperkalemia, hypomagnesemia, hypophosphatemia, and metabolic acidosis. In a study of 109 transplant recipients, 33 % were found to have RTA on the basis of plasma HCO_3, arterial pH, and urine and serum anion gap measurements. There was no increased incidence of osteoporosis or osteopenia in the patients with RTA but bone mineral density is a relative insensitive measure of skeletal complications particularly over a short period [187]. Changing to a non-calcineurin inhibitor immunosuppressive regimen may be appropriate in selected patients and could improve electrolyte imbalance and acidosis [188]. Oral base replacement therapy is frequently required to achieve a serum HCO_3 >22 mEq/L. However, no specific guidelines for the post-transplant patients exist, and no trials on particular outcome measures (e.g., bone disease) are available in the literature.

In summary, on the treatment of metabolic acidosis in patients with CKD—pre-dialysis, dialysis, post-transplant—there remains an overall paucity of information to guide the clinician, though more recently, some promising data has emerged, in particular in patients in advanced pre-dialysis stages of CKD [177]. Though close monitoring of blood pressure and weight is recommended, $NaHCO_3$ has furthermore proven to be surprisingly safe, probably because of its larger volume of distribution. Sodium salts other than sodium chloride appear to have a negligible effect on blood pressure. If confirmed in a larger trial, sodium bicarbonate could represent a simple and highly cost-effective intervention that might become another instrument in the armamentarium to treat CKD.

Pancreatic Transplant

In pancreatic transplantation, exocrine drainage via duodenocystostomy was commonly performed in the past. It has been largely replaced by enteric drainage (duodenojejunostomy), because of a reduced rate of complications with enteric drainage, including pancreatitis, urinary tract infections, volume depletion, and a non-anion gap metabolic acidosis (loss of HCO_3-rich pancreatic secretions). In 71 simultaneous pancreas–kidney transplant recipients (37 bladder drainage and 34 bowel drainage), metabolic acidosis was found in 41 % in the former, and none in the latter. Also, volume depletion was observed in 34 and 3 %, respectively [189]. There is a minimal difference in serum HCO_3^- between patients with stable renal function and acute renal dysfunction (25.2 mEq/L vs. 23.2 mEq/L) with enteric drainage. Conversely, in patients with bladder drainage, a dramatic drop was observed, from 21.7 to 12.5 mEq/L in the setting of acute renal dysfunction. It is suggested that with normal renal function, the renal allograft is able to compensate for the heavy urinary HCO_3^- losses with enhanced net acid excretion, but is unable to do so with acute dysfunction [190].

Renal Tubular Acidosis

The term RTA refers to a defect in urinary acidification in the absence of low GFR. Three different types are distinguished. Classic distal RTA type I has an inappropriately high urine pH (typically >5.5), hypokalemia, and hypocitraturia. This promotes both parenchymal calcifications (nephrocalcinosis) and nephrolithiasis. Children exhibit stunted growth due to the effects of chronic metabolic acidosis, in particular, growth hormone resistance. Hypercalciuria and osteoporosis are common. Classic distal RTA type I has a variety of etiologies, ranging from congenital mutations to acquired defects due to inflammatory disease (systemic lupus erythematosus, rheumatoid arthritis, and Sjogren's syndrome) or drugs (amphotericin and topiramate). Hypokalemic RTA responds well to alkali therapy, and with early detection and continuous monitoring, the prognosis is excellent [191]. Aggressive replacement is needed in children to restore normal growth and to avoid bone demineralization and progressive nephrocalcinosis. Incomplete correction with ongoing low-grade acidosis is inadequate [36]. Potassium citrate is preferred, because sodium aggravates hypercalciuria and the risk of kidney stones. Conversely, correction of hypokalemia enhances citrate excretion. In children, the daily potassium citrate requirement is higher than in adults (about 4 mmol/kg BW), because of release of protons during the process of skeletal growth [192]. Bone biopsies reveal low turnover bone disease. Base therapy corrects hypokalemia and hypophosphatemia, and levels of intact PTH increase [193]. Monitoring of serum HCO_3^- and urinary calcium and citrate is essential. Excess base replacement leads to volume expansion, especially if a sodium-based alkali therapy is chosen, with an attendant calciuric effect. In addition, inducing metabolic alkalosis increases the propensity for calcium phosphorus precipitation and the risk of nephrocalcinosis.

Incomplete distal RTA (idRTA) may have normal appearing resting urine pH and normal serum HCO_3^- but the patient is unable to acidify the urine pH below 5.3 in response to an acid load (NH_4Cl). Marked hypocitraturia is the hallmark of this disorder. If untreated, patients develop kidney stones and bone loss and bone demineralization [194]. Primary (idiopathic) osteoporosis may be the only clinical sign [195]. Treatment is correction of hypocitraturia preferably with potassium citrate, as it corrects hypercalciuria and hypocitraturia, reduces the rate of kidney stone formation, increases fractional intestinal calcium absorption, and increases bone mineral density while only minimally increasing serum bicarbonate levels [196, 197]. It is speculated that a low-grade "eubicarbonatemic" metabolic acidosis may exist in certain persons with idRTA. In 13 surgically treated children with posterior urethral valve and persistent incomplete distal RTA based on urinary acidification testing, sodium bicarbonate therapy increased height standard deviation scores by 66 %, compared to 3 % in the control group, after a mean follow-up of 24.7 ± 8.3 months [198].

The *trade-off hypothesis* states that an organism responds with both beneficial and detrimental defense mechanisms in response to chronic exposure to a (nonvolatile) dietary acid load. Compensatory mechanisms contribute to bone demineralization, loss of bone mass, kidney stones, and reduction of lean body mass (LBM) due to enhanced protein degradation [38]. Thus, correction of a diet-dependent, low-grade metabolic acidosis may counteract these compensatory changes, including an acidosis-induced protein degradation in skeletal muscle. In 18 postmenopausal women treated with $KHCO_3$ (60–120 mmol/day) to neutralize production of endogenous nonvolatile acid, a reversal of a negative calcium and phosphorus balance was observed, with reduced bone resorption and increased bone formation [40]. In a study of osteopenic women receiving 30 mEq KCitrate vs. 30 mEq KCl over 12 months, there was a significant increase in bone mineral density in the KCitrate group, a reduction in calciuria, increase in citraturia, and reduced urinary bone resorption markers [39]. A placebo-controlled, randomized and double-blinded study in 19 adults (ages 54–82 years) on two metabolic diets containing low (0.5 g/kg) or high (1.5 g/kg) protein over 41 days, $KHCO_3$ attenuated the urinary nitrogen excretion on the high-protein diet. $KHCO_3$ on the low-protein diet had higher IGF-1 levels, and higher fraction absorption of calcium [199].

The treatment of proximal RTA is much more daunting. Fanconi syndrome refers to a generalized defect of proximal tubular reabsorption including proximal RTA. Fanconi syndrome can be complete or partial, congenital, or acquired [191]. Short stature is a prominent feature in children; rickets and osteomalacia develop in adults due to phosphate wasting and vitamin D deficiency. Metabolic acidosis contributes to the osteomalacia, but due to the massive proximal HCO_3^- leak, enormous amount of base is required. A mixture of potassium and sodium salts is used because of ECFV contraction and K^+ deficiency. Total daily base requirement is up to 10–20 mmol/kg BW, split in multiple doses both during the day and at night. Addition of a loop or thiazide diuretic may aggravate hypokalemia but reduces base requirement as volume contraction enhances proximal tubular absorption of HCO_3^-. K^+ supplements or a combination with a K^+-sparing diuretic is helpful.

Hyperkalemic distal RTA is by far the most common type. It is usually due to hyporeninemic hypoaldosteronism in the setting of diabetes mellitus or other types of CKD, in particular interstitial nephritis, chronic allograft nephropathy after transplantation, or any of a long list of drugs that directly or indirectly affects the renin–angiotensin–aldosterone axis. Reduced renin may be a consequence of nonsteroidal anti-inflammatory drugs, beta-blockers, or the calcineurin inhibitors cyclosporine and tacrolimus. Aliskiren is the first of a new class of drugs of renin inhibitors. This agent increases renin production but plasma renin activity is inhibited and angiotensin I generation suppressed. The effect on serum potassium is likely similar to that of an ACE-inhibitor. Renin and ACE inhibition may be clinically very similar, but to date data on its effect on distal tubular transport is not available. Heparin and ketoconazole inhibit aldosterone *synthesis*, while spironolactone and eplerenone inhibit aldosterone *binding* to its receptor. The potassium-sparing diuretics amiloride and triamterene, and the antimicrobial agents trimethoprim and pentamidine block the epithelial sodium channel in the principal cell of the collecting duct [200]. Regardless of the mechanism, hyperkalemia inhibits both renal ammoniagenesis (proximal tubule) [201–204] and NH_3/NH_4^+ transport (renal medulla) [205, 206]. Managing hyperkalemia is thus important in managing these patients. It is best achieved by stopping or reducing the dosage of the culprit drug, a low potassium diet, or a thiazide or loop diuretic which act by promoting distal Na^+ delivery and enhance distal acidification [207]. Patients who have hypoaldosteronism with intact end-organ sensitivity respond to pharmacologic doses of fludrocortisones, typically combined with a loop diuretic [208].

Patients with CKD and co-existing metabolic acidosis usually benefit from base therapy. It corrects underlying metabolic acidosis and improves hyperkalemia by cellular translocation and renal excretion. A diuretic is typically added to the alkali regimen to counter the volume effect of sodium. Managing insulinopenia or insulin resistance in poorly controlled individuals with diabetes mellitus with adequate amounts of exogenous insulin aids in treating hyperkalemia and acidosis. Hyperkalemic distal RTA may be associated with obstructive uropathy. In this situation, a defect in the distal proton secretion impedes urinary acidification, resulting in a urine pH of 5.5 or greater [186]. Relief of the obstruction typically normalizes the disorder within days, unless prolonged obstruction has led to irreversible damage.

Chronic Diarrhea

Unlike RTA where the principal aberration is impaired renal acid excretion, chronic diarrheal states generate *augmented* renal ammonium excretion due to a net loss of base. Urine pH may be unexpectedly high due to high ammonium excretion. Patients with surreptitious laxative use are thus misdiagnosed with distal RTA. Under normal conditions, alkaline pancreatic and biliary secretions neutralize acidic gastric secretions. Robust HCO_3^- absorption in the small intestine also keeps bicarbonate loss in normal stool to a minimum.

Osmotic diarrhea originates from incompletely absorbed, water-soluble solutes, such as magnesium (hydroxide, sulfate) or sodium phosphate salts, polyethylene glycol, or lactulose. It may also occur in individuals with lactose intolerance, or after ingesting excessive amounts of certain fruits. The stool contains high solutes but low electrolytes. Net base loss is minor and acidosis is not observed. In contrast, secretory diarrhea results from active secretion of electrolytes and malabsorption of sodium and bicarbonate. Daily bicarbonate loss may be several hundred millimoles. A rough estimate is the difference between the sum of stool sodium plus potassium minus stool chloride ($Na^+ + K^+ - Cl^-$). Some of this loss is not bicarbonate itself, as stool pH remains neutral or even acidic. Rather, it reflects titration of bicarbonate with organic acids generated by intestinal flora (lactic acid, acetic acid, butyric acid, and others) [209]. Causes of secretory diarrhea include laxatives (cathartics), most commonly senna, bisacodyl, or castor oil; bacterial toxins (cholera, toxigenic *E. coli*) or enteropathogenic viruses; bile acids or fatty acids (short-bowel syndrome); drugs (colchicine, quinidine, and protease inhibitors), or rarely endocrine tumors.

Patients with ureterosigmoidostomy may develop severe hyperchloremic metabolic acidosis due to a prolonged contact of colonic epithelium with urine. An epithelial chloride/bicarbonate exchanger leads to bicarbonate loss and a high urine pH, which dissociates ammonium to ammonia. The final urine contains sodium and potassium bicarbonate, but little ammonium or chloride, and thus, the urine anion gap becomes highly positive. Patients may be misdiagnosed with RTA. Metabolic acidosis is much less likely with ureteroileostomy or ileal conduits as the contact time of the urine with the intestinal mucosa is brief before emptying externally into an ileostomy bag. No significant exchange of electrolytes or ammonia occurs.

Treatment of diarrhea, or excessive stool output through fistulas or drains, includes correction of the underlying pathology, discontinuation of offending drug, or a change of diet with specific avoidance (e.g., gluten in celiac sprue, lactose in lactase deficiency). Anti-motility agents, antisecretory drugs, and intraluminal agents (psyllium, bismuth, methylcellulose, and polycarbophil) are useful [210]. Chronic base replacement is needed to correct metabolic acidosis. In severe cases, oral rehydration solution may be required. The World Health Organization (WHO) Oral Rehydration Solution contains sodium (90 mEq/L), potassium (20 mEq/L), chloride (80 mEq/L), glucose (111 mmol/L), and citrate at 30 mEq/L. Importantly, oral rehydration solutions do not reduce stool volume output, and may actually increase it. However, in chronic diarrhea, these solutions may enable a patient to maintain adequate electrolyte and acid–base balance and avoid therapy with intravenous fluids. An excellent review was recently published [211].

Oral Base Therapy

A common formula to calculate the amount of HCO_3^- required to correct the metabolic acidosis uses the volume of distribution (Vd) for HCO_3^-, which is 0.5 × LBM. This formula is valid with an acute infusion of HCO_3^- under eubicarbonatemic conditions. With worsening acidosis, the apparent Vd expands due to increasing buffering by other constituents such as phosphate, albumin, intracellular proteins, and bone. It is estimated that the Vd for bicarbonate is 60 % LBM in mild-to-moderate acidosis, and 70 % LBM in severe states, typically when bicarbonate drops below 10 mEq/L [212]. Chronicity of the acidosis also increases Vd. A common example is initiation of oral alkali therapy in a patient with chronic metabolic acidosis from CKD or RTA; the rise in serum HCO_3^- may be zero after 1 week or 2, without urinary loss of base, most likely due to replacement of bone alkali.

Table 8.6 provides a summary of the most commonly used types of oral base replacement. A cheap and highly effective way of delivering oral base is baking soda, providing 12 mEq HCO_3^-/g. A flat teaspoon provides roughly 6 g or 72 mEq. The main drawback is the high sodium load, which promotes fluid retention and puts the patient at risk for heart failure and pulmonary congestion. The effect is less than with an equivalent amount of NaCl because of its larger Vd. An excess sodium load leads to calciuria and hypocitraturia and should be avoided in patients with a history of kidney stones. Abdominal bloating and cramping can be lessened by taking it after a meal, and adding the powder to a glass of water. $NaHCO_3$ in pill form is better tolerated but provides much less base (3.8 mEq/325 mg tablet). An alternative is sodium citrate (with citric acid for dissolution), such as in Shohl's solution and Bicitra. It adds better taste and gastrointestinal tolerance. One tablespoon (15 mL) provides 15 mEq HCO_3^- equivalents. Citrate containing preparations should be avoided in patients with advanced kidney disease, as citrate enhances gastrointestinal absorption of aluminum with the risk of toxicity. Polycitra syrup is a combination of Na citrate and K citrate; one tablespoon provides 15 mEq K^+, 15 mEq Na^+, and 30 mEq HCO_3^-. Polycitra-K contains only K^+ and citrate; it comes as a liquid or powder in several different flavors. The solution contains 10 mEq HCO_3^- and 10 mEq K^+/5 mL; the powder comes in packets providing 30 mEq HCO_3^- and 30 mEq K^+ each. The K^+ load is significant and is contraindicated in patients with hyperkalemia or advanced stages of CKD. Conversely, the combination of metabolic acidosis and hypokalemia often indicates a significant potassium deficit, and treatment with K containing base is preferred. Furthermore, a rising pH may aggravate hypokalemia by intracellular translocation. Two more K^+ containing preparations are available. K-lyte is an effervescent tablet of both K^+ citrate and HCO_3^-, providing 25 or 50 mEq (double strength) bicarbonate equivalent. It is especially useful in patients with hypokalemia and typically used for this purpose. Finally, Urocit-K is potassium citrate in 5 or 10 mEq strength. Overall, K citrate appears to be less well tolerated than Na citrate (Shohl's, Bicitra), with more frequent complaints of heartburn, abdominal cramps, and diarrhea. Conversely, potassium bicarbonate or citrate is preferred over the sodium moiety in patients with kidney stones, as it reduces urinary calcium excretion [213].

Acknowledgments The authors are grateful to Ms. Vicki Perkins for her expert assistance in the preparation of the chapter. The authors are supported by the National Institutes of Health, The National Kidney Foundation, the Charles and Jane Pak Foundation, and the Simmons Family Foundation.

References

1. Narins RG, Emmett M. Simple and mixed acid-base disorders: a practical approach. Medicine (Baltimore). 1980;59:161–87.
2. Alpern RJ, Sakhaee K. The clinical spectrum of chronic metabolic acidosis: homeostatic mechanisms produce significant morbidity. Am J Kidney Dis. 1997;29:291–302.
3. Bleich HL, Tannen RL, Schwartz WB. The induction of metabolic alkalosis by correction of potassium deficiency. J Clin Invest. 1966;45:573–9.
4. Ramsay AG. Clinical application of the Henderson–Hasselbalch equation. Appl Ther. 1965;7:730–6.
5. Severinghaus JW, Astrup PB. History of blood gas analysis. II. pH and acid-base balance measurements. J Clin Monit. 1985;1:259–77.
6. Madison LL, Seldin DW. Ammonia excretion and renal enzymatic adaptation in human subjects, as disclosed by administration of precursor amino acids. J Clin Invest. 1958;37:1615–27.

7. Haussinger D. Liver regulation of acid-base balance. Miner Electrolyte Metab. 1997;23:249–52.
8. Bean ES, Atkinson DE. Regulation of the rate of urea synthesis in liver by extracellular pH. A major factor in pH homeostasis in mammals. J Biol Chem. 1984;259:1552–9.
9. Mackenzie W. Roles of urea production, ammonium excretion, and amino acid oxidation in acid-base balance. Am J Physiol. 1986;250:F181–8.
10. Halperin ML, Chen CB, Cheemadhadli S, West ML, Jungas RL. Is urea formation regulated primarily by acid-base-balance in vivo. Am J Physiol. 1986;250: F605–12.
11. Cheema-Dhadli S, Jungas RL, Halperin ML. Regulation of urea synthesis by acid-base balance in vivo: role of NH3 concentration. Am J Physiol. 1987;252:F221–5.
12. Hosch M, Muser J, Hulter HN, Krapf R. Ureagenesis: evidence for a lack of hepatic regulation of acid-base equilibrium in humans. Am J Physiol Renal Physiol. 2004;286:F94–9.
13. Yatani A, Fujino T, Kinoshita K, Goto M. Excess lactate modulates ionic currents and tension components in frog atrial muscle. J Mol Cell Cardiol. 1981;13:147–61.
14. Mitchell JH, Wildenthal K, Johnson Jr RL. The effects of acid-base disturbances on cardiovascular and pulmonary function. Kidney Int. 1972;1: 375–89.
15. Cingolani HE, Faulkner SL, Mattiazzi AR, Bender HW, Graham Jr TP. Depression of human myocardial contractility with "respiratory" and "metabolic" acidosis. Surgery. 1975;77:427–32.
16. Poole-Wilson PA, Langer GA. Effect of pH on ionic exchange and function in rat and rabbit myocardium. Am J Physiol. 1975;229:570–81.
17. Shapiro JI. Functional and metabolic responses of isolated hearts to acidosis: effects of sodium bicarbonate and Carbicarb. Am J Physiol. 1990; 258:H1835–9.
18. Wildenthal K, Mierzwiak DS, Myers RW, Mitchell JH. Effects of acute lactic acidosis on left ventricular performance. Am J Physiol. 1968;214:1352–9.
19. Campbell HDB, Crisp Jr NW, Weil MH, Brown Jr EB. Depressed response to intravenous sympathicomimetic agents in humans during acidosis. Dis Chest. 1958;33:18–22.
20. Marsh JD, Margolis TI, Kim D. Mechanism of diminished contractile response to catecholamines during acidosis. Am J Physiol. 1988;254:H20–7.
21. Nakanishi T, Okuda H, Kamata K, Seguchi M, Nakazawa M, Takao A. Influence of acidosis on inotropic effect of catecholamines in newborn rabbit hearts. Am J Physiol. 1987;253:H1441–8.
22. Shepherd JT, Vanhoutte PM. George E. Brown memorial lecture. Local modulation of adrenergic neurotransmission. Circulation. 1981;64:655–66.
23. Bygdeman S. Vascular reactivity in cats during induced changes in the acid-base balance of the blood. Acta Physiol Scand. 1963;61 Suppl 222:1–65.
24. Gerst PH, Fleming WH, Malm JR. A quantitative evaluation of the effects of acidosis and alkalosis upon the ventricular fibrillation threshold. Surgery. 1966;59:1050–60.
25. Kerber RE, Pandian NG, Hoyt R, et al. Effect of ischemia, hypertrophy, hypoxia, acidosis, and alkalosis on canine defibrillation. Am J Physiol. 1983; 244:H825–31.
26. Kette F, Weil MH, von Planta M, Gazmuri RJ, Rackow EC. Buffer agents do not reverse intramyocardial acidosis during cardiac resuscitation. Circulation. 1990;81:1660–6.
27. von Planta I, Weil MH, von Planta M, Gazmuri RJ, Duggal C. Hypercarbic acidosis reduces cardiac resuscitability. Crit Care Med. 1991;19:1177–82.
28. Sharpey-Schafer EP, Semple SJ, Halls RW, Howarth S. Venous constriction after exercise; its relation to acid-base changes in venous blood. Clin Sci. 1965; 29:397–406.
29. Bellingham AJ, Detter JC, Lenfant C. Regulatory mechanisms of hemoglobin oxygen affinity in acidosis and alkalosis. J Clin Invest. 1971;50:700–6.
30. Ditzel J, Andersen H, Peters ND. Oxygen affinity of haemoglobin and red cell 2,3-diphosphoglycerate in childhood diabetes. Acta Paediatr Scand. 1975;64: 355–61.
31. Krieger NS, Sessler NE, Bushinsky DA. Acidosis inhibits osteoblastic and stimulates osteoclastic activity in vitro. Am J Physiol. 1992;262:F442–8.
32. Lemann Jr J, Litzow JR, Lennon EJ. The effects of chronic acid loads in normal man: further evidence for the participation of bone mineral in the defense against chronic metabolic acidosis. J Clin Invest. 1966;45:1608–14.
33. Langman CB, Bushinsky DA, Favus MJ, Coe FL. Ca and P regulation of 1,25(OH)2D3 synthesis by vitamin D-replete rat tubules during acidosis. Am J Physiol. 1986;251:F911–8.
34. Graham KA, Hoenich NA, Tarbit M, Ward MK, Goodship TH. Correction of acidosis in hemodialysis patients increases the sensitivity of the parathyroid glands to calcium. J Am Soc Nephrol. 1997;8: 627–31.
35. Domrongkitchaiporn S, Pongsakul C, Stitchantrakul W, et al. Bone mineral density and histology in distal renal tubular acidosis. Kidney Int. 2001;59: 1086–93.
36. McSherry E, Morris Jr RC. Attainment and maintenance of normal stature with alkali therapy in infants and children with classic renal tubular acidosis. J Clin Invest. 1978;61:509–27.
37. Wachman A, Bernstein DS. Diet and osteoporosis. Lancet. 1968;1:958–9.
38. Alpern RJ. Trade-offs in the adaptation to acidosis. Kidney Int. 1995;47:1205–15.
39. Jehle S, Zanetti A, Muser J, Hulter HN, Krapf R. Partial neutralization of the acidogenic Western diet with potassium citrate increases bone mass in postmenopausal women with osteopenia. J Am Soc Nephrol. 2006;17:3213–22.

40. Sebastian A, Harris ST, Ottaway JH, Todd KM, Morris Jr RC. Improved mineral balance and skeletal metabolism in postmenopausal women treated with potassium bicarbonate. N Engl J Med. 1994;330:1776–81.
41. Challa A, Chan W, Krieg Jr RJ, et al. Effect of metabolic acidosis on the expression of insulin-like growth factor and growth hormone receptor. Kidney Int. 1993;44:1224–7.
42. Isozaki U, Mitch WE, England BK, Price SR. Protein degradation and increased mRNAs encoding proteins of the ubiquitin-proteasome proteolytic pathway in BC3H1 myocytes require an interaction between glucocorticoids and acidification. Proc Natl Acad Sci U S A. 1996;93:1967–71.
43. Ballmer PE, McNurlan MA, Hulter HN, Anderson SE, Garlick PJ, Krapf R. Chronic metabolic acidosis decreases albumin synthesis and induces negative nitrogen balance in humans. J Clin Invest. 1995;95:39–45.
44. Brungger M, Hulter HN, Krapf R. Effect of chronic metabolic acidosis on the growth hormone/IGF-1 endocrine axis: new cause of growth hormone insensitivity in humans. Kidney Int. 1997;51:216–21.
45. Brungger M, Hulter HN, Krapf R. Effect of chronic metabolic acidosis on thyroid hormone homeostasis in humans. Am J Physiol. 1997;272:F648–53.
46. Litzow JR, Lemann Jr J, Lennon EJ. The effect of treatment of acidosis on calcium balance in patients with chronic azotemic renal disease. J Clin Invest. 1967;46:280–6.
47. Blum WF, Ranke MB, Kietzmann K, Tonshoff B, Mehls O. Growth hormone resistance and inhibition of somatomedin activity by excess of insulin-like growth factor binding protein in uraemia. Pediatr Nephrol. 1991;5:539–44.
48. Haffner D, Schaefer F, Girard J, Ritz E, Mehls O. Metabolic clearance of recombinant human growth hormone in health and chronic renal failure. J Clin Invest. 1994;93:1163–71.
49. Fouque D, Peng SC, Kopple JD. Impaired metabolic response to recombinant insulin-like growth factor-1 in dialysis patients. Kidney Int. 1995;47:876–83.
50. Lim VS, Fang VS, Katz AI, Refetoff S. Thyroid dysfunction in chronic renal failure. A study of the pituitary-thyroid axis and peripheral turnover kinetics of thyroxine and triiodothyronine. J Clin Invest. 1977;60:522–34.
51. Mak RH. Effect of metabolic acidosis on insulin action and secretion in uremia. Kidney Int. 1998;54:603–7.
52. Owen Jr WF, Lew NL, Liu Y, Lowrie EG, Lazarus JM. The urea reduction ratio and serum albumin concentration as predictors of mortality in patients undergoing hemodialysis. N Engl J Med. 1993;329:1001–6.
53. Pifer TB, McCullough KP, Port FK, et al. Mortality risk in hemodialysis patients and changes in nutritional indicators: DOPPS. Kidney Int. 2002;62:2238–45.
54. Movilli E, Zani R, Carli O, et al. Correction of metabolic acidosis increases serum albumin concentrations and decreases kinetically evaluated protein intake in haemodialysis patients: a prospective study. Nephrol Dial Transplant. 1998;13:1719–22.
55. Uribarri J, Levin NW, Delmez J, et al. Association of acidosis and nutritional parameters in hemodialysis patients. Am J Kidney Dis. 1999;34:493–9.
56. Wiederkehr MR, Kalogiros J, Krapf R. Correction of metabolic acidosis improves thyroid and growth hormone axes in haemodialysis patients. Nephrol Dial Transplant. 2004;19:1190–7.
57. Williams AJ, Dittmer ID, McArley A, Clarke J. High bicarbonate dialysate in haemodialysis patients: effects on acidosis and nutritional status. Nephrol Dial Transplant. 1997;12:2633–7.
58. Emmett M, Narins RG. Clinical use of the anion gap. Medicine (Baltimore). 1977;56:38–54.
59. Moe OW, Fuster D. Clinical acid-base pathophysiology: disorders of plasma anion gap. Best Pract Res Clin Endocrinol Metab. 2003;17:559–74.
60. Oh MS, Carroll HJ. The anion gap. N Engl J Med. 1977;297:814–7.
61. Kraut JA, Kurtz I. Metabolic acidosis of CKD: diagnosis, clinical characteristics, and treatment. Am J Kidney Dis. 2005;45:978–93.
62. Carlisle EJ, Donnelly SM, Vasuvattakul S, Kamel KS, Tobe S, Halperin ML. Glue-sniffing and distal renal tubular acidosis: sticking to the facts. J Am Soc Nephrol. 1991;1:1019–27.
63. Goldstein MB, Bear R, Richardson RM, Marsden PA, Halperin ML. The urine anion gap: a clinically useful index of ammonium excretion. Am J Med Sci. 1986;292:198–202.
64. Hilton JG, Vandenbroucke AC, Josse RG, Buckley GC, Halperin ML. The urine anion gap: the critical clue to resolve a diagnostic dilemma in a patient with ketoacidosis. Diabetes Care. 1984;7:486–90.
65. Batlle DC, Hizon M, Cohen E, Gutterman C, Gupta R. The use of the urinary anion gap in the diagnosis of hyperchloremic metabolic acidosis. N Engl J Med. 1988;318:594–9.
66. Halperin ML, Margolis BL, Robinson LA, Halperin RM, West ML, Bear RA. The urine osmolal gap: a clue to estimate urine ammonium in "hybrid" types of metabolic acidosis. Clin Invest Med. 1988;11:198–202.
67. Kamel KS, Ethier JH, Richardson RM, Bear RA, Halperin ML. Urine electrolytes and osmolality: when and how to use them. Am J Nephrol. 1990;10:89–102.
68. Hood VL, Tannen RL. Protection of acid-base balance by pH regulation of acid production. N Engl J Med. 1998;339:819–26.
69. Nakashima K, Yamashita T, Kashiwagi S, Nakayama N, Kitahara T, Ito H. The effect of sodium bicarbonate on CBF and intracellular pH in man: stable Xe-CT and 31P-MRS. Acta Neurol Scand Suppl. 1996;166:96–8.

70. Ritter JM, Doktor HS, Benjamin N. Paradoxical effect of bicarbonate on cytoplasmic pH. Lancet. 1990;335:1243–6.
71. Shapiro JI, Whalen M, Kucera R, Kindig N, Filley G, Chan L. Brain pH responses to sodium bicarbonate and Carbicarb during systemic acidosis. Am J Physiol. 1989;256:H1316–21.
72. Cooper DJ, Walley KR, Wiggs BR, Russell JA. Bicarbonate does not improve hemodynamics in critically ill patients who have lactic acidosis. A prospective, controlled clinical study. Ann Intern Med. 1990;112:492–8.
73. Mathieu D, Neviere R, Billard V, Fleyfel M, Wattel F. Effects of bicarbonate therapy on hemodynamics and tissue oxygenation in patients with lactic acidosis: a prospective, controlled clinical study. Crit Care Med. 1991;19:1352–6.
74. Graf H, Leach W, Arieff AI. Evidence for a detrimental effect of bicarbonate therapy in hypoxic lactic acidosis. Science. 1985;227:754–6.
75. Klepper ID, Kucera RF, Kindig NB, Sherrill DL, Filley GF. A comparative study of sodium bicarbonate and carbicarb in the treatment of metabolic acidosis induced by hemorrhagic shock. J Crit Care. 1988;3:256–61.
76. Cooper DJ, Herbertson MJ, Werner HA, Walley KR. Bicarbonate does not increase left ventricular contractility during L-lactic acidemia in pigs. Am Rev Respir Dis. 1993;148:317–22.
77. Makisalo HJ, Soini HO, Nordin AJ, Hockerstedt KA. Effects of bicarbonate therapy on tissue oxygenation during resuscitation of hemorrhagic shock. Crit Care Med. 1989;17:1170–4.
78. Fraley DS, Adler S, Bruns FJ, Zett B. Stimulation of lactate production by administration of bicarbonate in a patient with a solid neoplasm and lactic acidosis. N Engl J Med. 1980;303:1100–2.
79. Gevers W, Dowdle E. The effect of pH on glycolysis in vitro. Clin Sci. 1963;25:343–9.
80. Hood VL, Schubert C, Keller U, Muller S. Effect of systemic pH on pHi and lactic acid generation in exhaustive forearm exercise. Am J Physiol. 1988;255:F479–85.
81. Levraut J, Labib Y, Chave S, Payan P, Raucoules-Aime M, Grimaud D. Effect of sodium bicarbonate on intracellular pH under different buffering conditions. Kidney Int. 1996;49:1262–7.
82. Levraut J, Garcia P, Giunti C, et al. The increase in CO2 production induced by NaHCO3 depends on blood albumin and hemoglobin concentrations. Intensive Care Med. 2000;26:558–64.
83. Levraut J, Giunti C, Ciebiera JP, et al. Initial effect of sodium bicarbonate on intracellular pH depends on the extracellular nonbicarbonate buffering capacity. Crit Care Med. 2001;29:1033–9.
84. Lang RM, Fellner SK, Neumann A, Bushinsky DA, Borow KM. Left ventricular contractility varies directly with blood ionized calcium. Ann Intern Med. 1988;108:524–9.
85. John M, Mallal S. Hyperlactatemia syndromes in people with HIV infection. Curr Opin Infect Dis. 2002;15:23–9.
86. Arieff AI, Leach W, Park R, Lazarowitz VC. Systemic effects of NaHCO3 in experimental lactic acidosis in dogs. Am J Physiol. 1982;242: F586–91.
87. Luft D, Schmulling RM, Eggstein M. Lactic acidosis in biguanide-treated diabetics: a review of 330 cases. Diabetologia. 1978;14:75–87.
88. Standards and guidelines for Cardiopulmonary Resuscitation (CPR) and Emergency Cardiac Care (ECC). National Academy of Sciences—National Research Council. JAMA 1986;255:2905–89.
89. Guidelines 2000 for Cardiopulmonary Resuscitation and Emergency Cardiovascular Care. Part 6: advanced cardiovascular life support: 7D: the tachycardia algorithms. The American Heart Association in collaboration with the International Liaison Committee on Resuscitation. Circulation 2000;102:I158–65.
90. Bonhomme L, Benhamou D, Comoy E, Preaux N. Stability of epinephrine in alkalinized solutions. Ann Emerg Med. 1990;19:1242–4.
91. Grillo JA, Gonzalez ER, Ramaiya A, Karnes HT, Wells B. Chemical compatibility of inotropic and vasoactive agents delivered via a multiple line infusion system. Crit Care Med. 1995;23:1061–6.
92. Kette F, Weil MH, Gazmuri RJ. Buffer solutions may compromise cardiac resuscitation by reducing coronary perfusion pressure. JAMA. 1991;266:2121–6.
93. Zipes DP, Camm AJ, Borggrefe M, et al. ACC/AHA/ESC 2006 Guidelines for Management of Patients With Ventricular Arrhythmias and the Prevention of Sudden Cardiac Death: a report of the American College of Cardiology/American Heart Association Task Force and the European Society of Cardiology Committee for Practice Guidelines (writing committee to develop Guidelines for Management of Patients With Ventricular Arrhythmias and the Prevention of Sudden Cardiac Death): developed in collaboration with the European Heart Rhythm Association and the Heart Rhythm Society. Circulation. 2006;114:e385–484.
94. Vukmir RB, Bircher N, Safar P. Sodium bicarbonate in cardiac arrest: a reappraisal. Am J Emerg Med. 1996;14:192–206.
95. Bar-Joseph G, Weinberger T, Castel T, et al. Comparison of sodium bicarbonate, Carbicarb, and THAM during cardiopulmonary resuscitation in dogs. Crit Care Med. 1998;26:1397–408.
96. Vukmir RB, Bircher NG, Radovsky A, Safar P. Sodium bicarbonate may improve outcome in dogs with brief or prolonged cardiac arrest. Crit Care Med. 1995;23:515–22.
97. Federiuk CS, Sanders AB, Kern KB, Nelson J, Ewy GA. The effect of bicarbonate on resuscitation from cardiac arrest. Ann Emerg Med. 1991;20:1173–7.

98. Guerci AD, Chandra N, Johnson E, et al. Failure of sodium bicarbonate to improve resuscitation from ventricular fibrillation in dogs. Circulation. 1986; IV74:75–9.
99. Minuck M, Sharma GP. Comparison of THAM and sodium bicarbonate in resuscitation of the heart after ventricular fibrillation in dogs. Anesth Analg. 1977; 56:38–45.
100. Adrogue HJ, Wilson H, Boyd 3rd AE, Suki WN, Eknoyan G. Plasma acid-base patterns in diabetic ketoacidosis. N Engl J Med. 1982;307:1603–10.
101. Adrogue HJ, Eknoyan G, Suki WK. Diabetic ketoacidosis: role of the kidney in the acid-base homeostasis re-evaluated. Kidney Int. 1984;25:591–8.
102. Beech JS, Williams SC, Iles RA, et al. Haemodynamic and metabolic effects in diabetic ketoacidosis in rats of treatment with sodium bicarbonate or a mixture of sodium bicarbonate and sodium carbonate. Diabetologia. 1995;38:889–98.
103. Hood VL, Danforth Jr E, Horton ES, Tannen RL. Impact of hydrogen ion on fasting ketogenesis: feedback regulation of acid production. Am J Physiol. 1982;242:F238–45.
104. Hale PJ, Crase J, Nattrass M. Metabolic effects of bicarbonate in the treatment of diabetic ketoacidosis. Br Med J (Clin Res Ed). 1984;289:1035–8.
105. Morris LR, Murphy MB, Kitabchi AE. Bicarbonate therapy in severe diabetic ketoacidosis. Ann Intern Med. 1986;105:836–40.
106. Gamba G, Oseguera J, Castrejon M, Gomez-Perez FJ. Bicarbonate therapy in severe diabetic ketoacidosis. A double blind, randomized, placebo controlled trial. Rev Invest Clin. 1991;43:234–8.
107. Okuda Y, Adrogue HJ, Field JB, Nohara H, Yamashita K. Counterproductive effects of sodium bicarbonate in diabetic ketoacidosis. J Clin Endocrinol Metab. 1996;81:314–20.
108. Assal JP, Aoki TT, Manzano FM, Kozak GP. Metabolic effects of sodium bicarbonate in management of diabetic ketoacidosis. Diabetes. 1974;23:405–11.
109. Green SM, Rothrock SG, Ho JD, et al. Failure of adjunctive bicarbonate to improve outcome in severe pediatric diabetic ketoacidosis. Ann Emerg Med. 1998;31:41–8.
110. Lever E, Jaspan JB. Sodium bicarbonate therapy in severe diabetic ketoacidosis. Am J Med. 1983;75: 263–8.
111. Viallon A, Zeni F, Lafond P, et al. Does bicarbonate therapy improve the management of severe diabetic ketoacidosis? Crit Care Med. 1999;27:2690–3.
112. Yaucher NE, Fish JT, Smith HW, Wells JA. Propylene glycol-associated renal toxicity from lorazepam infusion. Pharmacotherapy. 2003;23:1094–9.
113. Speth PA, Vree TB, Neilen NF, et al. Propylene glycol pharmacokinetics and effects after intravenous infusion in humans. Ther Drug Monit. 1987;9:255–8.
114. Parker MG, Fraser GL, Watson DM, Riker RR. Removal of propylene glycol and correction of increased osmolar gap by hemodialysis in a patient on high dose lorazepam infusion therapy. Intensive Care Med. 2002;28:81–4.
115. Wilson KC, Reardon C, Farber HW. Propylene glycol toxicity in a patient receiving intravenous diazepam. N Engl J Med. 2000;343:815.
116. Wilson KC, Reardon C, Theodore AC, Farber HW. Propylene glycol toxicity: a severe iatrogenic illness in ICU patients receiving IV benzodiazepines: a case series and prospective, observational pilot study. Chest. 2005;128:1674–81.
117. Bedichek E, Kirschbaum B. A case of propylene glycol toxic reaction associated with etomidate infusion. Arch Intern Med. 1991;151:2297–8.
118. Demey HE, Daelemans RA, Verpooten GA, et al. Propylene glycol-induced side effects during intravenous nitroglycerin therapy. Intensive Care Med. 1988;14:221–6.
119. Hayman M, Seidl EC, Ali M, Malik K. Acute tubular necrosis associated with propylene glycol from concomitant administration of intravenous lorazepam and trimethoprim-sulfamethoxazole. Pharmacotherapy. 2003;23:1190–4.
120. Arroliga AC, Shehab N, McCarthy K, Gonzales JP. Relationship of continuous infusion lorazepam to serum propylene glycol concentration in critically ill adults. Crit Care Med. 2004;32:1709–14.
121. Fenves AZ, Kirkpatrick 3rd HM, Patel VV, Sweetman L, Emmett M. Increased anion gap metabolic acidosis as a result of 5-oxoproline (pyroglutamic acid): a role for acetaminophen. Clin J Am Soc Nephrol. 2006;1:441–7.
122. Bonham JR, Rattenbury JM, Meeks A, Pollitt RJ. Pyroglutamicaciduria from vigabatrin. Lancet. 1989;1:1452–3.
123. Croal BL, Glen AC, Kelly CJ, Logan RW. Transient 5-oxoprolinuria (pyroglutamic aciduria) with systemic acidosis in an adult receiving antibiotic therapy. Clin Chem. 1998;44:336–40.
124. Pitt JJ, Brown GK, Clift V, Christodoulou J. Atypical pyroglutamic aciduria: possible role of paracetamol. J Inherit Metab Dis. 1990;13:755–6.
125. Merten GJ, Burgess WP, Gray LV, et al. Prevention of contrast-induced nephropathy with sodium bicarbonate: a randomized controlled trial. JAMA. 2004;291:2328–34.
126. Brar SS, Hiremath S, Dangas G, Mehran R, Brar SK, Leon MB. Sodium bicarbonate for the prevention of contrast induced-acute kidney injury: a systematic review and meta-analysis. Clin J Am Soc Nephrol. 2009;4:1584–92.
127. Zoungas S, Ninomiya T, Huxley R, et al. Systematic review: sodium bicarbonate treatment regimens for the prevention of contrast-induced nephropathy. Ann Intern Med. 2009;151:631–8.
128. Sun S, Weil MH, Tang W, Fukui M. Effects of buffer agents on postresuscitation myocardial dysfunction. Crit Care Med. 1996;24:2035–41.
129. Kallet RH, Jasmer RM, Luce JM, Lin LH, Marks JD. The treatment of acidosis in acute lung injury with

tris-hydroxymethyl aminomethane (THAM). Am J Respir Crit Care Med. 2000;161:1149–53.
130. Weber T, Tschernich H, Sitzwohl C, et al. Tromethamine buffer modifies the depressant effect of permissive hypercapnia on myocardial contractility in patients with acute respiratory distress syndrome. Am J Respir Crit Care Med. 2000;162: 1361–5.
131. Nahas GG, Sutin KM, Fermon C, et al. Guidelines for the treatment of acidaemia with THAM. Drugs. 1998;55:191–224.
132. Dybvik T, Strand T, Steen PA. Buffer therapy during out-of-hospital cardiopulmonary resuscitation. Resuscitation. 1995;29:89–95.
133. Stacpoole PW, Moore GW, Kornhauser DM. Metabolic effects of dichloroacetate in patients with diabetes mellitus and hyperlipoproteinemia. N Engl J Med. 1978;298:526–30.
134. Stacpoole PW, Kerr DS, Barnes C, et al. Controlled clinical trial of dichloroacetate for treatment of congenital lactic acidosis in children. Pediatrics. 2006;117:1519–31.
135. Graf H, Leach W, Arieff AI. Effects of dichloroacetate in the treatment of hypoxic lactic acidosis in dogs. J Clin Invest. 1985;76:919–23.
136. Wahr JA, Ullrich K, Bolling SF. The use of dichloroacetate in the treatment of overwhelming hypoxic acidosis. J Cardiothorac Vasc Anesth. 1994;8:64–9.
137. Stacpoole PW, Harman EM, Curry SH, Baumgartner TG, Misbin RI. Treatment of lactic acidosis with dichloroacetate. N Engl J Med. 1983;309:390–6.
138. Stacpoole PW, Lorenz AC, Thomas RG, Harman EM. Dichloroacetate in the treatment of lactic acidosis. Ann Intern Med. 1988;108:58–63.
139. Stacpoole PW, Wright EC, Baumgartner TG, et al. A controlled clinical trial of dichloroacetate for treatment of lactic acidosis in adults. The Dichloroacetate-Lactic Acidosis Study Group. N Engl J Med. 1992;327:1564–9.
140. Bersin RM, Arieff AI. Improved hemodynamic function during hypoxia with Carbicarb, a new agent for the management of acidosis. Circulation. 1988;77:227–33.
141. Rhee KH, Toro LO, McDonald GG, Nunnally RL, Levin DL. Carbicarb, sodium bicarbonate, and sodium chloride in hypoxic lactic acidosis. Effect on arterial blood gases, lactate concentrations, hemodynamic variables, and myocardial intracellular pH. Chest. 1993;104:913–8.
142. Benjamin E, Oropello JM, Abalos AM, et al. Effects of acid-base correction on hemodynamics, oxygen dynamics, and resuscitability in severe canine hemorrhagic shock. Crit Care Med. 1994;22: 1616–23.
143. Beech JS, Nolan KM, Iles RA, Cohen RD, Williams SC, Evans SJ. The effects of sodium bicarbonate and a mixture of sodium bicarbonate and carbonate ("Carbicarb") on skeletal muscle pH and hemodynamic status in rats with hypovolemic shock. Metabolism. 1994;43:518–22.
144. Shapiro JI, Whalen M, Chan L. Hemodynamic and hepatic pH responses to sodium bicarbonate and Carbicarb during systemic acidosis. Magn Reson Med. 1990;16:403–10.
145. Gazmuri RJ, von Planta M, Weil MH, Rackow EC. Cardiac effects of carbon dioxide-consuming and carbon dioxide-generating buffers during cardiopulmonary resuscitation. J Am Coll Cardiol. 1990;15: 482–90.
146. Leung JM, Landow L, Franks M, et al. Safety and efficacy of intravenous Carbicarb in patients undergoing surgery: comparison with sodium bicarbonate in the treatment of mild metabolic acidosis. SPI Research Group. Study of Perioperative Ischemia. Crit Care Med. 1994;22:1540–9.
147. Halperin ML, Cheema-Dhadli S, Halperin FA, Kamel KS. Rationale for the use of sodium bicarbonate in a patient with lactic acidosis due to a poor cardiac output. Nephron. 1994;66:258–61.
148. Gudis SM, Mangi S, Feinroth M, Rubin JE, Friedman EA, Berlyne GM. Rapid correction of severe lactic acidosis with massive isotonic bicarbonate infusion and simultaneous ultrafiltration. Nephron. 1983; 33:65–6.
149. Levraut J, Ciebiera JP, Jambou P, Ichai C, Labib Y, Grimaud D. Effect of continuous venovenous hemofiltration with dialysis on lactate clearance in critically ill patients. Crit Care Med. 1997;25: 58–62.
150. Hilton PJ, Taylor J, Forni LG, Treacher DF. Bicarbonate-based haemofiltration in the management of acute renal failure with lactic acidosis. QJM. 1998;91:279–83.
151. Barrueto F, Meggs WJ, Barchman MJ. Clearance of metformin by hemofiltration in overdose. J Toxicol Clin Toxicol. 2002;40:177–80.
152. Mariano F, Benzi L, Cecchetti P, et al. Efficacy of continuous venovenous haemofiltration (CVVH) in the treatment of severe phenformin-induced lactic acidosis. Nephrol Dial Transplant. 1998;13:1012–5.
153. Reeker W, Schneider G, Felgenhauer N, Tempel G, Kochs E. Metformin-induced lactic acidosis. Dtsch Med Wochenschr. 2000;125:249–51.
154. Phu NH, Hien TT, Mai NT, et al. Hemofiltration and peritoneal dialysis in infection-associated acute renal failure in Vietnam. N Engl J Med. 2002;347: 895–902.
155. Ewaschuk JB, Naylor JM, Zello GA. D-Lactate in human and ruminant metabolism. J Nutr. 2005;135:1619–25.
156. Halperin ML, Kamel KS. D-Lactic acidosis: turning sugar into acids in the gastrointestinal tract. Kidney Int. 1996;49:1–8.
157. Uribarri J, Oh MS, Carroll HJ. D-Lactic acidosis. A review of clinical presentation, biochemical features, and pathophysiologic mechanisms. Medicine (Baltimore). 1998;77:73–82.
158. Loughnan P, Mullins GC. Brain damage following a hypertonic phosphate enema. Am J Dis Child. 1977;131:1032.

159. McConnell TH. Fatal hypocalcemia from phosphate absorption from laxative preparation. JAMA. 1971;216:147–8.
160. Gonlusen G, Akgun H, Ertan A, Olivero J, Truong LD. Renal failure and nephrocalcinosis associated with oral sodium phosphate bowel cleansing: clinical patterns and renal biopsy findings. Arch Pathol Lab Med. 2006;130:101–6.
161. Ma KK, Ng CS, Mui LM, Chan KC, Ng EK, Chung SC. Severe hyperphosphatemia and hypocalcemia following sodium phosphate bowel preparation: a forgotten menace. Endoscopy. 2003;35:717.
162. Kirschbaum B. The acidosis of exogenous phosphate intoxication. Arch Intern Med. 1998;158:405–8.
163. Lieberman DA, Ghormley J, Flora K. Effect of oral sodium phosphate colon preparation on serum electrolytes in patients with normal serum creatinine. Gastrointest Endosc. 1996;43:467–9.
164. Markowitz GS, Stokes MB, Radhakrishnan J, D'Agati VD. Acute phosphate nephropathy following oral sodium phosphate bowel purgative: an underrecognized cause of chronic renal failure. J Am Soc Nephrol. 2005;16:3389–96.
165. Desmeules S, Bergeron MJ, Isenring P. Acute phosphate nephropathy and renal failure. N Engl J Med. 2003;349:1006–7.
166. Dorhout-Mees EJ, Machado M, Slatopolsky E, Klahr S, Bricker NS. The functional adaptation of the diseased kidney. 3. Ammonium excretion. J Clin Invest. 1966;45:289–96.
167. Kopple JD. National kidney foundation K/DOQI clinical practice guidelines for nutrition in chronic renal failure. Am J Kidney Dis. 2001;37:S66–70.
168. K/DOQI clinical practice guidelines for bone metabolism and disease in chronic kidney disease. Am J Kidney Dis. 2003;42:S1–201.
169. Wrong OM, Harland CE. Sevelamer-induced acidosis. Kidney Int. 2005;67:776–7. author reply 7.
170. Qunibi WY, Hootkins RE, McDowell LL, et al. Treatment of hyperphosphatemia in hemodialysis patients: The Calcium Acetate Renagel Evaluation (CARE Study). Kidney Int. 2004;65:1914–26.
171. Soudan K, Ricanati ES, Leon JB, Sehgal AR. Determinants of metabolic acidosis among hemodialysis patients. Hemodial Int. 2006;10:209–14.
172. Kirschbaum BB, Schoolwerth AC. Acute aluminum toxicity associated with oral citrate and aluminum-containing antacids. Am J Med Sci. 1989;297:9–11.
173. Walker JA, Sherman RA, Cody RP. The effect of oral bases on enteral aluminum absorption. Arch Intern Med. 1990;150:2037–9.
174. Mehta BR, Fischer D, Ahmad M, Dubose Jr TD. Effects of acetate and bicarbonate hemodialysis on cardiac function in chronic dialysis patients. Kidney Int. 1983;24:782–7.
175. Oettinger CW, Oliver JC. Normalization of uremic acidosis in hemodialysis patients with a high bicarbonate dialysate. J Am Soc Nephrol. 1993;3:1804–7.
176. Shah SN, Abramowitz M, Hostetter TH, Melamed ML. Serum bicarbonate levels and the progression of kidney disease: a cohort study. Am J Kidney Dis. 2009;54:270–7.
177. de Brito-Ashurst I, Varagunam M, Raftery MJ, Yaqoob MM. Bicarbonate supplementation slows progression of CKD and improves nutritional status. J Am Soc Nephrol. 2009;20:2075–84.
178. Szeto CC, Wong TY, Chow KM, Leung CB, Li PK. Oral sodium bicarbonate for the treatment of metabolic acidosis in peritoneal dialysis patients: a randomized placebo-control trial. J Am Soc Nephrol. 2003;14:2119–26.
179. Lefebvre A, de Vernejoul MC, Gueris J, Goldfarb B, Graulet AM, Morieux C. Optimal correction of acidosis changes progression of dialysis osteodystrophy. Kidney Int. 1989;36:1112–8.
180. Brady JP, Hasbargen JA. Correction of metabolic acidosis and its effect on albumin in chronic hemodialysis patients. Am J Kidney Dis. 1998;31:35–40.
181. Mendoza FJ, Lopez I, Montes de Oca A, Perez J, Rodriguez M, Aguilera-Tejero E. Metabolic acidosis inhibits soft tissue calcification in uremic rats. Kidney Int. 2008;73:407–14.
182. Lowrie EG, Lew NL. Death risk in hemodialysis patients: the predictive value of commonly measured variables and an evaluation of death rate differences between facilities. Am J Kidney Dis. 1990;15:458–82.
183. Bommer J, Locatelli F, Satayathum S, et al. Association of predialysis serum bicarbonate levels with risk of mortality and hospitalization in the Dialysis Outcomes and Practice Patterns Study (DOPPS). Am J Kidney Dis. 2004;44:661–71.
184. Kirschbaum B. Spurious metabolic acidosis in hemodialysis patients. Am J Kidney Dis. 2000;35:1068–71.
185. Zazra JJ, Jani CM, Rosenblum S. Are the results of carbon dioxide analysis affected by shipping blood samples? Am J Kidney Dis. 2001;37:1105–6.
186. Batlle DC, Arruda JA, Kurtzman NA. Hyperkalemic distal renal tubular acidosis associated with obstructive uropathy. N Engl J Med. 1981;304:373–80.
187. Keven K, Ozturk R, Sengul S, et al. Renal tubular acidosis after kidney transplantation—incidence, risk factors and clinical implications. Nephrol Dial Transplant. 2007;22:906–10.
188. Gonwa TA, Hricik DE, Brinker K, Grinyo JM, Schena FP. Improved renal function in sirolimus-treated renal transplant patients after early cyclosporine elimination. Transplantation. 2002;74:1560–7.
189. Bloom RD, Olivares M, Rehman L, Raja RM, Yang S, Badosa F. Long-term pancreas allograft outcome in simultaneous pancreas-kidney transplantation: a comparison of enteric and bladder drainage. Transplantation. 1997;64:1689–95.
190. Nghiem DD, Gonwa TA, Corry RJ. Metabolic effects of urinary diversion of exocrine secretions in pancreatic transplantation. Transplantation. 1987;43:70–3.

191. Rodriguez Soriano J. Renal tubular acidosis: the clinical entity. J Am Soc Nephrol. 2002;13:2160–70.
192. Domrongkitchaiporn S, Khositseth S, Stitchantrakul W, Tapaneya-olarn W, Radinahamed P. Dosage of potassium citrate in the correction of urinary abnormalities in pediatric distal renal tubular acidosis patients. Am J Kidney Dis. 2002;39:383–91.
193. Disthabanchong S, Domrongkitchaiporn S, Sirikulchayanonta V, Stitchantrakul W, Karnsombut P, Rajatanavin R. Alteration of noncollagenous bone matrix proteins in distal renal tubular acidosis. Bone. 2004;35:604–13.
194. Osther PJ, Bollerslev J, Hansen AB, Engel K, Kildeberg P. Pathophysiology of incomplete renal tubular acidosis in recurrent renal stone formers: evidence of disturbed calcium, bone and citrate metabolism. Urol Res. 1993;21:169–73.
195. Weger M, Deutschmann H, Weger W, Kotanko P, Skrabal F. Incomplete renal tubular acidosis in 'primary' osteoporosis. Osteoporos Int. 1999;10:325–9.
196. Preminger GM, Sakhaee K, Pak CY. Hypercalciuria and altered intestinal calcium absorption occurring independently of vitamin D in incomplete distal renal tubular acidosis. Metabolism. 1987;36:176–9.
197. Preminger GM, Sakhaee K, Skurla C, Pak CY. Prevention of recurrent calcium stone formation with potassium citrate therapy in patients with distal renal tubular acidosis. J Urol. 1985;134:20–3.
198. Sharma AP, Singh RN, Yang C, Sharma RK, Kapoor R, Filler G. Bicarbonate therapy improves growth in children with incomplete distal renal tubular acidosis. Pediatr Nephrol. 2009;24:1509–16.
199. Ceglia L, Harris SS, Abrams SA, Rasmussen HM, Dallal GE, Dawson-Hughes B. Potassium bicarbonate attenuates the urinary nitrogen excretion that accompanies an increase in dietary protein and may promote calcium absorption. J Clin Endocrinol Metab. 2009;94:645–53.
200. Palmer BF. Managing hyperkalemia caused by inhibitors of the renin-angiotensin-aldosterone system. N Engl J Med. 2004;351:585–92.
201. Sastrasinh S, Tannen RL. Effect of potassium on renal NH3 production. Am J Physiol. 1983;244:F383–91.
202. Tannen RL. Relationship of renal ammonia production and potassium homeostasis. Kidney Int. 1977;11:453–65.
203. Tannen RL, Kunin AS. Effect of potassium on ammoniagenesis by renal mitochondria. Am J Physiol. 1976;231:44–51.
204. Tannen RL, McGill J. Influence of potassium on renal ammonia production. Am J Physiol. 1976;231:1178–84.
205. DuBose Jr TD, Good DW. Effects of chronic hyperkalemia on renal production and proximal tubule transport of ammonium in rats. Am J Physiol. 1991;260:F680–7.
206. DuBose Jr TD, Good DW. Chronic hyperkalemia impairs ammonium transport and accumulation in the inner medulla of the rat. J Clin Invest. 1992;90:1443–9.
207. Sebastian A, Schambelan M, Sutton JM. Amelioration of hyperchloremic acidosis with furosemide therapy in patients with chronic renal insufficiency and type 4 renal tubular acidosis. Am J Nephrol. 1984;4:287–300.
208. Sebastian A, Schambelan M, Lindenfeld S, Morris Jr RC. Amelioration of metabolic acidosis with fludrocortisone therapy in hyporeninemic hypoaldosteronism. N Engl J Med. 1977;297:576–83.
209. Fordtran JS. Speculations on the pathogenesis of diarrhea. Fed Proc. 1967;26:1405–14.
210. Schiller LR. Diarrhea. Med Clin North Am. 2000;84:1259–74.
211. Atia AN, Buchman AL. Oral rehydration solutions in non-cholera diarrhea: a review. Am J Gastroenterol. 2009;104:2596–604. quiz 605.
212. Fernandez PC, Cohen RM, Feldman GM. The concept of bicarbonate distribution space: the crucial role of body buffers. Kidney Int. 1989;36:747–52.
213. Lemann Jr J, Gray RW, Pleuss JA. Potassium bicarbonate, but not sodium bicarbonate, reduces urinary calcium excretion and improves calcium balance in healthy men. Kidney Int. 1989;35:688–95.

Metabolic Alkalosis

9

F. John Gennari

Introduction

Metabolic alkalosis is perhaps the most common clinical acid–base disorder, due in part to the widespread use of diuretic drugs to treat edema. This disorder is initiated by any event, with the exception of hypercapnia, that causes an increase in bicarbonate concentration ($[HCO_3^-]$) in the extracellular fluid. Such an event raises pH, which in turn induces hypoventilation, producing a secondary increase in arterial PCO_2. Metabolic alkalosis is thus characterized by an increase in serum $[HCO_3^-]$, and in arterial pH and PCO_2. Only when the increase in $[HCO_3^-]$ is sustained, however, does metabolic alkalosis become clinically manifest. Maintenance of a high $[HCO_3^-]$ requires a second event, a failure or disruption of the normal renal regulatory mechanisms to excrete the excess HCO_3^-. This chapter reviews the pathophysiology of the events that cause a sustained primary increase in serum $[HCO_3^-]$, the nature of the secondary response, and the various clinical presentations of this disorder, all with an eye to treatment and prevention.

F.J. Gennari, M.D. (✉)
Department of Medicine, University of Vermont, Burlington, VT 05401, USA
e-mail: fgennari@uvm.edu

Pathophysiology

Table 9.1 lists the settings in which sustained metabolic alkalosis occurs. The simplest setting to understand is alkali administration in patients with renal failure. If alkali is added to the extracellular fluid of a patient with no functioning kidneys, the excess cannot be excreted and serum $[HCO_3^-]$ will remain elevated until the HCO_3^- is consumed over time by endogenous acid production [1]. In patients with functioning kidneys, however, excess HCO_3^- is normally excreted quickly, restoring serum $[HCO_3^-]$ to normal. Metabolic alkalosis persists only when tubule ion transport is altered in a way that limits or prevents excretion of the excess HCO_3^-. Virtually all clinical causes of sustained metabolic alkalosis are the result of abnormal stimulation of H^+ and K^+ secretion in the collecting duct, secondary either to electrolyte losses or to abnormal primary activation of ion transport [2]. The most common setting, by far, is when body chloride stores are depleted due either to Cl^- losses from the gastrointestinal tract or to diuretic drugs that inhibit renal Cl^- reabsorption. Potassium depletion can also cause metabolic alkalosis, although only to a very modest degree in the absence of either primary stimulation of collecting duct H^+ secretion or depletion of body chloride stores. Although often categorized separately, Cl^- and K^+ depletion interact in a complex and complementary way to sustain most forms of metabolic alkalosis.

D.B. Mount et al. (eds.), *Core Concepts in the Disorders of Fluid, Electrolytes and Acid-Base Balance*, DOI 10.1007/978-1-4614-3770-3_9, © Springer Science+Business Media New York 2013

Table 9.1 Pathophysiological classification of causes of sustained metabolic alkalosis

Kidney failure
Secondary stimulation of collecting duct H^+ and K^+ secretion
Extrarenal chloride losses and secondary renal potassium losses
Renal chloride losses with secondary renal potassium losses
Pharmacological (diuretics)
Inactivating genetic mutations of Cl^-—linked Na^+ cotransporters
Primary stimulation of collecting duct H^+ and K^+ secretion
Mineralocorticoid induced
Activating genetic mutations of ENaC[a] or its signal pathway

[a] Epithelial sodium channel

Secondary Stimulation of Collecting Duct Ion Secretion

Chloride Depletion

The features of metabolic alkalosis initiated by Cl^- depletion have been elucidated by classic studies in normal human subjects [3, 4]. In one of these studies (Fig. 9.1), subjects were given a diet containing very little chloride and then underwent nocturnal nasogastric (NG) suction for several days after histamine stimulation of gastric acid secretion [3]. All the electrolytes lost in the collected gastric fluid were replaced with the exception of hydrogen and chloride. These experimental maneuvers caused a characteristic sequence of events to occur. Metabolic alkalosis developed rapidly during the period of suctioning, with plasma [HCO_3^-] rising to almost 40 mmol/L. This change in extracellular fluid (ECF) composition was associated with a brief period of natriuresis and bicarbonaturia, followed by an increase in renal K^+ excretion and a return in net acid excretion towards normal despite the sustained alkalemia. After cessation of the NG drainage, metabolic alkalosis and K^+ depletion persisted despite a normal dietary K^+ intake, until sufficient Cl^- was given to replete the losses induced [4].

In additional studies, induction and maintenance of the disorder was found to be independent of ECF volume and not mediated by increased aldosterone levels [4–6]. In addition, correction of the disorder by Cl^- administration occurred without repletion of body K^+ stores and despite mineralocorticoid administration [4, 6]. Nonetheless, secondary K^+ depletion likely plays a contributing role in sustaining the disorder. In the absence of K^+ supplements much larger amounts of Cl^- must be given to correct the metabolic alkalosis induced by chloride depletion [4, 7].

Chloride depletion alkalosis is often associated with some degree of ECF volume depletion. This association has led to the unfortunate term "contraction alkalosis" to describe this form of metabolic alkalosis. The term is inappropriate because it implies that volume contraction is *responsible* for the disorder. Although suggested to play a pathogenetic role, the weight of the evidence indicates that a reduction in ECF volume is neither necessary nor sufficient to induce or sustain the disorder [5, 8].

Most forms of chloride-depletion alkalosis are associated with a reduction in glomerular filtration rate (GFR), and such a change was proposed to be instrumental in sustaining the disorder by limiting HCO_3^- excretion [9]. Against this possibility, GFR increases above normal in a rat model of sustained chloride-depletion alkalosis [10, 11]. The increase in GFR is likely due to the associated K^+ depletion, which stimulates renal growth and hypertrophy. In this model, proximal tubule HCO_3^- reabsorption increases in direct relation to the increase in GFR, despite an alkaline pH. Because HCO_3^- is preferentially reabsorbed in the proximal tubule, the continued selective recapture of most of the filtered HCO_3^- in this segment of the nephron clearly contributes to sustaining the alkalosis. Nonetheless, alterations in distal tubule and collecting transport are likely the key factors in this disorder as in most other forms of metabolic alkalosis.

Potassium Depletion

The role of K^+ depletion as opposed to Cl^- depletion in the pathogenesis of metabolic alkalosis has been a subject of debate for many years, primarily because of species differences in the effects of K^+ depletion on acid–base homeostasis

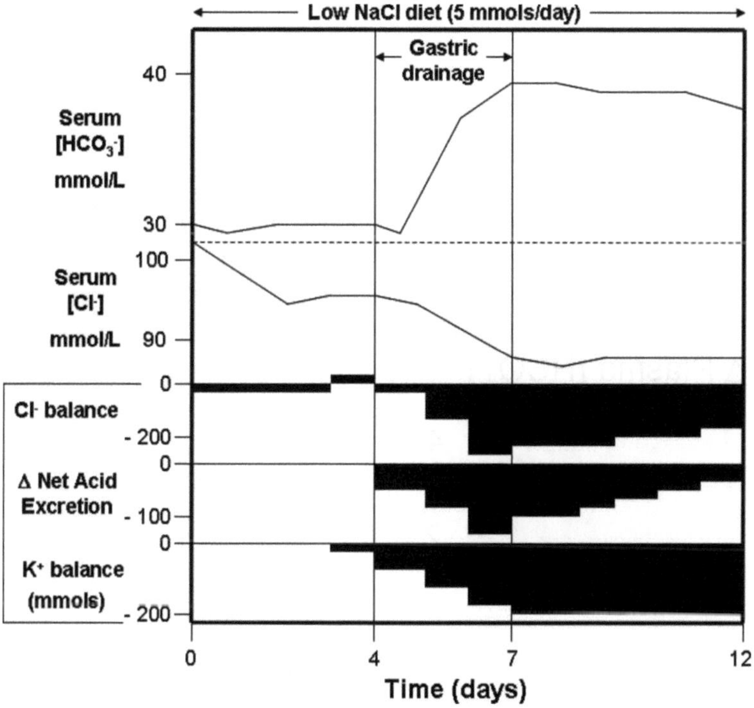

Fig. 9.1 Effect of gastric drainage on serum composition, chloride and potassium balance, and renal net acid excretion in a normal human subject ingesting a low NaCl diet. See text for full description of study

[12]. The question of whether K^+ depletion, independent of Cl^- depletion, can cause metabolic alkalosis in humans, however, has been answered in the affirmative by a well-designed study in normal subjects [7]. Potassium depletion was induced by placing the subjects on a synthetic diet very low in K^+ with either a low or normal Cl^- content. Even in the subjects with adequate Cl^- intake and no evidence of any depletion of body Cl^- stores, serum [HCO_3^-] rose significantly, by 2 mmol/L, after induction of moderate K^+ depletion (Fig. 9.2). In the presence of concomitant dietary Cl^- restriction, however, the increase in serum [HCO_3^-] was 7.5 mmol/L. This experiment in humans underscores the interplay between K^+ and Cl^- depletion in determining the severity of metabolic alkalosis.

The effects of K^+ depletion that induce and sustain a metabolic alkalosis are (1) a shift of H^+ into cells that raises ECF [HCO_3^-] and (2) renal effects leading to an increase in H^+ secretion and in ammonium excretion, facilitating acid excretion and sustaining the increase in ECF [HCO_3^-]. In addition, K^+ depletion downregulates chloride-linked Na^+ reabsorption in the loop and early distal tubule [13], facilitating continued delivery of sufficient Na^+ delivery to the collecting duct for ongoing stimulation of H^+ and K^+ secretion at that site in the nephron.

Induction of K^+ Depletion in Cl^- Depletion States

Years before specific ion transport proteins were identified, Schwartz and coworkers postulated that both Cl^- and K^+ depletion alkalosis were sustained by a shift in Na^+ reabsorption from proximal sites along the nephron, where it was linked to Cl^- reabsorption, to more distal sites, where its reabsorption was somehow linked to K^+ and H^+ secretion [14]. This postulate was subsequently substantiated in its essential features, after specific membrane ion transporters in various tubule segments were identified and their regulation delineated. The alkalosis induced by

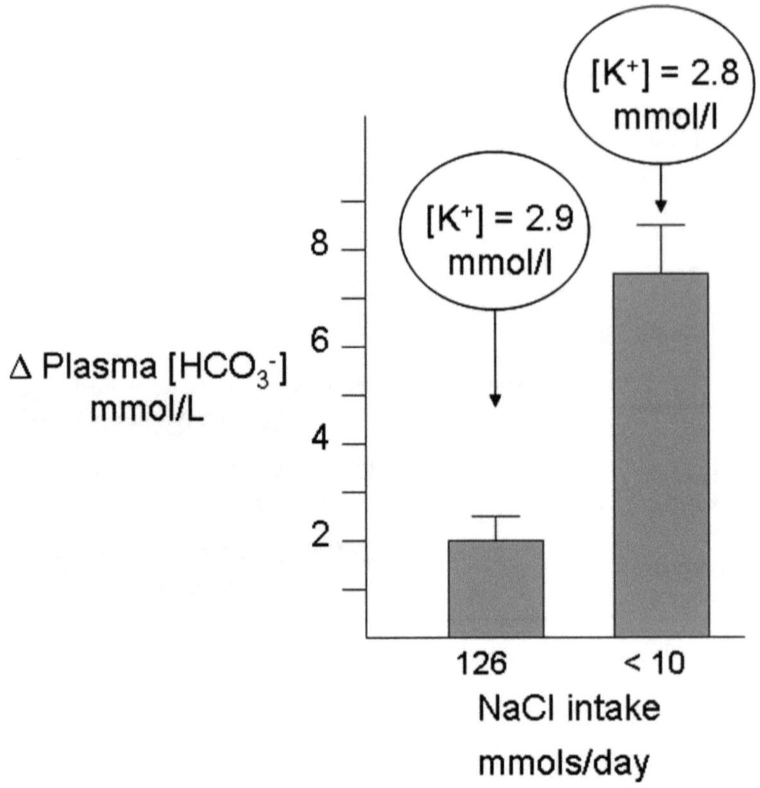

Fig. 9.2 Effect of K^+ depletion (400–500 mmol, induced by dietary K^+ restriction for 2 weeks) on plasma $[HCO_3^-]$ in normal human subjects. The *left-hand bar* depicts the increase with no dietary Cl^- restriction. The *right-hand bar* depicts the increase when dietary Cl^- intake was also markedly restricted. In both instances the increase is significant ($p=0.02$ in the normal NaCl group, and 0.001 in the low NaCl group). As indicated in the figure, plasma $[K^+]$ was essentially the same in both groups. Data from Hernandez et al. [7]. See text for a full description of study

chloruretic diuretics, primary aldosteronism and by certain genetic disorders is clearly associated with such a shift in transport, as discussed below. Although it is presumed that the alkalosis caused by gastrointestinal Cl^- losses is due to a similar shift, such a change cannot be detected in segmental studies of Na^+ and Cl^- reabsorption along the nephron, and the specific pathophysiology of metabolic alkalosis in this setting remains to be completely explained [15]. The key transporters in the loop and distal nephron whose function is altered in sustained metabolic alkalosis, and their proposed role in sustaining the disorder, are discussed below.

Effects of Cl^- and K^+ Depletion on Specific Ion Transporters

Na^+–K^+–$2Cl^-$ cotransporter. In the thick ascending limb of the loop of Henle, Na^+ reabsorption is linked to K^+ and Cl^- reabsorption, via the epithelial membrane Na^+–K^+–$2Cl^-$ cotransporter (Fig. 9.3). Impairment of its function, either by the loop diuretics or by one of several mutations in Bartter syndrome (see later), invariably leads to metabolic alkalosis by increasing delivery of Na^+ to the collecting duct where its reabsorption stimulates both H^+ and K^+ excretion. Chloride depletion per se has been postulated to impair Na^+ uptake via this transporter, although this effect cannot be detected using micropuncture technique [15]. Concomitant K^+ depletion has several potential effects on this transporter as well. It can contribute to impaired Na^+ uptake because K^+ recycling across the epithelial membrane is necessary for optimal transporter function. In addition, K^+ depletion in rats decreases both the activity of this transporter and mRNA levels for its synthesis [13]. Because NH_4^+ com-

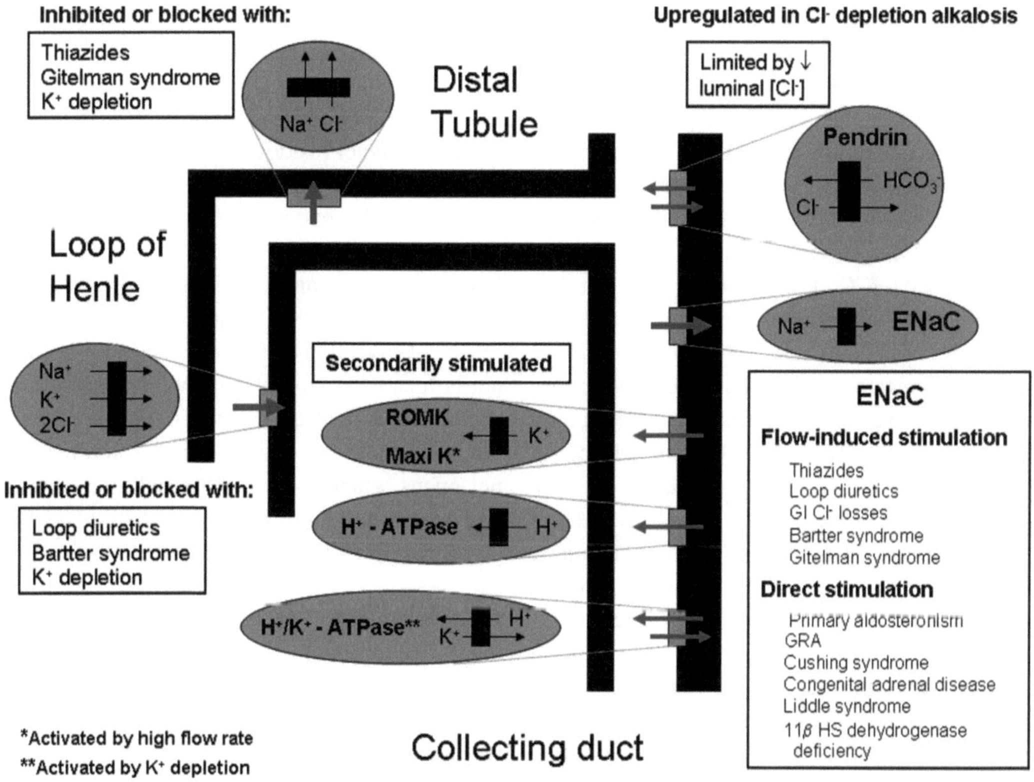

Fig. 9.3 Schematic depiction of the key apical membrane ion transport proteins in the Loop of Henle and distal nephron, and the ways in which their function is altered both to impair the excretion of excess HCO_3^- and to sustain K^+ losses in various forms of metabolic alkalosis. GRA = Glucocorticoid remediable aldosteronism

petes with K^+ binding to the transporter, K^+ depletion may allow for increased NH_4^+ uptake by the loop, facilitating an increase in NH_4^+ excretion.

Na^+–Cl^- cotransporter. The Na^+–Cl^- cotransporter is located on the apical membrane of epithelial cells in the early distal tubule (Fig. 9.3). Blockade of this transporter either by thiazide diuretics or by mutations in Gitelman syndrome causes metabolic alkalosis. The activity of this transporter and the mRNA for its synthesis are also downregulated by K^+ depletion [13]. In Cl^- depletion states, it is proposed, but unproven, that a decrease in Cl^- delivery to this site in the nephron impairs Na^+ uptake by this transporter, contributing to an increase in Na^+ delivery to the collecting duct.

Cl^-/HCO_3^- exchanger (Pendrin). This anion transporter, named pendrin when it was identified as the transporter whose mutation was the cause of Pendred's syndrome in humans [16], is located on apical membrane of the β(beta) intercalated cells of the connecting tubule and cortical collecting duct (Fig. 9.3). Its orientation is such that HCO_3^- is secreted into the tubule urine and Cl^- is reabsorbed. Although the activity of this transporter is more closely linked to Cl^- balance rather than to acid–base balance, a linkage between its activity and H^+ secreting transporter function in the collecting duct appears to play an important role in sustaining metabolic alkalosis. Pendrin is upregulated by dietary Cl^- restriction in experimental animals, allowing for maximal Cl^- conservation [17, 18]. It is also upregulated in an animal model of Cl^- depletion alkalosis, and thus potentially poised to facilitate HCO_3^- secretion [19, 20]. Removal of Cl^- from distal tubule fluid blocks HCO_3^- secretion by this transporter [19, 21], but this situation does not occur in vivo in any form of metabolic alkalosis. In pendrin-null homozygous mice, HCO_3^- secretion does not

occur, but metabolic alkalosis develops only when they are placed on a Cl^- restricted diet [17]. In the absence of Cl^- restriction, these mutant animals downregulate H^+ secreting transport proteins in the collecting duct, apparently compensating for the lack of HCO_3^- secretion, and as a result have no acid–base disturbance [22]. Recent data suggest that the activity of ENaC is directly related to the [HCO_3^-] in the tubule lumen and in the peritubular interstitium providing a potential mechanism for cross talk between pendrin and ENaC [23]. Humans with Pendred's syndrome also do not have metabolic alkalosis [16]. In normal animals with metabolic alkalosis induced by Cl^- depletion, the Cl^-/HCO_3^- exchanger is fully functional and upregulated [8]. Because no HCO_3^- appears in the urine in these animals, secretion of HCO_3^- via pendrin is apparently counterbalanced by continued high rates of H^+ secretion in the collecting duct [8, 24]. Chloride administration in this model must allow for enough of an increase in Cl^- delivery to shift the balance so that HCO_3^- secretion exceeds collecting duct H^+ secretion, facilitating excretion of the excess HCO_3^-. Pendrin is also upregulated when metabolic alkalosis is induced by mineralocorticoid administration [25]. Strikingly, pendrin is downregulated in a mouse model where K^+ depletion is induced by dietary K^+ restriction [26]. The role of pendrin in sustaining metabolic alkalosis and its functional linkage with collecting duct H^+ secretion remains an evolving story.

Epithelial Na^+ channel (ENaC). The epithelial Na^+ channel resides on the apical membrane of principal cells in the collecting duct (Fig. 9.3), and its activity is regulated principally by flow rate (and thus Na^+ delivery) and by aldosterone [27, 28]. Impairment of Na^+ uptake earlier in the nephron, for example, by chloruretic diuretics, results in increased delivery of Na^+ to this transporter, leading to increased Na^+ uptake via ENaC. An increase in Na^+ reabsorption at this site increases the electrochemical driving forces favoring both K^+ and H^+ secretion. Primary stimulation of this transporter also causes K^+ depletion and metabolic alkalosis in primary aldosteronism and in a variety of genetic and acquired disorders (see later).

Epithelial K^+ channels (ROMK and Maxi-K). The ROMK channel resides on the apical membrane of the principal cells of the collecting tubule and allows for K^+ movement down its electrochemical gradient into the tubule urine (Fig. 9.3). Potassium secretion is increased whenever Na^+ reabsorption via ENaC is increased, even in the setting of overall K^+ depletion. The maxi-K channel is located on the apical membranes of both principal and intercalated cells. This channel is not open under normal conditions, but the channel opens when flow is increased at either site and it facilitates K^+ secretion with higher conductance than ROMK [29].

H^+-ATPase and H^+/K^+-ATPase. H^+ secretion in the collecting duct can occur either via the H^+-ATPase or the H^+/K^+-ATPase transporter on the apical membrane of intercalated cells in the collecting tubule (Fig. 9.3). The first of these H^+ transporters is active all the time, although it requires some aldosterone for effective function. Secretion of H^+ via this transporter shows flow dependence, presumably in response to flow-dependent Na^+ reabsorption creating a favorable electrochemical gradient for H^+ secretion. In metabolic alkalosis induced by chloruretic diuretics and by Bartter and Gitelman syndrome, H^+ secretion is increased by the increase in Na^+ delivery to the collecting duct and reabsorption via ENaC. In an experimental model of chloride-depletion metabolic alkalosis, distal nephron H^+ secretion is increased as well for any given level of luminal [HCO_3^-] [24]. Two isoforms of an additional H^+ secretory transporter, the H^+/K^+-ATPase, are present in the collecting duct, and the activity of at least one of these is increased by K^+ depletion [30], providing an addition route for H^+ secretion into the tubule in metabolic alkalosis. As noted earlier, in animals lacking pendrin who are ingesting adequate salt, these H^+ secreting transporters are apparently downregulated, suggesting a functional linkage between HCO_3^- and H^+ secretion in the distal nephron.

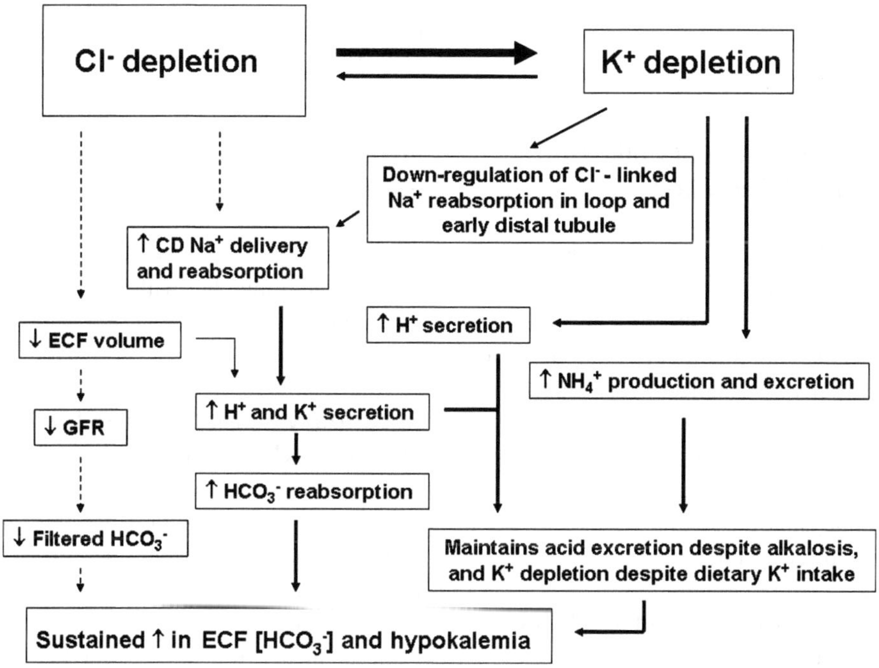

Fig. 9.4 Schematic representation of the interactions between Cl^- and K^+ depletion in sustaining metabolic alkalosis. *Hatched arrows* indicate potential contributing effects. Depletion of Cl^- invariably leads to K^+ losses and sustained K^+ depletion, while primary K^+ depletion leads to Cl^- losses and depletion only when very severe. Depletion of K^+ stimulates collecting duct H^+ secretion, downregulates Cl^--linked Na^+ reabsorption and increases renal ammonium excretion. See text for more detailed description of effects. CD = collecting duct

Summary of Effects of Cl^- and K^+ Depletion on Tubule Ion Transport

Although Cl^- and K^+ depletion can be shown to produce metabolic alkalosis independently of each other, depletion of either of these ions influences the renal handling of the other ion through a series of linked transport events in the loop of Henle and distal nephron (Figs. 9.3 and 9.4). Severe K^+ depletion actually leads to renal Cl^- wasting, presumably through inhibition of the Na^+–K^+–$2Cl^-$ and Na^+–Cl^- cotransporters [13]. In addition to the linked transport events, K^+ depletion stimulates NH_4^+ production in the renal cortex facilitating net acid excretion. If ECF volume depletion is present, as it commonly is in clinical states of metabolic alkalosis, this event reduces GFR, limiting HCO_3^- filtration and excretion as well.

Aldosterone

It is unlikely that aldosterone plays anything more than a facilitating role, if that, in the maintenance of metabolic alkalosis. As discussed earlier, aldosterone levels actually fall in the alkalosis caused by Cl^- losses, and rise during correction with potassium chloride treatment [5, 6]. In addition, Cl^- depletion alkalosis can be induced and sustained in adrenalectomized rats [31]. Although not essential, ample aldosterone is secreted in patients with sustained Cl^- depletion metabolic alkalosis, facilitating Na^+ uptake via ENaC [5, 6]. It seems likely that in all forms of Cl^- depletion metabolic alkalosis, some increase in Na^+ delivery occurs in a setting in which a continued signal for reabsorption is present—e.g., the absence of ECF volume expansion.

Role of PCO_2

The secondary increase in PCO_2 that occurs in metabolic alkalosis paradoxically is an additional stimulus to increase H^+ secretion in the collecting duct [32]. As a result, a small increment in serum $[HCO_3^-]$ can be attributed solely to the rise in

PCO_2 that normally occurs when metabolic alkalosis is induced.

Primary Stimulation of Collecting Duct H^+ and K^+ Secretion

Although different in the specifics of its pathophysiology, metabolic alkalosis induced by primary stimulation of collecting duct ion secretion shares the common theme of an increase in distal Na^+ delivery coupled with stimulation of ion transport in the collecting duct. A major difference is that it does not feature chloride depletion and is typically associated with hypertension. The pathophysiology of this type of metabolic alkalosis is discussed below.

Mineralocorticoid-Induced and Direct Stimulation of ENaC

Aldosterone and other mineralocorticoids stimulate Na^+ reabsorption in the cortical collecting duct directly by upregulating ENaC and stimulating Na^+/K^+ ATPase activity (Fig. 9.3). When secretion of these hormones is unlinked from ECF volume, primary Na^+ retention and sustained ECF volume expansion results unless NaCl intake is severely restricted. Expansion of ECF volume by continuous mineralocorticoid secretion or administration, by triggering signals that both increase GFR and reduce Na^+ reabsorption in the proximal tubule and loop of Henle, causes a sustained increase in delivery of Na^+ to the collecting duct. This sequence of events redistributes Na^+ reabsorption from proximal to distal sites in the nephron in the steady state, where its uptake stimulates K^+ and H^+ secretion, leading to K^+ depletion and metabolic alkalosis. In this regard, the pathophysiology of mineralocorticoid-induced metabolic alkalosis is similar to Cl^- and K^+ depletion metabolic alkalosis. A significant difference, however, is that in mineralocorticoid-induced alkalosis the shift is initiated by a primary increase in Na^+ reabsorption in the collecting duct, rather than by a decrease in Na^+ reabsorption more proximally. Thus, ECF volume is expanded, leading to associated hypertension. Moreover, no depletion of body Cl^- stores occurs, and the severity of the alkalosis is determined primarily by the degree of K^+ depletion [33]. As discussed earlier, K^+ depletion promotes alkalosis by causing a shift of H^+ into cells and by causing changes in renal H^+secretion and ammonium excretion (Figs. 9.3 and 9.4). A variety of rare genetic and acquired disorders, discussed later, leads to abnormal direct stimulation of collecting duct Na^+ reabsorption and produces the same clinical syndrome, but with suppressed aldosterone secretion.

Secondary Response to an Increase in Blood pH and $[HCO_3^-]$

Regardless of the specific pathophysiology that causes an increase in pH and serum $[HCO_3^-]$, the resultant alkalemia induces hypoventilation, increasing arterial PCO_2. In uncomplicated metabolic alkalosis, the increase in PCO_2 virtually always prevents blood pH from exceeding 7.60. The ventilatory response is rapid and potent, occurring despite arterial PO_2 values falling to less than 50 mmHg. Studies in animals and in humans indicate that the rise is roughly linear, increasing PCO_2, on average, by 0.7 mmHg for every mmol/L increase in serum $[HCO_3^-]$ [34]. These observations form the basis for the "rule of thumb" formula used to evaluate the secondary response to metabolic alkalosis (see later under Diagnosis).

Clinical Manifestations

Effects of Alkalemia

Unless serum $[HCO_3^-]$ rises to >40 mmol/L, the resultant alkalemia and hypercapnia produce few clinically significant changes in body functions, and patients are typically asymptomatic. When symptoms do occur in patients with mild to moderate metabolic alkalosis, they are usually attributable to either the associated volume depletion or to hypokalemia (see below). With more severe metabolic alkalosis, central nervous system dysfunction, including agitation, disorientation, stupor, and coma, has been noted. The central nervous system effects have been attributed to the combined effects of alkalemia and hypoxemia.

The former decreases cerebral blood flow and both decrease oxygen delivery to the cerebral tissues. Rarely, the alkalemia causes muscle twitching, tetany, and seizures. The latter effects are assumed to be due to a decrease in ionized calcium concentration caused by alkalemia, although the Chvostek and Trousseau signs in these patients are usually negative. There is little effect of alkalemia and hypercapnia per se on cardiac output or rhythm. Any cardiac effects are dominated by hypokalemia.

Metabolic alkalosis has minor effects on body metabolism. It increases lactic acid production, but this effect is rarely significant unless alkalosis is severe. The increase in lactic acid production is triggered by an increase in cell pH, but may be exacerbated by severe vasoconstriction or hypovolemia. Metabolic alkalosis increases muscle glycogen utilization and increases urinary citrate excretion.

Effects of Hypokalemia

The symptoms in patients with metabolic alkalosis are usually dominated by those caused by hypokalemia. Mild hypokalemia (serum [K^+] 3.0–3.5 mmol/L) usually produces few symptoms, but when serum [K^+] falls to less than 3.0 mmol/L, fatigue, weakness, and constipation are commonly present. With more severe hypokalemia, muscle breakdown can occur and when the value falls to <2.0 mmol/L, an ascending paralysis can occur. In patients with coronary artery disease or congestive heart failure, even mild hypokalemia increases the likelihood of cardiac arrhythmias. In patients without heart disease, however, arrhythmias are extremely rare even in patients with severe hypokalemia.

Table 9.2 Metabolic alkalosis: specific causes

Secondary stimulation of collecting duct H^+ and K^+ secretion
Chloride depletion syndromes (blood pressure normal or low)
Gastrointestinal and other nonrenal Cl^- losses
Vomiting, nasogastric (NG) drainage
Congenital chloridorrhea
Some villous adenomas
High-volume ileostomy drainage
Cystic fibrosis
Renal Cl^- losses
Chloruretic diuretic drugs[a]
Recovery from chronic hypercapnia
Genetic disorders
Bartter syndrome
Gitelman syndrome
Isolated potassium depletion
Laxative abuse
Severe K^+ depletion
Primary stimulation of collecting duct H^+ and K^+ secretion
Mineralocorticoid excess syndromes (blood pressure ↑)
Primary aldosteronism
Glucocorticoid remediable aldosteronism
Cushing syndrome
Congenital adrenal hyperplasia
Renin-secreting tumors
Medications
Fludrocortisone
9 α(alpha)-fluoroprednisolone (inhaled)
Apparent mineralocorticoid excess syndromes (blood pressure ↑)
Liddle syndrome
11 β(beta)-OH steroid dehydrogenase inhibition or deficiency
Other causes
Alkali intake or administration
Milk–alkali syndrome

[a] Blood pressure may be elevated in patients with associated hypertension

Specific Causes of Metabolic Alkalosis

The major causes of metabolic alkalosis have traditionally been divided into two groups, depending on whether or not they are reversed by chloride administration. While useful for considering the appropriate management in some cases, this classification adds confusion by placing causes of metabolic alkalosis that have the same pathophysiology into two separate categories, obscuring their commonality (e.g., Bartter and Gitelman syndrome are separated from diuretic-induced metabolic alkalosis). Table 9.2 presents a new classification based on pathophysiology rather than response to treatment. Using this classification, diagnosis of the specific cause of metabolic alkalosis focuses on the history and physical examination (Fig. 9.5). A history of gastrointestinal losses or diuretic usage points to the

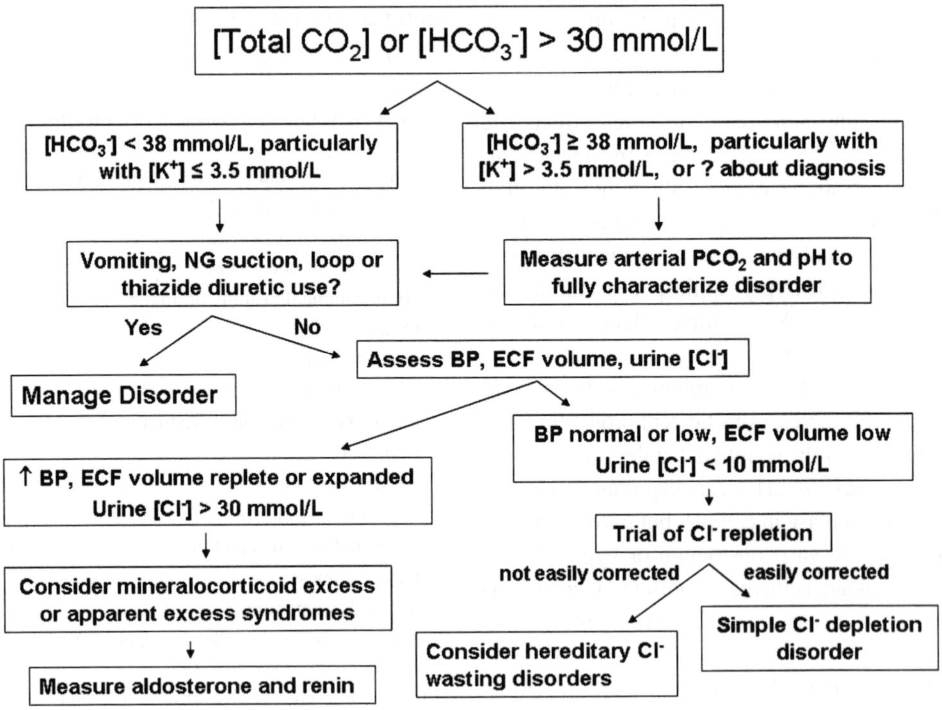

Fig. 9.5 Approach to the patient found to have an elevated serum [Total CO_2] or [HCO_3^-]. Steps in identifying the disorder and determining the underlying cause

most common causes of metabolic alkalosis. Obtaining a good history is coupled with an assessment of ECF volume and blood pressure. Complementing this assessment, when appropriate, is measurement of plasma aldosterone and renin levels. Only in rare instances is the measurement of urine chloride concentration or a diagnostic trial of saline or potassium chloride administration necessary to make the diagnosis. The causes of metabolic alkalosis are discussed below.

Secondary Stimulation of Collecting Duct Ion Secretion

Gastrointestinal and Other Nonrenal Chloride Losses

Vomiting or nasogastric drainage. Loss of stomach secretions either from vomiting or NG drainage causes disproportionate Cl^- losses, accompanied by varying amounts of H^+ depending on the pH of the gastric contents. To the extent that H^+ is lost, serum [HCO_3^-] rises immediately, but even if the losses are primarily NaCl, the resultant Cl^- losses induce changes in renal HCO_3^- reabsorption and acid excretion that lead to sustained metabolic alkalosis. With continued emesis or NG suction, serum [HCO_3^-] may rise to as high as 80 mmol/L [35]. This cause of metabolic alkalosis is virtually always present, at least as a contributing factor, when the serum [HCO_3^-] is >45 mmol/L. The disorder is completely reversed by repletion of body Cl^- stores. The use of drugs that inhibit the gastric H^+/K^+ ATPase ameliorates this form of metabolic alkalosis and may reverse it completely in some instances [36, 37]. In patients with end-stage kidney failure, HCl losses from vomiting will cause a sustained metabolic alkalosis independent of body Cl^- and K^+ stores [1]. In the absence of kidney function, hypokalemia does not occur.

Congenital chloridorrhea. This autosomal recessive inherited disorder causes large-volume watery diarrhea that is rich in chloride, producing metabolic alkalosis. The alkalosis is associated with volume depletion and hypokalemia, as Na^+ and K^+

is lost in the stool as well. The renal response is characterized by continued delivery to and stimulation of Na^+ reabsorption in the collecting duct, leading to urinary K^+ losses and maintained acid excretion. Thus, the pathophysiology is identical to that seen with upper gastrointestinal Cl^- losses. The disorder is caused by a mutation in the *down-regulated in adenoma* (DRA) gene, leading to a loss of function defect in the apical membrane Cl^-/HCO_3^- exchanger in the distal ileum and colon [38]. Although the alkalosis responds to vigorous NaCl and KCl administration, management is difficult as the losses continue unabated. In order to counter the hypovolemia and alkalosis, dietary potassium and chloride intake must exceed losses, even though the volume of diarrhea may increase. Recent data provide a new hope for treatment using a proton-pump inhibitor. This class of drugs reduces gastric Cl^- secretion, and as a result stool volume falls dramatically [39].

Villous adenoma of the colon. These tumors, almost all of which are found in the rectosigmoid portion of the colon, typically secrete 1–3 L/day of fluid that is rich in Na^+, Cl^- and K^+. As a result of these secretions, diarrhea occurs and can sometimes lead to clinically significant hypovolemia. Surprisingly, less than half of these tumors cause metabolic alkalosis despite the disproportionate Cl^- and K^+ losses [40]. The remaining tumors are associated with either no acid–base abnormality or metabolic acidosis. The specific acid–base abnormality that occurs in a given patient does not correlate with the composition of the secretions, but may be related to the balance between Na^+, Cl^-, and K^+ intake and excretion.

High volume ileostomy drainage. In patients with Crohn's disease who have ileostomy drainage after small bowel resection, severe metabolic alkalosis may occur in association with a major increase in drainage [41]. The ileostomy fluid in these cases contains abnormally high concentrations of Cl^-, accounting for the acid–base disorder.

Gastrocystoplasty. The use of gastric tissue to augment bladder size can occasionally lead to mild metabolic alkalosis as a result of gastrin-induced Cl^- secretion into the urine. In no instances is the metabolic alkalosis sustained in long-term follow-up studies [42].

Cystic Fibrosis. Cystic fibrosis, caused by mutations in the cystic fibrosis transmembrane regulator (CFTR), is characterized by high $[Cl^-]$ in sweat and other body secretions. With excess sweating, these Cl^- losses can produce metabolic alkalosis. Metabolic alkalosis can be the presenting symptom of the disease in adolescence [43].

Renal Chloride Losses

Chloruretic diuretics. Diuretic drugs that inhibit chloride-linked Na^+ reabsorption in the kidney are the most common cause of metabolic alkalosis. These drugs include the thiazide diuretics and metolazone, which inhibit the Na^+–Cl^- cotransporter in the early distal tubule, and the so-called "loop diuretics", furosemide, torsamide, bumetinide, and ethacrynic acid, which inhibit the Na^+–K^+–$2Cl^-$ cotransporter in the thick ascending limb of the loop of Henle. Both classes of drugs induce disproportionate Cl^- losses and shift Na^+ reabsorption to the collecting duct, where its uptake facilitates K^+ and H^+ secretion (see earlier discussion and Figs. 9.3 and 9.4). The alkalosis produced is typically mild (serum $[HCO_3^-] < 36$ mmol/L), but it can be more severe, particularly in patients who continue to take in excess NaCl and have a continued stimulus for Na^+ reabsorption. In such individuals, ingestion of NaCl simply promotes more Na^+ delivery to the collecting duct where its reabsorption leads to the secretion of more K^+ and H^+. Hypokalemia due to K^+ depletion is typically more prominent than the alkalosis and is the major management problem.

Recovery from chronic hypercapnia. The renal response to sustained hypercapnia causes a disproportionate loss of Cl^- into the urine. In the new steady state, serum $[HCO_3^-]$ is increased and serum $[Cl^-]$ is decreased. Restoration of a normal serum $[HCO_3^-]$ after recovery from hypercapnia requires repletion of the Cl^- stores lost during the secondary renal response to hypercapnia. If they are not, the same changes in renal electrolyte transport ensue that are seen with Cl^- depletion from gastrointestinal losses, resulting in sustained metabolic alkalosis. Normally, dietary Cl^- intake is more than sufficient to replete body Cl^- stores when renal Cl^- reabsorption returns to normal. As a result this form of metabolic alkalosis is unusual, only occurring in patients who are unable to ingest a normal diet.

Bartter syndrome. Bartter syndrome is a hereditary disorder that causes Na^+ and Cl^- wasting with metabolic alkalosis and hypokalemia in infants and young children [44]. This disorder is now known to be caused by one of several mutations that inactivate or misregulate the Na^+–K^+–$2Cl^-$ cotransporter in the thick ascending limb of Henle's loop [44–46]. The pathophysiology of the disorder is identical therefore to that seen with chronic loop diuretic therapy, although it is more severe and not easily corrected by treatment with sodium or potassium chloride. ECF volume depletion is a common presenting feature, and patients typically have low blood pressure and symptomatic hypokalemia that is difficult to correct.

Gitelman syndrome. Gitelman syndrome is a hereditary disorder that causes a milder degree of hypokalemia and metabolic alkalosis than does Bartter syndrome, and is accompanied by hypomagnesemia and and hypocalciuria [44, 47]. Patients typically first present with symptoms as adults, and these symptoms are primarily due to hypomagnesemia and hypokalemia (muscle cramps, weakness, and fatigue). The disorder is caused by mutations that inactivate or interfere with the function of the Na^+–Cl^- cotransporter in the early distal tubule [44–46]. As a result, the pathophysiology of the metabolic alkalosis is similar to that seen with chronic thiazide therapy. Treatment is primarily directed at treating K^+ and magnesium deficiencies, but the symptoms are rarely cleared by treatment.

Isolated Potassium Depletion

Laxative abuse. Laxative abuse leads to excessive K^+ loss in the stool. When this loss of K^+ is not balanced by dietary K^+ intake, body K^+ stores are depleted [48]. The major clinical feature of laxative abuse without associated bulimia is hypokalemia; clinically significant metabolic alkalosis, if present, is extremely mild.

Severe K^+ deficiency. Mild to moderate K^+ depletion causes a modest increase in serum [HCO_3^-] even when dietary Cl^- intake is adequate (Fig. 9.2). When K^+ losses are more severe and prolonged, clinically significant metabolic alkalosis (sometimes with serum [HCO_3^-] greater than 40 mmol/L) can occur, independent of dietary Cl^- intake or administration [49]. In such instances, serum [K^+] is typically less than 2.0 mmol/L. Partial correction of the K^+ deficit results in restoring the ability of Cl^- to correct the alkalosis. The mechanism of the so-called "Cl^- wasting" with severe K^+ depletion may be inhibition of both the Na^+–K^+–$2Cl^-$ and the Na^+–K^+ cotransporters in the loop and early distal tubule (Fig. 9.3).

Primary Stimulation of Collecting Duct Ion Secretion

Mineralocorticoid Excess Syndromes

Primary aldosteronism. The clinical presentation of primary aldosteronism is dominated by hypertension and hypokalemia, with only a mild increase in serum [HCO_3^-] (30–35 mmol/L). The severity of the metabolic alkalosis, in fact, is inversely correlated with serum [K^+], presumably reflecting the degree of K^+ depletion [33]. As discussed earlier, Cl^- depletion plays no role in the pathogenesis and ECF volume is increased, causing the hypertension. As a result, urine Cl^- excretion reflects dietary intake, and the disorder is not affected by Cl^- balance. The alkalosis can be corrected by aggressive potassium supplementation, or by inhibiting the effects of aldosterone in collecting duct cells with spironolactone or epleronone.

Glucocorticoid remediable aldosteronism. Glucocorticoid remediable aldosteronism (GRA) is caused by a genetic mutation that results in aldosterone secretion being regulated by ACTH rather than angiotensin II, and is transmitted in an autosomal dominant pattern [50]. As a result of this mutation, aldosterone is no longer controlled by changes in ECF volume, but rather by signals regulating glucocorticoid secretion. This change in control leads to the development of a mineralocorticoid excess syndrome with hypertension and with elevated aldosterone and low renin levels, a pattern that is indistinguishable from primary aldosteronism. Hypokalemia and metabolic alkalosis are variable, however, and may be less common than in primary aldosteronism. Early onset hypertension and a strong family history are key features that should lead one to suspect the diagnosis. Both the hypertension and electrolyte abnormalities are reversed by administering dexamethasone, which suppresses ACTH and thereby reduces aldosterone secretion. Correction of the hypertension and alkalosis by dexamethasone is diagnostic of the disorder. Genetic testing and identification of the specific mutations involved remains a research enterprise.

Cushing syndrome. Hyperadrenocorticism secondary to autonomous adrenocorticotropin (ACTH) or corticotropin-releasing hormone (CRH) secretion can occur as a result of a pituitary or hypothalamic tumor, or from a malignancy that produces ACTH or CRH elsewhere in the body. These tumors cause a marked increase in the synthesis and secretion of glucocorticoids, with only minor increases in mineralocorticoid production. Not surprisingly, hypokalemia and metabolic alkalosis occur only in a small minority of patients with primary pituitary or hypothalamic tumors. When present, metabolic alkalosis is typically very mild. By contrast, over 50 % of patients with malignancies producing ectopic ACTH have hypokalemia and metabolic alkalosis, and both abnormalities may be more severe [51]. The pathophysiology of the hypokalemia and metabolic alkalosis in Cushing's syndrome is unclear, as the primary abnormality is elevated glucocorticoid secretion by the adrenal glands. One postulate is that the very high cortisol levels seen with ectopic ACTH secretion saturate the enzyme that inactivates cortisol at the mineralocorticoid receptor (11 β(beta)-hydroxysteroid dehydrogenase, see below), resulting in cortisol binding to the receptor and producing mineralocorticoid effects [51]. Supporting this view, the presence of hypokalemia is associated with higher urine cortisol levels in patients with ectopic ACTH secretion. Although corticosterone and deoxycorticosterone levels are increased in Cushing's syndrome, the levels are not correlated with hypokalemia and are not high enough to account for the mineralocorticoid features seen. The metabolic alkalosis in this syndrome can be reversed by aggressive potassium repletion [52].

Congenital adrenal hyperplasia. Two forms of congenital adrenal hyperplasia are associated with hypertension, hypokalemia, and metabolic alkalosis. In both forms, the hypertension and changes in electrolyte composition are caused by excess production and secretion of mineralocorticoids [53]. One form is caused by 17-hydroxylase deficiency and is now known to be secondary to a mutation in the CYP17 gene that encodes P450c17, the 17-hydroxylase enzyme. This defect causes increased production and secretion of 11-deoxycorticosterone (DOC), 18 hydroxydeoxycorticosterone, and corticosterone, all of which have mineralocorticoid activity, and it is also associated with defective androgen production. The other form is due to 11-hydroxylase deficiency, which leads only to excess DOC production and secretion, and is associated with increased androgen production. Management is directed at decreasing mineralocorticoid production by cortisol administration.

Renin-secreting tumors. Renin-secreting tumors arising either within the kidney or at extrarenal sites are an extremely rare cause of hypokalemia and metabolic alkalosis. These tumors are manifested by severe hypertension and hypokalemia. Serum [K^+] is typically very low, with values <2.5 mmol/L. By contrast, metabolic alkalosis is usually very mild. The hypokalemia and metabolic alkalosis are presumed to be due to secondary hyperaldosteronism.

Malignant and renovascular hypertension. Both malignant and renovascular hypertension are associated with secondary increases in aldosterone secretion, but these disorders are only rarely associated with hypokalemia and metabolic alkalosis. In such patients, the finding of metabolic alkalosis should prompt a search for another cause.

Medications. Fludrocortisone is an oral mineralocorticoid drug used primarily to treat mineralocorticoid deficiency, but also postural hypotension. In the usual dosage, it does not cause metabolic alkalosis, but can cause this disorder if taken in excessive amounts. Habitual use of a nasal spray that contains 9 α(alpha)-fluoroprednisolone for chronic rhinitis has been reported to cause hypertension, hypokalemia and metabolic alkalosis [54]. This drug is no longer available in inhalers in the United States, but is still available in other countries. Glucocorticoids when administered in very high doses increase renal K^+ excretion nonspecifically and can result in a mild increase in serum [HCO_3^-].

Syndromes of Apparent Mineralocorticoid Excess

Liddle syndrome. This rare familial hereditary disorder is caused by a gene mutation that truncates the intracellular tail of the collecting duct epithelial Na^+ channel, ENaC, blocking its normally regulated removal from the epithelial membrane and degradation [55]. As a result, collecting duct Na^+ reabsorption is continually stimulated, leading to Na^+ retention, and K^+ and H^+ losses in the urine. The phenotypic result is early onset hypertension, with variable hypokalemia and metabolic alkalosis. The pathophysiology of the disorder is identical to that caused by mineralocorticoid excess (see earlier), but because the ECF volume expansion is caused by a regulatory defect in ENaC rather than by any abnormality in aldosterone secretion, serum aldosterone and renin levels are vanishingly low. Hence, the syndrome is one of apparent mineralocorticoid excess. The hypertension, hypokalemia and metabolic alkalosis are all corrected by blocking ENaC function with amiloride or triamterene.

11 β(beta)-hydroxysteroid dehydrogenase inhibition or deficiency. The mineralocorticoid receptor in collecting duct epithelial cells binds with equal affinity to cortisol and aldosterone. Its selectivity for aldosterone is controlled enzymatically, through degradation of cortisol by 11 β(beta)-hydroxysteroid dehydrogenase. Even though cortisol levels are normally 1,000-fold greater than aldosterone levels, the enzyme rapidly inactivates cortisol before it can bind to the receptor, allowing aldosterone to be the primary ligand. Inhibition of this enzyme by glycyrrhizic acid, a component of natural licorice, allows the abundant cortisol to bind to and activate the receptor, continually stimulating Na^+ reabsorption independent of ECF [56]. This abnormal activation produces a syndrome identical to primary aldosteronism (see above), except that aldosterone levels are vanishingly low due to the sustained ECF volume expansion that occurs. Sustained hypokalemia and metabolic alkalosis occur only in individuals who consume licorice in large amounts on a daily basis. As with primary aldosteronism, the clinical presentation is dominated by hypertension and hypokalemia, with only mild elevations in serum [HCO_3^-]. Carbenoxolone, a component of chewing tobacco, and gossypol (a drug that inhibits spermatogenesis and has been used for birth control) also inhibit the enzyme and can produce the same clinical picture.

In addition to pharmacologic blockade, a rare genetic mutation inactivates the enzyme, causing the same clinical syndrome [57]. In families with this disorder, hypertension, hypokalemia, and metabolic alkalosis are present in the affected individuals [57]. In some patients with the disorder, renal damage from nephrocalcinosis occurs, presumably due to metabolic alkalosis promoting calcium phosphate deposition in the renal parenchyma. The familial form of the disorder is called *the syndrome of apparent mineralocorticoid excess*, because, as in the case of Liddle syndrome, its clinical presentation is identical to primary aldosteronism, but aldosterone levels are low instead of high. Given the pathophysiology of this disorder, treatment with either amiloride or spironolactone should be effective in ameliorating the hypertension, hypokalemia and metabolic alkalosis.

Other Causes

Alkali Intake or Administration

Ingested alkali (e.g., sodium or potassium bicarbonate) or alkali precursors (e.g., sodium or potassium citrate or acetate) transiently increases serum [HCO_3^-], but the excess alkali is normally excreted rapidly and the increase is not sustained. In individuals placed on a diet that contains very little Cl^- (less than 20 mmol/day), however, ingestion of as little as 4 mmol/Kg of sodium bicarbonate a day will cause a sustained increase in serum [HCO_3^-] [58]. In patients with preexisting Cl^- or K^+ depletion, alkali ingestion or administration will also result in a sustained increase in serum [HCO_3^-]. Although calcium carbonate is a potential source of alkali, only a fraction is normally absorbed and thus it has little impact on serum [HCO_3^-] unless ingested in large amounts (see later under milk–alkali syndrome). In patients with renal insufficiency of failure, ingested or administered alkali is retained independently of body Cl^- or K^+ stores. In hospitalized patients with renal failure receiving daily hemodialysis treatments, for example, metabolic alkalosis invariably develops unless bath [HCO_3^-] is adjusted downward. In such patients, administration of a wide variety of alkali precursors, including acetate, lactate, citrate (either as a bicarbonate precursor or as an anticoagulant), and amino acid anions, will also cause metabolic alkalosis. Although rarely used now, aluminum hydroxide given in combination with sodium polystyrene sulfonate (kayexelate) can cause metabolic alkalosis in patients with kidney failure [59]. This occurs because aluminum binds to the kayexelate resin in exchange for Na^+. As a result, the HCO_3^- normally secreted into the duodenum is neither neutralized by H^+ secreted into the stomach (which was neutralized by the aluminum hydroxide) nor does it form an insoluble salt with aluminum, and so it is reabsorbed and retained.

Milk–Alkali Syndrome

This syndrome is characterized by the concomitant presence of metabolic alkalosis and renal insufficiency in individuals ingesting alkali in combination with excess calcium (milk or calcium carbonate) [60]. The renal damage is caused by the excess calcium intake, which precipitates with phosphate in the renal parenchyma in the presence of alkalemia. The resultant fall in GFR, in turn, facilitates retention of ingested alkali. The metabolic alkalosis in milk–alkali syndrome is usually mild, unless there is concomitant vomiting. Although this syndrome almost vanished with the replacement of calcium carbonate by aluminum-containing antacids, there has been a resurgence due to the more widespread use of calcium carbonate both for esophageal reflux disease and also to improve body calcium stores [60].

Hyperparathyroidism, Vitamin D Intoxication, and Hypercalcemia

Administration of parathyroid hormone acutely decreases proximal tubule HCO_3^- reabsorption and reduces serum [HCO_3^-], but when continued for more than 24 h, causes an increase in serum [HCO_3^-] of 2–3 mmol/L above normal [61]. The increase in serum [HCO_3^-] is accounted for by a transient increase in net acid excretion followed by a sustained increase in HCO_3^- reabsorption, indicating a primary renal response. The mechanisms responsible for this renal effect remain undefined. Administration of either vitamin D or parathyroid hormone to thyroparathyroidectomized dogs also causes an increase in [HCO_3^-], but without any detectable changes in net acid excretion, suggesting that carbonate release from bone may also play a role in generating the disorder. Even in this model, however, the kidney must be a contributor as renal HCO_3^- reabsorption increased and net acid excretion did not fall despite the presence of alkalemia. Paradoxically, early clinical reports of primary hyperparathyroidism (in which both parathyroid hormone and vitamin D are elevated) found the disorder to be associated not with metabolic alkalosis but with a mild metabolic acidosis. One possible explanation is that patients with hyperparathyroidism were diagnosed later in the course of their disease before hormone assays were available, and they may have already suffered renal damage from nephrocalcinosis, causing the metabolic acidosis. Hypercalcemia and vitamin D intoxication are sometimes associated with clinically significant metabolic alkalosis, but when present the alkalosis is most likely due to the vomiting that accompanies these disorders.

Miscellaneous

Individuals exposed to prolonged starvation (e.g., prisoners of war, voluntary fasting) characteristically develop a metabolic acidosis, due to increased ketogenesis. When these individuals are fed again, serum [HCO_3^-] increases abruptly, and sometimes rises transiently above normal. The causes of this mild and short-lived metabolic alkalosis are multiple, including rapid HCO_3^- generation from metabolism of organic anions when their production is stopped by insulin, and by K^+ and Cl^- depletion that may be present at the time of refeeding. Metabolic alkalosis, if present, is never a significant clinical issue.

Based on in vitro observations and theoretic considerations, hypoalbuminemia has been proposed as a cause of metabolic alkalosis, due to a decrease in the anionic contribution of albumin to the strong ion charge. While reducing albumin concentration in a test tube in which Na^+, Cl^-, and K^+ concentrations are fixed and PCO_2 is kept constant will increase both pH and [HCO_3^-], the same changes will not cause a sustained increase in serum [HCO_3^-] in intact organisms unless renal regulatory mechanisms are also disrupted. In a single report of seven patients with low serum albumin concentrations, mild elevations in serum [HCO_3^-] were noted [62]. In this report, however, insufficient information is given about the patients to exclude known causes of metabolic alkalosis. In the absence of further evidence, the finding of an elevated serum [HCO_3^-] in a patient with a low serum albumin concentration should prompt a search for other causes.

Diagnosis

Identifying the Disorder

Detection of the presence of metabolic alkalosis is usually very straightforward. The finding of a serum [total CO_2] > 30 mmol/L in association with a serum [K^+] < 3.5 mmol/L in a venous blood sample is virtually pathognomonic (Fig. 9.5). The only other cause for an elevated serum [total CO_2] is chronic respiratory acidosis, and hypokalemia is not a feature of that acid–base disorder. Full characterization of metabolic alkalosis, however, requires measurement of arterial pH and PCO_2, and calculation of serum [HCO_3^-]. The presence of a pH > 7.40 and a PCO_2 > 45 mmHg along with an elevated arterial serum [HCO_3^-] (>30 mmol/L) indicate with certainty that the disorder is present. Metabolic alkalosis is so common that when it is mild, arterial blood measurements are not usually needed unless a mixed disorder is suspected. When the disorder is severe (serum [total CO_2] ≥ 38 mmol/L), arterial blood measurements are necessary to manage the disorder appropriately.

Evaluation of the Secondary Response

To evaluate whether an uncomplicated metabolic alkalosis is present or there is a mixed disorder, one must assess whether the secondary response (hypoventilation) is appropriate for the degree of elevation in serum [HCO_3^-]. This assessment requires measurement of arterial pH and PCO_2. As discussed earlier, the expected increase in PCO_2 is 0.7 mmHg for each mmol/L increase in serum [HCO_3^-]. Assuming the normal arterial serum [HCO_3^-] to be 24 mmol/L and PCO_2 to be 40 mmHg, the predicted arterial PCO_2 for any given serum [HCO_3^-] in metabolic alkalosis can be estimated using the following formula:

$$\text{Predicted } PCO_2 = 40 + 0.7 \times \left(\left[HCO_3^-\right] - 24\right)$$

In this formula, PCO_2 is in mmHg and [HCO_3^-] is in mmol/L. The formula should only be considered as a helpful tool, not a precise estimate. The variability is large, particularly when metabolic alkalosis is severe [34]. Variations of as much as 5–7 mmHg between the observed and predicted PCO_2 may occur in uncomplicated metabolic alkalosis. Nonetheless, the finding of a measured PCO_2 that is more than 8 mmHg less than or greater than the expected value for the serum [HCO_3^-] indicates the presence of a complicating respiratory acid–base disorder (see Chap. 10).

Anion Gap in Metabolic Alkalosis

The anion gap ($[Na^+]-([Cl^-]+[HCO_3^-])$) is usually normal in uncomplicated mild to moderate metabolic alkalosis but may increase when alkalosis is more severe, sometimes exceeding 20 mmol/L [63]. The increase is due both to a rise in serum albumin concentration (due to hemoconcentration) and to an increase in its anion equivalency as the pH rises. Severe metabolic alkalosis is also associated with an increase in organic anion accumulation. As in the case of any acid–base disorder, the normal value for the anion gap should be adjusted for the serum albumin concentration to estimate whether the anion gap is increased and to evaluate whether a mixed disorder is present (see Chap. 11).

Determining the Cause

The final step in assessing a patient with metabolic alkalosis is to determine the specific cause (Fig. 9.5). In most instances this step is straightforward. Over 95 % of metabolic alkalosis is caused either by diuretic therapy or by vomiting or NG drainage. This information is usually easily obtainable, and attention can be directed towards appropriate treatment. When the cause is not clear, one should carefully evaluate the patient's ECF volume status and blood pressure. The presence of hypertension is suggestive of a mineralocorticoid excess or apparent mineralocorticoid excess syndrome. In these individuals, measurement of serum aldosterone and renin levels, as well as a careful family history, can be helpful to separate primary aldosteronism from familial genetic disorders. The presence of normal or low blood pressure or of ECF volume depletion is more suggestive of renal or extrarenal Cl^- losses. When the diagnosis is not straightforward, measurement of urine $[Cl^-]$ in a random urine sample *in the absence of diuretic therapy* can be helpful. If the disorder is due to Cl^- depletion from an extrarenal cause or from prior diuretic-induced renal losses, the urine $[Cl^-]$ should be low (<10 mmol/L). If the disorder is not caused by extrarenal or *reversible* renal Cl^- losses, urine $[Cl^-]$ should reflect intake, and will usually be >30 mmol/L. In patients suspected of surreptitious diuretic use, a urine screen for diuretic agents may be needed to identify the cause of the metabolic alkalosis. Patients with bulimia should have a low urine $[Cl^-]$ unless the urine sample is obtained immediately following emesis.

Management

Management of metabolic alkalosis depends upon the pathophysiology of the specific form encountered (Table 9.3). As with most disorders, removal of the offending agent or taking steps to stop the initiating event (e.g., vomiting) is the first approach to management, but in most instances repletion of body electrolyte stores is needed for reversal of the alkalosis in a timely fashion. Specific approaches to management are discussed below.

Specific Forms

Gastrointestinal Cl^- Losses

Patients with metabolic alkalosis as a result of gastrointestinal losses require Cl^- repletion to fully correct the serum $[HCO_3^-]$. These patients are usually volume depleted on presentation, and in such instances intravenous saline is the first line of treatment. Extracellular fluid volume and serum creatinine should be monitored carefully during saline administration to assure that renal failure, if present, is prerenal in nature and that ECF volume overload does not occur. In most instances, serum $[HCO_3^-]$ will fall rapidly as body Cl^- stores and ECF volume are restored to normal. Because secondary K^+ depletion invariably occurs with Cl^- depletion alkalosis, KCl should be administered as well. If gastrointestinal Cl^- losses cannot be stopped, treatment with a proton-pump inhibitor such as omeprazole should be initiated to minimize gastric Cl^- secretion. As noted earlier, this pharmacologic intervention not only is effective in minimizing upper tract losses but also shows great promise for managing the ongoing stool Cl^- losses in congenital chloridorrhea [39].

Table 9.3 Management strategies in metabolic alkalosis

For all causes, remove offending agent or underlying cause if possible	
Cause	Recommended treatment
Secondary stimulation of collecting duct ion secretion	
Gastrointestiinal Cl^- losses	Intravenous NaCl Oral or intravenous KCl
Congenital chloridorrhea	Oral NaCl, KCl Proton-pump inhibitor
Diuretic-induced Cl^- losses	Discontinue diuretic when possible Oral KCl, reduce dietary salt intake Add K^+ sparing diuretic
Bartter syndrome	Oral KCl, often in large amounts Prostaglandin inhibitors ACE inhibitors, K^+ sparing diuretics
Gitelman syndrome	Oral KCl, often in large amounts Oral magnesium supplement Prostaglandin inhibitors ACE inhibitors, K^+ sparing diuretics
Isolated K^+ losses	Oral or intravenous potassium
Primary stimulation of collecting duct ion secretion	
Primary Hyperaldosteronism	Oral KCl Spironolactone, epleronone Surgery
GRA[a]	Dexamethasone
Cushing syndrome	Oral KCl
Congenital adrenal hyperplasia	Cortisol
Renin secreting tumor	KCl Surgery
Liddle syndrome	Amiloride, triamterene
↓ 11 β(beta)-HS dehydrogenase[b]	Spironolactone, amiloride
Other causes	
Milk–alkali syndrome	Discontinue calcium supplements
Special considerations	
Alkalosis + ECF volume overload	Acetazolamide
Alkalosis + renal failure	Continuous renal replacement therapy

[a]Glucocorticoid remediable aldosteronism
[b]Decreased or absent 11 β(beta)-hydroxysteroid dehydrogenase activity

Diuretic-Induced Cl^- Losses

Management of metabolic alkalosis that is induced by diuretic therapy presents a different set of issues. In these patients, a reduction in ECF volume is the goal of the therapy, and therefore volume repletion is not usually indicated. Discontinuation of the offending diuretic agent will spontaneously correct the disorder if dietary Cl^- intake is adequate, but this approach is not always feasible. A modest degree of metabolic alkalosis is usually well tolerated, and often not treated when diuretic therapy is needed for fluid volume control. The primary management is to replace urinary K^+ losses and minimize the hypokalemia. When metabolic alkalosis is present, the appropriate replacement therapy is potassium chloride. In patients with hypokalemia who have not yet developed a metabolic alkalosis, potassium citrate or bicarbonate is a useful alternative therapy. Unless emergency treatment is necessary, K^+ repletion should always be undertaken with an oral preparation. Potassium-sparing diuretics, such as amiloride or spironolactone, have also been used to manage this form of metabolic alkalosis, allowing for continued diuresis while ameliorating hypokalemia and alkalosis. An often overlooked but effective maneuver is to encourage the patient to reduce dietary salt consumption, which will decrease Na^+ delivery to the collecting duct. Regardless of the intervention, some degree of K^+ depletion and metabolic alkalosis is likely to persist until the chloruretic diuretic agent is discontinued.

Bartter and Gitelman Syndromes

Of all the causes of metabolic alkalosis, Barter and Gitelman syndromes present the greatest therapeutic challenge. Early studies describing attempts at treatment did not distinguish between the two disorders, as Gitelman syndrome was not recognized as a separate disorder [45]. Although many of the papers are entitled Bartter syndrome, most of the patients reported appear in retrospect to have Gitelman syndrome. The mainstay of treatment for both disorders is oral potassium chloride, sometimes as much as 500 mmol/day. While this therapy may lessen the severity of the K^+ depletion, it almost never fully corrects the hypokalemia or the metabolic alkalosis. A second approach, used in conjunction with dietary K^+ supplementation, is drug therapy with prostaglandin inhibitors. These agents appear to have a beneficial effect by reducing renin and aldosterone levels, while at the same time reducing GFR and thereby decreasing K^+, Na^+, and Cl^- losses. Other treatments used less frequently include spironolactone or amiloride to inhibit Na^+ reabsorption via ENaC, and angiotensin-converting enzyme inhibitors to reduce aldosterone levels. The latter treatments have limited utility because of their blood pressure lowering effects, and their potential to worsen ECF volume depletion. As noted earlier, a key component of therapy in patients with Gitelman syndrome is repletion of magnesium as well as potassium stores. Despite all these interventions, patients with Bartter and Gitelman syndromes continue to have metabolic alkalosis and hypokalemia often with low blood pressure and continued symptoms.

Mineralocorticoid and Apparent Mineralocorticoid Excess

As discussed earlier, syndromes associated with unregulated aldosterone excess all respond well to treatment with KCl supplements or spironolactone. The metabolic alkalosis that occurs with Cushing syndrome also responds well to aggressive treatment with KCl supplements. In patients with glucocorticoid remediable aldosteronism, the alkalosis and hypokalemia are both reversed by dexamethasone. In Liddle syndrome, where the genetic defect causes continued abnormal stimulation of Na^+ reabsorption via ENaC, blockade of this epithelial membrane ion channel using either amiloride or triamterene corrects the metabolic alkalosis. When the apparent mineralocorticoid excess is due to inhibition of the enzyme 11 β(beta)-hydroxysteroid dehydrogenase, a search for the offending agent is the first step in management. In the rare familial form caused by the lack of a functioning enzyme, either amiloride or spironolactone is likely to be effective.

Special Considerations in Treatment

Patients with ECF fluid volume overload and/or renal failure with concomitant metabolic alkalosis represent a special challenge. In most instances the metabolic alkalosis itself is not severe enough to warrant specific treatment, and none is recommended. When serum $[HCO_3^-]$ is >40 mmol/L and/or is producing symptoms or problems with ventilator management, however, it should be reduced. In patients with residual renal function, oral or intravenous treatment with the carbonic anhydrase inhibitor acetazolamide is effective in reducing serum $[HCO_3^-]$ by inducing renal HCO_3^- losses. A single daily oral dose of 500 mg appears to be as effective as several 250 mg doses a day. Acetazolamide is also effective as an adjunct to furosemide and spironolactone. When this agent is given, serum $[K^+]$ should be monitored carefully as it promotes renal K^+ losses and concomitant K^+ replacement therapy is often needed.

In patients with renal failure, serum [HCO_3^-] can be reduced easily and safely using any of several forms of continuous renal replacement therapy. The most effective method is sustained low efficiency dialysis. Using this technique with a bath [HCO_3^-] of 23–25 mmol/L, serum [HCO_3^-] can be reduced to normal levels over 24 h. With continuous venovenous hemofiltration, using saline as the replacement, serum [HCO_3^-] can also be reduced effectively. Conventional hemodialysis is also effective, although less so, because bath [HCO_3^-] can only be reduced to ~30 mmol/L without making a totally new bath solution. Because of the ready availability of renal replacement therapies, the potentially dangerous use of intravenous HCl, or arginine or ammonium chloride to lower serum [HCO_3^-] in patients with metabolic alkalosis is no longer recommended.

References

1. Huber L, Gennari FJ. Severe metabolic alkalosis in a hemodialysis patient. Am J Kidnes Dis. 2011;58(1): 144–9.
2. Gennari FJ, Pathophysiology of metabolic alkalosis: A new classification based on the centrality of stimulated collecting duct ion transport. Am J Kidney Dis. 2011;58(4):626–636.
3. Kassirer JP, Schwartz WB. The response of normal man to selective depletion of hydrochloric acid. Factors in the genesis of persistent gastric alkalosis Am J Med. 1966;40(1):10–8.
4. Kassirer JP, Schwartz WB. Correction of metabolic alkalosis in man without repair of potassium deficiency. A re-evaluation of the role of potassium Am J Med. 1966;40(1):19–26.
5. Rosen RA, Julian BA, Dubovsky EV, Galla JH, Luke RG. On the mechanism by which chloride corrects metabolic alkalosis in man. Am J Med. 1988;84(3 Pt 1):449–58.
6. Kassirer JP, Appleton FM, Chazan JA, Schwartz WB. Aldosterone in metabolic alkalosis. J Clin Invest. 1967;46(10):1558–71.
7. Hernandez RE, Schambelan M, Cogan MG, Colman J, Morris Jr RC, Sebastian A. Dietary NaCl determines severity of potassium depletion-induced metabolic alkalosis. Kidney Int. 1987;31(6): 1356–67.
8. Galla JH, Gifford JD, Luke RG, Rome L. Adaptations to chloride-depletion alkalosis. Am J Physiol. 1991;261(4 Pt 2):R771–81.
9. Berger BE, Cogan MG, Sebastian A. Reduced glomerular filtration and enhanced bicarbonate reabsorption maintain metabolic alkalosis in humans. Kidney Int. 1984;26(2):205–8.
10. Wesson DE. Augmented bicarbonate reabsorption by both the proximal and distal nephron maintains chloride-deplete metabolic alkalosis in rats. J Clin Invest. 1989;84(5):1460–9.
11. Maddox DA, Gennari FJ. Load dependence of proximal tubular bicarbonate reabsorption in chronic metabolic alkalosis in the rat. J Clin Invest. 1986;77(3): 709–16.
12. Gennari FJ. Hypokalemia in metabolic alkalosis. A new look at an old controversy. In: Hatano M, editor. Nephrology (proceedings, XIth International Society of Nephrology). Tokyo: Springer-Verlag; 1991. p. 262–9.
13. Amlal H, Wang Z, Soleimani M. Potassium depletion downregulates chloride-absorbing transporters in rat kidney. J Clin Invest. 1998;101(5):1045–54.
14. Schwartz WB. Pathogenesis and replacement of diuretic-induced potassium and chloride loss. Ann N Y Acad Sci. 1966;139(2):506–11.
15. Galla JH, Bonduris DN, Luke RG. Effects of chloride and extracellular fluid volume on bicarbonate reabsorption along the nephron in metabolic alkalosis in the rat. Reassessment of the classical hypothesis of the pathogenesis of metabolic alkalosis J Clin Invest. 1987;80(1):41–50.
16. Royaux IE, Wall SM, Karniski LP, et al. Pendrin, encoded by the Pendred syndrome gene, resides in the apical region of renal intercalated cells and mediates bicarbonate secretion. Proc Natl Acad Sci U S A. 2001;98(7):4221–6.
17. Wall SM, Kim YH, Stanley L, et al. NaCl restriction upregulates renal Slc26a4 through subcellular redistribution: role in Cl- conservation. Hypertension. 2004;44(6):982–7.
18. Verlander JW, Kim YH, Shin W, et al. Dietary Cl(-) restriction upregulates pendrin expression within the apical plasma membrane of type B intercalated cells. Am J Physiol Renal Physiol. 2006;291(4): F833–9.
19. Gifford JD, Sharkins K, Work J, Luke RG, Galla JH. Total CO2 transport in rat cortical collecting duct in chloride-depletion alkalosis. Am J Physiol. 1990;258(4 Pt 2):F848–53.
20. Verlander JW, Madsen KM, Galla JH, Luke RG, Tisher CC. Response of intercalated cells to chloride depletion metabolic alkalosis. Am J Physiol. 1992;262(2 Pt 2):F309–19.
21. Levine DZ, Vandorpe D, Iacovitti M. Luminal chloride modulates rat distal tubule bidirectional bicarbonate flux in vivo. J Clin Invest. 1990;85(6): 1793–8.
22. Kim YH, Verlander JW, Matthews SW, et al. Intercalated cell H+/OH- transporter expression is reduced in Slc26a4 null mice. Am J Physiol Renal Physiol. 2005;289(6):F1262–72.
23. Pech V, Pham TD, Hong S, et al. Pendrin modulates ENaC function by changing luminal HCO3. J Am Soc Nephrol. 2010;21(11):1928–41.

24. Wesson DE, Dolson GM. Augmented bidirectional HCO3 transport by rat distal tubules in chronic alkalosis. Am J Physiol. 1991;261(2 Pt 2):F308–17.
25. Verlander JW, Hassell KA, Royaux IE, et al. Deoxycorticosterone upregulates PDS (Slc26a4) in mouse kidney: role of pendrin in mineralocorticoid-induced hypertension. Hypertension. 2003;42(3): 356–62.
26. Wagner CA, Finberg KE, Stehberger PA, et al. Regulation of the expression of the Cl-/anion exchanger pendrin in mouse kidney by acid-base status. Kidney Int. 2002;62(6):2109–17.
27. Satlin LM, Carattino MD, Liu W, Kleyman TR. Regulation of cation transport in the distal nephron by mechanical forces. Am J Physiol Renal Physiol. 2006;291(5):F923–31.
28. Bhalla V, Hallows KR. Mechanisms of ENaC regulation and clinical implications. J Am Soc Nephrol. 2008;19(10):1845–54.
29. Woda CB, Bragin A, Kleyman TR, Satlin LM. Flow-dependent K+secretion in the cortical collecting duct is mediated by a maxi-K channel. Am J Physiol Renal Physiol. 2001;280(5):F786–93.
30. Ahn KY, Park KY, Kim KK, Kone BC. Chronic hypokalemia enhances expression of the H(+)-K(+)-ATPase alpha 2-subunit gene in renal medulla. Am J Physiol. 1996;271(2 Pt 2):F314–21.
31. Luke RG. Effect of adrenalectomy on the renal response to chloride depletion in the rat. J Clin Invest. 1974;54(6):1329–36.
32. Madias NE, Adrogue HJ, Cohen JJ. Maladaptive renal response to secondary hypercapnia in chronic metabolic alkalosis. Am J Physiol. 1980;238(4):F283–9.
33. Kassirer JP, London AM, Goldman DM, Schwartz WB. On the pathogenesis of metabolic alkalosis in hyperaldosteronism. Am J Med. 1970;49(3):306–15.
34. Javaheri S, Kazemi H. Metabolic alkalosis and hypoventilation in humans. Am Rev Respir Dis. 1987;136(4):1011–6.
35. Javaheri S, Nardell EA. Severe metabolic alkalosis: a case report. Br Med J (Clin Res Ed). 1981;283(6298):1016–7.
36. Eiro M, Katoh T, Watanabe T. Use of a proton-pump inhibitor for metabolic disturbances associated with anorexia nervosa. N Engl J Med. 2002;346(2):140.
37. Kirsch BM, Sunder-Plassmann G, Schwarz C. Metabolic alkalosis in a hemodialysis patient—successful treatment with a proton pump inhibitor. Clin Nephrol. 2006;66(5):391–4.
38. Hoglund P, Haila S, Socha J, et al. Mutations of the Down-regulated in adenoma (DRA) gene cause congenital chloride diarrhoea. Nat Genet. 1996;14(3): 316–9.
39. Aichbichler BW, Zerr CH. Santa Ana CA, Porter JL. Fordtran JS Proton-pump inhibition of gastric chloride secretion in congenital chloridorrhea N Engl J Med. 1997;336(2):106–9.
40. Babior BM. Villous adenoma of the colon. Study of a patient with severe fluid and electrolyte disturbances Am J Med. 1966;41(4):615–21.
41. Weise WJ, Serrano FA, Fought J, Gennari FJ. Acute electrolyte and acid-base disorders in patients with ileostomies: a case series. Am J Kidney Dis. 2008;52(3):494–500.
42. DeFoor W, Minevich E, Reeves D, Tackett L, Wacksman J, Sheldon C. Gastrocystoplasty: long-term followup. J Urol. 2003;170(4 Pt 2):1647–9.
43. Bates CM, Baum M, Quigley R. Cystic fibrosis presenting with hypokalemia and metabolic alkalosis in a previously healthy adolescent. J Am Soc Nephrol. 1997;8(2):352–5.
44. Shaer AJ. Inherited primary renal tubular hypokalemic alkalosis: a review of Gitelman and Bartter syndromes. Am J Med Sci. 2001;322(6):316–32.
45. Simon DB, Lifton RP. The molecular basis of inherited hypokalemic alkalosis: Bartter's and Gitelman's syndromes. Am J Physiol. 1996;271(5 Pt 2):F961–6.
46. Zelikovic I, Szargel R, Hawash A, et al. A novel mutation in the chloride channel gene, CLCNKB, as a cause of Gitelman and Bartter syndromes. Kidney Int. 2003;63(1):24–32.
47. Cruz DN, Shaer AJ, Bia MJ, Lifton RP, Simon DB. Gitelman's syndrome revisited: an evaluation of symptoms and health-related quality of life. Kidney Int. 2001;59(2):710–7.
48. Schwartz WB, Relman AS. Metabolic and renal studies in chronic potassium depletion resulting from overuse of laxatives. J Clin Invest. 1953;32(3): 258–71.
49. Garella S, Chazan JA, Cohen JJ. Saline-resistant metabolic alkalosis or "chloride-wasting nephropathy". Report of four patients with severe potassium depletion Ann Intern Med. 1970;73(1):31–8.
50. Lifton RP, Dluhy RG, Powers M, et al. A chimaeric 11 beta-hydroxylase/aldosterone synthase gene causes glucocorticoid-remediable aldosteronism and human hypertension. Nature. 1992;355(6357):262–5.
51. Torpy DJ, Mullen N, Ilias I, Nieman LK. Association of hypertension and hypokalemia with Cushing's syndrome caused by ectopic ACTH secretion: a series of 58 cases. Ann N Y Acad Sci. 2002;970:134–44.
52. Islam M, Paul RV. Correction of metabolic alkalosis by potassium chloride in ectopic adrenocorticotropic hormone syndrome. Am J Kidney Dis. 1996;28(4): 610–3.
53. Auchus RJ. The genetics, pathophysiology, and management of human deficiencies of P450c17. Endocrinol Metab Clin North Am. 2001;30(1):101–19.
54. Mantero F, Armanini D, Opocher G, et al. Mineralocorticoid hypertension due to a nasal spray containing 9 alpha-fluoroprednisolone. Am J Med. 1981;71(3):352–7.
55. Warnock DG. Liddle syndrome: genetics and mechanisms of Na+channel defects. Am J Med Sci. 2001;322(6):302–7.
56. Stewart PM, Wallace AM, Valentino R, Burt D, Shackleton CH, Edwards CR. Mineralocorticoid activity of liquorice: 11-beta-hydroxysteroid dehydrogenase deficiency comes of age. Lancet. 1987;2(8563):821–4.

57. Morineau G, Sulmont V, Salomon R, et al. Apparent mineralocorticoid excess: report of six new cases and extensive personal experience. J Am Soc Nephrol. 2006;17(11):3176–84.
58. Cogan MG, Carneiro AV, Tatsuno J, et al. Normal diet NaCl variation can affect the renal set-point for plasma pH-(HCO3-) maintenance. J Am Soc Nephrol. 1990;1(2):193–9.
59. Madias NE, Levey AS. Metabolic alkalosis due to absorption of "nonabsorbable" antacids. Am J Med. 1983;74(1):155–8.
60. Beall DP, Scofield RH. Milk-alkali syndrome associated with calcium carbonate consumption. Report of 7 patients with parathyroid hormone levels and an estimate of prevalence among patients hospitalized with hypercalcemia. Medicine (Baltimore). 1995; 74(2):89–96.
61. Hulter HN, Peterson JC. Acid-base homeostasis during chronic PTH excess in humans. Kidney Int. 1985;28(2):187–92.
62. McAuliffe JJ, Lind LJ, Leith DE, Fencl V. Hypoproteinemic alkalosis. Am J Med. 1986;81(1): 86–90.
63. Madias NE, Ayus JC, Adrogue HJ. Increased anion gap in metabolic alkalosis: the role of plasma-protein equivalency. N Engl J Med. 1979;300(25):1421–3.

10 Respiratory Acid–Base Disorders

Biff F. Palmer

Introduction

In order to ensure normal function of cellular enzymes the acid–base status of the body is carefully regulated to maintain the arterial pH between 7.35 and 7.45. Similarly, cell pH is regulated within normal limits that vary from cell to cell, but are generally between 7.0 and 7.3. This regulation occurs in the setting of continuous production of acidic metabolites and is accomplished by intracellular and extracellular buffering processes in conjunction with respiratory and renal regulatory mechanisms. This chapter discusses the respiratory regulatory mechanisms and the pathologic disturbances that arise when such mechanisms go awry.

Buffer Systems in Regulation of pH

Under normal circumstances, humans are confronted by an ongoing acid challenge. The normal diet contains components which upon metabolism are converted to acid or alkali. In addition, there is a small daily production of organic acids such as acetic acid, lactic acid, and pyruvic acid. Lastly, there is a small amount of acid generated by the excretion of alkali into the stool. Under normal circumstances, daily net acid production is approximately 1 mEq of H^+ per kilogram body weight.

The most immediate defense against the addition of acid or alkali to the body is intracellular and extracellular buffers. Buffer systems serve to minimize the change in pH during the addition of acid or base equivalents, but do not remove acid/alkali from the body. The most important buffer system is that of HCO_3/CO_2. The pivotal role of this system stems from its high concentration. The HCO_3/CO_2 system is an open buffer system, which means that one of the members of the buffer pair can enter or leave the system. A closed buffer system, by contrast, is one in which neither member of the buffer pair can enter or leave, such that the concentration of total buffer is fixed. In the case of the HCO_3/CO_2 buffer system, the CO_2 concentration is maintained at a constant level set by respiratory control. Addition of acid leads to conversion of HCO_3 to CO_2 according to the reaction:

$$HA + NaHCO_3 = NaA + H_2O + CO_2.$$

HCO_3 is consumed, but CO_2 concentration does not change because this is maintained constant by respiration. The net result is that the H^+ generated is no longer free and pH changes are minimal.

While buffers minimize the changes in pH upon acid/alkali addition, they do not serve to

B.F. Palmer, M.D. (✉)
UT Southwestern Medical Center,
5323 Harry Hines Blvd, Dallas, TX 75390, USA
e-mail: biff.palmer@utsouthwestern.edu

D.B. Mount et al. (eds.), *Core Concepts in the Disorders of Fluid, Electrolytes and Acid-Base Balance*,
DOI 10.1007/978-1-4614-3770-3_10, © Springer Science+Business Media New York 2013

remove the acid or alkali from the body. This is accomplished by the lungs and kidneys working in concert. The lungs regulate the CO_2 tension, while the kidneys regulate the HCO_3 concentration. While the HCO_3/CO_2 system is not the only buffer system, all buffer systems in the extracellular system are in equilibrium at a common pH. Because the concentration of HCO_3 is far greater than that of other buffers, changes in the HCO_3/CO_2 buffer pair can easily titrate other buffer systems and thus set pH. To understand how the lungs and kidneys function in concert, it is useful to look at the Henderson-Hasselbalch equation:

$$\text{pH} = 6.1 + \log\left[\frac{\text{HCO}_3}{0.03} \times \text{pCO}_2\right].$$

From this equation, it can be seen that pH is determined by the ratio of HCO_3–CO_2. Thus, an increase in the pCO_2 of the blood will lead to a decrease in the blood pH which is called a respiratory acidosis. Conversely, a decrease in the pCO_2 will increase the pH of the blood leading to respiratory alkalosis. A decrease in the HCO_3 concentration lowers pH (metabolic acidosis) and an increase in the HCO_3 concentration raises pH (metabolic alkalosis). It can also be seen from the Henderson-Hasselbalch equation that similar proportional changes in HCO_3 concentration and pCO_2 will have no effect on the logarithm term and thus have no effect on pH. Thus, if HCO_3 concentration is halved from 24 to 12 and pCO_2 is halved from 40 to 20, pH remains unchanged.

In general, changes in CO_2 production by peripheral tissues do not affect the pCO_2 because of the lung's ability to markedly increase or decrease the rate of pCO_2 removal. Thus, a primary alteration in the pCO_2 is generally attributable to some change in ventilation. The kidney then responds to this, in an attempt to defend cell pH by moving the HCO_3 concentration in the same direction as the pCO_2. Thus, a primary decrease in pCO_2 causing a primary respiratory alkalosis, will cause the kidney to develop a compensatory metabolic acidosis by lowering the plasma HCO_3 concentration (decreased renal acid excretion).

The lungs serve to defend pH by altering alveolar ventilation which serves to control the pCO_2 of body fluids. An increase in nonvolatile acid production lowers blood pH and HCO_3 concentration (metabolic acidosis). The lungs respond to this fall in pH by lowering the pCO_2 (compensatory respiratory alkalosis). As a result, the fall in blood pH will be less than that which would have occurred in the absence of respiratory compensation. The opposite happens with metabolic alkalosis. If the fractional change in CO_2 tension were similar to that in HCO_3 concentration, blood pH would not change. However, respiratory compensations generally do not return blood pH to normal, and thus the fractional change in CO_2 tension will be less than that in HCO_3 concentration. The normal response of the respiratory system in metabolic acidosis is approximately a 1.2 mmHg decrease in pCO_2 for every 1 mEq/L fall in HCO_3 concentration, while the response to metabolic alkalosis is a 0.6 mmHg increase in pCO_2 for every 1 mEq/L rise in HCO_3 concentration.

The contribution of the respiratory tract in maintaining acid–base homeostasis becomes obvious in view of the large amount of daily cellular CO_2 production. Each day approximately 15,000 mmol of CO_2 are produced by cellular metabolism. Under physiologic conditions, CO_2 produced during cellular metabolism matches CO_2 excretion by the lungs and arterial CO_2 tension ($PaCO_2$) is maintained relatively constant between 35 and 45 mmHg. Even during exercise, when the amount of CO_2 production increases many fold per unit of time, the respiratory system is able to maintain acid–base balance by increasing minute ventilation.

Respiratory Acidosis

Minute ventilation is the product of tidal volume and respiratory rate. As only the volume of air that reaches the alveoli participates in gas exchange, it is more accurate to use the term alveolar ventilation to describe how the respiratory system participates in acid–base regulation.

$$\text{Alveolar ventilation} = (\text{tidal volume} - \text{dead space}) \times \text{respiratory rate}.$$

The concept of the matching of alveolar ventilation to CO_2 production is central to the understanding of respiratory acidosis:

$$PaCO_2 = \frac{V_{CO_2} k}{V_A}.$$

$$PaCO_2 = \frac{V_{CO_2} k}{V_E - V_D}.$$

where k is a constant, V_E is minute ventilation, and V_D is dead space ventilation. Increased $PaCO_2$ can be the result of increased CO_2 production (V_{CO2}), a decrease in alveolar ventilation (V_A), or both. Both pulmonary and non-pulmonary derangements can lead to an increase in $PaCO_2$ since normal lung function requires the integrated actions of the central and peripheral nervous systems, the musculoskeletal system, and the cardiovascular system.

Respiratory acidosis develops as a result of ineffective alveolar ventilation. This acid–base disorder, which is also called primary hypercapnia, needs to be differentiated from secondary hypercapnia, which develops as a compensatory mechanism in the setting of primary metabolic alkalosis.

Before discussing the different etiologies of hypercapnia, it is helpful to review the basic mechanisms of ventilatory regulation. Arterial hypoxemia and hypercapnia have been recognized as the main physiologic stimuli to respiration [1]. Changes in $PaCO_2$ are sensed as cerebral interstitial pH changes in the chemosensitive areas of the medulla. Changes in arterial oxygen tension are sensed by chemoreceptors in the carotid bodies, which are located close to the carotid artery bifurcation [2]. Among these two, the medullary chemoreceptors are more sensitive and respond to subtle CO_2 tension changes as low as 1 mmHg with stimulation of the respiratory drive [3]. Due to the sensitive regulatory mechanism of medullary chemoreceptors, hypercapnia is almost always due to ineffective alveolar ventilation, and not a result of increased metabolic $PaCO_2$ production.

Primary hypercapnia is clinically recognized by the presence of $PaCO_2$ levels of greater than 45 mmHg on arterial blood gas analysis. Yet, $PaCO_2$ levels of less than 45 mmHg might still be indicative of respiratory acidosis, if a primary metabolic acidosis is not adequately compensated by alveolar ventilation.

A state of chronic CO_2 retention eventually leads to chronic respiratory acidosis [4]. After approximately 24–48 h of acidemia, the kidneys start to compensate for the primary respiratory acid–base disorder by elevating the serum bicarbonate concentration. This is accomplished by increasing H^+ secretion in the proximal and distal nephron segments [5–7]. In chronic respiratory acidosis, each increase of 1 mmHg in $PaCO_2$ leads to an approximately 0.3 mEq/L compensatory increment of plasma bicarbonate level by the kidneys [7].

Etiology of Respiratory Acidosis

The development of respiratory acidosis is usually multifactorial. Major causes of CO_2 retention include diseases or malfunction within any element of the respiratory system, including the central and peripheral nervous systems, the respiratory muscles, the thoracic cage, the pleural space, the airways, and the lung parenchyma. The following six factors should be considered in the differential diagnosis of acute and chronic respiratory acidosis: inhibition of the medullary respiratory center, disorders of the chest wall and the respiratory muscles, airway obstruction, disorders affecting gas exchange across the pulmonary capillary, increased CO_2 production and mechanical ventilation.

Increased CO_2 Production

Increased levels of CO_2 can be found in physiological as well as pathophysiological settings. Physical activity, shivering, fever, hyperthyroidism, as well as prolonged seizure activity can lead to increased CO_2 production. Yet, increased metabolic CO_2 production alone rarely leads to hypercapnia. Chemosensitive areas of the medulla respond to elevated CO_2 levels, which are sensed as interstitial pH changes, by increasing the respiratory drive. The large ventilatory reserve of most patients allows alveolar ventilation to increase in proportion to the amount of additional CO_2 produced. Increased production can only play a role in the pathophysiology of respiratory acidosis when alveolar ventilation is fixed as in a patient receiving controlled mechanical ventilation.

The administration of large amounts of carbohydrates to a mechanically ventilated patient can lead to increased CO_2 production particularly when glycogen stores are replete. In this setting pyruvate generated from the metabolism of glucose coupled with acetylcoenzyme A leads to increased lipogenesis. The shunting of these metabolites toward fatty acid synthesis increases the activity of the tricarboxylic acid cycle with resultant increased generation of CO_2 [8].

Inhibition of the Medullary Respiratory Center

Anesthetics, sedatives, and opiates cause hypercapnia by decreasing the respiratory drive. Patients with chronic hypercapnia may develop worsening hypercapnia and respiratory failure if they use high flow rates of supplemental oxygen, as hypoxemia serves as an important stimulus for respiratory drive in these patients.

Disorders of the Respiratory Muscles and Chest Wall

Electrolyte disturbances such as severe hypokalemia or hypophosphatemia may lead to hypercapnia secondary to muscle weakness. Neurologic diseases like spinal cord injury, myasthenia gravis, Guillain–Barré syndrome, poliomyelitis, amyotrophic lateral sclerosis, and multiple sclerosis are other causes that may lead to hypercapnia due to respiratory muscle weakness.

Airway Obstruction

Hypercapnia can result in the setting of acute upper airway obstruction with foreign bodies as frequently observed in the pediatric age range or with vomitus in patients who cannot control their airways due to altered mental status, unconsciousness, or neurologic diseases.

Disorders Affecting Gas Exchange Across the Pulmonary Capillary

Any clinical disorder that impairs gas exchange in the alveoli can lead to hypoxemia and hypercapnia. Exacerbation of underlying lung disease, acute pulmonary edema, pneumonia, and adult respiratory distress syndrome are the most common causes.

Mechanical Ventilation

In the intensive care setting, mechanically ventilated patients can develop primary respiratory acidosis if the ventilator settings do not allow proper exhalation of CO_2. Increasing the respiratory rate or the tidal volume both increases alveolar ventilation and corrects primary hypercapnia. Table 10.1 presents the causes of acute and chronic respiratory acidosis in accordance with their usual mode of onset and duration.

Clinical Manifestations of Respiratory Acidosis

Acute respiratory acidosis manifests with a variety of neurologic symptoms [9]. The severity of symptoms depends on the magnitude of hypercapnia and hypoxemia as well as the rapidity with which the respiratory acidosis develops. All patients with hypercapnia will also be hypoxemic when breathing room air as a result of decreased oxygen uptake. In disease states, hypoxemia often occurs earlier and is more prominent than hypercapnia due to the fact that CO_2 diffuses much more rapidly across the alveolar capillaries than does oxygen. In the setting of parenchymal disease of the lung, there is also preferential ventilation of less involved areas allowing for more CO_2 excretion. Additional oxygen cannot be taken up since hemoglobin is nearly saturated in these areas.

Table 10.1 Causes of acute and chronic respiratory acidosis

1. Increased CO_2 production
2. Inhibition of the medullary respiratory center
(a) Drugs: opiates, anesthetics, sedatives
(b) Administration of oxygen in chronic hypercapnia
(c) Central sleep apnea
(d) Extreme obesity (Pickwickian syndrome)
(e) Central nervous system lesions
(f) Metabolic alkalosis (although hypercapnia is an appropriate response to the rise in pH)
3. Disorders of the respiratory muscles and chest wall
(a) Acute
• Muscle weakness: myasthenia gravis crisis, Guillain-Barré syndrome, severe hypokalemia or hypophosphatemia
(b) Chronic
• Muscle weakness: spinal cord injury, poliomyelitis, amyotrophic lateral sclerosis, multiple sclerosis, myxedema
• Kyphoscoliosis
• Extreme obesity
4. Upper airway obstruction
(a) Acute
• Aspiration of foreign body or vomitus
• Obstructive sleep apnea
• Laryngospasm
5. Disorders affecting gas exchange across the pulmonary capillary bed
(a) Acute
• Exacerbation of underlying lung disease
• Adult respiratory distress syndrome
• Acute pulmonary edema
• Severe asthma or pneumonia
• Pneumothorax or hemothorax
(b) Chronic
• Chronic obstructive pulmonary disease
• Extreme obesity

Hypercapnic encephalopathy is a clinical syndrome that usually starts with irritability, headache, mental cloudiness, apathy, confusion, anxiety, restlessness, and can progress to asterixis, transient psychosis, delirium, and somnolence, and coma. Papilledema and other manifestations of increased intracranial pressure that are collectively named pseudotumor cerebri are occasionally observed in patients with either acute or chronic hypercapnia. The increase in intracranial pressure is in part due to cerebral vasodilation resulting from acidemia. Acute respiratory acidosis is typically much more symptomatic that is acute metabolic acidosis since CO_2 diffuses and equilibrates across the blood-brain barrier much more rapidly than does HCO_3 resulting in a more rapid fall in cerebral spinal fluid and cerebral interstitial pH.

Severe respiratory acidosis may have life-threatening effects on the cardiovascular system. Severe hypercapnia can lead to decreased myocardial contractility, arrhythmias, and peripheral vasodilatation particularly when the blood pH falls to <7.1.

Diagnosis

The diagnosis of primary respiratory acidosis can be made by the presence of acidemia and hypercapnia on arterial blood gas analysis. Sometimes the differentiation between acute and chronic hypercapnia can be a challenging task. Obtaining a detailed clinical history and performing a physical exam not only helps to make this distinction, but will also elicit the underlying etiology.

Changes in the serum chemistries can aid in the diagnosis of respiratory acidosis. Acute hypercapnia is associated with several effects that lead to an immediate small rise in the serum HCO_3 concentration. First, the decrease in pH that accompanies acute respiratory acidosis increases H^+ binding to albumin. This effect will cause a fall in the anion gap and a slight rise in the serum HCO_3 concentration. Second, a small amount of H^+ enters parenchymal cells in exchange for Na^+ and K^+ also contributing to a small increase in extracellular HCO_3 concentration. Third, the high CO_2 tension is immediately transmitted into red blood cells, where in the presence of carbonic anhydrase, H_2CO_3 is generated. This acid dissociates and the H^+ binds to hemoglobin leaving HCO_3 in the cytoplasm of the red cell. Hemoglobin can bind a considerable amount of H^+ due to the rich histidine content of the molecule. As the HCO_3 concentration rises, it exits from the cell in exchange for plasma Cl^-, a process termed the red cell $HCO_3^-Cl^-$ shift. The net effect of these changes is that in acute respiratory acidosis the plasma HCO_3 concentration increases by 1 mM for each 10 mmHg elevation in $PaCO_2$.

In chronic respiratory acidosis, the increase in plasma HCO_3 concentration is higher due to compensatory renal mechanisms. The chronic elevation in CO_2 leads to intracellular acidosis in proximal tubular cells increasing H^+ secretion resulting in accelerated HCO_3 reabsorption. The retention of $NaHCO_3$ leads to slight expansion of the extracellular fluid compartment and causes increased renal excretion of NaCl so as return volume back to normal. The net effect is an increase in serum HCO_3 and decreased Cl^- concentration. In chronic respiratory acidosis, there is a 3–4 mEq/L increase in HCO_3 for each 10 mmHg elevation in $PaCO_2$. Higher or lower plasma HCO_3 concentrations suggest the presence of mixed respiratory and metabolic acid–base disorders.

Treatment of Acute Respiratory Acidosis

The mainstay of treatment in acute respiratory acidosis is to recognize and treat the underlying cause whenever possible [10]. Patients with acute respiratory acidosis are primarily at risk of hypoxemia rather than hypercapnia or acidemia. Thus, immediate therapeutic efforts should focus on establishing and securing a patent airway in order to provide adequate oxygenation. If the patient is in coma, severely obtunded, extremely hypercapnic ($PaCO_2$ greater than 80 mmHg), or severely acidemic (blood pH less than 7.10), assisted ventilation should be initiated promptly. In emergency situations, the clinician should provide a high inspired oxygen tension to all patients with acute respiratory acidosis; concerns that this measure will further depress ventilation are unfounded. Indeed, maximal PaO_2 levels must be assured for those found apneic, in cardiac arrest, or unconscious from carbon monoxide poisoning.

Although the primary aim of therapy is to restore ventilation in acute respiratory acidosis, the administration of $NaHCO_3$ may allow the pH to be partially corrected in settings where the pCO_2 cannot be rapidly corrected. In patients with status asthmaticus, a lower ventilatory rate and peak inspiratory pressure may be required to minimize barotrauma to the lung but at the expense of a persistently higher pCO_2. Small amounts of $NaHCO_3$ can help prevent excessive falls in blood pH in this setting. The downside of such therapy is infusion of $NaHCO_3$ can result in increased CO_2 production causing a further increase in pCO_2 when ventilation cannot be increased.

Treatment of Chronic Respiratory Acidosis

Patients with chronic respiratory acidosis suffer from hypoxemia in addition to hypercapnia. The primary therapeutic goal in these patients is to ensure adequate oxygenation. Unfortunately, in most cases the underlying disease cannot be removed. The appropriate treatment of chronic respiratory acidosis depends on the underlying disease.

Clinicians should be careful in prescribing drugs, which might suppress the central ventilatory drive.

Excessive oxygen should be avoided as it might lead to worsening hypoventilation. Chronic respiratory acidosis is accompanied by a progressive insensitivity to the stimulatory effect of CO_2 and hypoxemia becomes an increasingly important factor in driving ventilation. In general, the hypoxic drive to ventilation remains adequate as long as the PaO_2 does not exceed 60 mmHg. Oxygen flow rates of 2 L/min by nasal canula deliver an inspired oxygen concentration of 23–28 % and improve PaO_2 values to levels of 50–60 mmHg in many patients with chronic respiratory failure. Use of continuous low-flow oxygen therapy is indicated in patients with severe hypoxemia (PaO_2 less than 55 mmHg) as it has been shown to diminish the severity of cor pulmonale, and improve the quality of life [11, 12].

Many patients with chronic respiratory acidosis have an underlying lung disease and are at risk of developing worsening hypercapnia and hypoxia during episodes of acute worsening of pulmonary functions as with the development of pneumonia. In case mechanical ventilation is required to ensure adequate ventilation, care should be taken to lower the $PaCO_2$ carefully and slowly as there is the risk of overshoot alkalemia due to the presence of a high HCO_3. The kidneys must excrete the HCO_3 in order to normalize the acid–base status. This excretion will not occur when effective arterial blood volume is reduced either because of salt depletion owing to restricted intake or diuretic therapy or a salt retentive state such as heart failure and cirrhosis. Under such circumstances, increased proximal reabsorption of HCO_3 prevents renal HCO_3 clearance despite the fall in pCO_2. Chronic respiratory acidosis is converted to metabolic alkalosis in a process called posthypercapnic metabolic alkalosis. A high pH in the central nervous system can lead to severe neurologic abnormalities such as seizure and coma [13, 14].

Correction of the superimposed metabolic alkalosis can usually be achieved with saline and discontinuation of loop diuretics if they are being utilized. In edematous patients with heart failure, this is not possible and acetazolamide may have to be used to correct the alkalosis. Acetazolamide inhibits HCO_3 reabsorption due to its ability to inhibit luminal carbonic anhydrase. This enzyme normally catalyzes the dehydration of carbonic acid (produced when filtered bicarbonate reacts with secreted H^+) to water and CO_2 thereby maintaining a favorable concentration gradient for further H^+ secretion. The uncatalyzed dehydration of carbonic acid occurs very slowly. By inhibiting the activity of this enzyme, acetazolamide allows for the concentration of luminal carbonic acid to increase. The resultant increase in H^+ concentration creates an unfavorable concentration gradient for further H^+ secretion. Due to the lipid solubility of acetazolamide, inhibition of intracellular carbonic anhydrase may also contribute to the impairment in proximal HCO_3 reabsorption. Inhibition of the intracellular enzyme will decrease the supply of H^+ available for the secretory process. In either case, decreased secretion of H^+ will inhibit reabsorption of filtered HCO_3 and thus cause the kidney to at least partially correct the metabolic alkalosis. The magnitude of the bicarbonaturia is directly related to the serum HCO_3 concentration. As the HCO_3 concentration falls, the clinical effectiveness of the drug declines in a parallel fashion. As a result, only rarely does the plasma HCO_3 concentration return to normal.

A potential problem that is associated with the use of carbonic anhydrase inhibitors in patients with lung disease is a worsening of hypercapnia. Carbonic anhydrase is normally present within red blood cells and is involved in CO_2 movement into red cells in peripheral tissues and movement from red cells into the alveoli in the lungs. Thus, carbonic anhydrase inhibition can prevent red cell uptake of pCO_2 in peripheral tissues and can prevent pCO_2 release in the lung. The latter can lead to an increase in pCO_2 of the arterial blood, while the former leads to an even further increase in pCO_2 in peripheral tissues. Generally, patients with normal lungs can respond to this by increasing respiration and preventing the increase in the pCO_2 of the arterial blood. However, patients with lung disease cannot respond adequately and further increases in arterial pCO_2 as well as even larger increases in tissue pCO_2 may be dangerous to the patient.

Respiratory Alkalosis

Primary respiratory alkalosis results from hypocapnia and is defined by a $PaCO_2$ of less than 35 mmHg in the setting of alkalemia. Primary respiratory alkalosis needs to be differentiated from secondary hypocapnia, which is a compensatory mechanism in the setting of primary metabolic acidosis.

Etiology

An increase in alveolar ventilation relative to CO_2 production gives rise to respiratory alkalosis (Table 10.2). Since changes in CO_2 production are negligible almost all cases of hypocapnia result from increased CO_2 elimination which is the equivalent of increased alveolar hyperventilation.

Table 10.2 Causes of hypocapnia

1. Hypoxemia	
	(a) High altitudes
	(b) Pulmonary disease
2. Pulmonary disorders	
	(a) Pneumonia
	(b) Interstitial pneumonitis
	(c) Fibrosis
	(d) Pulmonary edema
	(e) Pulmonary embolism
	(f) Vascular disease
	(g) bronchial asthma
	(h) Pneumothorax
3. Cardiovascular disorders	
	(a) Congestive heart failure
	(b) Hypotension
4. Metabolic disorders	
	(a) Acidosis (diabetic, renal, or lactic)
	(b) Hepatic failure
5. Central nervous system disorders	
	(a) Psychogenic or anxiety-induced hyperventilation
	(b) Central nervous system infection
	(c) Central nervous system tumors
6. Drugs	
	(a) Salicylates
	(b) Methylxanthines
	(c) β(Beta)-adrenergic agonist
	(d) Progesterone
7. Miscellaneous	
	(a) Fever
	(b) Sepsis
	(c) Pain
	(d) Pregnancy

In the large majority of cases, primary hypocapnia reflects pulmonary hyperventilation due to increased ventilatory drive. The latter might result from signals arising from the lung, the peripheral chemoreceptors (carotid and aortic), the brain stem chemoreceptors, or influences originating in other centers of the brain. The response to CO_2 of the brain stem chemoreceptors can be augmented by systemic diseases (e.g., sepsis, liver disease), pharmacological agents, anxiety, volition, and other influences. Hypoxemia is a major stimulus to pulmonary ventilation, but PaO_2 values less than 60 mmHg are required to elicit this effect consistently.

Primary hypocapnia is probably the most frequent acid–base disturbance encountered. In critically ill patients, its presence might be a grave prognostic sign, especially if pCO_2 levels are below 20–25 mmHg [15]. Furthermore, respiratory alkalosis is the most common acid–base abnormality in patients hospitalized in intensive care units, occurring either as the simple disorder or as a component of mixed disturbances.

Hepatic failure is a common and important cause of primary hypocapnia [16]. The severity of hypocapnia correlates with the level of blood ammonia and has prognostic significance. Systemic infections arising from gram-positive and gram-negative bacteria are also a major cause of respiratory alkalosis. Direct stimulation of central chemoreceptors by bacterial toxins from gram-negative organisms accounts, at least in part, for the hyperventilation observed in some patients with sepsis. Thus, unexplained respiratory alkalosis in a hospitalized patient calls for evaluation for the presence of gram-negative sepsis. The presence of respiratory alkalosis can be an important clue to the presence of salicylate intoxication. High progesterone levels (pregnancy) can also cause respiratory alkalosis.

A cause of decreased pCO_2 worth mentioning that is of historical interest is that which occurs during use of acetate containing dialysate. In this setting, there are large fluxes of both acetate and bicarbonate across the dialyzer with little overall net gain in base [17]. Since the acetate dialysate lacks HCO_3, there is diffusion of actual HCO_3 from the blood into the dialysate. In addition, potential HCO_3 is lost from the blood in the form of organic anions such as citrate, lactate, pyruvate, beta-hydroxy-butyrate, and acetoacetate as these anions diffuse across the dialyzer and into the dialysate [18]. The pH of blood exiting the dialysis cartridge does not fall because CO_2 diffuses from the blood as well. Despite this large efflux of potential and actual HCO_3 from the body, there is net gain of alkali due to the greater influx of acetate as it diffuses from the dialysate into the blood and is later metabolized by skeletal muscle and the liver to HCO_3. In response to the diffusive loss of soluble CO_2 and in an attempt to maintain normal blood CO_2 concentration, pulmonary hypoventilation occurs resulting in hypoxemia.

Clinical Manifestation of Respiratory Alkalosis

Mild respiratory alkalosis causes lightheadedness, palpitations, as well as paresthesias of the extremities and the circumoral area [19]. Acute hypocapnia decreases cerebral blood flow and produces decreased acidity in all body fluids as well as hypocalcemia, hypokalemia, and a pH-induced shift of oxyhemoglobin dissociation curve; all these alterations have been implicated as determinants of the clinical manifestations of this acid–base disorder [20, 21]. The acute hypocapnia-induced reduction in cerebral blood flow might reach values lower than 50 % of normal, resulting in an increased lactate output by the brain due to cerebral hypoxia. A reduction in intracranial pressure, which is generally not harmful, and electroencephalographic changes consisting of generalized slowing and high-voltage waves are also present in acute respiratory alkalosis. The effects of acute hypocapnia on the cerebral circulation have been used in the treatment of brain edema resulting from neurosurgical procedures, head trauma, meningitis, and encephalitis. Unfortunately, the hypocapnia-induced reduction in intracranial pressure is short-lasting, and blood flow returns to normal in sustained hypocapnia.

Hypocapnia leads to alkalemia which causes binding of free calcium to albumin in the blood. Thus, patients with acute respiratory alkalosis might present clinically in a similar way to patients with hypocalcemia. Chvostek's and Trousseau's sign are well-known clinical tests, which can be occasionally elicited in patients with acute respiratory alkalosis.

The cardiovascular manifestations of respiratory alkalosis might be also very prominent [22]. A major reduction in cardiac output accompanied by arteriolar vasoconstriction, tissue hypoperfusion, and a large increment in plasma lactate is frequently attributed to severe acute hypocapnia. This syndrome is typically observed in surgical patients under general anesthesia or those having depression of the central nervous system and receiving mechanical respiratory assistance; in all likelihood, it reflects the effects of passive hyperventilation. Normal volunteers with active hyperventilation do not develop clinical manifestations of coronary insufficiency or cardiac arrhythmias. Patients with ischemic heart disease might occasionally develop cardiac arrhythmias, ischemic electrocardiographic changes, and even angina pectoris during acute hypocapnia. None of the previously described hemodynamic effects seems to be present in uncomplicated chronic hypocapnia.

Diagnosis

The diagnosis of respiratory alkalosis is made by evaluating the patient's history, performing a physical exam, and obtaining laboratory data including a blood gas analysis.

Tachypnea or Kussmaul breathing can be detected on physical exam and be the first clue to the presence of a primary respiratory alkalosis or a compensatory respiratory mechanism in the setting of a primary metabolic acidosis. In order to assess if a respiratory alkalosis is adequately compensated, a detailed history needs to be obtained.

Changes in serum electrolytes can aid in the diagnosis of respiratory alkalosis. An acute fall in pCO_2 causes plasma and red blood cell CO_2 tensions to fall. In response, albumin and other non-HCO_3 buffers release H^+ to decrease the plasma HCO_3 concentration. Within red cells the fall in pCO_2 causes hemoglobin to release H^+ and red blood cell HCO_3 concentration also falls. Plasma HCO_3 will enter the red cell in exchange for Cl^-. This HCO_3^--Cl^- shift accounts for the small initial compensatory response in acute respiratory alkalosis in which the HCO_3 concentration falls by 2 mEq/L for every 10 mmHg decrease in pCO_2.

In chronic respiratory alkalosis, the renal HCO_3 reabsorptive capacity decreases and there is a transient HCO_3 diuresis. This process takes 2–3 days to become fully manifest. Once a new steady state is achieved the HCO_3 concentration will have decreased by 4–5 mEq/L for each 10 mmHg fall in pCO_2. A higher or lower value for the plasma HCO_3 concentration suggests the presence of an additional metabolic disorder.

In order to defend extracellular fluid volume in the setting of increased urinary loss of $NaHCO_3$, the kidney retains NaCl. These changes are reflected in the serum electrolytes of patients with chronic respiratory alkalosis in which the Cl^- is typically increased with respect to the serum Na^+ concentration. Another characteristic finding is an increase of 3–5 mEq/L in the serum anion gap. The increased gap is due to the greater fixed negative charge on serum albumin as well as an increase in serum lactate concentration. Lactate production is increased due to a stimulatory effect of high pH on phosphofructokinase, the rate limiting step in the glycolytic pathway.

Treatment

Primary respiratory alkalosis is treated by correcting the underlying cause. A patient with anxiety-hyperventilation syndrome should be treated by providing reassurance. Rebreathing into a paper bag or any other closed system will cause the pCO_2 to increase with each breath taken and lead to a partial correction of hypocapnia and improvement of symptoms. In the rare case where there is no response to conservative management sedatives can be used.

References

1. Berger AJ, Mitchell RA, Severinghaus JW. Regulation of respiration (first of three parts). N Engl J Med. 1977;297:92–7.
2. Fencl V, Miller TB, Pappenheimer JR. Studies on the respiratory response to disturbances of acid–base balance, with deductions concerning the ionic composition of cerebral interstitial fluid. Am J Physiol. 1966;210:459–72.
3. Weinberger SE, Schwartzstein RM, Weiss JW. Hypercapnia. N Engl J Med. 1989;321:1223–31.
4. Brackett Jr NC, Wingo CF, Muren O, Solano JT. Acid–base response to chronic hypercapnia in man. N Engl J Med. 1969;280:124–30.
5. Cogan MG. Chronic hypercapnia stimulates proximal bicarbonate reabsorption in the rat. J Clin Invest. 1984;74:1942–7.
6. Laski ME, Kurtzman NA. Collecting tubule adaptation to respiratory acidosis induced in vivo. Am J Physiol. 1990;258:F15–20.
7. Madias NE, Wolf CJ, Cohen JJ. Regulation of acid–base equilibrium in chronic hypercapnia. Kidney Int. 1985;27:538–43.
8. Covelli HD, Black JW, Olsen MS, Beekman JF. Respiratory failure precipitated by high carbohydrate loads. Ann Intern Med. 1981;95:579–81.
9. Kilburn KH. Neurologic manifestations of respiratory failure. Arch Intern Med. 1965;116:409–15.
10. McFadden Jr ER, Gilbert IA. Asthma. N Engl J Med. 1992;327:1928–37.
11. Anthonisen NR. Long-term oxygen therapy. Ann Intern Med. 1983;99:519–27.
12. Palevsky HI, Fishman AP. Chronic cor pulmonale. Etiology and management. JAMA. 1990;263:2347–53.
13. Rotheram Jr EB, Safar P, Robin E. CNS disorder during mechanical ventilation in chronic pulmonary disease. JAMA. 1964;189:993–6.
14. Kilburn KH. Shock, seizures, and coma with alkalosis during mechanical ventilation. Ann Intern Med. 1966;65:977–84.
15. Mazzara JT, Ayers SM, Grace WJ. Extreme hypocapnia in the critically ill patient. Am J Med. 1974;56:450–6.
16. Mulhausen R, Eichenholz A, Blumentals A. Acid–base disturbances in patients with cirrhosis of the liver. Medicine. 1967;46:185–9.
17. Gotch FA, Sargent JA, Keen ML. Hydrogen ion balance in dialysis therapy. Artif Organs. 1982;6:388–95.
18. Gennari FJ. Acid–base balance in dialysis patients. Kidney Int. 1985;28:678–88.
19. Laffey JG, Kavanagh BP. Hypocapnia. N Engl J Med. 2002;347:43–53.
20. Nevin M, Colchester AC, Adams S, Pepper JR. Evidence for involvement of hypocapnia and hypoperfusion in aetiology of neurological deficit after cardiopulmonary bypass. Lancet. 1987;2:1493–5.
21. Ayres SM, Grace WJ. Inappropriate ventilation and hypoxemia as causes of cardiac arrhythmias. The control of arrhythmias without antiarrhythmic drugs. Am J Med. 1969;46:495–505.
22. Lenfant C, Sullivan K. Adaptation to high altitude. N Engl J Med. 1971;284:1298–309.

Mixed Acid–Base Disorders

11

Jeffrey A. Kraut and Ira Kurtz

Introduction

Mixed acid–base disorders are commonly encountered clinically, particularly in seriously ill patients [1, 2]. If the disturbances have additive effects on blood pH, they can produce more profound alterations in blood pH than single disturbances and therefore have a greater negative impact on organ function [1, 3]. In addition, because of their complexity, their diagnosis and appropriate treatment are more challenging. Thus, it is essential that the clinician is able to recognize when the acid–base parameters reflect a mixed disturbance, and also understand the benefits and complications of treatment.

The present chapter summarizes a systematic approach to the diagnosis of acid–base disorders propounded by the authors and others that facilitates the rapid recognition and precise diagnosis of mixed acid–base disorders [4, 5]. It also presents a structured approach to treatment that takes into account potential complications of therapy.

Approach to Diagnosis of Mixed Acid–Base Disorders

We utilize a systematic approach to the diagnosis of acid–base disorders summarized in Table 11.1 which is based in physiologic principles [4, 6, 7]. As is commonly done, we utilize acid–base parameters obtained from arterial blood in the evaluation of mixed acid–base disorders. Recent studies indicate that when available central venous blood can provide the same information as arterial blood [8]. In addition if the patient manifests a marked decrease in tissue perfusion, acid–base parameters obtained from central venous blood might more truly reflect the acid–base milieu of the cell [9]. Therefore, in patients with a central line, central venous blood gases might be better for monitoring the acid–base status of the patient. However, this remains to be determined.

When analyzing acid–base disorders, it is important to assess the accuracy of the acid–base data which can be accomplished by inserting values for the individual parameters into the mass action equation for the bicarbonate/carbonic acid buffer system. Two forms of the equation exist, the linear (Henderson) and logarithmic (Henderson–Hasselbalch):

$$\text{Henderson} - H^+\left(\text{nEq}/1\right) = 24 \times PaCO_2 / HCO_3^-$$

J.A. Kraut, M.D. (✉)
Dialysis Unit and Department of Nephrology, VHAGLA Healthcare System, David Geffen School of Medicine at UCLA, 11301 Wilshire Blvd, Los Angeles, CA 90073, USA
e-mail: jkraut@ucla.edu

I. Kurtz, M.D., F.R.C.P.(C)
Department of Medicine, Division of Nephrology, University of California at Los Angeles, 10833 Le Conte Ave, Los Angeles, CA 90095, USA

D.B. Mount et al. (eds.), *Core Concepts in the Disorders of Fluid, Electrolytes and Acid-Base Balance*,
DOI 10.1007/978-1-4614-3770-3_11, © Springer Science+Business Media New York 2013

Table 11.1 Stepwise approach to diagnosis of mixed acid–base disorders

1.	Determine if the acid–base parameters available appear correct by inserting values for each of the parameters in either the linear Henderson or logarithmic form (Henderson–Hasselbalch) of the mass action equation for the bicarbonate–carbonic acid buffer system at equilibrium. Henderson: H^+ (nEq/l) = $24 \times PaCO_2/HCO_3^-$ Henderson–Hasselbalch: pH = $6.1 + HCO_3^-/0.03\ PaCO_2$
2.	Obtain a good history and perform a complete physical examination searching for clues to the presence of particular acid–base disorder
3.	Determine, if possible, the dominant acid–base disturbance present. Then assess whether the secondary response or compensatory response to the disturbance is appropriate.
4.	Calculate the serum anion gap: $Na^+ - HCO_3^- + Cl^-$ using the value for the individual obtained when there was no acid–base abnormality. If not available use mean for particular clinical laboratory.
5.	Examine serum potassium concentration to quickly subcategorize causes of normal anion gap metabolic acidosis and assess potassium stores to gauge the impact of treatment of acid–base disorder.
6.	Measure urinary Na^+, K^+, Cl^- to determine urine anion gap for assessment of ammonium excretion in the presence of hyperchloremic acidosis. If urine anion gap is positive, confirm low urine ammonium excretion by assessment of urine osmolal gap[a]. Measure urine pH to exclude certain renal tubular acidoses.
7.	Measure urine Cl^- in patients with dominant metabolic alkalosis to quickly subcategorize causes of metabolic alkalosis into Cl^--responsive and Cl^--resistant forms[a].

[a] These studies are not necessary to determine the type of mixed acid–base disorder present but will be helpful in further evaluation of individual components of the mixed acid–base disorder

$$\text{Henderson–Hasselbalch} - \text{pH} = 6.1 + \log HCO_3^- / 0.03 \times PaCO_2$$

Values for blood pH and $PaCO_2$ are obtained from the blood gas laboratory, while serum total CO_2 concentration is determined in the chemistry laboratory. Total CO_2 is measured by acidifying the specimen and determining the total CO_2 released. Since HCO_3^- represents ~95 % of the total CO_2 concentration, total CO_2 can be substituted for HCO_3^- in the equation. Errors can occur during the sampling or measuring process of any of the individual parameters [10].

The Henderson formula can be used at the bedside, but requires the translation of blood pH into hydrogen ion concentration [4, 11]. The Henderson–Hasselbalch equation requires the use of logarithms, but the common availability of calculators or smart phones with the formula embedded makes utilization of this form of the equation a reasonable alternative.

Next, a good history should be obtained and a careful physical examination performed looking for clues to the presence of a particular acid–base disorder or combination of acid–base disorders. This is valuable since a particular set of acid–base parameters can be the result of either a single disturbance or a combination of more than one disturbance. For example, patients with poorly controlled diabetes receiving diuretics or subject to gastric drainage might be expected to have both metabolic acidosis and metabolic alkalosis. Individuals taking aspirin or who are septic commonly will have metabolic acidosis and respiratory alkalosis. Patients with severe congestive heart failure in the presence of hypoxemia and impaired tissue perfusion can have metabolic and respiratory acidosis.

Each of the primary acid–base disturbances elicits a compensatory or adaptive response which is an integral part of the disturbance. Therefore, one must know the time course and nature of the compensatory responses for each of the primary disturbances. Values falling outside the appropriate range suggest the presence of a mixed acid–base disturbance.

The compensatory responses to each of the primary acid–base disorder, with the exception of mild chronic hypocapnia and hypercapnia, are thought to return blood pH towards, but not completely to, normal. Therefore, a normal blood pH in the face of abnormal values for either $PaCO_2$ or serum [HCO_3^-] should alert the clinician to the possibility that a mixed metabolic and respiratory acid–base disturbance is present. With both mild chronic hypocapnia and chronic hypercapnia, blood pH can fall within the normal range in the absence of a coexisting acid–base disturbance [12].

The next step is to calculate the serum anion gap and if elevated the rise in the serum anion gap termed the delta anion gap. The serum anion gap which represents the difference between unmeasured anions and unmeasured cations can be calculated by subtracting the sum of $HCO_3^- + Cl^-$ from that of Na^+. The serum anion gap is useful in detecting errors in the measurement of electrolytes, or the presence of hematological malignancies, and bromide or iodide intoxication [13, 14]. However, it is most frequently utilized for the diagnosis of acid–base disturbances, and is of particular value in the diagnosis of mixed metabolic acid–base disturbances.

Examination of the serum potassium concentration is used in the determination of the cause of normal anion gap (hyperchloremic) metabolic acidosis [15] since the disorders causing this form of metabolic acidosis often have differing effects on serum potassium concentration. In addition, since treatment of mixed acid–base disorders will often have an impact on total potassium stores and/or the serum potassium concentration, it is necessary to assess potassium homeostasis with all acid–base disorders [16].

Impairment of renal bicarbonate generation underlies several of the disorders producing normal anion gap metabolic acidosis. Direct measurement of urine NH_4^+ is the best way of assessing alterations in renal bicarbonate generation. However, a simple inexpensive method of measuring urine NH_4^+ is not available in most clinical laboratories. Therefore two indirect methods have been developed to assess urinary NH_4^+ excretion: the urine anion [17] and urine osmolal gap [7, 17].

The urine anion gap, analogous to the serum anion gap, represents the difference between unmeasured anions and unmeasured cations in the urine. It is given by

$$\text{Urine anion gap} = Na^+ + K^+ - Cl^-$$

During metabolic acidosis, normally, the urine anion gap is negative by ~30 mEq/l reflecting the excretion of ample quantities of positively charged NH_4^+ in the urine [18]. When the urine anion gap is positive, this reflects reduced urinary ammonium excretion and is commonly seen in disorders with impaired renal acid excretion.

A positive value for the urine anion gap, while consistent with reduced urine NH_4^+ excretion, can also be observed in the presence of the large urinary excretion of anions such as ketones [19–21]. Therefore, the urinary osmolal gap was derived to circumvent this problem. The urine osmolal gap will give an assessment of urinary NH_4^+ excretion even in the face of large urinary anion excretion. It is therefore a valuable tool to confirm impaired urinary NH_4^+ excretion. However, it is not generally utilized as the initial assessment of urinary NH_4 because of the additional urinary parameters that have to be measured for its calculation.

The urine osmolal gap is determined as follows:

$$\text{Measured urine osmolality} - 2'[Na^+ + K^+] + \text{urine urea nitrogen}\left(\text{mg/dl}\right)/2.8 + \text{glucose}\left(\text{mg/dl}\right)/18$$

Dividing the value obtained by 2 will give an approximation of urinary ammonium excretion.

Measurement of urine pH can also be of use in confirming defective urinary acidification in some cases of renal tubular acidosis. In individuals with fully intact renal acidification, urine pH should fall below 5.5 when serum [HCO_3^-] is reduced to ≤20 mEq/l [22]. Therefore, a value above this level can indicate impaired renal acidification. However, many clinicians do not routinely use the urine pH to assess renal acid excretion, because it can be elevated with chronic

Table 11.2 Primary acid–base disorders

Disorder	Initiating mechanism	Time course and limits of compensatory response	Comments
Metabolic acidosis	Decreased serum HCO_3^-	($PaCO_2$ mmHg) Acute: ~8 h or less 0.8 × Δ(DELTA) Serum [HCO_3^-] Chronic > 24 h 1–1.3 Δ(DELTA) Serum [HCO_3^-] or 1.5 Serum [HCO_3^-] + 8 ± 2	$PaCO_2$ < 10 mmHg rare
Metabolic alkalosis	Increased serum HCO_3^-	Chronic > 24 h or more 0.4–0.7 Δ(DELTA) Serum [HCO_3^-]	Change in $PaCO_2$ less consistent than with metabolic acidosis
Respiratory acidosis	Increased $PaCO_2$	(Δ serum [HCO_3^-] mEq/l) Acute ~10 min 0.1 Δ(DELTA) $PaCO_2$ Chronic 3–5 days 3.5–5 Δ(DELTA) $PaCO_2$	In some human studies values different from those found in animals
Respiratory alkalosis	Decreased $PaCO_2$	Acute ~10 min 0.2 Δ(DELTA) $PaCO_2$ Chronic 3–5 days 0.5 Δ(DELTA) $PaCO_2$	Blood pH may be within normal limits as a result of compensation

metabolic acidosis even in the face of appropriate urinary NH_4^+ excretion. Conversely, it can be reduced appropriately despite impaired renal acid excretion as seen with hyporeninemic hypoaldosteronism [23].

In patients with metabolic alkalosis, measurement of urinary Cl^- will be effective in categorizing the causes of the metabolic alkalosis. Based on the urine chloride, metabolic alkalosis can be divided into Cl^--responsive (urine Cl^- < 20 mEq/l) or Cl^--resistant forms (urine Cl > 20 mEq/l) [24].

In summary, this systematic approach integrates information obtained from the history and physical examination, examines the appropriateness of the compensatory responses to individual primary acid–base disorders, assesses changes in the serum anion gap, and utilizes ancillary information obtained from the measurement of serum potassium concentration, urinary electrolytes, and urine pH as necessary to facilitate the rapid diagnosis of mixed acid–base disorders.

Definition of Simple and Mixed Acid–Base Disorders

As shown in Table 11.2, there are four primary acid–base disturbances. Metabolic disturbances are initiated by changes in serum [HCO_3^-], whereas respiratory disturbances are initiated by changes in $PaCO_2$. Metabolic acidosis is due to a primary reduction in serum [HCO_3^-] and metabolic alkalosis is initiated by a primary elevation in serum [HCO_3^-]. Respiratory acidosis is due to a primary elevation in $PaCO_2$, whereas respiratory alkalosis is due to a primary reduction in $PaCO_2$.

Soon after initiation of either metabolic or respiratory acid–base disturbances, there is a change in the same direction of the other variable (i.e., with metabolic disturbances a compensatory change in $PaCO_2$ and with respiratory disturbances a compensatory change in serum [HCO_3^-]) termed the secondary adaptive or compensatory response. As noted previously, this response tends to return blood pH towards but not completely to normal with the exception of some cases of mild chronic hypocapnia or chronic hypercapnia [12] in which blood pH can fall within the normal range.

The temporal characteristics and the magnitude of the adaptive responses for each of the primary acid–base disturbances have been determined empirically [25–28] and are indicated in Table 11.2. Although the adaptive response is assumed to attenuate the change in blood pH induced by the primary change in serum [HCO_3^-] or $PaCO_2$, studies by Madias et al. [29, 30] have shown that under certain circumstances the ventilatory response to metabolic acidosis and alkalosis can actually exacerbate the underlying deviation in blood pH. These data are intriguing, and indicate that changes in ventilation in response to metabolic disturbances may in some cases be maladaptive. Further discussion of this issue is beyond the scope of this chapter.

A single or simple acid–base disturbance is diagnosed when the compensatory response to either a metabolic or respiratory disorder falls within the predicted range. Mixed metabolic and respiratory acid–base disturbances are present when the compensatory response to the primary acid–base disturbance falls outside of the expected range for that disturbance. It is important to emphasize, however, that even when a set of acid–base parameters are consistent with a simple acid–base disturbance, this does not exclude the presence of a mixed acid–base disorder.

Since acute and chronic forms of the primary acid–base disturbances have been described, mixed acid–base disorders can also be due to the combination of acute and chronic forms of a particular acid–base disturbance [31]. Acute and chronic respiratory acidosis and acute and chronic respiratory alkalosis are the most frequent combination of acute and chronic acid–base disorders usually described [31]. Recent studies indicate that metabolic acidosis can also be divided into acute and chronic forms, suggesting that acute and chronic metabolic acidosis is an additional mixed acid–base disturbance.

Mixed disturbances comprising two or more metabolic disturbances can be present. Examples include normal and high anion gap metabolic acidosis and high anion gap metabolic acidosis and metabolic alkalosis. As noted above, and described in detail below, assessment of the serum anion gap will be useful in detecting these mixed metabolic acid–base disturbances [2, 14]. More than two disturbances can also be present and this situation is most commonly due to the concordance of more than one metabolic acid–base disturbance in association with a respiratory acid–base disturbance. These complex acid–base disorders are relatively common in seriously ill patients.

Compensatory Responses to Primary Acid–Base Disorders

As noted above, recognition of a mixed metabolic and respiratory acid–base disturbance or acute and chronic forms of a respiratory or metabolic disturbance requires knowledge of the time course and limits of the compensatory response to each of the primary acid–base disturbances [4].

Metabolic Acidosis

Within minutes of the development of metabolic acidosis, there is an increase in ventilation resulting in a reduction in $PaCO_2$ [28, 32]. Studies performed both in animals and humans have delineated the nature of the relationship between serum bicarbonate and $PaCO_2$ in uncomplicated metabolic acidosis during its evolution, in the acute and chronic steady state, and during its repair [27, 32–36]. In the seminal human studies of Albert et al. [27], the relationship between serum bicarbonate and $PaCO_2$ was established in children with diarrhea or ketoacidosis of more than 24 h in duration. An analysis of the data revealed a linear relationship between the severity of the acidosis as reflected by serum bicarbonate concentration and level of ventilation as reflected by $PaCO_2$. An equation including the 95 % confidence limits for the data revealed that expected $PaCO_2$ for any given value of serum HCO_3^- could be derived using the formula

$$1.5\left[HCO_3^-\right] + 8 \pm 2$$

familiarly referred to as the Winters formula. This relationship has been confirmed by several other studies [32]. Studies by others of patients with metabolic acidosis associated with chronic renal failure and diabetic ketoacidosis have indicated that the appropriate $PaCO_2$ can be calculated by multiplying $1.2 \times \Delta$(DELTA) HCO_3^- [37].

The importance of a steady state for serum $[HCO_3^-]$ for a period of ~24 h or greater to elicit the maximal ventilatory response was established by Pierce et al. [32]. They studied 35 patients with cholera during the development, steady state, and repair of metabolic acidosis. They found a delay in the development of the maximum ventilatory response during the rapid development of metabolic acidosis and a similar delay during the rapid correction with base administration. Formulae for determining the relationship between serum [HCO_3^-] and $PaCO_2$ during the development and recovery phase were not given. However, the relationship between $PaCO_2$ and serum [HCO_3^-] in the steady-state phase reported in this study was similar to that of other investigators.

In a careful study of six patients with metabolic acidosis of 8 h or less duration (mean arterialized HCO_3 of 19 mEq/l) induced by oral administration of ammonium chloride the slope of the relationship between Δ(DELTA)$PaCO_2$ and Δ(DELTA)HCO_3 was 0.85 [28] suggesting that the ventilatory response to acute metabolic acidosis was less brusque than with chronic metabolic acidosis, consistent with the observations of Pierce et al. [32].

These data have been criticized by Adrogue and Madias because differences between control and experimental data were not used [38]. Indeed, in their animal studies, Adrogue and Madias found that the slope of the relationship between serum [HCO_3^-] and $PaCO_2$ was less than 1 [33]. They suggested that further studies are necessary to delineate the nature of the ventilatory response to metabolic acidosis.

In the absence of experimental studies in humans that encompass the full range of serum [HCO_3^-] likely to be encountered clinically and in which differences between control and experimental phases are used to determine the ventilatory response, it will be impossible to reconcile the differences between the clinical studies in the literature and experimental results of Madias and Adrogue [33].

In summary, it is reasonable to assume that with both short-term and chronic metabolic acidosis, the relationship between changes in HCO_3^- and $PaCO_2$ will be ~1:1. With more acute metabolic acidosis (~8 h or less) it can be slightly less than 1 (0.85:1) and with more chronic acidosis it can be 1 or greater (1–1.3:1). The $PaCO_2$ in the chronic steady state can also be obtained using the Winters formula which results in values similar to that achieved by multiplying 1–1.3 × Δ(DELTA) serum [HCO_3^-].

Metabolic Alkalosis

With the onset of metabolic alkalosis, changes in interstitial hydrogen concentration in the cerebrospinal fluid are associated with suppression of ventilation and a rise in $PaCO_2$ [39, 40]. Although it is presumed this response occurs immediately, the nature of the respiratory response to acute increments in serum [HCO_3^-] concentration is not well established. Indeed, some of the acute studies of metabolic alkalosis induced by sodium bicarbonate infusion or gastric drainage showed a minimal hypoventilation [41]. The failure to detect hypoventilation in these studies was attributed to other factors inducing an increase in ventilation, since several of the patients did manifest an increase in $PaCO_2$ 2–3 h after development of the alkalosis. However, a full time course similar to that described for metabolic acidosis was not established, so it is difficult to determine the length of time necessary for the maximal ventilatory response to be expressed. In the absence of data, it is reasonable to assume that the evolution of the ventilatory response with metabolic alkalosis is similar to that of metabolic acidosis, requiring several hours of steady-state values till the maximal respiratory response is established.

The nature of the respiratory response to steady-state elevations in serum HCO_3^- of >24 h has been determined both in animals and humans [33, 39, 40, 42]. The bulk of the studies show consistent hypoventilation, although some have indicated that the hypoventilation can be minimal or even absent [33, 39, 41, 42]. In studies in which suppression of ventilation was absent, this was attributed to changes in serum potassium concentration affecting the respiratory response or stimulation of ventilation by factors such as anxiety.

Javeheri et al. [39] studied six normal patients with mild to moderate metabolic alkalosis (serum HCO_3^-, 34–42 mEq/l) induced by diuretic administration for 7 days. In all patients $PaCO_2$

rose and the relationship between steady-state $PaCO_2$ and serum HCO_3^- was 0.7 + 20 ± 1.5. Similarly, Ypersalle de Stihou examined the ventilatory response to metabolic alkalosis induced in dialysis patients for more than a week [42]. These investigators found a slope of the relationship of 0.9. Madias and Adrogue studied the respiratory response to metabolic alkalosis in dogs with alkalosis produced by different methods for several days. They found that the slope of the relationship between $PaCO_2$ and HCO_3 was 0.7 [33]. Interestingly, in both the studies of Madias and Adrogue [33] and Yperselle de Strihou [42] the slope of the relationship was similar to that described for chronic metabolic acidosis. Although experimental data were not available to assess the ventilatory response in normal individuals with serum HCO_3^- concentrations above 45 mEq/l, Javaheri and Kazemi [40] examined the ventilatory response in a number of patients reported in the literature with values as high as 62 mEq/l. They found that the slope of the relationship between $PaCO_2$ and HCO_3^- was also ~0.7.

At present, most clinicians estimate the expected $PaCO_2$ by multiplying 0.5–0.7 × Δ(DELTA) serum [HCO_3^-] [43]. If the increment in $PaCO_2$ is greater than this a coexisting respiratory acidosis is said to be present. By contrast, if the $PaCO_2$ is less than predicted from this relationship, then a coexisting respiratory alkalosis is said to be present. As with chronic metabolic acidosis, this relationship assumes a steady-state hyperbicarbonatemia for a defined period of time, and therefore use of any of the formula describing the predicted changes in $PaCO_2$ may not hold either during the generation or during the correction of the alkalosis [39].

Respiratory Acidosis

A rise in $PaCO_2$ elicits compensatory changes in serum [HCO_3^-]. This increment in serum HCO_3^- occurs in two steps [25, 43, 44]. Acutely, a rise in serum [HCO_3^-] occurs which is complete within 5–15 min of the elevation in $PaCO_2$ [26]. This increment arises from titration of non-bicarbonate buffers. As the hypercapnia persists, generation of bicarbonate by the kidney causes serum [HCO_3^-] to rise further and this process is complete within 3–5 days [45]. Careful studies in experimental animals have shown that serum [HCO_3^-] rises acutely by ~2 mEq/l for every 10 mmHg increase in $PaCO_2$ [46] and by an average of ~3.5 mEq/l [45] with more prolonged hypercapnia. Data from humans is conflicting. Early studies had indicated that the adaptation to respiratory acidosis in man was similar to that of dogs [26, 47]. Other investigators have found slight deviation from this relationship. Martinu et al. evaluated 18 stable patients with chronic obstructive lung disease and CO_2 retention ($PaCO_2$ 45–78 mmHg) [12]. These investigators found that for every 10 mmHg increment in $PaCO_2$, serum [HCO_3^-] rose by ~5.1 mEq/l. Although it is not possible to reconcile these results, at present most clinicians utilize the relationship established in the earlier studies of humans and animals to assess whether the appropriate compensatory response to acute and chronic respiratory acidosis is appropriate.

The previous studies involved examination of a relatively small number of patients with chronic hypercapnia, but it is conceivable that studies involving larger numbers of patients could give us further insight into the biological variability in the compensatory response to respiratory acidosis.

The rise in serum [HCO_3^-] in response to acute changes in $PaCO_2$ may vary depending on the starting level of serum [HCO_3^-]: for example, in dogs, the relationship between Δ(DELTA) serum [HCO_3^-] and Δ(DELTA) $PaCO_2$ was steeper the lower the starting serum [HCO_3^-] whether this was caused by metabolic acidosis or chronic hypocapnia [48]. Similar studies have not been performed in humans.

Mixed respiratory disturbances can result when acute respiratory acidosis is superimposed upon chronic respiratory acidosis. Acid–base parameters can also appear to represent the combination of acute and chronic respiratory acidosis if acid–base parameters are sampled at a time point intermediate between the achievement of the acute and chronic steady state, i.e., between 10 and 15 min and 3 days [31, 44, 49].

Respiratory Alkalosis

Similar to the compensatory response to a rise in $PaCO_2$, the response to a fall in $PaCO_2$ occurs in two steps [44]. Data from animal studies indicated that initially, alkaline titration of non-bicarbonate buffers results in a fall in serum [HCO_3^-] which is complete within 5–10 min and results in a fall of ~2 mEq/l for every 10 mmHg decrement in $PaCO_2$ [46]. Subsequently, as the hypocapnia persists, suppression of renal net acid excretion causes retention of protons and a further reduction in serum [HCO_3^-] that averages ~5 mEq/l [50]. This adaptive response is complete within 3–5 days. As noted, blood pH may be minimally perturbed with mild chronic hypocapnia and therefore, a normal blood pH in a patient with chronic hypocapnia does not necessarily indicate a mixed acid–base disorder.

Studies in humans with chronic hypocapnia induced by hyperbaric hypoxia gave similar results: serum [HCO_3^-] was reduced by ~4.1 mEq/l for every 10 mmHg decrement in $PaCO_2$ [51]. Interestingly, the nature of the relationship between changes in $PaCO_2$ and serum [HCO_3^-] remained the same in individuals made acidotic prior to induction of hypocapnia (4.2 vs. 4.1 mEq/l).

Mixed acute and chronic respiratory alkalosis can result when acute hypocapnia is superimposed upon chronic hypocapnia. Also, acid–base parameters consistent with the combination of acute and chronic hypocapnia can also be present if acid–base data is obtained at points intermediate between the completion of the acute and chronic adaptive phases.

Mixed Metabolic and Respiratory Acid-Base Disturbances

From the forgoing discussion, recognition of mixed metabolic and respiratory disturbances necessitates identification of the primary disturbance followed by determination of the appropriateness of the compensatory response. Either the metabolic or respiratory disorder can be the dominant disorder; however, in some cases it will be difficult to dissect out which is the dominant disturbance. Be that as it may, metabolic and respiratory acid–base disturbances frequently coexist in hospitalized patients [1, 52]. In one study, ~8 % of 110 consecutive patients admitted to a general medical ward had the combination of metabolic acidosis or alkalosis and respiratory acidosis or alkalosis [53]. By contrast, in an analysis of more than 10,000 consecutive blood gases, Anderson et al. [1] found approximately 409 (4 %) with alkalemia. Over 30 % of these had mixed acid–base disturbances. A classification of mixed metabolic and respiratory disturbances and the common clinical situations in which they are encountered are shown in Table 11.3.

Metabolic Acidosis and Respiratory Acidosis

This combination of acid–base disorders is diagnosed in patients with dominant metabolic acidosis, if the ventilatory response to the metabolic acidosis is less than expected. Again, it is important to emphasize that to correctly identify that a mixed metabolic acidosis and respiratory acidosis is present one must be cognizant of the duration of the disorder: The fall in $PaCO_2$ with very acute metabolic acidosis is less than with chronic metabolic acidosis and the increment in serum [HCO_3^-] with acute respiratory acidosis is less than with chronic respiratory acidosis.

This combination of acid–base disorders is often found in seriously ill patients in the intensive care unit with lactic acidosis accompanied by respiratory failure, in those with cardiorespiratory failure undergoing cardiopulmonary resuscitation [54], and in those with severe congestive heart failure [52].

If respiratory acidosis is the dominant disturbance, the presence of concomitant metabolic acidosis can be surmised by finding that the serum [HCO_3^-] is lower than predicted for the respiratory disturbance. The finding of an elevated serum anion gap will also point to the coexistence of a high anion gap metabolic acidosis (see below).

Whether metabolic acidosis or respiratory acidosis is the dominant disturbance, this

Table 11.3 Common mixed metabolic and respiratory acid–base disorders

Disorders	Common causes	Effect on blood pH	Relative frequency
Metabolic acidosis and respiratory acidosis	Shock with respiratory distress syndrome; severe congestive heart failure	Additive	+++
Metabolic acidosis and respiratory alkalosis	Aspirin intoxication; sepsis	Counterbalancing	+++
Metabolic alkalosis and respiratory acidosis	COPD with right-sided heart failure	Counterbalancing	+++
Metabolic alkalosis and respiratory alkalosis	Decompensated liver disease; mild congestive heart failure	Additive	++
Acute and chronic respiratory acidosis	Acute on chronic respiratory failure	Additive	+++
Acute and chronic respiratory alkalosis	Decompensated liver disease; sepsis	Additive	++
High anion gap metabolic acidosis and metabolic alkalosis	Metabolic alkalosis due to vomiting with hypotensive-induced lactic acidosis	Counterbalancing	+++
High anion gap and normal anion gap metabolic acidosis	Diabetic ketoacidosis; metabolic acidosis of chronic kidney disease	Additive	+++

combination of acid–base disturbances often produces the most severe degrees of acidemia and represents a difficult therapeutic challenge.

Metabolic Acidosis and Respiratory Alkalosis

This combination is frequent in patients with sepsis associated with lactic acidosis [55], those with aspirin intoxication [56], or in hypotensive patients with decompensated liver disease [57]. Circulating factors found with sepsis or decompensated liver disease and metabolites of aspirin independently stimulate the respiratory center producing respiratory alkalosis. If metabolic acidosis is the dominant disturbance, a coexisting respiratory alkalosis can be diagnosed by finding that the fall in $PaCO_2$ is greater than expected in patients with uncomplicated metabolic acidosis. Conversely, if respiratory alkalosis is the dominant disturbance, a coexisting metabolic acidosis can be detected by evidence that the fall in serum [HCO_3^-] is greater than expected. As noted above, use of formulae for determining the appropriateness of the compensatory response requires knowledge of the duration of the acid–base disturbances.

An additional clue to the presence of a coexisting metabolic acidosis is a substantial elevation in the serum anion gap (see below). Although the increment in blood pH with respiratory alkalosis causes a rise in the serum anion gap, this value is low: ~15 mEq/l for every 0.1 unit change in blood pH [58]. This value might be slightly greater with chronic respiratory alkalosis, but still results in a minor change in the serum anion gap [50].

Metabolic Alkalosis and Respiratory Acidosis

This combination is common in patients with chronic obstructive lung disease and complicating heart failure receiving diuretics and in patients with metabolic alkalosis who develop some pulmonary process [59, 60]. Of note, in patients with dominant respiratory acidosis, the development of a superimposed metabolic alkalosis can worsen the hypercapnia. Therefore, amelioration of the metabolic alkalosis is of benefit in improving pulmonary function [59]. This combination of acid–base disturbance can be diagnosed in a patient with dominant metabolic alkalosis, if the compensatory increment in $PaCO_2$ is greater than anticipated. Conversely, in an individual with dominant respiratory acidosis, this combination can be diagnosed if the rise in serum [HCO_3^-] for any given increment in $PaCO_2$ is greater than expected.

Metabolic Alkalosis and Respiratory Alkalosis

The frequent combination of respiratory alkalosis and metabolic alkalosis in these patients is often due to the presence of infection or liver disease that can cause respiratory alkalosis [57], and the common use of diuretics, gastric drainage, and administration of blood containing citrate, factors that can produce metabolic alkalosis [61].

This combination of acid–base disorders is diagnosed in a patient with metabolic alkalosis if the rise in $PaCO_2$ is less than anticipated for the degree of hypercarbonatemia. Conversely, this combination of acid–base disorders can also be diagnosed when the degree of hypocarbonatemia for a given reduction in $PaCO_2$ is less than anticipated [1].

Whatever the dominant primary acid–base disturbance, this combination of acid–base disorders produces the most severe alkalemia and can have an important impact on morbidity and mortality [1].

Mixed Acute and Chronic Respiratory Acidosis

This combination is extremely frequent in patients with chronic respiratory acidosis who develop acute exacerbations of their lung disease [62]. Prior knowledge of the presence of chronic hypercapnia will be important in detecting this combination. The serum [HCO_3^-] at a given level of $PaCO_2$ will be lower than anticipated for a patient with chronic elevations in $PaCO_2$. Similar acid–base parameters can be found in patients with chronic hypercapnia and metabolic acidosis, emphasizing the value of historical information in detecting this combination. As noted previously, the change in serum [HCO_3^-] in response to acute hypercapnia will be affected by the preexisting level of serum [HCO_3^-] [48]. However, precise formulae to derive the expected change at any given value of serum [HCO_3^-] are not available.

Acute and Chronic Respiratory Alkalosis

This combination is less common than acute and chronic respiratory acidosis. As with acute and chronic respiratory acidosis, a history of prior chronic hypocapnia will be useful in detecting this combination of disorders. The decrement in serum [HCO_3^-] will be less than anticipated for the degree of hypocapnia in a patient with chronic respiratory alkalosis. A similar set of acid–base parameters can be observed in patients with chronic hypocapnia and metabolic alkalosis.

Mixed Metabolic Acid–Base Disturbances

Mixed metabolic disturbances including normal and high anion gap metabolic acidosis or metabolic alkalosis and high anion gap metabolic acidosis are frequent. Calculation of serum anion gap and the Δ(Delta) serum anion gap will be useful in the diagnosis of either combination of metabolic acid–base disturbances. However, examination of the serum anion gap will not be useful in detecting the combination of a normal anion gap acidosis and metabolic alkalosis since with this combination the changes in electrolyte pattern are the mirror images of each other.

Serum Anion Gap

Metabolic acidosis is classically divided into normal (hyperchloremic acidosis) and high anion gap metabolic acidosis based on the impact on the accumulating acid on the serum anion gap [63]. The concept of the serum anion gap was derived from the recognition that total serum cations and total serum anions in the blood must always remain equal to ensure charge balance. Thus, the sum of circulating cations—sodium, potassium, calcium, magnesium, and cationic proteins—must equal the sum of circulating anions—chloride, bicarbonate, anionic proteins, inorganic phosphate, sulfate, and organic anions:

$$Na^+ + K^+ + Ca^{++} + Mg^{++} + Protein^+ + OC^+ = Cl^- + HCO_3^- + Protein^- + HPO_{4-}^{\ 2} / HPO_4^- + SO_{4-}^{\ 2} + OA^-$$

Since routinely only sodium, potassium, chloride, and bicarbonate were measured, the remaining circulating cations (UC) and anions (UA) were unmeasured:

$$Na^{+} + K^{+} + UC = Cl^{-} + HCO_3^{-} + UA$$

Rearranging the equation to highlight the known electrolytes, we obtain

$$Na^{+} + K^{+} - \left(Cl^{-} + HCO_3^{-}\right) = UA - UC$$

Under normal circumstances, the total unmeasured anions exceed the total unmeasured cations; therefore there is an anion gap. Serum potassium concentration is often omitted from the formula so that the serum anion gap is most commonly given as

$$Na^{+} - \left(Cl^{-} + HCO_3^{-}\right)$$

The serum anion gap in healthy subjects measured in mEq/l is variable both between individuals and among different laboratories with values varying from 11±2.5 (range, 6–16) [64] to as low as 6±3 mEq/l (range, 3–9) [13, 65]. Low values are reported in clinical laboratories using ion-specific electrodes to measure serum chloride [65]. Given that the average anion gap and range of normal values vary among different clinical laboratories, the clinician should know the range of normal for the particular clinical laboratory [65]. Furthermore, even within a specific clinical laboratory the value for the serum anion gap among individuals can differ. Therefore, to use the serum anion gap correctly it is necessary to know the baseline value for a particular individual.

Several factors can affect the serum anion gap. Most frequently, a reduction in serum albumin concentration will cause a decrease in the serum anion gap that averages 2.3 mEq/l for every 1 g/dl reduction in serum albumin concentration [66]. Less commonly, the serum anion gap can be reduced and rarely even be negative in the presence of certain hematological malignancies, and bromide or iodide intoxication [14].

An increment in the serum anion gap has been reported with severe hyperphosphatemia [67] and an increase in serum albumin concentration resulting from hemoconcentration [68]. Indeed, the presence of a marked elevation in the serum anion gap (>45 mEq/l) is usually accompanied by increases in both parameters [69]. Rarely, accumulation of anionic paraproteins can also raise the serum anion gap [14].

However, far and away the most common cause of an elevated serum anion gap is accumulation in the blood of the anion of a non-chloride containing acid such as lactate or beta hydroxybutyrate [17] and therefore it is worthwhile to briefly explore the impact of different accumulating acids on the serum anion gap.

When the acid accumulating in blood is hydrochloric acid, then no change in the serum anion gap would be expected, since the number of chloride ions retained in the blood is equivalent to the number of protons (as reflected by the decrement in serum bicarbonate concentration). This type of metabolic acidosis is termed normal anion gap (hyperchloremic). The serum anion gap in this type of acidosis actually can fall slightly reflecting titration of circulating proteins [70]. On the other hand, if the accumulating acid contains an anion other than chloride such as one of the ketones, then the fall in serum [HCO_3^-] is associated with an equivalent elevation in serum anion gap and this acidosis is termed a high anion gap acidosis. [14]. This simple concept enabled the clinician to divide the metabolic acidoses into two apparently nonoverlapping categories. Also, because with high anion gap acidoses there were equivalent but opposite changes in the anion gap and serum bicarbonate concentration, when the decrement in the serum bicarbonate concentration (Δ(DELTA)HCO_3^-) exceeded the rise in the serum anion gap (Δ(DELTA)AG), it was possible to infer that a coexisting hyperchloremic acidosis was present. Conversely, if the Δ(DELTA) serum [HCO_3^-] was less than the Δ(DELTA)AG, then a coexisting metabolic alkalosis (or other hyperbicarbonatemic disorder) can be said to be present [2, 71, 72].

However, careful experimental studies have indicated that a 1:1 relationship between the Δ(DELTA)AG and Δ(DELTA) serum [HCO_3^-] does not always exist [73, 74]. Within first 60 min of accumulation of organic acids in the blood, the accumulating protons titrates serum bicarbonate and the accompanying anion is retained to

Table 11.4 Δ(DELTA)anion gap/Δ(DELTA)HCO_3^- in common metabolic acidoses

Disorder	Δ(DELTA)AG/Δ(DELTA)HCO_3^-	Type of metabolic acidosis
Ketoacidosis	<1:1 – 1:1	High anion gap, mixed, normal anion gap
L-lactic acidosis	1:1 – 1.6:1	High anion gap
D-lactic acidosis	<1:1 – 1.6:1	High anion gap, mixed, normal anion gap
Chronic renal failure	<1:1 – 1:1	High anion gap, mixed, normal anion gap
Salicylate intoxication[a]	1:1	High anion gap
Methanol/ethylene glycol intoxication[a]	1:1	High anion gap

[a]The nature of the Δ(DELTA)AG/Δ(DELTA)HCO_3^- and the type of acidoses observed have not been studied in detail in these disorders

maintain charge balance producing a 1:1 relationship between the Δ(DELTA) serum [HCO_3^-] and Δ(DELTA)AG [73, 75]. However, as the metabolic acidosis persists for more than a few hours a discontinuity between these variables can evolve as protons are buffered intracellularly while the accompanying anion can remain in the extracellular compartment. As a result, the ratio can rise to 1.6–1.8 [73]. This ratio can remain elevated, return to 1:1, or fall below 1:1 depending on whether excretion of the accompanying anion is equivalent to or is greater than the synthesis of bicarbonate. With the latter circumstances, some component of hyperchloremic metabolic acidosis can develop [74, 76, 77]. Infusion of saline during the treatment of the acid–base disorder can accelerate the urinary excretion of anions and thereby the conversion of the electrolyte pattern to that of a hyperchloremic acidosis [76, 77]. The presence of significant renal impairment or volume contraction might lessen excretion of the offending anions and tend to maintain a high anion gap metabolic acidosis.

As indicated in Table 11.4, L-lactic acidosis typically has a ratio above 1:1. By contrast, the ratio in diabetic ketoacidosis is usually 1:1 or can fall below 1:1 [74, 76]. Typical Δ(DELTA)AG/Δ(DELTA)HCO_3^- ratios seen in several common acid–base disorders associated with increased acid production or reduced acid and anion excretion are shown in Table 11.4. Knowledge of the type of organic acidosis present, its duration, and other important factors affecting the Δ(DELTA) AG/Δ(DELTA)HCO_3^- such as the level of renal function and type and quantity of fluids administered is important for interpreting these complex mixed metabolic acid–base disorders.

High Anion Gap and Normal Anion Gap Metabolic Acidosis

The coexistence of these acid–base disorders is suggested by a fall in serum [HCO_3^-] that exceeds the increment in the serum anion gap (Δ(DELTA)HCO_3^-/Δ(DELTA) anion gap > 1). This combination of acid–base disorders is frequently observed in patients with chronic kidney disease, those with diabetic ketoacidosis, and in some patients with toluene intoxication or D-lactic acidosis [14, 21, 78]. On the other hand, high and normal anion gap metabolic acidosis has also been described in patients with ketoacidosis or chronic kidney disease who develop diarrhea and in patients with severe diarrhea and associated volume contraction [68].

High Anion Gap Metabolic Acidosis and Metabolic Alkalosis

The coexistence of this combination of acid–base disorders is suggested by the presence of an increase in the serum anion gap that exceeds the fall in serum [HCO_3^-] (Δ(DELTA) anion gap/Δ(DELTA)HCO_3^- > 1) or an elevated serum anion gap in a patient with an elevated serum [HCO_3^-]. However, as described above, because the Δ(DELTA) serum anion gap can exceed the Δ(DELTA)HCO_3^- in some patients with lactic acidosis, the mere presence of a discordance between the Δ(DELTA) anion gap and Δ(DELTA)HCO_3^- in a patient with a metabolic acidosis does not always indicate the coexistence of metabolic alkalosis.

Also, in patients with chloride-responsive metabolic alkalosis a small increment in the serum anion gap (<6 mEq/l) has been described which has been ascribed to the combination of an increase in the total serum albumin concentration and the number of uncovered negative charges [79]. Thus, in the absence of an increment in the serum anion gap that exceeds the change in bicarbonate by more than 6 mEq/l, one cannot be sure that a coexisting high anion gap metabolic acidosis is present.

This combination of acid–base disorders is most commonly observed in patients with metabolic alkalosis complicated by lactic acidosis or in those with any type of high anion gap acidosis complicated by bicarbonate generating process such as vomiting.

Metabolic Alkalosis and Normal Anion Gap Metabolic Acidosis

Examination of the acid–base parameters and serum anion gap in isolation is not helpful in detecting this combination of acid–base disorders because the elevation in serum $[HCO_3^-]$ and concomitant reduction in serum Cl^- characterizing metabolic alkalosis are the exact opposite of changes in these parameters noted with normal anion gap acidosis. Particularly in patients in whom acid–base parameters are normal (which could result from this combination of disorders), it will be difficult to detect mixed metabolic alkalosis and metabolic acidosis. Historical information suggesting the coexistence of disorders such as vomiting and diarrhea that can produce this combination can be helpful in identifying this combination, although with current techniques it would be difficult to prove. Furthermore alterations in serum potassium concentration, either hypokalemia or hyperkalemia, which can occur with these disorders also could suggest the presence of covert acid–base disturbances.

Three or More Acid–Base Disorders

The presence of three independent acid–base disorders is not uncommon in seriously ill patients hospitalized in an intensive care unit. Patients with sepsis having high anion gap metabolic acidosis and respiratory alkalosis who are subject to gastric drainage are very likely to manifest these disorders. Also, patients with congestive heart failure treated with diuretics might manifest metabolic alkalosis, lactic acidosis, and respiratory acidosis [80]. It is of course conceivable that more than three independent acid–base disturbances can be present. For example, metabolic acidosis and metabolic alkalosis could exist with acute and chronic forms of the respiratory disturbances. Alternatively, acute and chronic forms of metabolic acidosis, metabolic alkalosis, and acute and chronic forms of the respiratory disturbances could be present. Identifying more than three acid–base disorders will be increasingly difficult, particularly without prior knowledge of the acid–base status of the patient, duration of the acid–base disorder, and potential contributory factors.

In summary, a careful history and physical examination and careful examination of the serum electrolytes, serum anion gap, and the relationship between serum bicarbonate and $PaCO_2$ will be helpful in detecting mixed acid–base disorders. A blood pH within the normal range (7.38–7.42) in an individual with serum $[HCO_3^-]$ or $PaCO_2$ values which are abnormal (with the possible exception of cases of mild chronic hypocapnia, $PaCO_2 \geq 34$ mmHg and mild chronic hypercapnia, $PaCO_2 \leq 55$ mmHg), should automatically raise the suspicion of a mixed acid–base disorder. Also, a marked elevation in the serum anion gap in a patient with a normal or elevated serum $[HCO_3^-]$ should also raise suspicion of a mixed acid–base disorder. Recognition of the presence of mixed acid–base disorders in the absence of these obvious clues requires careful adherence to the systematic approach to the diagnosis of acid–base disorders described above.

Treatment of Mixed Acid–Base Disorders

Treatment of mixed acid–base disorders is often more complicated than that of simple acid–base disorders, although the goals of therapy are very similar. Improvement in extracellular and intracellular acid–base parameters is usually the

Table 11.5 Treatment of common mixed acid–base disorders

Acid–base disorder	Therapy	Goals of therapy	Comments
Metabolic acidosis and respiratory acidosis	Sodium bicarbonate THAM Dialysis Controlled hyperventilation	Blood pH ~ 7.2 Improvement of intracellular acidosis	Controversy about goals of therapy Sodium bicarbonate therapy has counterproductive effects that may constrain use THAM particularly useful. Watch for hyperkalemia Dialysis helpful with renal failure Hyperventilation usually avoided because of concern about lung injury
Metabolic acidosis and respiratory alkalosis	Base therapy Dialysis	Blood pH ~ 7.2	Cautious use of base to avoid overshoot alkalemia
Metabolic alkalosis and respiratory acidosis	NaCl, KCl Carbonic anhydrase inhibitors Dilute HCl Dialysis	If respiratory acidosis dominant disturbance goal to achieve a $[HCO_3^-]$s which is appropriate for hypercapnia	Role in worsening of respiratory failure unclear Improvement in respiratory function and decrease in $PaCO_2$ important goal
Metabolic alkalosis and respiratory alkalosis	NaCl Carbonic anhydrase inhibitors Dilute HCl Dialysis Controlled ventilation	Blood pH < 7.5	Combination important cause of severe akalemia In intubated patients increase in $PaCO_2$ can be the most rapid way of lessening alkalemia

primary goal. Recent studies have indicated that some acid–base disorders can induce alterations in certain cellular cascades that can contribute to cellular injury [81, 82] and therefore therapy directed against these pathways might be beneficial. However, discussion of this topic is beyond the scope of this chapter. Treatment options for the most commonly observed mixed acid–base disorders are summarized in Table 11.5.

Metabolic and Respiratory Acidosis

The combination of metabolic and respiratory acidosis often produces the most severe degree of acidemia and intracellular acidosis. Studies done both in vitro and in vivo have shown that the decrement in extracellular and intracellular pH are the major factors in producing cellular dysfunction in patients with metabolic and respiratory acidosis [82, 83], although changes in CO_2, independent of its effects on pH, can have deleterious effects on cellular function [84]. The decreased extracellular pH affects binding of important hormones to their receptors [85], affects the concentration of ionized calcium, alters the flux through K channels in the heart and blood vessels, and activates acid-sensing ion channels, while the intracellular acidosis affects the function of critical enzymes and other important cellular proteins [86, 87]. Therefore, amelioration of the acidemia and intracellular acidosis is important. The optimal blood pH desired has been debated and there remains disagreement even among experts [88–91]. A goal of a blood pH ~7.2 seems reasonable since experimental studies show values below this result in reduced cardiac contractility and output, at least in normal animals [92]. Unfortunately, human studies of short duration have not demonstrated these beneficial effects possibly because of adverse effects of bicarbonate administration such as exacerbation of intracellular acidosis [93].

Sodium bicarbonate has been the mainstay of therapy of metabolic acidosis for more than 50 years. However, despite improvement in extracellular pH with bicarbonate therapy, there is no evidence in animal or human studies of significant benefit either in cellular function or outcome [94]. One of the major reasons postulated for this failure has included potential exacerbation of intracellular acidosis and worsening of cellular function resulting from generation of CO_2 during the titration of blood bicarbonate by accumulating protons; the CO_2 traverses the cell membrane more rapidly than bicarbonate leading to an intracellular respiratory acidosis [82, 95]. This complication appears to be more likely when the sodium bicarbonate is given as a bolus, in the presence of reduced tissue perfusion or with impaired respiratory function. Thus, some clinicians avoid bicarbonate administration in patients with metabolic acidosis, particularly when they have any component of respiratory failure.

Since improvement of the acid–base balance still was deemed important, alternatives to sodium bicarbonate have been developed or are under study to improve extracellular and intracellular acid–base parameters including alternative forms of base or base delivery. THAM, Tribonat, and Carbicarb have been developed to improve extracellular acid–base parameters while avoiding or attenuating the generation of CO_2 [96–98]. Various modes of dialysis have been recommended to prevent volume excess from the administered sodium, to attenuate hyperosmolality, and to stabilize extracellular ionized calcium, a modulator of cardiac output and vascular tone that is reduced by an elevation in extracellular pH.

THAM was introduced into clinical practice in 1960 [96]. It buffers protons by virtue of an ammonia side chain and therefore does not generate CO_2. Animal studies had shown that it had less depressive effect on cardiac contractility than bicarbonate and in some cases actually caused an improvement in contractility [99]. Also, in patients with acute metabolic acidosis, it has been shown to be as effective in raising systemic pH and serum $[HCO_3^-]$ as sodium bicarbonate [100]. It can be particularly useful in the treatment of mixed metabolic and respiratory acidosis, since its administration will not generate CO_2, despite impaired pulmonary function [101]. In this regard, this agent has been utilized with success in people with permissive hypercapnia to alleviate the acidemia. Studies of permissive hypercapnia revealed that improvement in blood pH caused a rise in cardiac contractility [101]. Studies of patients with respiratory distress syndrome have also shown the effectiveness of this agent. Paradoxically, one of the complications of THAM therapy reported has been CO_2 retention, the mechanism of which is not clear. However, a study in patients with lactic acidosis in the intensive care unit given either sodium bicarbonate or THAM to those not on respiratory support revealed no difference in $PaCO_2$ [100].

Tribonat is a mixture of THAM, sodium bicarbonate, acetate, and sodium phosphate available only outside the United States [97]. It has been shown to successfully improve acid–base parameters with various acid–base disorders, but has not been shown to be superior to other forms of base.

Carbicarb is a 1:1 mixture of sodium bicarbonate and sodium carbonate [102]. It has been shown to produce substantially less CO_2 than administration of sodium bicarbonate. Animal studies had confirmed more rapid and effective improvement in acid–base parameters, better stabilization of blood pressure, and improved contractility [103]. However, the only published study in humans revealed improvement in cardiac output in a small subset of patients [98]. It has never been approved for clinical use and apparently has been abandoned for further study.

Dialysis

Anecdotal cases of improvement of lactic acidosis when base is provided via various dialytic modalities has led to interest to using dialysis to treat patients with severe metabolic acidosis [104]. Limited large uncontrolled studies of patients with lactic acidosis treated with continuous venovenous hemofiltration demonstrated rapid correction of the metabolic acidosis (within 12h) without severe morbidity [105]. Randomized controlled studies are necessary to demonstrate the benefit of this therapy.

Controlled Hyperventilation

Since lowering of $PaCO_2$ in patients with combined metabolic and respiratory acidosis will attenuate the acidemia and presumably also lessen the degree of intracellular acidosis, on the surface this seems as reasonable option. However, many pulmonologists caution against increased ventilation because of the danger of producing lung injury [106]. Thus, this therapy should be utilized infrequently.

Metabolic Acidosis and Respiratory Alkalosis

Since the respiratory alkalosis causes a rise in intracellular and blood pH, the clinician should be cautious in administering base to patients with this combination of acid-base disorders so as not to produce an overshoot alkalemia. Similarly, the benefits of the prevailing hypocapnia should not be ignored. Intubated patients in whom hypocapnia is lessened will have exacerbation of their acidemia. Elimination of the causes of these disturbances is obviously extremely important.

Metabolic Alkalosis and Respiratory Acidosis

This combination is most commonly observed in patients with chronic lung disease and CO_2 retention treated with diuretics for secondary heart failure. Although the alkalosis will tend to lessen the degree of acidemia, studies by several groups have demonstrated that the superimposition of metabolic alkalosis upon a stable respiratory acidosis can worsen the degree of CO_2 retention [60]. Therefore correction of this acid–base abnormality is important. Since, Cl-responsive forms of metabolic alkalosis are the most common types encountered clinically, administration of sodium and or potassium chloride will result in significant amelioration of the hypercarbonatemia [3]. In patients with significant congestive heart failure or renal impairment in whom sodium chloride administration is deleterious, administration of carbonic anhydrase inhibitors will reduce the bicarbonate reabsorptive threshold and speed the improvement in the metabolic alkalosis [24].

Other options include administration of dilute concentration of hydrochloric acid (0.1 N) [59] and dialysis with a low bicarbonate dialysate [107]. The former is effective, but the acid must be administered via a central vein to avoid venous sclerosis [108] and has potentially serious complications. Dialysis has proved to be useful particularly in patients with coexisting renal failure as it can improve acid–base parameters while removing extracellular fluid and should be considered with severe alkalosis and compromised renal function [107].

Metabolic Alkalosis and Respiratory Alkalosis

The coexistence of these acid–base abnormalities gives rise to the most severe alkalemia. In a study of more than 300 patients with more than 10,000 blood values, overall mortality was ~44 % in patients with metabolic and respiratory alkalosis [1]. Moreover, there was a direct correlation between the severity of the alkalemia and mortality, with mortality approaching 49 % when the blood pH exceeded 7.60. Therefore, aggressive treatment of this combination of acid–base disorders seems warranted. Diuretic administration, infusion of blood products containing citrate as a preservative, or gastric drainage are factors contributing to the development of metabolic alkalosis, whereas infection, hypoxemia, and decompensated liver disease are associated with respiratory alkalosis.

Measures to treat the metabolic akalosis such as administration of sodium or potassium chloride described above can be used, but will take time to be effective. Administration of HCl will be more rapid as would dialysis with a low bicarbonate dialysate as described previously [108, 109]. In intubated patients, increasing dead space or reducing the frequency of ventilation can lead to an increment in CO_2 to reduce blood pH <7.5, values considered safe.

In summary, combinations of various primary acid–base disorders particularly when they have similar effects on blood pH can represent medical emergencies. Therefore, aggressive treatment with frequent monitoring of acid–base parameters is warranted.

References

1. Anderson LE, Henrich WL. Alkalemia-associated morbidity and mortality in medical and surgical patients. South Med J. 1987;80:729–33.
2. Narins RG, Emmett M. Simple and mixed acid-base disorders: a practical approach. Medicine. 1980;59:161–87.
3. Adrogue HJ, Madias NE. Management of life-threatening acid-base disorders 1. N Engl J Med. 1998; 338:107–10.
4. Kraut JA, Madias NE. Approach to the diagnosis of acid-base disorders. Respir Care. 2001;46:392–403.
5. Maccari C, Kamel KS, Davids MR, Halperin ML. The patient with a severe degree of metabolic acidosis: a deductive analysis. Q J Med. 2006;99:475–85.
6. Kurtz I. Acid-base Case Studies. Trafford publishing, Victoria, Canada. 2004;1–143.
7. Kamel KS, Halperin ML. An improved approach to the patient with metabolic acidosis: a need for four amendments. J Nephrol. 2006;S9:S76–85.
8. Treger R, Pirouz S, Kamangar N, Corry D. Agreement between central venous and arterial blood gas measurements in the intensive care unit. Clin J Am Soc Nephrol. 2010;5:390–4.
9. Adrogue HJ, Rashad MN, Gorin AB, Yacoub J, Madias NE. Assessing acid-base status in circulatory failure—differences between arterial and central venous-blood. N Engl J Med. 1989;320:1312–6.
10. Bloom SA, Canzanello VJ, Strom JA, Madias NE. Spurious assessment of acid-base status due to dilutional effect of heparin. Am J Med. 1985;79:528–30.
11. Kassirer JP, Bleich HL. Rapid estimation of plasma carbon dioxide tension from pH and total carbon dioxide content. N Engl J Med. 1965;272:1067–8.
12. Martinu T, Menzies D, Dial S. Re-evaluation of acid-base prediction rules in patients with chronic respiratory acidosis. Can Respir J. 2003;10:311–5.
13. Gabow PA. Disorders associated with an altered anion gap. Kidney Int. 1985;27:472–83.
14. Kraut JA, Madias NE. Serum anion gap: its uses and limitation in clinical medicine. Clin J Am Soc Nephrol. 2006;2:162–74.
15. Adrogue HJ, Madias NE. Changes in plasma potassium concentration during acute acid-base disturbances. Am J Med. 1981;71:456–67.
16. Kamel KS, Quaggin S, Scheich A, Halperin ML. Disorders of potassium homeostasis—an approach based on pathophysiology. Am J Kidney Dis. 1994; 24:597–613.
17. Kim GH, Han JS, Kim YS, et al. Evaluation of urine acidification by urine anion gap and urine osmolal gap in chronic metabolic acidosis. Am J Kidney Dis. 1996;27:42–7.
18. Battle D, Hizon M, Cohen E, Gutterman C, Gupta R. The use of the urinary anion gap in the diagnosis of hyperchloremic metabolic acidosis. N Engl J Med. 1988;318:594–9.
19. Kamel KS, Ethier JH, Richardson RM, Bear RA, Halperin ML. Urine electrolytes and osmolality: when and how to use them. Am J Nephrol. 1990;10: 89–102.
20. Meregalli P, Luthy C, Oetliker OH, Bianchetti MG. Modified urine osmolal gap: an accurate method for estimating urinary ammonium concentration. Nephron. 1995;69:98–101.
21. Carlisle EJF, Donnelly SM, Vasuvattakul S, Kamel KS, Tobe S, Halperin ML. Glue-sniffing and distal renal tubular-acidosis—sticking to the facts. J Am Soc Nephrol. 1991;1:1019–27.
22. Halperin ML, Vasuvattakul S, Bayoumi A. A modified classification of metabolic acidosis. A pathophysiologic approach. Nephron. 1992;60:129–33.
23. Oster JR, Preston RA, Materson BJ. Fluid and electrolyte disorders in congestive heart failure. Semin Nephrol. 1994;14:485–505.
24. Galla JH. Metabolic alkalosis. J Am Soc Nephrol. 2000;11:369–75.
25. Schwartz WB, Brackett NC, Cohen JJ. Defense of the hydrogen ion concentration during acute and chronic hypercapnia: the response to progressive elevation of carbon dioxide tension. Trans Assoc Am Physicians. 1964;77:182–7.
26. Brackett NC, Cohen JJ, Schwartz WB. Carbon dioxide titration curve of normal man—effect of Iicreasing degrees of acute hypercapnia on acid-base equilibrium. N Engl J Med. 1965;272:6–12.
27. Albert MS, Dell RB, Winters RW. Quantitative displacement of acid-base equlibrium in metabolic acidosis. Ann Intern Med. 1967;66:312–22.
28. Wiederseiner JM, Muser J, Lutz T, Hulter HN, Krapf R. Acute metabolic acidosis: characterization and diagnosis of the disorder and the plasma potassium response. J Am Soc Nephrol. 2004;15:1589–96.
29. Madias NE, Schwartz WB, Cohen JJ. The maladaptive renal response to secondary hypocapnia during chronic HCl acidosis in dog. J Clin Invest. 1977;60:1393–401.
30. Madias NE, Adrogue HJ, Cohen JJ. Maladaptive renal response to secondary hypercapnia in chronic metabolic alkalosis. Am J Physiol. 1980;238:F283–7.
31. Cohen JJ, Schwartz WB. Evaluation of acid-base equilibrium in pulmonary insufficiency. An approach to a diagnostic dilemma. Am J Med. 1966;41:163–7.
32. Pierce NF, Fedson DS, Brigham KL, Mitra RC, Sack RB, Mondal A. The ventilatory response to acute base deficit in humans. Ann Intern Med. 1979;72:633–40.
33. Madias NE, Bossert WH, Adrogue HJ. Ventilatory response to chronic metabolic acidosis and alkalosis in the dog. J Appl Physiol. 1984;56:1640–6.
34. Fulop M. A guide for predicting arterial CO2 tension in metabolic acidosis. Am J Nephrol. 1997;17: 421–4.
35. Winters RW, Lowder JA, Ordway NK. Observations on carbon dioxide tension during recovery from metabolic acidosis. J Clin Invest. 1958;37:640–5.

36. Asch MJ, Dell RB, Williams GS, Cohen M, Winters RW. Time course for development of respiratory compensation in metabolic acidosis. J Lab Clin Med. 1969;73:610–5.
37. Bushinsky DA, Coe FL, Katzenberg C, Szidon JP, Parks JH. Arterial PCO2 in chronic metabolic acidosis. Kidney Int. 1982;22:311–4.
38. Adrogue HJ, Madias NE. PCO2 (and [K+])(p) in metabolic acidosis: certainty for the first and uncertainty for the other. J Am Soc Nephrol. 2004;15:1667–8.
39. Javaheri S, Shore NS, Rose B, Kazemi H. Compensatory hypoventilation in metabolic alkalosis. Chest. 1982;81:296–301.
40. Javaheri S, Kazemi H. Metabolic alkalosis and hypoventilation in humans. Am Rev Respir Dis. 1987;136:1011–6.
41. Roberts KE, Poppell JW, Vanamee P, Beals R, Randall HT. Evaluation of respiratory compensation in metabolic alkalosis. J Clin Invest. 1956;35:261–6.
42. de Strihou Y. Frans A: the respiratory response to chronic metabolic alkalosis and acidosis in disease. Clin Sci Mol Med. 1973;45:439–48.
43. Kraut JA, Adrogue HJ, Madias NE. Respiratory and mixed acid-base disorders. In: Brady H, Wilcox C, editors. Therapy in nephrology and hypertension: companion to the kidney. Saunders Philadelphia Pennsylvania 1st ed. 1999;292–302.
44. Ackerman GL, Arruda JAL. Acid-base and electrolyte imbalance in respiratory failure. Med Clin North Am. 1983;67:645–56.
45. Schwartz WB, Brackett NCJ, Cohen JJ. Response of extracellular hydrogen ion concentration to graded degrees of chronic hypercapnia:physiologic limits of defense of pH. J Clin Invest. 1965;44:291–301.
46. Arbus GS, Hebert LA, Levesque PR, Etsten BE, Schwartz WB. Characterization and clinical application of significance band for acute respiratory alkalosis. N Eng J Med. 1969;280:117–23.
47. Brackett NCJ, Wingo CF, Muren O, Solano JT. Acid-base response to chronic hypercapnia in man. N Engl J Med. 1969;280:124–30.
48. Adrogue HJ, Madias NE. Influence of chronic respiratory acid-base disorders on acute CO2 titration curve. J Appl Physiol. 1985;58:1231–8.
49. Robin EG. Abnormalities of acid-base regulation in chronic pulmonary disease with special reference to hypercapnia and extracellular alkalosis. N Engl J Med. 2006;268:917–22.
50. Gennari FJ, Goldstein MB, Schwartz WB. The nature of the renal adaptation to chronic hypocapnia. J Clin Invest. 1972;51:1722–30.
51. Krapf R, Beeler I, Hertner D, Hulter HN. Chronic respiratory alkalosis—the effect of sustained hyperventilation on renal regulation of acid-base-equilibrium. N Engl J Med. 1991;324:1394–401.
52. Aberman A, Fulop M. The metabolic and respiratory acidosis of acute pulmonary edema. Ann Intern Med. 1972;76:173.
53. Palange P, Carlone S, Galassetti P, Felli A, Serra P. Incidence of acid-base and electrolyte disturbances in a general hospital: a study of 110 consecutive admissions. Recenti Prog Med. 1990;81:788–91.
54. Weil MH, Rackow EC, Trevino R, et al. Difference in acid-base state between venous and arterial blood during cardiopulmonary resusitation195. N Engl J Med. 1986;315:153–6.
55. Elisaf M, Theodrou J, Pappas H, Siamopoulos KC. Acid-base and electrolyte abnormalities in febrile patients with bacteremia. Eur J Med. 1993;2:404–7.
56. Gabow PA, Anderson RJ, Potts DE, Schrier RW. Acid-base disturbances in the salicylate intoxicated adult. Arch Intern Med. 1978;138:1481–4.
57. Oster JR, Perez GO. Acid-base disturbances in liver disease. J Hepatol. 1986;2:299–306.
58. Paulson WD. Effect of acute pH change on the serum anion gap. J Am Soc Nephrol. 1996;7:357–64.
59. Brimioulle S, Berre J, Dufaye P, Vincent JLDJP, Kahn RJ. Hydrochloric acid infusion for the treatment of metabolic alkalosis with respiratory acidosis. Crit Care Med. 1989;17:232–6.
60. Bear R, Goldstein M, Phillipson E, Ho M, Hammeke M, Feldman R, Handelsman S, Halperin M. Effect of metabolic alkalosis on respiratory function in patients with chronic obstructive lung disease. Can Med Assoc J. 1977;117:900–3.
61. Hodgkin JE, Soeprono FF, Chan DM. Incidence ofmetabolic alkalemia in hospitalized patients. Crit Care Med. 1980;8:725–8.
62. Cham GWM, Tan WP, Earnest A, Soh CH. Clinical predictors of acute respiratory acidosis during exacerbation of asthma and chronic obstructive pulmonary disease. Eur J Emerg Med. 2002;9:225–32.
63. Emmett M, Narins RG. Clinical use of the anion gap. Medicine. 1977;56:38–54.
64. Frohlich J, Adam W, Golbey MJ, Bernstein M. Decreased anion gap associated with monoclonal and pseudomonoclonal gammopathy. Can Med Assoc J. 1976;114:231–2.
65. Winter SD, Pearson R, Gabow PA, et al. The fall of the serum anion gap. Arch Intern Med. 1990;150:311–6.
66. Feldman M, Soni N, Dickson B. Influence of hypoalbuminemia or hyperalbuminemia on the serum anion gap. J Lab Clin Med. 2005;146:317–20.
67. Kirschbaum B. The acidosis of exogenous phosphate intoxication. Arch Intern Med. 1998;158:405–8.
68. Wang F, Butler T, Rabbani GH, Jones PK. The acidosis of cholera. Contributions of hyperproteinemia, lactic acidemia, and hyperphosphatemia to an increased serum anion gap. N Engl J Med. 1986;315:1591–5.
69. Oster JR, Singer I, Contreras GN, Ahmad HI, Vieira CF. Metabolic acidosis with extreme elevation of anion gap: case report and literature review. Am J Med Sci. 1999;317:38–49.
70. Adrogue HJ, Brensilver J, Madias NE. Changes in plasma anion gap during chronic metabolic acid-base disturbances. Am J Physiol. 1978;235: F291–7.
71. Goodkin DA, Krishna GG, Narins RG. The role of the anion gap in detecting and managing mixed

metabolic acid-base disorders. Clin Endocrinol Metab. 1984;13:333–49.
72. Emmett M. Anion gap interpretation: the old and the new. Nat Clin Pract Nephrol. 2006;2:4–6.
73. Madias NE, Homer SM, Johns CA, Cohen JJ. Hypochloremia as a consequence of anion gap metabolic acidosis. J Lab Clin Med. 1984;104:15–23.
74. Kim HY, Han JS, Jeon US, Joo KW, Earm JH, Ahn C, Kim S, Lee JS, Kim GH. Clinical signficiance of the fractional excretion of anions in metabolic acidosis. Clin Nephrol. 2001;55:448–52.
75. Oh MS, Carroll HJ, Uribarri J. Mechanism of normochloremic and hyperchloremic acidosis in diabetic ketoacidosis. Nephron. 1990;54:1–6.
76. Adrogue HJ, Ecknoyan G, Suki WN. Diabetic ketoacidosis role of the kidney in acid-base homeostasis reevaluated. Kidney Int. 1984;25:591–9.
77. Adrogue HJ, Wilson H, Boyd AE, Suki WN, Eknoyan G. Plasma acid-base patterns in diabetic ketoacidosis. N Engl J Med. 1982;307:1603–10.
78. Uribarri J, Oh MS, Carroll HJ. D-Lactic acidosis—a review of clinical presentation, biochemical features, and pathophysiologic mechanisms. Medicine. 1998;77:73–82.
79. Madias NE, Ayus JC, Adrogue HJ. Increased anion gap in metabolic alkalosis: the role of plasma protein equivalency. N Engl J Med. 1979;300:1421–3.
80. Greenberg A. Diuretic complications. Am J Med Sci. 2000;319:10–24.
81. Wu DM, Bassuk J, Arias J, Doods H, Adams JA. Cardiovascular effects of Na+/H+ exchanger inhibition with BIIB513 following hypovolemic circulatory shock. Shock. 2005;23:269–74.
82. Kraut JA, Kurtz I. Use of base in the treatment of severe acidemic states. Am J Kidney Dis. 2001;38:703–27.
83. Steenbergen C, Deleeuw G, Terrell R, Williamson JR. Effects of acidosis and ischemia on contractility and intracellular pH of rat heart. Circ Res. 1977;41:849–58.
84. Daniel SR, Morita SY, Yu MH, Dzierba A. Uncompensated metabolic acidosis: an underrecognized risk factor for subsequent intubation requirement. J Trauma. 2004;57:993–7.
85. Davies AO. Rapid desensitization and uncoupling of human b-adrenergic receptors in an in vitro model of lactic acidosis. J Clin Endocrinol Metab. 1984;59:398–404.
86. Halperin FA, Cheema-Dhadli S, Chen CB, Halperin MI. Alkali therapy extends the period of survival during hypoxia: studies in rats. Am J Physiol. 1996;271:R381–7.
87. Halperin ML, Cheema-Dhadli S, Halperin FA, Kamel KS. Rationale for the use of sodium bicarbonate in a patient with lactic acidosis due to a poor cardiac output. Nephron. 1994;66:258–61.
88. Narins RG, Cohen JJ. Bicarbonate therapy for organic acidosis: the case for its continued use. Ann Intern Med. 1987;106:615–8.
89. Forsythe S, Schmidt GA. Sodium bicarbonate for the treatment of lactic acidosis. Chest. 2000;117:260–7.
90. Sabatini S, Kurtzman NA. Bicarbonate therapy in severe metabolic acidosis. J Am Soc Nephrol. 2009;20:692–5.
91. Kraut JA, Madias N. Metabolic acidosis pathophysiology, diagnosis and management. Nat Rev Nephrol. 2010;6:274–85.
92. Widenthal K, Mierzwiak DS, Myers RW, Mitchell JH. Effects of acute lactic acidosis on left ventricular performance. Am J Physiol. 1968;214:1352–9.
93. Cooper DJ, Walley KR, Wiggs BR, Russell JA. Bicarbonate does not improve hemodynamics in critically ill patients who have lactic acidosis. Ann Intern Med. 1990;112:492–8.
94. Stacpoole PW. Lactic acidosis: the case against bicarbonate therapy. Ann Intern Med. 1986;105:276–9.
95. Levraut J, Labib Y, Chave S, et al. Effect of sodium bicarbonate on intracellular pH under different buffering conditions. Kidney Int. 1996;49:1262–7.
96. Nahas GG, Sutin KM, Fermon C. Guidelines for the treatment of acidaemia with THAM. Drugs. 1998;55:191–224.
97. Bjerneroth G. Tribonat (R)—a comprehensive summary of its properties. Crit Care Med. 1999;27:1009–13.
98. Leung JM, Landow L, Franks M, Soja-Strzepa D, Heard SO, Arieff AI, Mangano DT. Safety and efficacy of intravenous carbicarb in patients undergoing surgery: comparison with sodium bicarbonate in the treatment of metabolic acidosis. Crit Care Med. 1994;22:1540–9.
99. Mazer CD, Naser B, Kamel KS. Effect of alkali therapy with NaHCO3 or THAM on cardiac contractility. Am J Physiol. 1996;270:955–62.
100. Hoste EA, Colpaert K, Vanholder RC, Lameire NH, De Waele JJ, Blot SI, Colardyn FA. Sodium bicarbonate versus THAM in ICU patients with mild metabolic acidosis. J Nephrol. 2005;18:303–7.
101. Weber T, Tschernich H, Sitzwohl C, Ullrich RGP, Zimpfer M, Sladen RN, Huemer G. Tromethamine buffer modifies the depressant effect of permissive hypercapnia on myocardial contractility in patient with acute respiratory distress syndrome. Am J Respir Crit Care Med. 2000;162:1361–5.
102. Sun JH, Filley GF, Hord K, Kindig NB, Bartle EJ. Carbicarb: an effective substitute for NaHCO3. Surgery. 1987;102:835–9.
103. Bersin RM, Arieff AI. Improved hemodynamic function during hypoxia with carbicarb, a new agent for the management of acidosis. Circulation. 1988;77:227–33.
104. Lalau JD, Westeel PF, Debussche X, Dkissi H, Tolani M, Coevoet B, Temperville B, Fournier A, Ouichaud J. Bicarbonate haemodialysis: an adequate treatment for lactic acidosis in diabetics treated by metformin. Intensive Care Med. 1987;13:383–7.

105. Hilton PJ, Taylor LG, Forni LG, Treacher DF. Bicarbonate-based haemofiltration in the management of acute renal failure with lactic acidosis. Q J Med. 1998;91:279–83.
106. Kallet RH, Liu K, Tang J. Management of acidosis during lung protective ventilation in acute respiratory distress. Respir Care Clin N Am. 2003;9:437–56.
107. Hsu SC, Wang MC, Liu HL, Tsai MC, Huang JJ. Extreme metabolic alkalosis treated with normal bicarbonate hemodialysis. Am J Kidney Dis. 2001;37:e31.
108. Webster NR, Kulkarni V. Metabolic alkalosis in the critically ill. Crit Rev Clin Lab Sci. 1999;36:497–510.
109. Gerhardt RE, Koethe JD, Glickman JD, Ntoso KA, Hugo JP, Wolf CJ. Acid dialysate correction of metabolic alkalosis in renal-failure. Am J Kidney Dis. 1995;25:343–5.

12 Case Studies in Electrolyte and Acid–Base Disorders

David B. Mount

Introduction

Acid–base and electrolyte cases can be intimidating for both medical trainees and experienced clinicians. The underlying physiological principles can be difficult to grasp, diagnostic workup elusive, and management options obscure. Therapy can be a daunting prospect, for hyponatremia in particular, where the dueling leitmotivs are that one is "damned if you do" (osmotic demyelination in chronic hyponatremia) and "damned if you don't" (acute symptomatic hyponatremia) [1]. I have chosen a handful of real-life clinical vignettes to reinforce selected concepts covered elsewhere in this textbook and to provide a step-by-step analysis of the pathophysiology, differential diagnosis, and management of selected clinical problems.

Case 1: Recurrent Hyponatremia that Improves with Hospitalization

Clinical Scenario

A 56-year-old male veteran is seen in consultation in the renal clinic at a Veteran's Administration (VA) hospital. He has a long history of hyponatremia, with transient decreases in serum sodium [Na^+] (see Table 12.1). He has been admitted 50 times to the local VA since 1998, most frequently for alcohol withdrawal or alcohol-related problems, but also for various medical and psychiatric issues. In the past year, he has been admitted several times to the psychiatric campus of the local VA, with suicidal ideation, depression, and suicidal attempts; during his most recent admission, citalopram was stopped in response to hyponatremia, and bupropion and lamotrigine were initiated for management of his depression. He was discharged 2 weeks prior to this outpatient evaluation, and has been living at home since that time. Current medications include bupropion SA 300 mg PO daily, lamotrigine 100 mg PO daily, and quetiapine 200 mg PO daily.

On review of systems, he denies lightheadedness, dizziness, headache, blurry vision, chest pain, cough productive of sputum, nausea, or vomiting. In addition to six or eight beers a day, he states that he drinks six glasses of orange juice a day. He also states that he maintains an adequate diet, with at least two large meals a day.

Past medical history includes hypertension, atrial flutter, cerebrovascular event in 1998, alcoholism, cocaine abuse, Barrett's esophagus, and a diagnosis of bipolar disorder. He has no history of congestive heart failure, with an unremarkable echocardiogram 2 years prior to this evaluation. He was treated for pulmonary tuberculosis (TB) in 1991, with residual granulomata and apical scarring on chest imaging. He was briefly treated again

D.B. Mount, M.D. (✉)
Renal Division, VA Boston Healthcare System, and Brigham and Women's Hospital,
Harvard Medical School, Boston, MA, USA
e-mail: dmount@rics.bwh.harvard.edu
david.mount2@va.gov

D.B. Mount et al. (eds.), *Core Concepts in the Disorders of Fluid, Electrolytes and Acid-Base Balance*,
DOI 10.1007/978-1-4614-3770-3_12, © Springer Science+Business Media New York 2013

Table 12.1 Selected biochemical data for Case 1

Date (month/day/year)	Clinical disposition	Serum Na^+ (mM)	Serum Osm (mOsm/kg)	Urine Na^+ (mM)	Urine Osm (mOsm/kg)
8/1/06	In-hospital	130			
8/6/06	In-hospital	119	251	126	379
5/24/07	Admission	126	267	<20	217
5/28/07	In-hospital	129		142	413
12/17/07	In-hospital	137			
1/12/08, p.m.	Admission	117		<20	119
1/13/08, a.m.	In-hospital	126			
1/16/08	In-hospital	130			
3/30/08, p.m.	Admission	116	270	<20	120
3/31/08, a.m.	In-hospital	125			
4/2/08	In-hospital	128		88	
7/29/08	In-hospital			85	535
7/30/08	In-hospital	130	272	37	527
8/18/08	Renal clinic	124	281	<20	146
10/26/08	Admission	123	264	<20	101
10/30/08	In-hospital	129			
12/7/08	In-hospital	135			
2/6/09	In-hospital	133			

with four agents in 2005 for a new cavitary lesion. This regimen was stopped after bronchoscopy cultures were negative for TB; the cavitary lesion resolved with antibiotics.

Social history is notable for intermittent homelessness; he currently lives in a cabin in Maine with no telephone and minimal amenities. He has a long history of alcohol abuse, drinking as much as 30 beers a day in the past. He also has a history of cocaine abuse, recently inactive. A longtime smoker, he quit in 2002.

Physical exam is notable for moderate truncal obesity. Heart rate and blood pressure are 72 and 100/60 supine, 72 and 100/60 standing. He has no peripheral edema, with jugular venous pressure (JVP) seen at 7 cm. Chest is clear, heart sounds are normal with no murmurs. Neurological exam is non-focal.

Bloodwork in clinic shows serum sodium concentration ($[Na^+]$) of 124 mM, $[K^+]$ 4.8 mM, $[Cl^-]$ 93 mM, bicarbonate concentration ($[HCO_3^-]$) 20 mM, urea 5 mg/dL, and creatinine 0.8 mg/dL. Selected serum and urinary sodium values, etc., are shown in Table 12.1. A recent thyroid-stimulating hormone (TSH) was 1.7 IU/mL (0.3–5.5) and a recent cosyntropin test increased cortisol from 5.64 to 22.48 and 28.50 μ[mu]g/dL at 30 and 60 min. A recent head computed tomography (CT) scan was unremarkable, with a recent chest X-ray that showed stable evidence of his prior TB.

Discussion

In summary, this 55-year-old alcoholic has had multiple hospital admissions wherein he was noted to have hyponatremia (see Table 12.1 for selected lab values). He was hyponatremic at his outpatient nephrology consultation, with urine $[Na^+]$ <20 mM and urine osmolality of 100 mOsm/kg (see Table 12.1); notably, he was living at home at this point, rather than in the psychiatric ward. During an admission to psychiatry in July, 2008 he was noted to have mild hyponatremia, with serum $[Na^+]$ of 130 mM; urine $[Na^+]$ was generous—37 and 85 mEq/L—with urine osmolalities of 535 and 527 mOsm/kg. When available, serial data from his various hospitalizations show that he has typically presented for admission at the local VA with worsening of his chronic hyponatremia, very low urine [Na^+], and urine osmolalities that vary between 101 and 217 mOsm/Kg; subsequent in-hospital data are more consistent with syndrome of inappropriate antidiuretic hormone (SIADH), with lesser hyponatremia, generous urine [Na^+], and higher urine osmolalities. One exception was an admission in 2006 for atrial flutter, when hyponatremia worsened *after* admission due to probable SIADH and excess free water intake (Table 12.1).

This patient has demonstrated two hyponatremic syndromes at various points in his medical history: SIADH and beer potomania. Contributors to his recent SIADH when seen in renal consultation were considered to be his therapy with bupropion and lamotrigine [2, 3]. Pulmonary, military, and meningeal TB can lead to SIADH and hyponatremia [4, 5]; however, his chest X-rays have been stable with no evidence of recurrent TB, such that this was considered to be an unlikely cause of his SIADH. His most recent serum [Na^+] was 135 and 135 mM, off of bupropion and still on quetiapine and lamotrigine.

Beer potomania, the primary focus of this vignette, appears to have been his dominant outpatient syndrome. Surprisingly, he had not previously been seen by the VA nephrology service for this problem, perhaps because his hyponatremia tended to "spontaneously" improve after admission. Superficially, his history of alcoholism and excessive beer intake immediately suggests beer potomania as a cause of his hyponatremia; indeed, a chart review of his 50 admissions indicates that alcoholism was frequently blamed as causative of his hyponatremia, although beer potomania was often dismissed as the specific cause due to urine biochemistries that differed from expected values. As we will discuss, however, his clinical course and biochemical presentations over the years have been fully consistent with beer potomania.

The patient was clinically euvolemic on exam when seen in the outpatient clinic; using the classical diagnostic algorithm [6], one would consider him to have euvolemic hyponatremia. However, his urine electrolytes and osmolality are at first glance somewhat puzzling, given that most cases of euvolemic hyponatremia will have a urine [Na^+] >20 mEq/L [6]. Why then is his urine [Na^+] so low, in the absence of obvious hypovolemia or a hypervolemic cause of hyponatremia such as heart failure? Certainly, patients with hypovolemic hyponatremia may be *clinically* euvolemic, without physical evidence of hypovolemia on exam, but with a urine [Na^+] <20 mEq/L and an increase in serum [Na^+] after saline hydration [7, 8]. Regardless, one also expects a much higher urine osmolality in hypovolemic hyponatremia, certainly >2–300 mOsm/kg; why then is his urine osmolality so low when his hyponatremia acutely worsens (see Table 12.1)? Furthermore, if beer potomania and low solute excretion is the cause of his reduced water excretion, why are his urine osmolalities not always ≤100 mOsm/kg when he presents with worsening hyponatremia, as one classically expects in this diagnosis [9, 10]?

One can take an epidemiological approach to clarifying this diagnostic issue; what are the observed urinary values for sodium and osmolality in patients who are considered to have beer potomania? This approach is somewhat less than satisfying, in that most reports of this syndrome have not included measurement of urine electrolytes or osmolality [11]. However, in case reports with adequate data, urine [Na^+] is typically low, with urine osmolalities that often exceed 100 mOsm/kg [11, 12]; the limitations of the literature data notwithstanding, this patient's urinary biochemistries (Table 12.1) are certainly consistent with beer potomania. As noted by Sanghvi et al., the recognition that a *very* low urine osmolality (≤100 mOsm/kg [10]) is not a universal finding prevents the dismissal of beer potomania in the appropriate clinical setting [11].

What is the physiological explanation for hyponatremia in this and related syndromes? The fundamental abnormality in beer potomania is the inadequate dietary intake of solutes; the reduced urinary solute excretion limits water excretion, leading to hyponatremia from the associated excess ingestion of free water. Beer is very low in protein and salt content, containing only 1–2 mmol/L of Na^+. Were these patients to take in salt and other solutes from their diet it would not be an issue; however, large quantities of beer tend to be their major or only nutrient, such that hyponatremia ensues. Given that the lower limit of urinary osmolality is ~30–50 mOsm/kg, solute excretion becomes limiting for water clearance in these patients.

A more mathematical analysis has been provided by Berl et al. [9, 13], explaining this physiology in an ovalolactovegetarian patient with hyponatremia due to profound dietary restriction of salt and protein:

$$\text{Urine flow(V)} = \text{cH}_2\text{O}\left(\text{free water clearance}\right) + \text{Cosm}\left(\text{solute clearance}\right) \quad (12.1)$$

Substituting UosmV/Posm for Cosm yields

$$\text{cH}_2\text{O} = \text{V} - \text{UosmV/Posm} \quad (12.2)$$

Because V=Solute excretion/Uosm, one can derive that

$$\text{cH}_2\text{O} = \frac{\text{solute excretion}}{\text{Uosm}\ \left(1 - \text{Uosm/Posm}\right)} \quad (12.3)$$

This analysis helps highlight how at a given urinary osmolality, solute excretion determines how much free water can be excreted. This is shown in Fig. 12.1, from Berl et al. [9, 13]. At a urine osmolality of 80 mOsm/kg, free water clearance is 2.7 L daily for a solute excretion of 300 mOsm/day, 5.4 L daily at 600 mOsm/day, and 8.1 L at 900 mOsm/day [9, 13]. Therefore, in patients with profoundly low daily solute intake, hyponatremia results from the reduction in urinary solute excretion and the associated ceiling in free water excretion, combined with excessive fluid intake. Vasopressin (AVP) levels have not been reported in patients with beer potomania, but are expected to be suppressed or rapidly suppressible with saline hydration; this fits with the overly rapid correction in serum [Na^+] that can be seen with saline hydration in beer potomania [11]. Patients with beer potomania are also solute-depleted, with initial Na^+-Cl^- retention after treatment with normal saline [12]; this initially positive Na^+ balance may also contribute to the rapid correction in serum [Na^+] with saline. In this particular patient, serum [Na^+] increased by >1 mEq/h on two occasions in response to overnight saline hydration (January and March of 2008, see Table 12.1); presumably his baseline SIADH prevented further overcorrection.

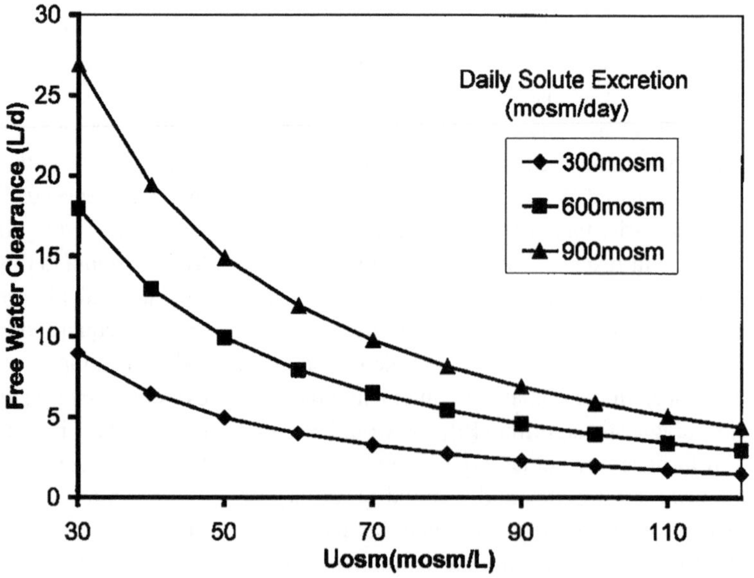

Fig. 12.1 Free water clearance as a function of urinary osmolality, at three different daily solute excretion levels. See text for details. From Thaler et al. [13]; used with permission

At steady state, ingested Na^+ contributes significantly to the ability to excrete a free water load [11], with a reduced capacity for water excretion after sodium restriction and increased capacity after high sodium diet [14]. To the extent that urea is for the most part not an effective osmole, one can derive the following equation for the effect of solute excretion on electrolyte-free water clearance [15]:

$$cH_2O = \frac{\text{solute excretion}(1 - U_{Na} + U_K)}{\text{Uosm } P_{Na}} \quad (12.4)$$

This equation helps understand the role of urinary urea in beer potomania [9, 13]. Protein metabolism generates ~50 mOsm of urea per 10 g of ingested protein; therefore, when patients with beer potomonia are admitted and fed, the increase in urinary urea will increase the ratio of solute excretion:Uosm (see (12.4) above) and increase electrolyte-free water clearance. Ingested urea can also apparently result in an increase in urinary Na^+ excretion [9], explaining in part the effect on free water clearance. Regardless, the combined effect of ingested Na^+ and protein on urinary solute excretion explains the longstanding observation that hyponatremia in beer potomania tends to improve with hospitalization [16]. This certainly fits with the clinical behavior of this particular patient during his various admissions over the years (see Table 12.1).

In summary, the available data from multiple admissions indicate that this patient has had recurrent hyponatremia due to beer potomania, a rare, AVP-independent cause. Urinary osmolalities on presentation were >100 mOsm/kg, the classical maximum in this diagnosis [9, 10]; as noted by Sanghvi et al., urinary osmolality is not universally <100 mOsm/kg in beer potomania, and awareness of this observation prevents the erroneous dismissal of the diagnosis [11]. Patients with beer potomania are prone to overcorrection (see also Table 12.1) and the development of osmotic demyelination syndrome (ODS); clinical management in the acute setting should take this into account [11]. As reviewed elsewhere [17], very low rates of correction in this and other syndromes may be required to avoid ODS. AVP levels are likely suppressed in this syndrome, such that "relowering" of serum [Na^+] will typically require desmopressin acetate (DDAVP) and free water administration [18]. Another strategy for controlled correction of serum [Na^+] in these and other hyponatremic patients is to utilize frequent doses of DDAVP (every 6–8 h) with constant infusion of hypertonic saline, to gradually increase serum [Na^+] [19]; this potentially avoids the erratic ups and downs in serum [Na^+] that are associated with DDAVP and free water administration [18]. In this particular case, education of the patient, in addition to psychiatric and medical staff, after a recurrent admission with hyponatremia (Table 12.1) resulted in a greater awareness of the importance of adequate nutrition, with no subsequent exacerbation in his hyponatremia.

Case 2: Persistent Hyponatremia After an Acute Presentation

Clinical Scenario

A 31-year-old woman, G2P2, 6 weeks postpartum, presents to the emergency room (ER) with nausea. The patient's past history is remarkable only for hypertension, initially noted at the time of her first delivery 3.5 years ago. She has subsequently been treated with atenolol, changed to labetalol after discovery of her second pregnancy. Her second pregnancy was not complicated by proteinuria or hypertension. The patient delivered a term infant by Caesarian section, with an uneventful postpartum course.

The patient recently developed intermittent severe headaches and leg cramps, with home blood pressure of 140/100; seen in her primary physician's office 4 days prior to admission, hydrochlorothiazide was added to her regimen. Within 2 days of starting the hydrochlorothiazide, the patient developed nausea, vomiting, and orthostatic dizziness. Review of systems is otherwise negative, except for some sinus symptoms throughout her recent pregnancy. Fluid intake has been maintained over the last 4 days.

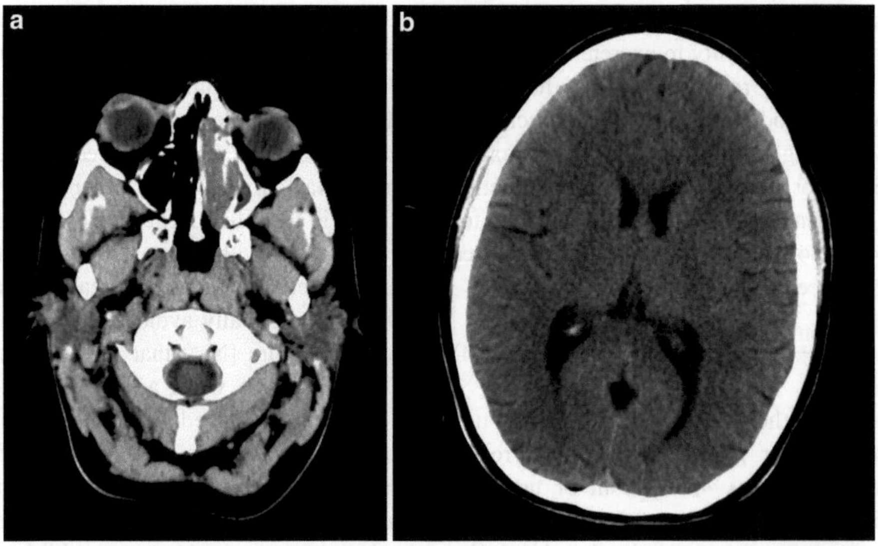

Fig. 12.2 Computed tomography (CT) scans of patients 2 and 3. (**a**) A head CT scan of the patient in case 2, performed at her presentation with acute hyponatremia. This shows a mass in the left nasal cavity, with thickening within the left maxillary sinus. (**b**) A head CT scan of the patient in case 3, performed after her generalized seizure. There is sulcal effacement consistent with cerebral edema

Medications include labetalol 200 mg twice a day, hydrochlorothiazide 12.5 mg daily, oral iron, a multivitamin, and occasional acetaminophen.

The patient is married. She previously worked in retail. There is no history of cigarette, alcohol, or drug abuse. Her family history is positive for hypertension in her father and brother.

On examination, the patient is in no acute distress. She is afebrile. Her blood pressure is 172/104, pulse 63. JVP is seen at 6 cm, with no peripheral edema. Lungs are clear. Heart sounds are unremarkable without an appreciable murmur. Abdominal exam is unremarkable, with no hepatosplenomgealy and no palpable masses. Neurological examination is non-focal, head and neck exam is unremarkable.

On admission, serum [Na^+] is 113 mM, potassium 4.1 mM, chloride 80 mM, CO_2 23 mM, BUN 10 mg/dL, creatinine 0.4 mg/dL. TSH is 1.58 IU/mL (0.3–5.5) and cortisol is 26.2 μ[mu]g/dL. Urine [Na^+] is 130 mM, urine osmolality 649 mOsm/kg; serum osmolality is ordered but not performed. A chest X-ray is unremarkable; CT scan of the head shows "no acute intracranial pathology." The patient's euvolemic hyponatremia is felt to be due to the alteration in osmotic sensitivity of AVP release associated with pregnancy [20] and thiazide-associated hyponatremia. The nausea is felt to be secondary to her acute hyponatremia. She is treated with 3 % saline and furosemide. Her serum [Na^+] increases to 117 mM within 1 day, 120 mM the second day, and 130 mM at the time of hospital discharge 4 days after admission. Serum [Na^+] is repeated 10 weeks later and found to be 132 mM.

The patient is seen in office follow up 26 weeks after her initial presentation. On review of systems, her only complaint is left-sided rhinorrhea. She is now on metoprolol 100 mg PO daily and loratidine 10 mg qd. She is euvolemic on physical exam, with a blood pressure of 114/82. Bloodwork now shows serum [Na^+] 128 mM; urine [Na^+] is 210 mM and a urine osmolality 1,093 mOsm/kg. Because of the suspicion of tumor-associated hyponatremia, her previous CT scan is again reviewed; this shows thickening seen in the left nasal cavity, and a suggestion of left nasal polyp (see Fig. 12.2a). Biopsy of the mass reveals an esthesioneuroblastoma (olfactory neuroblastoma). She undergoes craniofacial resection followed by a course of radiation therapy. One year after initial presentation, she is doing well clinically, with the exception of alterations in taste and smell; serum [Na^+] is 138 mM.

Discussvion

This case illustrates the frequent multifactorial causality of hyponatremia and the need for longitudinal follow up of patients with hyponatremia that does not completely resolve. A residual pregnancy-associated increase in the sensitivity of AVP release to osmolality [20] is conceivable but perhaps unlikely, given that her delivery was 6 weeks prior to her presentation with hyponatremia. However, although the osmotic threshold for thirst and AVP release certainly reverts to pre-pregnancy values within 10–12 weeks of delivery [21], published studies have not excluded a residual effect 6 weeks postpartum. Preeclampsia can also be complicated by hyponatremia [22]; however, this patient did not develop excessive proteinuria during her pregnancy. Sheehan's syndrome with pituitary failure and hyponatremia after delivery is also a concern in this setting [23]; however, the clinical presentation, clinical course, and robust cortisol level do not fit with this diagnosis.

This patient's initial presentation was entirely consistent with thiazide-associated hyponatremia, which can occur within days of starting the drug [24]. The female preponderance for this complication is more marked in elderly patients [25], and perhaps less likely to play a predisposing role in this case. Regardless, urine [Na^+] is often >20 mM on presentation, as in this case, with subsequent sodium-avid urine studies after stopping the drug [24]. Thiazide-associated hyponatremia is classically attributed to volume depletion, with drug-associated impairment in urinary dilution but not countercurrent multiplication (versus loop diuretics, which impair maximal urinary concentration via their effect on countercurrent multiplication) [6]. Polydipsia may also play an important role [26], perhaps due to the effect of hypokalemia on water intake [27]. Indeed, knockout mice with targeted deletion of the thiazide-sensitive Na^+-Cl^- cotransporter, one of the major pharmacological targets of thiazides, develop hypokalemia and polydipsia on a potassium-restricted diet [28]. Finally, thiazides directly increase water transport in perfused collecting ducts [29], and have a modest inductive effect on the aquaporin-2 water channel in lithium-associated nephrogenic diabetes insipidus [30]. The stimulatory effect of thiazide on water transport is blocked by prostaglandins [29]. Of note, indirect evidence suggests a relative deficiency in intra-renal prostaglandin generation in elderly patients with thiazide-associated hyponatremia [31]; this is perhaps due to a relative deficiency in medullary cyclo-oxygenase-2 (COX2), which is conversely *upregulated* in models of nephrogenic diabetes insipidus [32, 33].

Follow up values of this patient's serum [Na^+] at 10 and 26 weeks after initial presentation were 132 and 128 mM, with urinary indices consistent with SIADH. A review of systems indicated unilateral rhinorrhea; review of her previous CT scan showed a left nasal mass (see Fig. 12.2). Biopsy revealed an olfactory neuroblastoma, with resolution of her hyponatremia after resection. There are more than ten reported cases of SIADH associated with olfactory neuroblastoma [34–37], with two additional cases in association with the related tumor sinonasal neuroendocrine carcinoma [38, 39]. A common theme is the substantial delay, of as much as 6 [35] to 8 [37] years, between the onset of hyponatremia and diagnosis of olfactory neuroblastoma as the cause [35–37]; the delayed diagnosis in this case is thus not atypical. As in small-cell lung cancer, the most common cause of malignancy-associated SIADH [40], tumor cells in these cases stain positive for both vasopressin and vasopressin neurophysin [35, 36].

Although approximately 75 % of malignancy-associated SIADH is caused by small-cell lung cancer (SCLC) [40], a considerable number of other malignancies can be causative [41]. Head and neck cancers are an important cause, typically due to squamous cell carcinoma [42]. An important general question in the workup of patients with SIADH is the choice and extent of imaging necessary to exclude malignant causes. In most patients, we will request a chest X-ray and head CT scan; due to anecdotal experience of patients with SCLC that was not detected on chest X-ray, we also typically request a chest CT in patients with a negative chest X-ray. It should be noted that many elderly patients may demonstrate hyponatremia from "idiopathic" SIADH, with no evidence on extensive evaluation for an obvious cause [43]. Regardless, even elderly patients with SIADH who fail to respond to vasopressin antagonists should be screened for nephrogenic SIADH due to activating mutations of the V2 vasopressin receptor [44].

Case 3: Acute Symptomatic Hyponatremia

Clinical Scenario

A 28-year-old woman is admitted with nausea and vomiting. The patient has been in her usual state of health. In the afternoon of the day of admission, she went to the gym and exercised heavily for 30 min on a treadmill, much greater than her usual exertion. She took four Advils after exercising and then drank three 1-L bottles of water, out of concern that she was "dehydrated." She subsequently went to a baseball game with family members, where she drank another three bottles of water, along a bottle of Powerade. At the baseball game she noticed a headache, then felt "shaky", with difficulty walking and paresthesias in her legs. She was brought to the ER, arriving at 10:33 p.m. On arrival to the triage area she vomited.

On review of systems, she denies illness prior to the day of admission. Specifically, she denies prior diarrhea, headache, or fever. She denies ingesting alcohol at the ball game, and denies drug use. She exclaims that "I'm drowning" and "I've made a terrible mistake"; it is subsequently documented that she had a friend who had died of water intoxication.

Past medical history is unremarkable. Medications include an oral contraceptive, four tablets of Advil on the day of admission. She denies drug abuse, including ecstasy.

Examination by ER staff shows that her heart rate is 104, respiratory rate 38, blood pressure is 146/70, O_2 saturation is 100 % on room air, and weight is 80 kg. Chest is clear, abdomen benign. On neurological examination, cranial nerves II–XII are intact, and she has a slight tremor on finger-to-nose cerebellar testing, left greater than right. Motor examination is normal. Initial bloodwork (see also Table 12.2) demonstrates a serum [Na^+] of 121 mM, potassium of 3.4, chloride of 89 mM, bicarbonate of 16 mM, anion gap (AG) of 16, BUN of 10 mg/dL, creatinine of 0.75 mg/dL, glucose of 165 mg/dL, and a normal complete blood count.

Nursing notes 2.5 h after presentation document that the patient "continues to shake and have nausea." A chest X-ray is performed

Table 12.2 Biochemical data for Case 3

Day	Time	Na^+ (mM)	Cl (mM)	HCO_3 (mM)	Anion gap	Serum Osm (mOsm/kg)	Urine Osm (mOsm/kg)	Urine Na^+ (mM)
1	23:30	121	89	16	16	252		
2	1:55						702	124
	4:00	129	91	9	29			
	6:00	124	93	19	12	256	581	97
	8:00	125	98	18	9			
	10:00	133	104	19	10			
	12:00	135	106	20	9			
	13:00						71	19
3	5:00	136	108	21	7	268		

(unremarkable, without pulmonary edema), and a decision is made to admit the patient to a medical floor; admission diagnoses are hyponatremia and water intoxication. While the patient is awaiting transfer to the floor, 4.5 h after presentation, the ER nurse is called to bedside by patient's father. The patient is incoherent and twitching. This myclonic activity escalates to clonic activity of arms/legs, lasting ~1 min. She was given 2 mg of intravenous lorazepam while the generalized seizure was resolving. A CT scan of the head performed, non-contrast: the report states "No acute intracranial abnormality is seen. Specifically, no edema."

At 6 h after presentation the renal service is consulted, and hypertonic saline is advised, beginning at 70 mL/h. At 7 h after admission, the renal and neurology attending physicians examine the patient. Note is made of anisocoria, right pupil larger than the left, with no relative afferent pupillary defect. There is also a grade II out of VI apical pan-systolic murmur; chest is clear. Review of the head CT suggests the presence of sulcal effacement consistent with cerebral edema (see Fig. 12.2b). Hypertonic saline is reduced to 60 mL/h by the second hour of infusion. The renal attending speaks to the admitting ER physician, with respect to initial management in the ER; the ER physician had been reluctant to administer hypertonic saline due to the perceived risk of osmotic demyelination.

Discussion

This patient developed acute, symptomatic hyponatremia in the setting of overexertion and polydipsia. She also presented with hyperglycemic ketoacidosis, in the absence of admitted alcohol intake or known insulinopenia or insulin resistance. Before this presumptive acidosis resolved she suffered a generalized seizure, with a further increase in her anion gap; subsequent to this event, her anion gap quickly normalized (see Table 12.2).

Exercise-associated hyponatremia is an important cause of acute symptomatic hyponatremia [45]. This is more commonly seen in endurance sports, such as marathons, due to a combination of non-osmotic AVP release and excessive water intake [45–47]. In this particular case, there were some indications that the water intoxication was deliberate (see the clinical scenario above). One interesting aspect is the acute consumption of an NSAID, which is expected to amplify the renal response to circulating AVP. It has thus been known for more than four decades that prostaglandins inhibit the effect of AVP on water transport in the collecting duct [48]. Prostaglandins also downregulate expression and activity of NKCC2 [49], the apical Na^+-K^+-$2Cl^-$ cotransporter of the thick ascending limb, thus inhibiting the countercurrent mechanism. Urinary excretion of prostaglandin metabolites in rats correlates with hydration status, with very low excretion in "dehydrated" animals with high urinary osmolality and higher than normal excretion in "hydrated" animals with low urine osmolality [50]. Finally, animal models of nephrogenic diabetes insipidus demonstrate an upregulation of medullary COX2, with improved water excretion after COX2 inhibition [32, 33]; a relative deficit in medullary COX2 conceivably plays a role in the genesis of some forms of hyponatremia [31] (see also discussion of Case 2). This physiological background notwithstanding, it should be noted that all but one study of exercise-associated hyponatremia [51] have failed to detect an association with NSAID use [45].

Acute hyponatremic encephalopathy ensues when volume regulatory mechanisms in the brain are overwhelmed by a rapid decrease in tonicity, resulting in acute cerebral edema [20]. As in this case, early symptoms can include nausea, headache, and vomiting. However, severe complications can rapidly evolve, encompassing seizure activity, brainstem herniation, coma, and death [52]. This particular patient was fortunate to not suffer severe sequelae of her acute hyponatremia, despite the initial failure to administer hypertonic saline.

A key complication of acute hyponatremia is normocapneic or hypercapneic respiratory failure [53]. Normocapneic respiratory failure in this setting is typically due to noncardiogenic pulmonary edema [53]. This particular case was not complicated by pulmonary edema or hypoxia. Notably, however, it can be particularly difficult to persuade other physicians to administer hypertonic saline in the setting of acute hyponatremia with associated pulmonary edema [54].

As shown in Table 12.2, at the time of the nephrology assessment at 6:00 a.m. on the morning after admission, the patient's serum [Na^+] had settled after her acute seizure at 124 mM, i.e., 3 mM greater than on presentation. The renal and neurology services felt that her CT scan showed evidence of cerebral edema (see Fig. 12.2b), with unequal pupils concerning for impending herniation. How should one decide on the therapeutic approach in a situation such as this? The primary consideration is the need to increase serum [Na^+] by an amount sufficient to reduce the acute, severesymptomsofhyponatremicencephalopathy; this evidently requires a modest increase of only 4–6 mM [41, 55]. The subsequent rate of correction in acute hyponatemia is not well established [41]; some authorities recommend that the total increase in serum [Na^+] should be less 12 mmol/L in the first 24 h, i.e., within widely accepted guidelines for the correction of chronic, "asymptomatic" hyponatremia [56].

A variety of published algorithms can be utilized to calculate the rate of administered hypertonic saline (see Table 4 of reference [41]). In this particular case, the "traditional" [41] sodium deficit was calculated, as 0.6 times body weight, times the difference between actual and desired serum [Na^+]. This deficit was estimated at 144 mmol of Na^+, aiming for an increase of 3 mM; if corrected over 3 h the rate of hypertonic saline would be approximately 90 mL/h. A more quantitative approach to therapy of dysnatremias has also been developed [57]. Notably, however, some authorities discourage the use of formulas to predict the response of serum [Na^+] to hypertonic saline, in part because these algorithms tend to underestimate the effect of treatment [58]; this is because serum AVP levels may change in response to hypertonic saline and/or other treatment measures, resulting in a water diuresis and a greater than expected rise serum [Na^+]. In this particular case, a decision was made to reduce the rate of hypertonic saline, with the expectation that her AVP levels would quickly plummet with a rapid water diuresis; this prediction was borne out by the reduction in urine osmolality to 581 and then subsequently to 71 mOsm/kg, consistent with an evolving water diuresis (see Table 12.2).

Case 4: A Microgram of Prevention

Clinical Scenario

A 76-year-old woman presents with a several-month history of diarrhea, with marked worsening over the last 2–3 weeks. Over the last 2–3 days, she has been having 12 stools a day. She has no systemic symptoms, specifically no fever, no myalgias, and no upper respiratory symptoms. She does not recollect having had antibiotics over the last few months. Review of systems is negative for orthostatic dizziness, nausea, and vomiting, and headache. Family members have not noticed recent confusion.

Past medical history is notable for knee replacement, cutaneous melanoma resection 3 years ago, hypertension treated with atenolol and spironolactone, and hypercholesterolemia for which she is on lovastatin. She also has a history of kidney stones, with lithotripsy in October 2007. Of note, a metabolic study demonstrated decreased urinary volume and hypocitraturia; she has since increased her daily water intake to five to six glasses of water a day. Medications include atenolol 50 mg PO daily, spironolactone 25 mg PO daily, and lovastatin.

She is a married, a retired school teacher with two children. She is a nonsmoker, nondrinker. Family history is positive for emphysema and heart failure.

On examination at 1:00 p.m. on March 23rd, 2008 (see Table 12.3), she is alert, oriented and

Table 12.3 Biochemical data for Case 4

Date (month/±day/±year)	4/05	3/23/08	3/23	3/23	3/23	3/23	3/23	3/24	3/25	3/26	1/09
Time		5:00	8:00	12:00	16:00	19:00	21:00	5:00	5:00		
Serum Na^+ (mM)	137	113	115	120	117	116	117	117	124	130	138
Creatinine (mg/dL)	1.2	2.35	2.10	2.02	1.97	1.79	1.78	1.53	1.20	1.13	1.2
Urine Osm (mOsm/kg)				319		415		397			
Urine Na^+ (mM)				17		23		47			

appropriate. Heart rate is 72 sitting and 90 standing; blood pressure is 105/50 lying and standing. Her JVP is indistinct. She has no peripheral edema; pulses are all present, with no bruits. Heart sounds are normal with no murmurs. Chest is clear to percussion and auscultation. On abdominal examination, she has a slight increase in her bowel sounds, with a non-tender exam and no organomegaly. On neurological exam, motor power is 4+/5, reflexes 1+ and symmetric, cranial nerves II–XII are normal.

Admission serum [Na^+] at 5:00 a.m. is 113 mM, with a creatinine of 2.35 (see Table 12.3). By 1:00 p.m. serum [Na^+] is 120 mM, with potassium of 5.4 mM, chloride 90 mM, bicarbonate 22 mM, BUN 32 mg/dL, creatinine 2.02 mg/dL, glucose 89 mg/dL, total protein 5.0, and albumin 1.9. Her hematocrit is 33.9, white count 7.6, platelets 405. An AM cortisol on 3/24 is 19.5, with TSH 1.7; serum osmolality is requested but not performed. Selected urinary and serum biochemistries are shown in Table 12.3.

The patient is treated with 1 μg of intravenous DDAVP, along with 75 mL/h of intravenous half-normal saline. When serum [Na^+] drops to 116 mM intravenous fluid is switched to normal saline at the same rate. Subsequent results are shown in Table 12.3. The patient's serum [Na^+] slowly increases to 130 mM by discharge; a subsequent serum [Na^+] is 138 mM.

Discussion

This patient presented with hypovolemic hyponatremia and a "pre-renal" reduction in glomerular filtration rate. As expected for hypovolemic hyponatremia, her urine [Na^+] was <20 mEq/L [7, 8], in the absence of congestive heart failure or other causes of "hypervolemic" hyponatremia; she responded to saline hydration with an increase in serum [Na^+] and a decrease in creatinine. Her baseline-free water intake was also increased, a habit ingrained from the management of her nephrolithiasis; this and an initial increase in free water excretion is presumably the explanation of the less-than-maximally concentrated urine 7 h after presentation (see Table 12.3).

Her initial hypovolemia would have increased the sensitivity of her AVP response to osmolality, both decreasing the osmotic threshold and increasing the slope of the osmolality response curve [20]. Reductions in blood volume and blood pressure are also potent stimuli for AVP release, albeit with a less sensitive profile than the osmotic response [20]. Regardless, AVP has a half-life of only 10–20 min [6]. Therefore, the acute increase in intravascular volume after a liter of intravenous saline led to a rapid reduction in circulating AVP; the ensuing water diuresis is the primary explanation for the rapid increase in serum [Na^+] in the first 7 h of her hospitalization.

The key concern in this case was the probable chronicity of the patient's hyponatremia [59], with several weeks of diarrhea followed by 2–3 days of acute exacerbation. This patient would be judged by most to have chronic hyponatremia, i.e., with a suspected duration of >48 h [59]; as such, she would be predisposed to osmotic demyelination were she to undergo too rapid a correction in her serum [Na^+], i.e., by more than 10 mM in 24 h, 18 mM in 48 h, or 20 mM in 72 h [17, 20, 60]. Notably, lesser reductions in serum [Na^+] may be advisable in patients who are otherwise predisposed to ODS [17]. Regardless, at presentation this patient had no symptoms that one would typically attribute to acute hyponatremia, and her serum [Na^+] had already increased by a sufficient amount to protect her from developing acute cerebral edema [17, 41, 55]. With these considerations in mind, a decision was made to intervene and prevent a further rapid rise in her serum [Na^+]. Therefore, she was given a microgram of intravenous DDAVP. Given her hypovolemia and resolving acute renal insufficiency, a decision was made to administer half-normal saline as her source of free water, rather than D5W [18]; this was switched to normal saline when serum [Na^+] acutely dropped to 117 mM (see Table 12.3).

Overcorrection of chronic hyponatremia is a major risk factor for the development of ODS [17, 20, 60]. Animal studies show a neurological and survival benefit in ODS of "re-lowering" serum [Na^+] with DDAVP and free water administration [61, 62], supported by a handful of clinical case reports [63–65]. Until recently, no larger studies of the safety and efficacy of this approach were available; legitimate concerns included the risk of cerebral edema and associated sequelae (seizures, etc.) when serum [Na^+] is relowered or reduced to a level less than that at presentation. The considerable literature on DDAVP-associated hyponatremic encephalopathy in patients administered the drug for enuresis or bleeding disorders has tended to confirm these fears; initially noted in children treated for nocturnal enuresis or von Willebrand's disease [66], DDAVP-induced hyponatremic seizures have also been described in adults [67, 68]. As a result, it has taken a considerable leap of faith to use DDAVP and free water to relower serum [Na^+] in patients who had overcorrected or were in the process of overcorrecting. However, a retrospective study of 20 hyponatremic patients treated with DDAVP has recently confirmed the safety and efficacy of this approach [18]. In six of these patients, DDAVP was given after patients had increased serum [Na^+] by greater than 12 mM over 24 h; in all but one, an increase greater than 18 mM over 48 h was prevented. In the other 14 cases, DDAVP was utilized to prevent an overcorrection, as in this particular case; none of these patients overcorrected over 48 h.

Many of the cases treated with DDAVP in Perianayagam et al. had begun a robust water diuresis prior to receiving the drug, with urine osmolalities of <150 mOsm/kg [18]. In this particular case, the urine was not maximally dilute before administration of DDAVP, suggesting that endogenous AVP was not yet fully suppressed; this may have contributed to the transient drop back to 116 mM after administration of the drug. Close monitoring of serum [Na^+] led to changing the intravenous fluid to normal saline, with subsequent stabilization then a slow increase (see Table 12.3); should serum [Na^+] have gone below 113 mM, the admission value, administration of hypertonic saline would have been considered, to prevent iatrogenic cerebral edema.

This patient's serum [Na^+] remained depressed for several days after receiving DDAVP. It is conceivable that residual hypovolemic hyponatremia attenuated the recovery in her serum [Na^+]. Alternatively, this slow increase in serum [Na^+] is due to persistent effects of the single dose of DDAVP. Of note, the plasma half-life of DDAVP is only 1–2 h [69]; however, the available pharmacodynamic studies indicate a much more prolonged effect on urine output and/or urine osmolality. See for example the effect of a single intravenous or oral dose on urinary volume and osmolality in healthy men aged 55–70 years, ingesting 35 mL/kg bodyweight of water per day; a 2 μg intravenous dose has persistent effects at the end of the 23-h study (see Fig. 12.3) [70]. There may also be substantial variability in the pharmacodynamic response to DDAVP, as shown in children treated for nocturnal enuresis [69]. Therefore, the attenuated recovery in serum [Na^+] (Table 12.3) may very well represent a prolonged pharmacodynamic effect of the drug. Another consideration is the effect of the patient's initial renal dysfunction on the pharmacokinetics and pharmacodynamics of the administered DDAVP, which is renally excreted [71]; DDAVP should be administered with caution for the re-induction of hyponatremia in patients with chronic kidney disease.

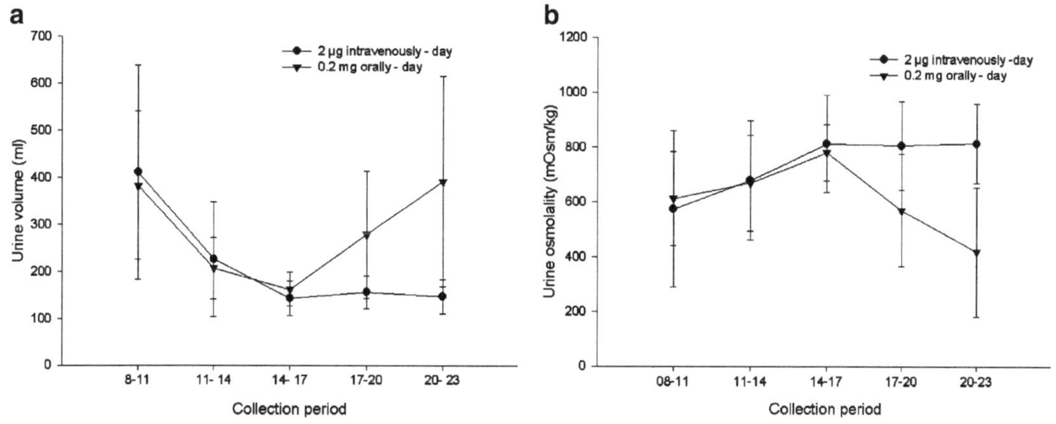

Fig. 12.3 Pharmacodynamics of oral and intravenous DDAVP in men aged 55–70 years. (**a**) The effect if a single 0.2 mg oral dose or a single intravenous 1 µg, given at 11:00 a.m., on urinary volume. (**b**) The effect if a single 0.2 mg oral dose or a single intravenous 1 µg, given at 11:00 a.m., on urinary osmolality. From Rembratt et al. [70]; used with permission

In this particular case, the serum [Na^+] initially corrected by 7 mM over 8 h, provoking the use of one dose of DDAVP, along with free water administration, to halt the subsequent rise in serum [Na^+]. An alternative approach is to administer frequent doses of DDAVP (every 6–8 h) with constant infusion of hypertonic saline, to increase serum [Na^+] at a steadier rate [19]; this potentially avoids an extended delay in subsequent correction of serum [Na^+], as occurred in this particular case.

Case 5: Overcorrection of Serum Sodium in a Patient with Pituitary Dysfunction

Clinical Scenario

A 55-year-old man presents with a 40-lb weight loss, fatigue, abdominal pain, decreased appetite, dizziness, headaches, myalgias, decreased libido, and depression with suicidal ideations. Three months prior to admission he was started on fluoxetine, when serum [Na^+] was 140 mM; 2 months later he was documented to have mild hyponatremia (133–135 mM). Admission medications include fluoxetine 20 mg daily, desipramine 25 mg daily, pyridium 100 mg three times a day, oxycodone 5 mg daily as needed.

Past medical history is notable for transsphenoidal resection of a pituitary macroadenoma in Puerto Rico 6 months prior to this admission, with no medical follow up prior to moving to the United States. He is also known to have a Chiari type I malformation and benign prostatic hypertrophy.

A urine culture is positive for Gram-negative bacteria, and the admission CT scan demonstrates mild thickening of the descending colon, thickened bladder wall consistent with cystitis, and an enlarged prostate; the patient receives levofloxacin and metronidazole. Admission serum [Na^+] is 120 mM, and the patient is considered to be volume depleted; he receives 150 mL/h of normal saline for the first 36 h of his admission, at which point a fluid restriction is initiated. Serum [Na^+] and osmolality drop to 109 mM and 235 mOsm/kg, respectively, by 60 h after admission; an urgent renal consult is requested. Hospital medications to that point include prednisone 5 mg daily, synthroid 100 mcg daily, salt tablets 1 g three times a day, omeprazole, enoxaparin, levofloxacin, metronidazole, colace, oxycodone prn, and pyridium. A nuclear magnetic resonance (NMR) study of the brain on hospital day 2 shows a large sella turcica with an inhomogeneously enhancing pituitary on the right with deviation of the infundibulum from the left side to the

Table 12.4 Biochemical data for Case 5

Hospital hour	Serum Na^+ (mM)	Urine Na^+ (mM)	Urine K^+ (mM)	Urine Osm (mOsm/kg)	Fluid intake	Urine output
1	120	190	74	598	2,000	0
21	119				3,020	1,460
35	115	100		459	1,410	1,450
58.5	109	101	89	602	1,020	4,190
62	112					
66	116					
72	122					
84	124				1,190	995
	128					
93	130					
	132				350	775
	131				1,560	2,200
	134	41	80	281		
	135	69	55	461	250	1,300

right side; no other radiological abnormality is reported.

On exam, he is in no apparent distress, but is considered moderately confused. Pulse is 89, with a blood pressure of 120/70. JVP is seen at 10 cm, with no edema. Heart sounds are normal, chest is clear. Abdomen is non-tender with no appreciable mass or organomegaly.

Selected biochemical and clinical data is shown in Table 12.4. A serum cortisol is 1.6 (6–24 μg/dL), TSH is 1.463, free T4 is 0.5 ng/dL (0.8–1.8), testosterone is 745 pg/mL (1,800–6,600), luteinizing and follicle-stimulating hormone are within normal limits, and prolactin is 4.6 ng/mL (2.6–13.1).

The renal consult service diagnoses acute hyponatremia due to secondary adrenal insufficiency, exacerbated perhaps by recent treatment with fluoxetine. His worsening hyponatremia after normal saline (versus improvement in the cerebral salt wasting syndrome) is felt to be consistent with SIADH. In response to the serum [Na^+] of 109 mM, the patient receives hypertonic saline from hospital hour 65 to 75; hydrocortisone 100 mg IV three times a day begins at hour 60. He rapidly increases his serum [Na^+] by almost 1 mM/h over the next 24 h. He suffers no neurological sequelae consistent with ODS, and has been doing well on thyroxine, glucocorticoid, and testosterone supplementation since discharge; serum [Na^+] has been stable, persistently higher than 140 mM.

Discussion

This patient developed hyponatremia from hypopituitarism and secondary adrenal insufficiency. Many of his seemingly unrelated presenting symptoms, including abdominal pain and headache, have been reported in other patients with hypopituitarism and hyponatremia [72]. Treatment with intravenous normal saline led to exacerbation of his hyponatremia; electrolyte-free water excretion for his second hospital day, calculated using the available urine electrolytes from hospital hour 58.5 (Table 12.4) and the relevant equation [15] (see also (12.4) for Case 1), was around −1,000 mL, i.e., a net gain of approximately 1 L for free water. In consequence, serum [Na^+] dropped to a nadir of 109 mM, from 120 mM on admission. Glucocorticoid repletion led to polyuria, unfortunately without documentation of urinary osmolality and electrolytes, and an increase in serum [Na^+] by almost 1 mM/h over 24 h.

Hypopituitarism and secondary adrenal dysfunction is an important and often overlooked cause of euvolemic hyponatremia. In this particular patient, levels of TSH, cortisol, and testosterone were all reduced, 6 months after undergoing trans-

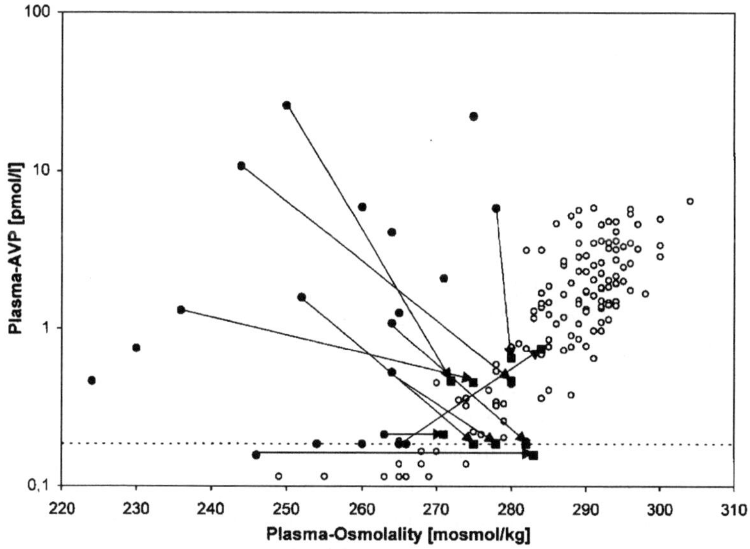

Fig. 12.4 Relationship between plasma osmolality and plasma AVP in 20 patients with hyponatremia and hypopituitarism (*solid circles*) in comparison with hydrated and dehydrated levels in normal subjects (*open circles*). In ten patients, AVP levels were remeasured after normalization of serum sodium following hydrocortisone treatment (*arrows* to *solid squares*), showing normalization of AVP levels. From Diederich et al. [72]; used with permission

sphenoidal resection of an anterior pituitary tumor. Not all patients with secondary adrenal dysfunction will have lower than normal cortisol levels, and dynamic testing of adrenal function may be required to make the diagnosis; this often consists of measuring the cortisol response to stimuli such as low-dose ACTH, hypoglycemia (insulin tolerance testing), or corticotrophin-releasing hormone [72]. Hyponatremia due to hypopituitarism and secondary adrenal dysfunction typically mimics SIADH, with a euvolemic presentation, generous urine [Na$^+$], and high urine osmolality. Unlike in primary adrenal failure, which causes hypovolemic hyponatremia due to renal salt wasting, plasma aldosterone levels, and plasma renin activity (PRA) are within normal range [72].

Glucocorticoids exert negative feedback on AVP release by the posterior pituitary [73] and downregulate AVP expression in magnocellular neurons [74]. Within the kidney, increases in circulating AVP in experimental glucocorticoid deficiency are associated with increased expression [75] and activation [76] of the AVP-regulated water channel aquaporin-2. As in SIADH, AVP release can demonstrate a variety of response patterns to increasing osmolality in patients with secondary adrenal failure [77], with levels that are not appropriately suppressed by baseline hypo-osmolality [72, 77]. Above a threshold dose [78], hydrocortisone replacement will rapidly suppress AVP, normalizing the AVP response to osmolality [72, 77] (see Fig. 12.4). This threshold requirement [78] explains perhaps why the oral prednisone this patient initially received had no effect on water excretion. Regardless, following administration of stress doses of hydrocortisone, AVP levels rapidly fell, with a marked water diuresis and rapid increase in serum [Na$^+$] (see Table 12.4).

The primary concern for the rapid increase in serum [Na$^+$] in this patient is the risk of ODS, although one can theorize that the relevant increase was in fact the lesser 10 mM difference between admission and hospital hour 93 (see Table 12.4). Regardless, ODS after the administration of hydrocortisone and rapid correction of serum [Na$^+$] is a known complication in patients with hyponatremia due to pituitary dysfunction [79, 80].

How might this "overcorrection" have been averted? First, hypertonic saline, infused between hospital hours 65 and 75, would ideally have been stopped at an earlier time point, as the patient began to overcorrect (a 1 mM/h correction between hospital hours 58.5, 62, and 66); alternatively, given the modest symptoms and an anticipated rapid drop in AVP levels with hydrocortisone, hypertonic saline was perhaps unnecessary. Second, a more controlled approach would have been to utilize a vasopressin antagonist such as conivaptan or tolvaptan to reduce serum [Na^+] by inhibiting circulating AVP, versus a rapid, uncontrolled reduction in AVP in response to glucocorticoid replacement. Glucocorticoids and thyroxine could have subsequently been started once serum [Na^+] had increased by a "safe" rate of 12 mM or less in 24 h. Notably, conivaptan and tolvaptan are United States Food and Drug Administration (FDA)-approved for the treatment of euvolemic hyponatremic due to pituitary dysfunction. However, vasopressin antagonists are not without their own risk of overcorrection; this occurred in 4 out of 233 patients in a large trial of tolvaptan [81], and in 4 out of 55 patients in a smaller trial of conivaptan [82]. This necessitates stopping the infusion, in the case of intravenous conivaptan, and administering free water to reduce the rate of rise in serum [Na^+].

Alternatively, once the patient in question had overcorrected (see Table 12.4), DDAVP and free water could have safely reduced serum [Na^+] back down to the low 120 s, as described by Perianayagam et al. [18]. This case thus demonstrates the need to frequently monitor serum [Na^+] after the initiation of therapy for hyponatremia and—most importantly—to rapidly make the necessary changes in therapy to avoid or respond to overcorrection.

Case 6: Hypernatremia and Polyuria

Clinical Scenario

A 58-year-old man is admitted to the ICU with severe pneumonia. Past medical history includes schizophrenia; treatment has included neuroleptics and intermittent lithium, the latter restarted 6 months prior to admission. The patient has been treated with antibiotics and intubated for several days, with the development of polyuria (3–5 L/day), hypernatremia, and acute renal insufficiency; the peak serum [Na^+] concentration is 156 mM and peak creatinine 2.6 mg/dL. Urine osmolality is measured once and reported as 157 mOsm/kg, with a coincident plasma osmolality of 318 mOsm/kg. Lithium was stopped on admission to the ICU.

Table 12.5 Water deprivation test for Case 6

Time (h)	0	+6	+8	AVP given at +9 h	+12	+18
Serum Na^+ (mM)	145	148	150		152	149
Serum K^+ (mM)	5.4	5.3	3.9		3.9	3.9
Serum Cl^- (mM)	111	110	118		120	114
Creatinine (mg/dL)	1.3	1.3	1.4		1.3	1.3
Serum Osm (mOsm/kg)	300	311	315			
Urine Osm (mOsm/kg)	132	140	201		237	257
AVP		8.4	6.3			

On physical exam, the patient is alert, extubated, and thirsty. Weight is 97.5 kg. Urine output for the last 24 h has been 3.4 L, with an IV intake of 2 L/day of D5W.

Laboratory data includes a serum [Na^+] of 150 mM, [K^+] of 3.9 mM, [Cl^-] of 114 mM, urea of 8 mg/dL, and creatinine 1.7 mg/dL. Plasma osmolality is 315 mOsm/kg, with urine [Na^+] 35 mM, urine [K^+] 5.2 mM, and urine osmolality 135 mOsm/kg. After 3 days of intravenous hydration, a water deprivation test is performed (Table 12.5). A single dose of 2 μ[mu]g IV DDAVP is given at 9 h (+9) after beginning water deprivation.

Discussion

This patient became polyuric after ICU admission for pneumonia, developing significant hypernatremia and acute renal insufficiency. Polyuria can result from either an osmotic diuresis or a water diuresis. An osmotic diuresis can be caused by excessive excretion of Na^+-Cl^-, mannitol, glucose, and/or urea, with a daily solute excretion of >750–1,000 mOsm/day (>15 mOsm/kg body water/day). This particular patient was excreting large volumes of very hypotonic urine, with a urine osmolality that was substantially lower than that of plasma; this was a water diuresis, resulting in excessive excretion of free water and hypernatremia. The appropriate response to hypernatremia and a plasma osmolality >295 mOsm/kg is an increase in circulating vasopressin (AVP) and the excretion of low volumes (<500 mL/day) of maximally concentrated urine, i.e., urine with osmolality >800 mOsm/kg; this patient's response to hypernatremia was clearly inappropriate, due to either a loss of circulating AVP (central diabetes insipidus, CDI) or renal resistance to AVP (nephrogenic diabetes insipidus, NDI). The ongoing loss of free water was sufficiently severe that absolute hypovolemia ensued, despite the fact that approximately two thirds of the excreted water was from the intracellular fluid compartment, rather than the extracellular fluid compartment. Hypovolemia led to an acute decrease in glomerular filtration, i.e., "pre-renal" acute renal insufficiency.

The patient was subjected to a water deprivation test followed by the administration of DDAVP, after correction of his hypernatremia and acute renal insufficiency with appropriate hydration. A water deprivation test helps determine whether an inappropriate water diuresis is caused by CDI or NDI. The patient was water restricted beginning in the early morning, with careful monitoring of vital signs and urine output; overnight water deprivation of patients with diabetes insipidus is unsafe, given the potential for severe hypernatremia. The serum [Na^+] was monitored hourly during water deprivation. A baseline AVP sample was drawn at the beginning of the test, with a second sample drawn once the serum [Na^+] reached 148–150 mM. At this point, a single 2 μg dose of the V2 vasopressin receptor agonist DDAVP was administered. An alternative approach would have been to measure AVP and administer DDAVP when the patient was initially hypernatremic; however, given the initial renal impairment the water deprivation test and administration was postponed until the patient had been adequately hydrated.

The patient's water deprivation test was consistent with NDI, with an AVP level within the normal range in the setting of hypernatremia (i.e., no evidence of CDI) and an inappropriately low urine osmolality that failed by increase by >50 % or >150 mOsm/kg after both water deprivation and the administration of DDAVP. This defect would be considered compatible with "complete" NDI; patients with "partial NDI" can achieve urine osmolalities of 500–600 mOsm/kg after DDAVP treatment, but will not maximally concentrate their urine to 800 mOsm/Kg or higher [83].

NDI has a number of genetic and acquired causes, which all share interference with some aspect of the renal concentrating mechanism [83]. This patient suffered from NDI due to lithium therapy, the most common cause of NDI in adult medicine. Lithium causes NDI via direct inhibition of renal glycogen synthase kinase-3 (GSK3), a kinase thought to be the pharmacological target of lithium in psychiatric disease; renal GSK3 is required for the response of principal cells to AVP [84]. Lithium also inhibits the activation of vasopressin-sensitive adenylate cyclase in renal epithelia by competing with magnesium for activation of the stimulatory GTP binding protein that couples to the V2 vasopressin receptor in principal cells [85]. Finally, lithium induces the expression of COX2 in the renal medulla via a GSK3-dependent mechanism [32]; COX2-derived prostaglandins inhibit AVP-stimulated salt transport by the thick ascending limb [49, 86]; and AVP-stimulated water transport by the collecting duct [48], thus exacerbating lithium-associated polyuria.

The entry of lithium through the amiloride-sensitive Na^+ channel ENaC is required for the effect of the drug on principal cells [87], such that combined therapy within lithium and amiloride can mitigate lithium-associated NDI [88, 89]. However, lithium causes chronic tubulointerstitial scarring and chronic kidney disease (CKD) after prolonged therapy, with a reduced therapeutic benefit from amiloride; patients may also have a persistent NDI long after stopping lithium [90]. Notably, this particular patient had been treated on and off for several years with lithium, leading to CKD (baseline creatinine of 1.3–1.4 mg/dL) and NDI that persisted after acute withdrawal of lithium.

Most patients with lithium-associated NDI are capable of compensating for the disorder by increasing water intake to match their polyuria.

For this patient, there were concerns about aspiration risk with aggressive oral hydration; a water deprivation test was pursued to determine if he had a partial NDI, with potential DDAVP treatment to reduce his obligatory daily free water intake. Other management options for lithium-associated NDI include treatment with thiazide diuretics, nonsteroidal anti-inflammatory drugs (NSAIDs), or COX2 inhibitors. Thiazides cause mild volume depletion and increase proximal tubular water reabsorption, in addition to increasing water transport within the distal nephron [29, 30]. A complicating issue for thiazide therapy in patients still taking lithium is the effect of diuresis on renal lithium excretion, with enhanced renal tubular absorption of lithium in volume depletion. NSAIDs and COX2 inhibitors reduce the negative effects of prostaglandins on renal concentrating ability [32, 48, 49, 86], thus ameliorating lithium-associated polyuria [91, 92]. However, these drugs must of course be utilized with caution in patients with lithium-associated CKD, given their potential to affect GFR, potassium excretion, and other renal functions. Finally, it should be noted that most of these measures for management of NDI are only rarely [92] appropriate for decompensated patients such as this one, in whom the initial management should focus on repletion with free water.

This patient developed severe hypernatremia due to a water diuresis; treatment of hypernatremia must include both replacement of the existing free water deficit and daily replacement of ongoing free water loss. The first step is to estimate total body water (TBW), estimated as 50 % of the body weight in women and 60 % in men. The free water deficit is then calculated as $[(Na^{+}-140)/140]\times TBW$. In this particular patient, the free water deficit was 4.2 L at a weight of 97.5 kg and serum [Na^+] of 150 mM. This free water deficit should be replaced slowly over 48–72 h, to avoid increasing the serum [Na^+] by >10 mM/24 h. A common mistake is to replace this deficit while neglecting to replace ongoing losses of free water, such that serum [Na^+] either fails to correct or in fact increases.

Ongoing losses of free water can be estimated using the equation for electrolyte-free water clearance [15]:

$$C_eH_2O = V(1 - U_{Na} + UK / P_{Na}, \quad (12.5)$$

where V is urinary volume, UNa is urinary [Na^+], UK is urinary [K^+], and PNa is serum [Na^+]. For this particular patient, the C_eH_2O was 2.5 L/day when initially evaluated, i.e., with urine [Na^+] and [K^+] 34 and 5.2 mM, respectively, serum [Na^+] of 150 mM, and a urinary volume of 3.4 L. Therefore, the patient was given 2.5 L of D5W over the first 24 h to replace ongoing free water losses, along with 2.1 L of D5W to replace half his free water deficit. Daily random urine electrolytes and urinary volume measurement can be utilized to monitor C_eH_2O and adjust daily fluid administration in this manner, while following serum [Na^+]. Physicians often calculate free water deficit to guide therapy of hypernatremia, providing half the deficit in the first 24 h. This approach is usually adequate in the majority of hypernatremic patients who do not have significant ongoing losses of free water, e.g., with hypernatremia due to decreased free water intake. However, this case illustrates how free water requirements can be grossly underestimated in hypernatremic patients if ongoing, daily free water losses are not taken into account in the management plan.

Case 7: Weakness and Hypokalemia

Clinical Scenario

A 37-year-old Hispanic man is admitted to hospital with weakness and hypokalemia. The patient had been very healthy until 2 months prior to admission, when he developed intermittent leg weakness. His review of systems is negative for symptoms other than weakness. He denies drug or laxative abuse, is on no medications. Past medical history is unremarkable. Family history is notable for a sister with thyroid disease. Physical exam is notable only for reduced deep tendon reflexes. Biochemical data is listed in Table 12.6.

Table 12.6 Laboratory data for Case 7

Laboratory data	Admission	Baseline	Units
Sodium	139	143	mM
Potassium	**2.0**	3.8	mM
Chloride	105	107	mM
Bicarbonate	26	29	mM
BUN	11	16	mg/dL
Creatinine	0.6	1.0	mg/dL
Calcium	8.8	8.8	mg/dL
Phosphate	**1.2**		mg/dL
Albumin	3.8		mg/dL
Plasma osmolality	290		mOsm/kg
Urine osmolality	590		mOsm/kg
Urine potassium	10		mEq/L

TSH 0.08 μIU/L (normal 0.2–5.39)
Free T4 41 pmol/L (normal 10–27)

Discussion

This patient developed hypokalemia due to a redistribution of potassium between intracellular and extracellular fluid space; this pathophysiology was readily apparent following calculation of the transtubular potassium gradient (TTKG). The TTKG is calculated as (POsm × UPotassium)/(PPotassium × UOsm) [93]. The expected values for the TTKG are <3 in the presence of hypokalemia and >7–8 in the presence of hyperkalemia [94]. In this case, the calculated TTKG was 2.5, consistent with appropriate renal conservation of K^+ and thus a non-renal cause for hypokalemia. In the absence of significant, gastrointestinal loss of K^+ the patient was diagnosed with a "redistributive" subtype of hypokalemia.

More than 98 % of total body potassium is intracellular; regulated buffering of extracellular K^+ by this large intracellular pool plays a crucial role in the maintenance of a stable plasma K^+ concentration. Clinically, changes in the exchange and distribution of intra- and extracellular K^+ can cause significant hypo- or hyperkalemia. Insulin, β[beta]2-adrenergic activity, thyroid hormone, and alkalosis promote cellular uptake of K^+ by multiple interrelated mechanisms, leading to hypokalemia [93]. In particular, alterations in the activity of the endogenous sympathetic nervous system can cause hypokalemia in several settings, including alcohol withdrawal, hyperthyroidism, acute myocardial infarction, and severe head injury [93].

Weakness is not uncommon in severe hypokalemia; hypokalemia causes hyperpolarization of muscle, thus impairing the capacity to depolarize and contract. In this particular patient, Grave's disease caused hyperthyroidism (see Table 12.6) and hypokalemic paralysis (thyrotoxic periodic paralysis, TPP). TPP develops more frequently in patients of Asian or Latin American origin. This shared predisposition has recently been linked to genetic variation in Kir2.6, a muscle-specific, thyroid hormone-induced K^+ channel [95]; however, the mechanisms that link dysfunction of this ion channel to TPP have yet to be elucidated in full.

The mechanisms through which hyperthyroidism causes TPP are not fully understood. However, direct and indirect activation of the Na^+/K^+-ATPase is thought to play a significant role, such that thyrotoxic patients with periodic paralysis have higher sodium pump activity than those without paralytic episodes [96]. Thyroid hormone directly induces the expression of Na^+/K^+-ATPase subunits in skeletal muscle [97], and also generates an increase in beta-adrenergic receptors [98], leading to additional, secondary activation of the Na^+/K^+-ATPase by circulating catecholamines. Insulin resistance and hyperinsulinemia, with downstream activation of Na^+/K^+-ATPase, have also been implicated in the pathogenesis [99, 100].

Clinically, patients with TPP present with weakness of the extremities and limb girdles, with paralytic episodes that occur most frequently between 1 and 6 a.m. Precipitants of weakness in TPP include high carbohydrate loads and strenuous exercise. Signs and symptoms of hyperthyroidism are not always present, often leading to delays in diagnosis. Hypokalemia is often profound and usually accompanied by redistributive hypophosphatemia and hypomagnesemia, as in this case. Patients with thyrotoxic periodic paralysis tend to be hypercalciuric and hypophosphaturic, such that a urine calcium:phosphate ratio of >1.7 mg/mg can be used to distinguish them from patients with non-thyrotoxic hypokalemic paralysis [101]. A TTKG of <2–3 in turn separates patients with redistributive hypokalemia from those with hypokalemia due to renal potassium wasting, who will have TTKG values that are >4 [102]. This latter distinction has considerable importance for therapy; patients with large potassium deficits require aggressive repletion with K^+-Cl^-, which has a significant risk of rebound hyperkalemia in TPP and related disorders.

Ultimately, definitive therapy for TPP requires treatment of the associated hyperthyroidism. In the short-term, however, potassium replacement is necessary to hasten muscle recovery and prevent cardiac arrhythmias. The average recovery time of an acute attack in TPP is reduced by ~50 % in patients treated with intravenous potassium chloride at a rate of 10 mEq/h; however, this incurs a significant risk of rebound hyperkalemia, with up to 70 % developing a plasma potassium concentration of >5.0 mEq/L [103]. Approximately 25 % of patients treated with 10 mEq/h of intravenous potassium chloride demonstrate a paradoxical *drop* in serum [K^+] of ~0.1 mM, after 3 h of therapy [104]. Patients with paradoxical worsening in hypokalemia take longer to recover, require more potassium chloride for recovery, and have greater rebound hyperkalemia (5.8±0.5 versus 5.1±0.4 mM peak [K^+]). The patients with paradoxical hypokalemic also have higher systolic blood pressures, heart, and free thyroxine levels, suggesting a greater severity of hyperthyroidism [104].

Rebound hyperkalemia is thus a major issue in the therapy of thyrotoxic hypokalemic paralysis, particularly in patients with paradoxical hypokalemia after intravenous potassium chloride [104]. There is the very real potential for fatal hyperkalemic arrhythmias following the administration of potassium chloride [105]; severe rebound hyperkalemia can also occur after replacement therapy for other causes of redistributive hypokalemia [106–108].

Case 8: Weakness, Hypokalemia, and Alkalosis

Clinical Scenario

A 68-year-old man is admitted to hospital with a serum [K^+] of 1.7 mEq/L and profound weakness of several days duration. His past medical history is notable for SCLC with metastases to brain, liver, and adrenals. He had been treated with one cycle of cisplatin/etoposide 1 year prior this admission, complicated by acute kidney injury (AKI) (peak creatinine of 5, with residual CKD) and three subsequent cycles of cyclophosphamide/doxorubicin/vincristine. He has also received 15 treatments with whole brain radiation.

On physical examination, the patient is jaundiced. BP is 130/70, increasing to 160/10 after a liter of saline, with a JVP at 8 cm. There is generalized muscle weakness. Laboratory data are listed in Table 12.7.

The patient's hospital course is complicated by acute respiratory failure attributed to pulmonary embolism; his clinical status is eventually changed to comfort care only, and he expires 2 weeks after admission.

Discussion

This patient suffered from metastatic small-cell lung cancer, persistent despite several rounds of chemotherapy and radiotherapy. He presented with profound hypokalemia, alkalosis, hypertension, severe weakness, jaundice, and worsening liver function tests.

With respect to the hypokalemia, there was no evident cause of non-renal potassium loss, e.g., diarrhea. The urinary TTKG was 11.7, at a plasma K^+ concentration of 1.7 mM; this TTKG value is consistent with inappropriate renal K^+ secretion, despite severe hypokalemia. The TTKG is calculated as (POsm × UPotassium)/(PPotassium × UOsm). The expected values for the TTKG are <3 in the presence of hypokalemia and >7–8 in the presence of hyperkalemia [94, 109].

The patient had several explanations for excessive renal excretion of potassium. First, he had a history of cisplatin-associated AKI, with residual CKD. Cisplatin can cause persistent renal tubular defects, with prominent hypokalemia and hypomagnesemia [110]; however, this patient had not previously required potassium or magnesium repletion, suggesting that cisplatin-associated renal tubular defects did not play a major role in

Table 12.7 Laboratory data for Case 8

Laboratory data	2 Months PTA	Admission	HD2	Units
Sodium	143	149	144	mM
Potassium	3.7	**1.7**	3.5	mM
Chloride	103	84	96	mM
Bicarbonate	26	**44**	34	mM
Venous pH		7.47		pH
Venous pCO_2		62		mmHg
BUN	21	41	40	mg/dL
Creatinine	2.8	2.9	2.3	mg/dL
Magnesium	1.3	1.6	2.4	mg/dL
CPK		183		U/L
ALT	8	75		U/L
Albumin	3.4	2.8	2.3	
Adjusted anion gap	15	24	18	
Total bilirubin	0.65	5.19		mg/dL
Alk phosphatase	93	217		U/L
Urine sodium		35	28	mM
Urine potassium		25	49	mM
Urine chloride		48	51	mM
Urine osmolality		391		mOsm/kg
Plasma osmolality		312		mOsm/kg
Urine pH		5.5		

Plasma ACTH: 185 pg/mL (7–50 pg/mL)
Plasma cortisol: 94 pg/mL (3–16 pg/mL)
24 h urine cortisol: 1,044 mcg/24 h (4–50 mcg/24 h)

this presentation. Second, he was hypomagnesemic on presentation, suggesting total body magnesium depletion. Magnesium depletion has inhibitory effects on muscle Na^+,K^+-ATPase activity [111], reducing influx into muscle cells and causing a secondary increase in K^+ excretion. Magnesium depletion also increases K^+ secretion by the distal nephron; this is attributed to a reduction in the magnesium-dependent, intracellular block of K^+ efflux through renal outer medullary K^+ channel (ROMK, see Fig. 12.5), the major secretory K^+ channel of principal cells [112, 113]. Clinically, hypomagnesemic patients are refractory to K^+ replacement in the absence of Mg^{2+} repletion [114, 115]. Again, however, this patient had not previously developed significant hypokalemia, despite periodic hypomagnesemia, such that other factors must have caused the severe hypokalemia.

The associated hypertension in this patient, which appeared following modest hydration, suggests an increase in mineralocorticoid activity,

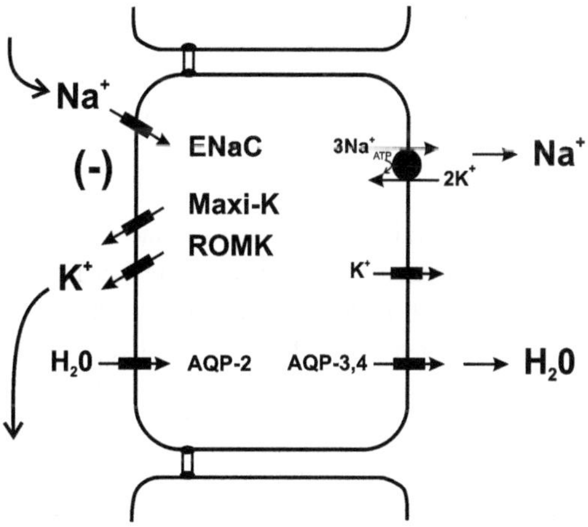

Fig. 12.5 Water, sodium, and potassium transport in principal cells. Water is absorbed down the osmotic gradient by principal cells, through the apical Aquaporin-2 (AQP-2) and basolateral Aquaporin-3 and Aquaporin-4. The absorption of Na^+ via the amiloride-sensitive epithelial sodium channel (ENaC) generates a lumen-negative potential difference, which drives K^+ excretion through the apical secretory K^+ channel renal outer medullary K^+ channel (ROMK) and/or the flow-dependent BK channel

causing increased activity of ENaC channels in principal cells, NaCl retention, hypertension, and hypokalemia. The increase in ENaC-mediated Na^+ transport in principal cells would have led to an increase in the lumen-negative potential difference in the connecting tubule and cortical collecting duct, driving an increase in K^+ secretion through apical K^+ channels (ROMK and BK channels—see Fig. 12.5). This explanation is compatible with the very high TTKG, i.e., an increase in K^+ excretion that is inappropriate for the plasma K^+ concentration.

What caused an increase in mineralocorticoid activity in this patient? The clinical presentation (hypokalemia, hypertension, and alkalosis) and the history of SCLC suggested Cushing's syndrome, with a massive increase in circulating glucocorticoid, stimulated by ectopic ACTH secretion by his SCLC tumor. Ectopic ACTH expression is associated primarily with neuroendocrine malignancies, most commonly bronchial carcinoid tumors, SCLC, and other neuroendocrine tumors [116]. Confirmation of this diagnosis was provided by a very high plasma cortisol level, high ACTH level, and increased urinary cortisol.

Why would an increase in circulating cortisol cause an apparent increase in mineralocorticoid activity? Cortisol has equal affinity for the mineralocorticoid receptor (MLR) to that of aldosterone, with resultant "mineralocorticoid-like" activity. However, cells in the aldosterone-sensitive distal nephron (the distal convoluted tubule (DCT), connecting tubule (CNT), and collecting duct) are protected from circulating cortisol by the enzyme 11β[beta]-hydroxysteroid dehydrogenase-2 (11β[beta]HSD-2), which converts cortisol to cortisone; cortisone has minimal affinity for the MLR [117]. Activation of the MLR causes activation of the basolateral Na^+/K^+-ATPase in multiple nephron segments, activation of the thiazide-sensitive Na^+-Cl^- cotransporter in the DCT [118], and activation of apical ENaC channels in principal cells of the CNT and collecting duct [119, 120]. Recessive loss-of-function mutations in the *11β[beta]HSD-2* gene lead to cortisol-dependent activation of the MLR and the "Syndrome of Apparent Mineralocorticoid Excess" (SAME), encompassing hypertension, hypokalemia, hypercalciuria, and metabolic alkalosis, with suppressed PRA and suppressed aldosterone [121]. A similar syndrome is caused by biochemical inhibition of 11β[beta]HSD-2 by glycyrrhetinic/glycyrrhizinic acid and/or carbenoxolone, typically encountered in patients who have ingested licorice or related substances [93].

In Cushing's syndrome caused by increases in pituitary ACTH, the incidence of hypokalemia is only 10 % [122], whereas it is ~70 % in patients with ectopic secretion of ACTH [122, 123], despite a similar incidence of hypertension. The activity of renal 11β[beta]HSD-2 is reduced in patients with ectopic ACTH compared with Cushing's syndrome, resulting in an SAME [124]; the prevailing theory is that the much greater cortisol production in ectopic ACTH syndromes overwhelms the renal 11β[beta]HSD-2 enzyme, resulting in activation of renal MLRs by unmetabolized cortisol.

The patient was profoundly weak, due to the combined effect of hypokalemia and increased cortisol. Hypokalemia causes hyperpolarization of muscle, thus impairing the capacity to depolarize and contract. Weakness and even ascending paralysis can frequently complicate severe hypokalemia [125, 126]. Hypokalemia also causes a myopathy and predisposes to rhabdomyolysis; notably, however, the patient had a normal CPK level. Cushing's syndrome is often accompanied by a proximal myopathy, due to the protein-wasting effects of cortisol excess.

The patient presented with a mixed acid–base disorder, with a significant metabolic alkalosis and a bicarbonate concentration of 44 mM. A venous blood gas was drawn soon after his presentation; venous and arterial blood gases demonstrate a high level of agreement in hemodynamically stable patients [127], allowing for the interpretation of acid–base disorders with venous blood gas results. In response to his metabolic alkalosis, the pCO_2 should have increased by 0.75 mmHg for each 1 mEq/L increase in bicarbonate; the expected pCO_2 should have been ~55 mmHg. Given the pCO_2 of 62 mmHg, he had an additional respiratory acidosis, likely caused by respiratory muscle dysfunction from his acute hypokalemia.

Calculation of the anion gap indicates an additional acid–base disorder. The anion gap must be corrected to account for the effect of reduced serum albumin, since albumin is a major unmeasured anion in serum; the anion gap drops by ~2.5 mM for every 1 mg/dL drop in serum albumin [128]. The patient's albumin-adjusted anion gap was $21+(4-2.8)\times 2.5=24$, indicating an anion gap acidosis. Notably, the measured anion gap can increase in alkalosis, due to both increases in plasma protein concentrations (in hypovolemic alkalosis) and to the alkalemia-associated increase in net negative charge of plasma proteins [128], both causing an increase in "unmeasured anions"; however, this patient was neither volume-depleted nor particularly alkalemic, suggesting that these effects played a minimal role in his increased anion gap. Alkalosis, be it respiratory or metabolic, also stimulates an increase in lactic acid production, due to activation of phosphofructokinase and accelerated glycolysis [129, 130]; unfortunately, however, a lactic acid level was not measured in this patient. It should be noted in this regard that alkalosis typically increases lactic acid levels by a mere 1.5–3 mM [129], and that the patient was not significantly alkalemic. However, regardless of the underlying pathophysiology, the increased anion gap was likely related to the metabolic alkalosis, given that the anion gap had decreased to 18 by hospital day 2, coincident with a reduction in plasma bicarbonate.

Why did the patient have a metabolic alkalosis? The activation of mineralocorticoid receptors in the distal nephron increases distal nephron acidification and net acid secretion. In consequence, mineralocorticoid excess causes a metabolic alkalosis, which is exacerbated significantly by the development of hypokalemia. Hypokalemia plays a key role in the generation of most forms of metabolic alkalosis, stimulating proximal tubular ammonium production, proximal tubular bicarbonate reabsorption, and distal tubular H^+,K^+-ATPase activity.

The first priority in management of this patient was to rapidly increase his serum [K^+] and magnesium concentrations; hypomagnesemic patients are refractory to K^+ replacement alone, hence the need to immediately correct hypomagnesemia. This was accomplished via the administration of both oral and intravenous K^+-Cl^-, giving a total of 240 mEq over the first 18 h; 5 g of intravenous magnesium sulfate was also administered. Multiple 100 mL "minibags" of saline containing 20 mEq each were infused, with cardiac monitoring and frequent measurement of plasma electrolytes. Of note, intravenous K^+-Cl^- should always be given in saline solutions, since dextrose-containing solutions can increase insulin levels and exacerbate hypokalemia [93].

This case illustrates the difficulty in predicting the whole body deficit of K^+ in hypokalemic patients. In the absence of abnormal K^+ redistribution, the total deficit correlates with plasma K^+ concentration, which drops by approximately 0.27 mM for every 100-mmol reduction in total body stores [93]; this would suggest a deficit of ~650 mEq of K^+ in this patient, at the admission plasma K^+ concentration of 1.7 mM. Notably, however, alkalemia induces a modest intracellular shift of circulating K^+, such that this patient's initial plasma K^+ concentration was not an ideal indicator of the total potassium deficit. Regardless of the underlying pathophysiology in this case, close monitoring of plasma K^+ concentration is always essential during the correction of severe hypokalemia, to gauge the adequacy of repletion and avoid overcorrection.

Subsequent management of this patient's Cushing's syndrome and ectopic ACTH secretion was complicated by his respiratory issues. The prognosis of this syndrome depends in large on the tumor histology and the presence or absence of distant metastases. This patient thus had an exceptionally poor prognosis, with widely metastatic SCLC that had failed treatment; other patients with ectopic ACTH secretion caused by more benign, isolated tumors, most commonly bronchial carcinoid tumors, have a much better prognosis [116]. In the absence of successful surgical resection of the causative tumor, management of this syndrome can include surgical adrenalectomy or medical therapy to block adrenal steroid production.

Case 9: Anion Gap Acidosis with Acute Kidney Injury

Clinical Scenario

A 50-year-old diabetic man presents with a 24-h history of nausea and vomiting. On the day prior to admission, he suddenly became nauseated at work, with the abrupt onset of vomiting. When this persisted for another 12 h, he presented to the emergency room. He has recently begun seeing a new primary care physician, who prescribed lisinopril 10 mg per day and metformin 1,000 mg twice a day 1 month prior to this admission. Other medications include rosuvastatin, lantus insulin, and humalog insulin. On review of systems, he denies any recent gastroenteritis or diarrhea. He admits to considerable alcohol intake, several beers per night. He denies intake of methanol or ethylene glycol.

Past medical history is notable for diabetes of 8 years duration, without retinopathy or significant proteinuria. He has a history of colon carcinoma, resected 4 years ago without recurrence on repeat colonoscopy. He also has hypercholesterolemia. Family history is positive for type II diabetes.

On exam, he is alert and appropriate. HR 90, blood pressure 135/70. He is anuric. JVP is seen at 6 cm with no peripheral edema. All pulses are palpable with no bruits. Heart sounds are normal with no murmurs. Abdomen is non-tender, without detectable organomegaly. Head and neck exam is unremarkable, neurological exam is non-focal.

Laboratory data includes a serum glucose of 137 mg/dL (70–99 mg/dL), [Na^+] of 136 mM, [K^+] of 5.0 mM, [Cl^-] of 74 mM, [HCO_3^-] of 15 mM, urea of 73 mg/dL, creatinine 17.36 mg/dL, calcium of 8.3 mg/dL, and phosphate 6.0 mg/dL; serum chemistries have been within normal range in the past, with a urea of 19 and creatinine of 1.0 mg/dL 1 month prior to this presentation. An arterial blood gas reveals pH 7.27, pCO_2 27 mmHg, pO_2 85 mmHg, and [HCO3$^-$] of 12 mM. The serum lactate is 10 mM. A qualitative serum acetone test is strongly positive, with a serum β[beta]-hydroxybutyrate level of 4.95 mM; metformin level, measured by high performance liquid chromatography, is 17 μ[mu]g/mL (therapeutic 1–2 μ[mu]g/mL). Liver function tests include an alkaline phosphatase of 76, ALT 109 IU/L (10–40 IU/L), AST 96 IU/L (10–40 IU/L), albumin 3.8, total bilirubin 0.63 (0.2–0.4 mg/dL), and prothrombin time 10.9 s (9.8–11.4 s). Creatinine phosphokinase (CPK) level is 180 U/L (21–232 U/L). Hemoglobin A1c was 9.5 % 1 month prior to this admission, with a urinary albumin:creatinine ratio of 76 (mg:mg).

The patient is dialyzed urgently for 4 h, with normalization of his lactate and anion gap within 24 h; serial lactate levels remain <2 mM over the next 48 h. He remains dialysis-dependent for 2 weeks, with a urea of 31 mg/dL, and creatinine 1.83 mg/dL 1 month after admission. His hospital admission is otherwise notable for the development of marked alcohol withdrawal 48 h after admission, requiring aggressive therapy with intravenous lorazepam.

Discussion

This diabetic male presented with AKI and anion gap acidosis. His recent history was notable for starting lisinopril and metformin 1 month prior to presentation. His AKI was attributed to the lisinopril, with probable volume depletion induced by his chronic alcoholism resulting in an angiotensin-II-dependent GFR, reduced renal perfusion from administration of lisinopril, and the development of acute tubular injury; unfortunately, he was anuric on presentation, hence urinary sediment analysis to assess for evidence of renal tubular injury was not feasible. The biochemical severity of his renal failure was greater than expected for primary hemodynamic or "prerenal" renal dysfunction induced by his ACE inhibitor. One diagnostic concern would be the possibility of ethylene glycol toxicity, given his wide anion gap acidosis and AKI; ethylene glycol toxicity is frequently accompanied by AKI [131]. However, the significant lactic acidosis would be unusual for ethylene glycol toxicity, he denied ingestion of ethylene glycol, and there were other explanations for his acidosis (see below).

This patient presented with a very wide anion gap, calculated at 47 on presentation. A qualitative serum acetone test was strongly positive, indicating the presence of acetoacetate and acetone. As at most institutions [132], direct testing for β[beta]-hydroxybutyrate was not immediately available; however, the β[beta]-hydroxybutyrate level was subsequently reported as 4.85 mM. At least part of his anion gap acidosis with due to ketoacidosis, given that his serum contained significant quantities of acetoacetate, acetone, and β[beta]-hydroxybutyrate. Although much more common in type I diabetics, diabetic ketoacidosis (DKA) can occur in patients with type II diabetes. DKA in type II diabetes typically occurs in the setting of extreme physiological stress (serious infection, trauma, etc.) and/or in patients with the so-called ketosis-prone subsets of type II diabetes [133]. DKA is however an unlikely cause for this patient's ketosis, given his modest hyperglycemia [134] on presentation and the lack of major physiological triggers for DKA.

This patient's presentation was at least partially consistent with alcoholic ketoacidosis (AKA). Classically, patients with AKA present with abdominal pain and vomiting, after abruptly stopping alcohol following a significant period of increased alcohol intake [135, 136]. Mild abnormalities in liver function tests (increased AST/ALT and hyperbilirubinemia) are very common in AKA, as in this case, likely due to ethanol-associated acute and chronic alcoholic hepatitis [135]. Pathogenesis of the ketosis in AKA is complex. Nutritional deficiencies result in a reduction in hepatic glycogen stores, with relative insulinopenia. Volume depletion from vomiting results in an increase in counter-regulatory hormones such as catecholamines, growth hormone, cortisol, and glucagon [134–136]. Metabolism of ethanol results in an increase in the ratio of reduced to oxidized nicotinamide adenine dinucleotide ($NADH:NAD^+$) (see Fig. 12.6), thus inhibiting gluconeogenesis [135]. The increased ratio of $NADH:NAD^+$ also tends to favor generation of β[beta]-hydroxybutyrate (see Fig. 12.6), with a ratio of β[beta]-hydroxybutyrate:acetoacetate of 7:1 in AKA versus 3:1 in DKA patients with equivalent β[beta]-hydroxybutyrate levels [134]. AKA typically responds to treatment with intravenous saline and intravenous glucose, with rapid clearance of the associated ketones due to reduction in counter-regulatory hormones and induction of endogenous insulin. In this particular case, however, the patient was immediately dialyzed, with clearance of ketones across the dialysis membrane and insulin-induced clearance of ketones due to absorption of glucose from the dialysate.

This patient also had a marked elevation of his serum lactate, with a level of 10 mM on presentation. Patients with AKA are predisposed to modest lactic acidosis, due to the elevated $NADH:NAD^+$ ratio, which favors lactate over pyruvate (see Fig. 12.6). Thiamine deficiency in AKA will also tend to block entry of pyruvate into the tricarboxylic acid cycle, wherein thiamine deficiency also inhibits the metabolism of α[alpha]-ketoglutarate (Fig. 12.6) [132]; this will also shunt glycolysis to anaerobic generation of lactate. Notably, however, in the absence of other causes of lactic acidosis (shock, etc.), hyperlactemia is rarely severe in AKA, with levels typically <6 mM [134–136]. This patient was hemodynamically stable, suggesting the need to search for an additional cause of his lactic acidosis.

This patient's presentation was consistent with metformin-associated lactic acidosis (MALA), provoked by his AKI and accumulation of metformin. Lactic acidosis is a rare complication of metformin use, typically occurring in the context of CKD or AKI [137]. The incidence of MALA has classically been considered to be low, in the range of three to nine cases per 100,000 patient years [138, 139]. More recent studies, however, have indicated a much higher incidence, of as much as 30–60 cases per 100,000 patient years [139]. The lactic acidosis in many patients with MALA may have been misattributed to other causes; measurement of metformin levels, as performed in this case, can confirm the causative role of the drug [139]. MALA is thus clearly related to metformin accumulation and the circulating concentration of the drug, with current recommendations to maintain therapeutic levels <2.5 μ[mu]g/mL to avoid toxicity [137].

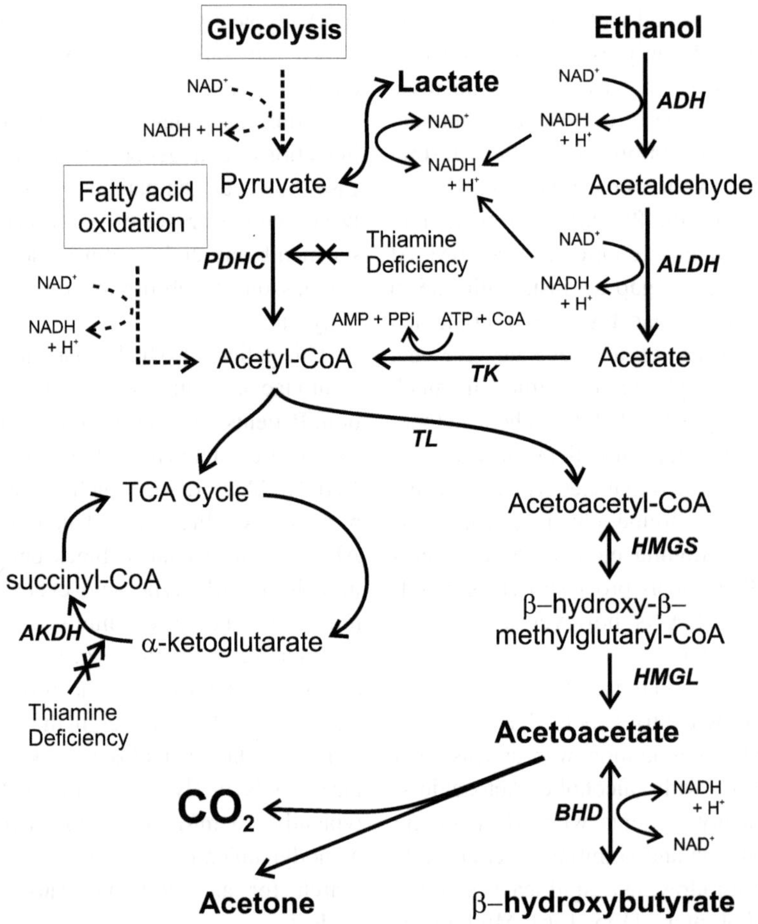

Fig. 12.6 Inter-relationships between ethanol and lactic, acetone, acetoacetate, and β[beta]-hydrobutyrate production. Ethanol metabolism by alcohol- and aldehyde dehydrogenase (ADH and ALDH, respectively) generates reduced nicotinamide adenine dinucleotide (NADH) from oxidized nicotinamide adenine dinucleotide (NAD^+). Glycolysis and acid oxidation, generating acetyl-coenzyme A (acetyl-CoA), also generate NADH. Thiamine is a required cofactor for α[alpha]-ketoglutarate dehydrogenase (AKDH) and the pyruvate dehydrogenase complex (PDHC), hence thiamine deficiency in alcoholism will tend to block oxidative phosphorylation and favor anaerobic glycolysis to lactate. β[beta]-hydrobutyrate dehydrogenase (BHD) and reduction of lactate to pyruvate both regenerate NAD^+. Increases in the ratio of NADH:NAD^+ induced by ethanol metabolism will tend to increase the ratio of lactate:pyruvate and β[beta]-hydrobutyrate:acetoacetate/acetone. See text for details. Other abbreviations include 3-hydroxy-3-methylglutaryl-CoA lyase (HMGL), HMG-CoA synthase (HMGS), thiokinase (TK), and thiolase (TL)

Metformin is excreted by the kidney and accumulates in renal insufficiency [137]. Most clinical guidelines suggest that metformin should be avoided at a creatinine of >1.4 mg/dL in female patients and 1.5 mg/dL in male patients. Notably, however, a substantial fraction of patients who are prescribed metformin have concomitant CKD, with eGFR of <60 mL/min/1.73 m^2 [140]. Dosage reductions in CKD are reasonable, however, prescribing <1.5 g/day in patients with eGFR of <60 mL/min/1.73 m^2 and <0.75 g/day in those with eGFR <30 mL/min/1.73 m^2 [137]. Monitoring of drug levels is not routine clinical practice, but may be appropriate in ensuring that patients with CKD are not exposed to an excessive risk of MALA [137]. Clearly, however, this does not protect patients taking metformin from the development of MALA in the context of AKI, as occurred in this particular patient.

The pathogenesis of MALA is not completely clear. Therapeutically, metformin exerts a hypoglycemic effect in diabetics by reducing hepatic glucose production. Metformin acts in part by stimulating phosphorylation of specific transcription factors, resulting in transcriptional repression of gluconeogenic enzymes [141, 142]. Many of these effects of metformin are mediated by the AMP-activated protein kinase (AMPK) and the upstream kinase STK11 (serine-threonine kinase-11, also known as LKB1) [142]. However, metformin has transcription- and STK11-independent effects on gluconeogenic enzymes, via inhibition of mitochondrial oxidative phosphorylation and a decrease in the ratio of ATP to ADP [143]. Metformin is known to inhibit complex I of the mitochondrial respiratory chain in hepatocytes and isolated hepatic mitochondria [144, 145], leading to a reduction in oxygen utilization, a decrease in the ratio of ATP to ADP and a secondary reduction in gluconeogenesis from lactate [145]. This inhibition of mitochondrial respiration is perhaps the most likely mechanism for MALA, given the recent finding that systemic oxygen consumption (VO_2) in patients with MALA is markedly reduced, with an increase in VO_2 and decrease in lactate following clearance of the drug [146].

Clinically, MALA has a high mortality, of as much as 30–50 % [146–148]. Notably, however, survival is considerably higher than in other patients with similar severity of lactic acidosis, underscoring the primary role for metformin accumulation in MALA. Patients with truly profound acidosis (pH of 6.62) and marked hyperlactemia (>30 mM) can survive an episode of MALA [146]. Liver dysfunction, manifested by an increased prothrombin time, is an important risk factor for mortality in MALA [148, 149]; notably, despite evidence of acute hepatitis, this patient had a normal prothrombin time. Metformin is removed by acute hemodialysis, which has become the standard of care in the management of MALA, providing both bicarbonate repletion and removal of the offending drug [146–150]. Prolonged hemodialysis is often required [149, 151], with serial measurement of lactate following dialysis to monitor for rebound lactic acidosis.

As discussed above, ethylene glycol toxicity was considered in this patient, given the combination of a wide anion gap acidosis and AKI. However, the high lactate level, other causes for AKI, and absence of reported ethylene glycol ingestion made this diagnosis clinically unlikely. In addition, given the anuric AKI and suspicion for MALA, urgent dialysis was pursued; this would be an appropriate therapy for ethylene glycol toxicity [131], i.e., management of ethylene glycol toxicity would have been similar. Classically, the presence of an osmolal gap, with a discrepancy between measured and calculated serum osmolality of >10 mOsm/kg, can indicate the presence of ethylene glycol [131]. However, osmolal gaps of as much as 30 mOsm/kg have been reported in AKA [152], due to retention of acetone and other neutral ketone metabolites, such that this test may have been misleading in this patient. Conversely, many patients with ethylene glycol toxicity will only manifest an elevated anion gap, due to late presentation with considerable metabolism of the ingested alcohol (and thus a lower osmolal gap) [131]. Notably, rapid measurement of β[beta]-hydroxybutyrate, osmolality, ethylene glycol, and metformin levels was not available at presentation; clinical diagnosis and the decision to pursue urgent dialysis hinged on the history, exam, the presence of AKI, the qualitative acetone test, and the elevated lactate level.

Careful analysis of the presenting laboratory data reveals another acid–base diagnosis. Classically, there should be a 1:1 correlation in anion gap acidosis between the drop in bicarbonate (consumed by titration of accumulated protons) and the increase in the measured AG; the limitations and caveats of this assumption are discussed elsewhere [128]. Deviations from this "Δ[delta]AG/Δ[delta]HCO_3^-" ratio of 1:1 can suggest the presence of an additional acid–base disorder. In this patient, the Δ[delta]HCO_3^- was only 9 mM (the median normal [HCO_3^-] of 24 minus the measured [HCO_3^-] of 15 mM), with a Δ[delta]AG of 37 mM (AG of 47 minus the median AG of 10 mM at the hospital in question). These data give an Δ[delta]AG/Δ[delta]HCO_3^- of approximately 4; this indicated the additional presence of a metabolic alkalosis, presumed to be due to his recent vomiting. Notably, assuming a β[beta]-hydroxybutyrate:acetoacetate ratio of ~7 [134], with a presenting β[beta]-hydroxybutyrate concentration of 4.85 mM, the acetoacetate concentration would have been 0.7 mM on presentation. The sum of the measured and calculated anions (~16–17 mM, including phosphate) is insufficient to explain the Δ[delta]AG of 37 mM. Such a discrepancy between measured organic anions and the AG is not uncommon in patients with very marked elevation in the AG [128]. Explanations in this particular case include the retention of other unmeasured anions (sulfate, etc.) due to AKI. Patients with lactic acidosis and DKA have also been shown to have elevations in the serum concentration of multiple anions from the tricarboxylic acid cycle (isocitrate, α[alpha]-ketoglutarate, etc.) [153, 154], albeit not at levels that would be expected to make up the discrepancy in the measured AG.

In summary, this patient presented with AKI and a marked elevation in the anion gap, with less than expected severity of academia due to concomitant metabolic alkalosis. His anion gap acidosis was attributed to a combination of AKA (with β[beta]-hydroxybutyrate concentration of 4.85 mM) and MALA (with lactate concentration of 10 mM and metformin concentration of 17 μ[mu]g/mL). His acidosis responded to acute hemodialysis, which can be curative in patients with metformin-associated severe lactic acidosis [146–150].

Case 10: Hypercalcemia and Renal Cell Carcinoma

Clinical Scenario

This 62-year-old man has been followed in renal clinic for several years for CKD stage IV with modest proteinuria. A recent abdominal CT for diverticulitis revealed bilateral renal cysts and a solid right superior renal pole mass; biopsy was positive for renal cell carcinoma, granular and clear cell variant. Ionized calcium had been 4.7 1 year ago, was recently found to be 5.5 with an increase in BUN and creatinine from 44 to 2.7 mg/dL 6 months ago to now 38 and 3.2 mg/dL. He was given 6 mg of intravenous ibandronate in an effort to control his hypercalcemia; ionized calcium was subsequently 6.1 with BUN and creatinine of 52 and 4.2 mg/dL (i.e., worsening renal function), hence he was given 45 mg of intravenous pamidronate. On follow-up 6 days later, his iCa was 6.3. On review of systems, he is asymptomatic. He denies excessive calcium intake (remote h/o milk alkali syndrome).

Past medical history is notable for CKD attributed to hypertensive nephrosclerosis. He has also had several episodes of AKI, with an episode of AKI due to milk alkali syndrome 15 years ago. He has a history of gout, peripheral vascular disease, and hypertension. Surgical history includes a left femoral-popliteal bypass. Family history is positive for prostate and ovarian cancer. He is a former smoker. Medications include atenolol, nifedipine, colchicine, ranitidine, and zolpidem tartrate.

On examination, he is obese, with heart 66 and blood pressure 130/70. He has chronic peripheral edema. Heart sounds are normal. Chest is clear. Abdomen is benign with no organomegaly. Head and neck examination is normal, with no lymphadenopathy.

Laboratory data include serum glucose of 98 mg/dL, [Na^+] of 142 mM, [K^+] of 5.40 mM, [Cl^-] of 106 mM, [HCO_3^-] of 25 mM, urea of 46 mg/dL, creatinine 4.3 mg/dL, total calcium of 11.3 mg/dL, ionized calcium 6.1 mg/dL (4.5–5.3), and phosphate 4.6 mg/dL. A complete blood count is normal, as are liver function tests. Serum protein electrophoresis is negative for a circulating paraprotein, serum-free light chains are within normal limits. His 25-dihydroxyvitamin D2 level is 27 ng/mL (30–100 ng/mL), with a 1,25-dihydroxyvitamin D3 level of <8 pg/mL (18–72 pg/mL). Parathyroid hormone is 11.1 pg/mL (12–88 pg/mL). A C-terminal PTH-related peptide (PTHRP) level is 49 pg/mL (14–27) but an N-terminal assay reveals a normal level of 0.8 pmol/L (<2.0). Serum angiotensin converting enzyme level is normal.

Imaging results include a normal bone scan, without evidence of bony metastases. CT and magnetic resonance imaging (MRI) of the abdomen reveal his right renal mass. A renal perfusion scan indicates that his left kidney accounts for 57 % of total renal function, the right kidney contributing 43 %.

The patient is admitted to hospital for management of his hypercalcemia and possible right nephrectomy. He is treated with indomethacin 25 mg PO tid, with rapid normalization of his ionized calcium. His creatinine falls to 3.0 mg/dL prior to an uncomplicated total right nephrectomy, after which creatinine stabilizes at 6.0 mg/dL with a urea of 80 mg/dL; calcium remains normal after nephrectomy, off of indomethacin. Pathology of the nephrectomy specimen reveals the expected renal cell carcinoma.

Discussion

In summary, this 62-year-old man with CKD developed progressive hypercalcemia with worsening in his renal function. An acute reduction in GFR is a common consequence of hypercalcemia [155]. The pathophysiology of this renal dysfunction includes salt and water loss due to activation of the intra-renal calcium receptor and inhibition of tubular salt and water transport [156, 157], downregulation of renal aquaporins [157, 158], and induction of medullary COX2 [159]. Hypercalcemia also reduces GFR due to direct and indirect vasoconstrictive effects on glomerular perfusion [160]. The subacute worsening in the patient's renal function was attributed to his progressive hypercalcemia, with a reduction in creatinine from a peak of 4.3 to 3.0 mg/dL following resolution of his hypercalcemia.

The patient was treated with intravenous bisphosphonates in an attempt to control his hypercalcemia. The patient's renal insufficiency strongly influenced the initial choice of agent. Pamidronate and zolendronate are thus associated with glomerular and tubular renal injury; pamidronate can cause a severe collapsing form of focal and segmental glomerulosclerosis, whereas zolendronate can worsen renal function in CKD and can cause a severe form of acute tubular injury [161]. The initial attempt was with intravenous ibandronate, which has lesser efficacy but less reported nephrotoxicity [161]. A subsequent attempt with renal-adjusted dosing of pamidronate was equally unsuccessful. The lack of success prompted admission for management of his hypercalcemia.

Why was this patient hypercalcemic? Bloodwork ruled out hypercalcemia from myeloma, with negative serum protein electrophoresis. His PTH was appropriately suppressed by the hypercalcemia, ruling out hyperparathyroidism as a cause. Notably, his level of 1,25-dihydroxyvitamin D3 (calcitriol) was also suppressed, with an almost normal level of 25-dihydroxyvitamin D2; hydroxylation of 25-dihydroxyvitamin D2 by the 1 α[alpha] hydroxylase enzyme in the proximal tubule is directly inhibited by increased extracellular calcium, providing feedback downregulation of the levels of physiologically active 1,25-dihydroxyvitamin D3 [162]. This physiological downregulation of 1,25-dihydroxyvitamin D3 rules out calcitriol-mediated hypercalcemia.

The patient was found to have a renal mass, with biopsy confirming renal cell carcinoma (RCC). Hypercalcemia is a common complication of RCC, occurring at some point during the course of disease in approximately 17 % of patients with this tumor [163]. The absence of bony metastases on bone scan indicated that osteolytic bony metastases were not involved. Secretion of PTRHP by the tumor cells is a common cause of RCC-associated hypercalcemia, and this patient had an elevated level of PTHRP when measured with a C-terminal radioimmunoassay (see labs above). However, the C-terminal fragment of PTHRP accumulates in renal insufficiency [164], and the patient had a normal PTHRP level when measured by N-terminal assay; therefore, this was not PTHRP-mediated hypercalcemia.

How else might the patient's RCC cause hypercalcemia, if not via secreted PTHRP? RCC cells may secrete osteoclast-activating cytokines such as interleukin-6, IL-1, tumor necrosis factor, and transforming growth factor; however, the role of these cytokines in RCC-associated hypercalcemia is unclear [163]. In this patient's case, however, there was pharmacological evidence for involvement of prostaglandins in his hypercalcemic syndrome, given his rapid response to treatment with indomethacin. Elevated prostaglandins are a well-characterized cause of refractory hypercalcemia in RCC, with a rapid response to NSAID therapy as in this case [165, 166]. Studies in mice reveal that COX2 plays a critical role in bone resorption stimulated by 1,25-dihydroxyvitamin D3 and PTH [167]. Prostaglandin E2 (PGE2) activates osteoclasts via the prostaglandin EP2 receptor [168], providing mechanistic explanation for the hypercalcemic effect of tumor-derived prostaglandins [165, 166].

In summary, this patient with biopsy-confirmed RCC developed refractory hypercalcemia, reversed by low-dose indomethacin. Tumor-secreted prostaglandins were the likely cause of his hypercalcemia [165, 166]. Renal function improved with indomethacin, due to resolution of his hypercalcemia, indomethacin would otherwise have been avoided in this patient with CKD and worsening renal function, underlining the importance of a literature- and physiologically based approach to patient care.

Acknowledgements Cases 1–5 are reproduced from Mount DB, Krahn TA. Hyponatremia: case vignettes. Semin Nephrol 2009;29:300–17, with permission of the publisher.

References

1. Berl T. Treating hyponatremia: damned if we do and damned if we don't. Kidney Int. 1990;37:1006–18.
2. Bagley SC, Yaeger D. Hyponatremia associated with bupropion, a case verified by rechallenge. J Clin Psychopharmacol. 2005;25:98–9.
3. Mewasingh L, Aylett S, Kirkham F, Stanhope R. Hyponatraemia associated with lamotrigine in cranial diabetes insipidus. Lancet. 2000;356:656.
4. Hill AR, Uribarri J, Mann J, Berl T. Altered water metabolism in tuberculosis: role of vasopressin. Am J Med. 1990;88:357–64.
5. Smith J, Godwin-Austen R. Hypersecretion of anti-diuretic hormone due to tuberculous meningitis. Postgrad Med J. 1980;56:41–4.
6. Verbalis JG, Berl T. Disorders of water balance. In: Brenner BM, editor. The kidney. 8th ed. Philadelphia: Saunders; 2008. p. 459–546.
7. Chung HM, Kluge R, Schrier RW, Anderson RJ. Clinical assessment of extracellular fluid volume in hyponatremia. Am J Med. 1987;83:905–8.
8. Milionis HJ, Liamis GL, Elisaf MS. The hyponatremic patient: a systematic approach to laboratory diagnosis. CMAJ. 2002;166:1056–62.
9. Berl T. Impact of solute intake on urine flow and water excretion. J Am Soc Nephrol. 2008;19:1076–8.
10. Liamis GL, Milionis HJ, Rizos EC, Siamopoulos KC, Elisaf MS. Mechanisms of hyponatraemia in alcohol patients. Alcohol Alcohol. 2000;35:612–6.
11. Sanghvi SR, Kellerman PS, Nanovic L. Beer potomania: an unusual cause of hyponatremia at high risk of complications from rapid correction. Am J Kidney Dis. 2007;50:673–80.
12. Musch W, Xhaet O, Decaux G. Solute loss plays a major role in polydipsia-related hyponatraemia of both water drinkers and beer drinkers. QJM. 2003;96:421–6.
13. Thaler SM, Teitelbaum I, Berl T. "Beer potomania" in non-beer drinkers: effect of low dietary solute intake. Am J Kidney Dis. 1998;31:1028–31.
14. Rosenbaum JD, Nelson 3rd WP, Strauss MB, Davis RK, Rossmeisl EC. Variation in the diurectic response to ingested water related to the renal excretion of solutes. J Clin Invest. 1953;32:394–404.
15. Rose BD. New approach to disturbances in the plasma sodium concentration. Am J Med. 1986; 81:1033–40.
16. Hilden T, Svendsen TL. Electrolyte disturbances in beer drinkers. A specific "hypo-osmolality syndrome". Lancet. 1975;2:245–6.
17. Sterns RH, Nigwekar SU, Hix JK. The treatment of hyponatremia. Semin Nephrol. 2009;29:282–99.
18. Perianayagam A, Sterns RH, Silver SM, et al. DDAVP is effective in preventing and reversing inadvertent overcorrection of hyponatremia. Clin J Am Soc Nephrol. 2008;3:331–6.
19. Sterns RH, Hix JK, Silver S. Treating profound hyponatremia: a strategy for controlled correction. Am J Kidney Dis. 2010;56:774–9.
20. Mount DB. The brain in hyponatremia: both culprit and victim. Semin Nephrol. 2009;29:196–215.
21. Davison JM, Shiells EA, Philips PR, Lindheimer MD. Serial evaluation of vasopressin release and thirst in human pregnancy. Role of human chorionic gonadotrophin in the osmoregulatory changes of gestation. J Clin Invest. 1988;81:798–806.
22. Hayslett JP, Katz DL, Knudson JM. Dilutional hyponatremia in pre-eclampsia. Am J Obstet Gynecol. 1998;179:1312–6.
23. Dokmetas HS, Kilicli F, Korkmaz S, Yonem O. Characteristic features of 20 patients with Sheehan's syndrome. Gynecol Endocrinol. 2006;22:279–83.
24. Fichman MP, Vorherr H, Kleeman CR, Telfer N. Diuretic-induced hyponatremia. Ann Intern Med. 1971;75:853–63.
25. Sharabi Y, Illan R, Kamari Y, et al. Diuretic induced hyponatraemia in elderly hypertensive women. J Hum Hypertens. 2002;16:631–5.
26. Friedman E, Shadel M, Halkin H, Farfel Z. Thiazide-induced hyponatremia. Reproducibility by single dose rechallenge and an analysis of pathogenesis. Ann Intern Med. 1989;110:24–30.
27. Berl T, Linas SL, Aisenbrey GA, Anderson RJ. On the mechanism of polyuria in potassium depletion. The role of polydipsia. J Clin Invest. 1977; 60:620–5.
28. Morris RG, Hoorn EJ, Knepper MA. Hypokalemia in a mouse model of Gitelman's syndrome. Am J Physiol Renal Physiol. 2006;290:F1416–20.

29. Cesar KR, Magaldi AJ. Thiazide induces water absorption in the inner medullary collecting duct of normal and brattleboro rats. Am J Physiol. 1999;277:F756–60.
30. Kim GH, Lee JW, Oh YK, et al. Antidiuretic effect of hydrochlorothiazide in lithium-induced nephrogenic diabetes insipidus is associated with upregulation of aquaporin-2, Na-Cl co-transporter, and epithelial sodium channel. J Am Soc Nephrol. 2004;15:2836–43.
31. Clark BA, Shannon RP, Rosa RM, Epstein FH. Increased susceptibility to thiazide-induced hyponatremia in the elderly. J Am Soc Nephrol. 1994;5: 1106–11.
32. Rao R, Zhang MZ, Zhao M, et al. Lithium treatment inhibits renal GSK-3 activity and promotes cyclooxygenase 2-dependent polyuria. Am J Physiol Renal Physiol. 2005;288:F642–9.
33. Norregaard R, Jensen BL, Li C, et al. COX-2 inhibition prevents downregulation of key renal water and sodium transport proteins in response to bilateral ureteral obstruction. Am J Physiol Renal Physiol. 2005;289:F322–33.
34. Plasencia YL, Cortes MB, Arencibia DM, et al. Esthesioneuroblastoma recurrence presenting as a syndrome of inappropriate antidiuretic hormone secretion. Head Neck. 2006;28:1142–6.
35. Osterman J, Calhoun A, Dunham M, et al. Chronic syndrome of inappropriate antidiuretic hormone secretion and hypertension in a patient with olfactory neuroblastoma. Evidence of ectopic production of arginine vasopressin by the tumor. Arch Intern Med. 1986;146:1731–5.
36. Cullen MJ, Cusack DA, O'Briain DS, Devlin JB, Kehely A, Lyons TA. Neurosecretion of arginine vasopressin by an olfactory neuroblastoma causing reversible syndrome of antidiuresis. Am J Med. 1986;81:911–6.
37. Renneboog B, Decaux G. Idiopathic hyponatremia in a young patient: look at the sinus. Am J Med. 2008;121:e5–6.
38. Ma AT, Lei KI. Small cell neuroendocrine carcinoma of the ethmoid sinuses presenting with generalized seizure and syndrome of inappropriate antidiuretic hormone secretion: a case report and review of literature. Am J Otolaryngol. 2009;30:54–7.
39. Vasan NR, Medina JE, Canfield VA, Gillies EM. Sinonasal neuroendocrine carcinoma in association with SIADH. Head Neck. 2004;26:89–93.
40. List AF, Hainsworth JD, Davis BW, Hande KR, Greco FA, Johnson DH. The syndrome of inappropriate secretion of antidiuretic hormone (SIADH) in small-cell lung cancer. J Clin Oncol. 1986;4:1191–8.
41. Ellison DH, Berl T. Clinical practice. The syndrome of inappropriate antidiuresis. N Engl J Med. 2007;356:2064–72.
42. Ferlito A, Rinaldo A, Devaney KO. Syndrome of inappropriate antidiuretic hormone secretion associated with head neck cancers: review of the literature. Ann Otol Rhinol Laryngol. 1997;106:878–83.
43. Anpalahan M. Chronic idiopathic hyponatremia in older people due to syndrome of inappropriate antidiuretic hormone secretion (SIADH) possibly related to aging. J Am Geriatr Soc. 2001;49:788–92.
44. Decaux G, Vandergheynst F, Bouko Y, Parma J, Vassart G, Vilain C. Nephrogenic syndrome of inappropriate antidiuresis in adults: high phenotypic variability in men and women from a large pedigree. J Am Soc Nephrol. 2007;18:606–12.
45. Rosner MH. Exercise-associated hyponatremia. Semin Nephrol. 2009;29(3):271–81.
46. Hew-Butler T, Jordaan E, Stuempfle KJ, et al. Osmotic and nonosmotic regulation of arginine vasopressin during prolonged endurance exercise. J Clin Endocrinol Metab. 2008;93:2072–8.
47. Hew-Butler T. Arginine vasopressin, fluid balance and exercise: is exercise-associated hyponatraemia a disorder of arginine vasopressin secretion? Sports Med. 2010;40:459–79.
48. Grantham JJ, Orloff J. Effect of prostaglandin E1 on the permeability response of the isolated collecting tubule to vasopressin, adenosine 3′,5′-monophosphate, and theophylline. J Clin Invest. 1968;47:1154–61.
49. Fernandez-Llama P, Ecelbarger CA, Ware JA, et al. Cyclooxygenase inhibitors increase Na-K-2Cl cotransporter abundance in thick ascending limb of Henle's loop. Am J Physiol. 1999;277:F219–26.
50. Sun R, Carlson NG, Hemmert AC, Kishore BK. P2Y2 receptor-mediated release of prostaglandin E2 by IMCD is altered in hydrated and dehydrated rats: relevance to AVP-independent regulation of IMCD function. Am J Physiol Renal Physiol. 2005;289:F585–92.
51. Wharam PC, Speedy DB, Noakes TD, Thompson JM, Reid SA, Holtzhausen LM. NSAID use increases the risk of developing hyponatremia during an ironman triathlon. Med Sci Sports Exerc. 2006;38:618–22.
52. Fraser CL, Arieff AI. Epidemiology, pathophysiology, and management of hyponatremic encephalopathy. Am J Med. 1997;102:67–77.
53. Ayus JC, Arieff AI. Pulmonary complications of hyponatremic encephalopathy. Noncardiogenic pulmonary edema and hypercapnic respiratory failure. Chest. 1995;107:517–21.
54. Kalantar-Zadeh K, Nguyen MK, Chang R, Kurtz I. Fatal hyponatremia in a young woman after ecstasy ingestion. Nat Clin Pract Nephrol. 2006;2:283–8. quiz 9.
55. Siegel AJ, Verbalis JG, Clement S, et al. Hyponatremia in marathon runners due to inappropriate arginine vasopressin secretion. Am J Med. 2007;120:461. e11–7.
56. Janicic N, Verbalis JG. Evaluation and management of hypo-osmolality in hospitalized patients. Endocrinol Metab Clin North Am. 2003;32:459–81. vii.
57. Nguyen MK. Quantitative approaches to the analysis and treatment of the dysnatremias. Semin Nephrol. 2009;29:216–26.
58. Mohmand HK, Issa D, Ahmad Z, Cappuccio JD, Kouides RW, Sterns RH. Hypertonic saline for

hyponatremia: risk of inadvertent overcorrection. Clin J Am Soc Nephrol. 2007;2:1110–7.
59. Lauriat SM, Berl T. The hyponatremic patient: practical focus on therapy. J Am Soc Nephrol. 1997;8:1599–607.
60. Sterns RH, Hix JK. Overcorrection of hyponatremia is a medical emergency. Kidney Int. 2009;76:587–9.
61. Soupart A, Penninckx R, Stenuit A, Perier O, Decaux G. Reinduction of hyponatremia improves survival in rats with myelinolysis-related neurologic symptoms. J Neuropathol Exp Neurol. 1996;55:594–601.
62. Soupart A, Penninckx R, Crenier L, Stenuit A, Perier O, Decaux G. Prevention of brain demyelination in rats after excessive correction of chronic hyponatremia by serum sodium lowering. Kidney Int. 1994;45:193–200.
63. Soupart A, Ngassa M, Decaux G. Therapeutic relowering of the serum sodium in a patient after excessive correction of hyponatremia. Clin Nephrol. 1999;51: 383–6.
64. Oya S, Tsutsumi K, Ueki K, Kirino T. Reinduction of hyponatremia to treat central pontine myelinolysis. Neurology. 2001;57:1931–2.
65. Goldszmidt MA, Iliescu EA. DDAVP to prevent rapid correction in hyponatremia. Clin Nephrol. 2000;53:226–9.
66. Smith TJ, Gill JC, Ambruso DR, Hathaway WE. Hyponatremia and seizures in young children given DDAVP. Am J Hematol. 1989;31:199–202.
67. Odeh M, Oliven A. Coma and seizures due to severe hyponatremia and water intoxication in an adult with intranasal desmopressin therapy for nocturnal enuresis. J Clin Pharmacol. 2001;41:582–4.
68. Pruthi RS, Kang J, Vick R. Desmopressin induced hyponatremia and seizures after laparoscopic radical nephrectomy. J Urol. 2002;168:187.
69. Dehoorne JL, Raes AM, van Laecke E, Hoebeke P, Vande Walle JG. Desmopressin toxicity due to prolonged half-life in 18 patients with nocturnal enuresis. J Urol. 2006;176:754–7. discussion 7–8.
70. Rembratt A, Graugaard-Jensen C, Senderovitz T, Norgaard JP, Djurhuus JC. Pharmacokinetics and pharmacodynamics of desmopressin administered orally versus intravenously at daytime versus nighttime in healthy men aged 55–70 years. Eur J Clin Pharmacol. 2004;60:397–402.
71. Fjellestad-Paulsen A, Hoglund P, Lundin S, Paulsen O. Pharmacokinetics of 1-deamino-8-D-arginine vasopressin after various routes of administration in healthy volunteers. Clin Endocrinol (Oxf). 1993;38: 177–82.
72. Diederich S, Franzen NF, Bahr V, Oelkers W. Severe hyponatremia due to hypopituitarism with adrenal insufficiency: report on 28 cases. Eur J Endocrinol. 2003;148:609–17.
73. Raff H. Glucocorticoid inhibition of neurohypophysial vasopressin secretion. Am J Physiol. 1987; 252:R635–44.
74. Erkut ZA, Pool C, Swaab DF. Glucocorticoids suppress corticotropin-releasing hormone and vasopressin expression in human hypothalamic neurons. J Clin Endocrinol Metab. 1998;83:2066–73.
75. Saito T, Ishikawa SE, Ando F, Higashiyama M, Nagasaka S, Sasaki S. Vasopressin-dependent upregulation of aquaporin-2 gene expression in glucocorticoid-deficient rats. Am J Physiol Renal Physiol. 2000;279:F502–8.
76. Wang W, Li C, Summer SN, et al. Molecular analysis of impaired urinary diluting capacity in glucocorticoid deficiency. Am J Physiol Renal Physiol. 2006;290:F1135–42.
77. Kamoi K, Tamura T, Tanaka K, Ishibashi M, Yamaji T. Hyponatremia and osmoregulation of thirst and vasopressin secretion in patients with adrenal insufficiency. J Clin Endocrinol Metab. 1993;77: 1584–8.
78. Agus ZS, Goldberg M. Role of antidiuretic hormone in the abnormal water diuresis of anterior hypopituitarism in man. J Clin Invest. 1971;50:1478–89.
79. Shoji M, Kimura T, Ota K, et al. Cortical laminar necrosis and central pontine myelinolysis in a patient with Sheehan syndrome and severe hyponatremia. Intern Med. 1996;35:427–31.
80. Lasheen I, Doi SA, Al-Shoumer KA. Glucocorticoid replacement in panhypopituitarism complicated by myelinolysis. Med Princ Pract. 2005;14:115–7.
81. Schrier RW, Gross P, Gheorghiade M, et al. Tolvaptan, a selective oral vasopressin V2-receptor antagonist, for hyponatremia. N Engl J Med. 2006; 355:2099–112.
82. Zeltser D, Rosansky S, van Rensburg H, Verbalis JG, Smith N. Assessment of the efficacy and safety of intravenous conivaptan in euvolemic and hypervolemic hyponatremia. Am J Nephrol. 2007;27:447–57.
83. Sands JM, Bichet DG. Nephrogenic diabetes insipidus. Ann Intern Med. 2006;144:186–94.
84. Rao R, Patel S, Hao C, Woodgett J, Harris R. GSK3beta mediates renal response to vasopressin by modulating adenylate cyclase activity. J Am Soc Nephrol. 2010;21:428–37.
85. Goldberg H, Clayman P, Skorecki K. Mechanism of Li inhibition of vasopressin-sensitive adenylate cyclase in cultured renal epithelial cells. Am J Physiol. 1988;255:F995–1002.
86. Takaichi K, Kurokawa K. Inhibitory guanosine triphosphate-binding protein-mediated regulation of vasopressin action in isolated single medullary tubules of mouse kidney. J Clin Invest. 1988;82:1437–44.
87. Christensen BM, Zuber AM, Loffing J, et al. alpha-ENaC-mediated lithium absorption promotes nephrogenic diabetes insipidus. J Am Soc Nephrol. 2011;22:253–61.
88. Batlle DC, von Riotte AB, Gaviria M, Grupp M. Amelioration of polyuria by amiloride in patients receiving long-term lithium therapy. N Engl J Med. 1985;312:408–14.
89. Bedford JJ, Weggery S, Ellis G, et al. Lithium-induced nephrogenic diabetes insipidus: renal effects of amiloride. Clin J Am Soc Nephrol. 2008;3: 1324–31.

90. Boton R, Gaviria M, Batlle DC. Prevalence, pathogenesis, and treatment of renal dysfunction associated with chronic lithium therapy. Am J Kidney Dis. 1987;10:329–45.
91. Allen HM, Jackson RL, Winchester MD, Deck LV, Allon M. Indomethacin in the treatment of lithium-induced nephrogenic diabetes insipidus. Arch Intern Med. 1989;149:1123–6.
92. Lam SS, Kjellstrand C. Emergency treatment of lithium-induced diabetes insipidus with nonsteroidal anti-inflammatory drugs. Ren Fail. 1997;19:183–8.
93. Mount DB, Zandi-Nejad K. Disorders of potassium balance. In: Brenner BM, editor. Brenner and Rector's the kidney. 8th ed. Philadelphia: W.B. Saunders Co.; 2008. p. 547–87.
94. Choi MJ, Ziyadeh FN. The utility of the transtubular potassium gradient in the evaluation of hyperkalemia. J Am Soc Nephrol. 2008;19:424–6.
95. Ryan DP, da Silva MR, Soong TW, et al. Mutations in potassium channel Kir2.6 cause susceptibility to thyrotoxic hypokalemic periodic paralysis. Cell. 2010;140:88–98.
96. Chan A, Shinde R, Chow CC, Cockram CS, Swaminathan R. In vivo and in vitro sodium pump activity in subjects with thyrotoxic periodic paralysis. BMJ. 1991;303:1096–9.
97. Azuma KK, Hensley CB, Tang MJ, McDonough AA. Thyroid hormone specifically regulates skeletal muscle Na(+)-K(+)-ATPase alpha 2- and beta 2-isoforms. Am J Physiol. 1993;265:C680–7.
98. Ginsberg AM, Clutter WE, Shah SD, Cryer PE. Triiodothyronine-induced thyrotoxicosis increases mononuclear leukocyte beta-adrenergic receptor density in man. J Clin Invest. 1981;67:1785–91.
99. Soonthornpun S, Setasuban W, Thamprasit A. Insulin resistance in subjects with a history of thyrotoxic periodic paralysis (TPP). Clin Endocrinol (Oxf). 2009;70:794–7.
100. Chan A, Shinde R, Chow CC, Cockram CS, Swaminathan R. Hyperinsulinaemia and Na^+, K(+)-ATPase activity in thyrotoxic periodic paralysis. Clin Endocrinol (Oxf). 1994;41:213–6.
101. Lin SH, Chu P, Cheng CJ, Chu SJ, Hung YJ, Lin YF. Early diagnosis of thyrotoxic periodic paralysis: spot urine calcium to phosphate ratio. Crit Care Med. 2006;34:2984–9.
102. Lin SH, Lin YF, Chen DT, Chu P, Hsu CW, Halperin ML. Laboratory tests to determine the cause of hypokalemia and paralysis. Arch Intern Med. 2004;164:1561–6.
103. Lu KC, Hsu YJ, Chiu JS, Hsu YD, Lin SH. Effects of potassium supplementation on the recovery of thyrotoxic periodic paralysis. Am J Emerg Med. 2004;22:544–7.
104. Shiang JC, Cheng CJ, Tsai MK, et al. Therapeutic analysis in Chinese patients with thyrotoxic periodic paralysis over 6 years. Eur J Endocrinol. 2009;161:911–6.
105. Ahmed I, Chilimuri SS. Fatal dysrhythmia following potassium replacement for hypokalemic periodic paralysis. West J Emerg Med. 2010;11:57–9.
106. Sigue G, Gamble L, Pelitere M, et al. From profound hypokalemia to life-threatening hyperkalemia: a case of barium sulfide poisoning. Arch Intern Med. 2000;160:548–51.
107. Zydlewski AW, Hasbargen JA. Hypothermia-induced hypokalemia. Mil Med. 1998;163:719–21.
108. Schaefer M, Link J, Hannemann L, Rudolph KH. Excessive hypokalemia and hyperkalemia following head injury. Intensive Care Med. 1995;21:235–7.
109. Ethier JH, Kamel KS, Magner PO, Lemann Jr J, Halperin ML. The transtubular potassium concentration in patients with hypokalemia and hyperkalemia. Am J Kidney Dis. 1990;15:309–15.
110. Panichpisal K, Angulo-Pernett F, Selhi S, Nugent KM. Gitelman-like syndrome after cisplatin therapy: a case report and literature review. BMC Nephrol. 2006;7:10.
111. Dorup I, Clausen T. Correlation between magnesium and potassium contents in muscle: role of Na(+)-K+ pump. Am J Physiol. 1993;264:C457–63.
112. Huang CL, Kuo E. Mechanism of hypokalemia in magnesium deficiency. J Am Soc Nephrol. 2007;18: 2649–52.
113. Yang L, Frindt G, Palmer LG. Magnesium modulates ROMK channel-mediated potassium secretion. J Am Soc Nephrol. 2010;21:2109–16.
114. Rodriguez M, Solanki DL, Whang R. Refractory potassium repletion due to cisplatin-induced magnesium depletion. Arch Intern Med. 1989;149:2592–4.
115. Whang R, Flink EB, Dyckner T, Wester PO, Aikawa JK, Ryan MP. Magnesium depletion as a cause of refractory potassium repletion. Arch Intern Med. 1985;145:1686–9.
116. Isidori AM, Kaltsas GA, Pozza C, et al. The ectopic adrenocorticotropin syndrome: clinical features, diagnosis, management, and long-term follow-up. J Clin Endocrinol Metab. 2006;91:371–7.
117. Funder JW, Pearce PT, Smith R, Smith AI. Mineralocorticoid action: target tissue specificity is enzyme, not receptor, mediated. Science. 1988;242: 583–5.
118. Kim GH, Masilamani S, Turner R, Mitchell C, Wade JB, Knepper MA. The thiazide-sensitive Na-Cl cotransporter is an aldosterone-induced protein. Proc Natl Acad Sci U S A. 1998;95:14552–7.
119. Soundararajan R, Melters D, Shih IC, Wang J, Pearce D. Epithelial sodium channel regulated by differential composition of a signaling complex. Proc Natl Acad Sci U S A. 2009;106:7804–9.
120. Zhang W, Xia X, Reisenauer MR, et al. Aldosterone-induced Sgk1 relieves Dot1a-Af9-mediated transcriptional repression of epithelial Na^+ channel alpha. J Clin Invest. 2007;117:773–83.
121. White PC, Mune T, Agarwal AK. 11 beta-Hydroxysteroid dehydrogenase and the syndrome of apparent mineralocorticoid excess. Endocr Rev. 1997;18: 135–56.
122. Howlett TA, Drury PL, Perry L, Doniach I, Rees LH, Besser GM. Diagnosis and management of ACTH-dependent Cushing's syndrome: comparison of the

features in ectopic and pituitary ACTH production. Clin Endocrinol (Oxf). 1986;24:699–713.
123. Torpy DJ, Mullen N, Ilias I, Nieman LK. Association of hypertension and hypokalemia with Cushing's syndrome caused by ectopic ACTH secretion: a series of 58 cases. Ann N Y Acad Sci. 2002;970: 134–44.
124. Stewart PM, Walker BR, Holder G, O'Halloran D, Shackleton CH. 11 beta-Hydroxysteroid dehydrogenase activity in Cushing's syndrome: explaining the mineralocorticoid excess state of the ectopic adrenocorticotropin syndrome. J Clin Endocrinol Metab. 1995;80:3617–20.
125. Tang NL, Hui J, To KF, Ng HK, Hjelm NM, Fok TF. Severe hypokalemic myopathy in Gitelman's syndrome. Muscle Nerve. 1999;22:545–7.
126. Wong KM, Chak WL, Cheung CY, et al. Hypokalemic metabolic acidosis attributed to cough mixture abuse. Am J Kidney Dis. 2001;38:390–4.
127. Treger R, Pirouz S, Kamangar N, Corry D. Agreement between central venous and arterial blood gas measurements in the intensive care unit. Clin J Am Soc Nephrol. 2010;5:390–4.
128. Kraut JA, Madias NE. Serum anion gap: its uses and limitations in clinical medicine. Clin J Am Soc Nephrol. 2007;2:162–74.
129. Korosi A, Kahn T, Kalb T, Uribarri J. Marked hyperlactatemia associated with severe alkalemia in a patient with thrombotic thrombocytopenic purpura. Am J Kidney Dis. 2000;36:E6.
130. Hood VL, Tannen RL. Protection of acid-base balance by pH regulation of acid production. N Engl J Med. 1998;339:819–26.
131. Kraut JA, Kurtz I. Toxic alcohol ingestions: clinical features, diagnosis, and management. Clin J Am Soc Nephrol. 2008;3:208–25.
132. Smith SW, Manini AF, Szekely T, Hoffman RS. Bedside detection of urine beta-hydroxybutyrate in diagnosing metabolic acidosis. Acad Emerg Med. 2008;15:751–6.
133. Balasubramanyam A, Nalini R, Hampe CS, Maldonado M. Syndromes of ketosis-prone diabetes mellitus. Endocr Rev. 2008;29:292–302.
134. Umpierrez GE, DiGirolamo M, Tuvlin JA, Isaacs SD, Bhoola SM, Kokko JP. Differences in metabolic and hormonal milieu in diabetic- and alcohol-induced ketoacidosis. J Crit Care. 2000;15:52–9.
135. Wrenn KD, Slovis CM, Minion GE, Rutkowski R. The syndrome of alcoholic ketoacidosis. Am J Med. 1991;91:119–28.
136. McGuire LC, Cruickshank AM, Munro PT. Alcoholic ketoacidosis. Emerg Med J. 2006;23:417–20.
137. Graham GG, Punt J, Arora M, et al. Clinical pharmacokinetics of metformin. Clin Pharmacokinet. 2011;50:81–98.
138. Prikis M, Mesler EL, Hood VL, Weise WJ. When a friend can become an enemy! Recognition and management of metformin-associated lactic acidosis. Kidney Int. 2007;72:1157–60.
139. van Berlo-van de Laar IR, Vermeij CG, Doorenbos CJ. Metformin associated lactic acidosis: incidence and clinical correlation with metformin serum concentration measurements. J Clin Pharm Ther. 2011;36:376–82.
140. Vasisht KP, Chen SC, Peng Y, Bakris GL. Limitations of metformin use in patients with kidney disease: are they warranted? Diabetes Obes Metab. 2011; 12:1079–83.
141. He L, Sabet A, Djedjos S, et al. Metformin and insulin suppress hepatic gluconeogenesis through phosphorylation of CREB binding protein. Cell. 2009;137:635–46.
142. Shaw RJ, Lamia KA, Vasquez D, et al. The kinase LKB1 mediates glucose homeostasis in liver and therapeutic effects of metformin. Science. 2005;310: 1642–6.
143. Foretz M, Hebrard S, Leclerc J, et al. Metformin inhibits hepatic gluconeogenesis in mice independently of the LKB1/AMPK pathway via a decrease in hepatic energy state. J Clin Invest. 2011;120: 2355–69.
144. El-Mir MY, Nogueira V, Fontaine E, Averet N, Rigoulet M, Leverve X. Dimethylbiguanide inhibits cell respiration via an indirect effect targeted on the respiratory chain complex I. J Biol Chem. 2000; 275:223–8.
145. Owen MR, Doran E, Halestrap AP. Evidence that metformin exerts its anti-diabetic effects through inhibition of complex 1 of the mitochondrial respiratory chain. Biochem J. 2000;348(Pt 3):607–14.
146. Protti A, Russo R, Tagliabue P, et al. Oxygen consumption is depressed in patients with lactic acidosis due to biguanide intoxication. Crit Care. 2010; 14:R22.
147. Friesecke S, Abel P, Roser M, Felix SB, Runge S. Outcome of severe lactic acidosis associated with metformin accumulation. Crit Care. 2010;14:R226.
148. Peters N, Jay N, Barraud D, et al. Metformin-associated lactic acidosis in an intensive care unit. Crit Care. 2008;12:R149.
149. Seidowsky A, Nseir S, Houdret N, Fourrier F. Metformin-associated lactic acidosis: a prognostic and therapeutic study. Crit Care Med. 2009;37:2191–6.
150. Finkle SN. Should dialysis be offered in all cases of metformin-associated lactic acidosis? Crit Care. 2009;13:110.
151. Guo PY, Storsley LJ, Finkle SN. Severe lactic acidosis treated with prolonged hemodialysis: recovery after massive overdoses of metformin. Semin Dial. 2006;19:80–3.
152. Renom G, Maisonneuve N, Kim I, Dehon B, Azar R. Major ketogenesis and the absence of an osmolar gap in an atypical case of alcoholic ketoacidosis. Ann Clin Biochem. 2003;40:424–6.
153. Forni LG, McKinnon W, Lord GA, Treacher DF, Peron JM, Hilton PJ. Circulating anions usually associated with the Krebs cycle in patients with metabolic acidosis. Crit Care. 2005;9:R591–5.

154. Forni LG, McKinnon W, Hilton PJ. Unmeasured anions in metabolic acidosis: unravelling the mystery. Crit Care. 2006;10:220.
155. Lins LE. Reversible renal failure caused by hypercalcemia. A retrospective study. Acta Med Scand. 1978;203:309–14.
156. Hebert SC. Calcium and salinity sensing by the thick ascending limb: a journey from mammals to fish and back again. Kidney Int Suppl. 2004;91:S28–33.
157. Procino G, Carmosino M, Tamma G, et al. Extracellular calcium antagonizes forskolin-induced aquaporin 2 trafficking in collecting duct cells. Kidney Int. 2004;66:2245–55.
158. Wang W, Li C, Kwon TH, Knepper MA, Frokiaer J, Nielsen S. AQP3, p-AQP2, and AQP2 expression is reduced in polyuric rats with hypercalcemia: prevention by cAMP-PDE inhibitors. Am J Physiol Renal Physiol. 2002;283:F1313–25.
159. Mangat H, Peterson LN, Burns KD. Hypercalcemia stimulates expression of intrarenal phospholipase A2 and prostaglandin H synthase-2 in rats. Role of angiotensin II AT1 receptors. J Clin Invest. 1997;100:1941–50.
160. Levi M, Ellis MA, Berl T. Control of renal hemodynamics and glomerular filtration rate in chronic hypercalcemia. Role of prostaglandins, renin-angiotensin system, and calcium. J Clin Invest. 1983; 71:1624–32.
161. Perazella MA, Markowitz GS. Bisphosphonate nephrotoxicity. Kidney Int. 2008;74:1385–93.
162. Bland R, Walker EA, Hughes SV, Stewart PM, Hewison M. Constitutive expression of 25-hydroxyvitamin D3-1alpha-hydroxylase in a transformed human proximal tubule cell line: evidence for direct regulation of vitamin D metabolism by calcium. Endocrinology. 1999;140:2027–34.
163. Pepper K, Jaowattana U, Starsiak MD, et al. Renal cell carcinoma presenting with paraneoplastic hypercalcemic coma: a case report and review of the literature. J Gen Intern Med. 2007;22:1042–6.
164. Burtis WJ, Brady TG, Orloff JJ, et al. Immunochemical characterization of circulating parathyroid hormone-related protein in patients with humoral hypercalcemia of cancer. N Engl J Med. 1990;322:1106–12.
165. Brereton HD, Halushka PV, Alexander RW, Mason DM, Keiser HR, DeVita Jr VT. Indomethacin-responsive hypercalcemia in a patient with renal-cell adenocarcinoma. N Engl J Med. 1974;291:83–5.
166. Seyberth HW, Raisz LG, Oates JA. Prostaglandins and hypercalcemic states. Annu Rev Med. 1978; 29:23–9.
167. Okada Y, Lorenzo JA, Freeman AM, et al. Prostaglandin G/H synthase-2 is required for maximal formation of osteoclast-like cells in culture. J Clin Invest. 2000;105:823–32.
168. Li X, Tomita M, Pilbeam CC, Breyer RM, Raisz LG. Prostaglandin receptor EP2 mediates PGE2 stimulated hypercalcemia in mice in vivo. Prostaglandins Other Lipid Mediat. 2002;67:173–80.

Index

D.B. Mount et al. (eds.), *Core Concepts in the Disorders of Fluid, Electrolytes and Acid-Base Balance*,
DOI 10.1007/978-1-4614-3770-3, © Springer Science+Business Media New York 2013

U

V

W

MIX
Papier aus verantwortungsvollen Quellen
Paper from responsible sources
FSC® C105338

If you have any concerns about our products,
you can contact us on
ProductSafety@springernature.com

In case Publisher is established outside the EU,
the EU authorized representative is:
Springer Nature Customer Service Center GmbH
Europaplatz 3, 69115 Heidelberg, Germany

Printed by Libri Plureos GmbH
in Hamburg, Germany